Vaccine Danger
Quackery and Sin

Edward Hendrie

O Timothy, keep that which is committed to thy trust, avoiding profane and vain babblings, and oppositions of science falsely so called: Which some professing have erred concerning the faith. Grace be with thee. Amen. (1 Timothy 6:20-21)

Put on the whole armour of God, that ye may be able to stand against the wiles of the devil. For we wrestle not against flesh and blood, but against principalities, against powers, against the rulers of the darkness of this world, against spiritual wickedness in high places. (Ephesians 6:11-12)

GREAT MOUNTAIN
PUBLISHING

ISBN: 978-1-943056-17-0
Other books from Great Mountain Publishing®

- 9/11-Enemies Foreign and Domestic
- Solving the Mystery of BABYLON THE GREAT
- The Anti-Gospel
- Bloody Zion
- What Shall I Do to Inherit Eternal Life?
- Murder, Rape, and Torture in a Catholic Nunnery
- Antichrist: The Beast Revealed
- The Greatest Lie on Earth
- The Greatest Lie on Earth (Expanded Edition)
- Rome's Responsibility for the Assassination of Abraham Lincoln
- The Damnable Heresy of Salvation by Dead Faith (Expanded Edition)
- The Sphere of Influence

Available at:
https://greatmountainpublishing.com
www.antichristconspiracy.com
www.911enemies.com
www.mysterybabylonthegreat.net
www.antigospel.com
https://play.google.com
www.barnesandnoble.com
www.amazon.com

Edward Hendrie rests on the authority of the Holy Bible alone for doctrine. He considers the Holy Bible to be the inspired and inerrant word of God. Favorable citation by Edward Hendrie to an authority outside the Holy Bible on a particular issue should not be interpreted to mean that he agrees with all of the doctrines and beliefs of the cited authority. All Scripture references are to the Authorized (King James) Version of the Holy Bible, unless otherwise indicated.

Table of Contents

Introduction 1

1 Religious Superstition 3

2 The Truth about the Polio Vaccine 27

3 Proof That the Measles Virus Does Not Exist. 38

4 Injecting Disease 44

5 Poisonous Magic Potions. 47

6 The American Medical Association 56

7 Dangerous Placebos. 59

8 Food Allergies 72

9 Vaccines Cause Autism. 76

10 Kangaroo Court 89

11 Toxic Excipients 99

12 Moral Hazard. 121

13 Edmund Massey's Sermon Against Vaccination. . . . 132

14 Vaccines Cause Diseases. 140

15 Unsafe and Ineffective Flu Vaccines 145

16 The Ends Do Not Justify the Means 158

17 The Sacrament of Vaccination. 169

18	Government Fraud	180
19	Vaccines Are Dangerous Medical Quackery	186
20	The AMA Cracks Down	226
21	Pediatricians Are Paid Bounties	232
22	Buying Influence to Injure and Kill	247
23	The Blind Leading the Blind	254
24	The Dangerous Quackery of the CDC	264
25	COVID-19 Vaccines are Ineffective	280
26	CDC Changes the Definition of Vaccine	322
27	Antibody Dependent Enhancement	330
28	COVID-19 Vaccines Are Dangerous	353
29	Increased All-Cause Mortality	379
30	Prion Disease	395
31	Myocarditis	398
32	Graphene	416
33	COVID-19 Vaccine Blood Clotting Danger	420
34	Scuttling the Control Group to Hide Injuries	423
35	Bait and Switch #1	428
36	Planned Obfuscation	460

37 Bait and Switch #2 467

38 Never-Ending Boosters 477

39 Killing Children to Save Them 481

40 Sudden Adult Death Syndrome 485

41 How the Vaccine Makers Scammed the Public 487

42 Hydroxychloroquine 509

43 Suppression of Hydroxychloroquine 532

44 Ivermectin 538

45 Fake News About Ivermectin 544

46 Operation Mockingbird Vaccine 548

47 Canceling Doctors 560

48 Child Abuse by Government Edict 563

49 None Dare Call it Genocide 567

50 The Emperor Has No Virus 586

51 The Spanish Flu of 1918 590

52 SARS-CoV-2 Virus Has Never Been Isolated 598

53 The Lie of Asymptomatic Virus Spread 607

54 Exosomes 611

55 Relocation Camps 616

56 Inflating COVID-19 Death Statistics 623

57 Closing Down Schools For No Good Reason. 668

58 None Dare Call It Conspiracy. 673

59 Anthony Fauci Predicts the Pandemic 689

60 5G Radiation Sickness 693

61 The Disappearing Flu 701

62 Veklury® (Remdesivir) 709

63 Ventilators. 728

64 Euthanasia. 734

65 Vaccine Passports 739

66 Your Legal Rights Under Vaccine Mandates 760

67 The Right of the People to Peaceably Assemble . . . 796

68 Social Distancing Is from the Mind of a Child. 804

69 Requiring Unsafe and Ineffective Masks 809

70 Compelling Symbolic Speech. 848

71 Abridging the Freedom of Speech 859

Appendix. 865

Endnotes 899

Introduction

This book reveals the most significant medical fraud in history. The theory that you can prevent illness by injecting poisons into the bodies of healthy people is dangerous quackery and sin. All true science has proven the practice of vaccination to be ineffective and unsafe. But the medical establishment has been lured into the superstitious practice, hook, line, and sinker.

It is not merely a matter of ignorance that the debilitating practice flourishes. It is, at its core, being promoted by those who know it is unsafe and ineffective. Dr. Archie Kalokerinos summarizes the reality of what he saw with the death and devastation caused by vaccinations among the aborigines in Australia:

> My final conclusion after forty years or more in this business is that the unofficial policy of the World Health Organisation and the unofficial policy of Save the Children's Fund and almost all those organisations is one of murder and genocide. They want to make it appear as if they are saving these kids, but in actual fact they don't. I am talking of those at the very top. Beneath that level is another level of doctors and health workers, like myself, who don't really understand what they are doing. But I cannot see any other possible

explanation: It is murder and it is genocide.[1]

There is a malevolent spirit behind vaccines. The practice of vaccination is part of a conspiracy against God and man. While most doctors are unwitting, some are willing minions of that old serpent, called the Devil, and Satan, who are quite happy to kill people for profit. Jesus describes such men:

> Ye are of your father the devil, and the lusts of your father ye will do. He was a murderer from the beginning, and abode not in the truth, because there is no truth in him. When he speaketh a lie, he speaketh of his own: for he is a liar, and the father of it. John 8:44.

All medical care and advice should be customized to the unique needs and characteristics of the patient. The author of this book is not a medical professional, and this book creates no physician-patient relationship. This book is for informational and educational purposes and does not constitute medical advice or professional services. The information provided in this book should not be used for diagnosing or treating a health problem or disease. That should only be done by a medical professional who knows your unique medical history and condition.

When seeking medical advice, you should find a medical professional who is not a quack. Seek a doctor who will not blindly follow the sometimes unsafe and ineffective edicts of incompetent government bureaucrats. Do your due diligence and take charge of your medical care by being informed and asking questions. When remedying a disease, a doctor should try to find the cause of that disease rather than treat only the symptoms. If you believe a vaccine or a pharmaceutical drug has injured you, find a doctor who will at least acknowledge that possibility and thus be able to treat the cause of your illness.

1 Religious Superstition

Many attribute the practice of vaccination to the quack doctor Edward Jenner (1749-1823).[2] The very word vaccine is from the Latin word for cow. Jenner pulled a trick. He renamed cowpox *variolae vaccinae,* from which we get the word vaccine. Jenner called the cowpox that he injected into humans *variolae vaccinae.* Jenner's theory was that it would make them immune from smallpox. While Jenner is often credited with the cowpox/smallpox hypothesis, it can be traced past Jenner's first experiments in 1796 to a farmer, Benjamin Jesty (1736-1816), who first used cowpox to innoculate against smallpox in 1774.[3] Cowpox is a disease of cows' udders and has no relation to smallpox, except they both have the suffix "pox" in their names. Indeed, *variolae vaccinae*, which means smallpox of the cow, is a made-up disease. There is a disease called cowpox and a disease called smallpox, but there is no such disease as smallpox of the cow.[4] Jenner was running a medical scam.

The esteemed Dr. Charles Creighton, writing in the Ninth Edition of the Encyclopedia Britannica, described Jenner's representation of cowpox as "smallpox of the cow" as "arbitrary and untenable."[5] He explained that cowpox and smallpox are infections that are quite unlike one another. Dr. Creighton further explained the dangers of Jenner's cowpox vaccination. He listed five diseases caused by vaccination: "1) erysipelas, (2) jaundice, (3) skin eruptions, (4) vaccinal ulcers, and (5) so-called vaccinal syphilis."[6] Dr. Creighton noted a 50% increase in infant deaths from syphilis after compulsory vaccination was instituted in England in 1853. Dr. Creighton opined that vaccination may predispose infants to be beset by illnesses because the vaccines "produce a considerable constitutional disturbance,"[7] rendering the infant's immature immune system unable to resist diseases. Tragically, this often caused the premature death of children or, if they survived, lifelong illness and frailty.

The practice of inoculation also involved using *variolae* (i.e., smallpox) as the inoculating antigen. But that practice was no more successful than using cowpox. Jenner was intimately aware of the ineffectiveness of both cowpox and smallpox vaccines. Thomas Morgan writes in his book, *Medical Delusions*, that "Jenner soon discovered that vaccination did not give immunity from smallpox, including some who had been vaccinated by himself and had died from it."[8] Eleanor McBean explains that "[i]t was not long ... before Jenner's cowpox vaccinations were followed by death and disease, and that practice was also branded as dangerous and deadly."[9] But Jenner convinced the world his cowpox vaccine worked because he lied about its efficacy and safety. Jenner's unceasing promotion of the practice and subsequent government funding of his research led to compulsory vaccination in England in 1853, unsurprisingly bringing death and disease to the population.[10] The smallpox vaccine was proven to be unsafe and ineffective. Morgan summarizes the fraudulent foundations of vaccines.

> From its inception until the present day, the vaccination scheme has been an endless record of lies, deception, fraud, juggling statistics, and falsifying death certificates in order to preserve vaccination from reproach and to secure its

> continuation. . . and all this after more than a century of terrible experience, which has demonstrated that vaccination has killed more than smallpox, besides crippling and disfiguring millions more.[11]

But those inconvenient historical details are ignored today. While "routine vaccination against smallpox among the general public was stopped ... the U.S. government has stockpiled enough smallpox vaccine to vaccinate everyone who would need it if a smallpox outbreak were to occur."[12] And the smallpox vaccine is still being administered on a case-by-case basis today. The Mayo Clinic reveals some of the risks of the smallpox vaccine and states that "the risks of the vaccine outweigh the benefits for most people."[13]

> The ACAM2000 vaccine uses a live virus that's like smallpox, but less harmful. It can sometimes cause serious side effects, such as infections in the heart or brain. That's why the vaccine is not given to everyone. Unless there is a smallpox outbreak, **the risks of the vaccine outweigh the benefits for most people**.[14]

The term vaccination did not exist until Edward Jenner (1749-1823). Before Edward Jenner, the method of gaining immunity from smallpox was called variolation, a name drawn from variola, the scientific name for smallpox.[15] The Chinese of the 15th century practiced a form of variolation where a practitioner would use nasal insufflation, where the recipient would suck powdered smallpox scabs into his lungs. The more common method was for the practitioner to dip a swab or other implement into a smallpox pustule and then introduce that smallpox material into a cut or poke a needle containing the material into the recipient's skin. This process was thought to give the recipient a mild case of smallpox but lifelong immunity from smallpox thereafter. This process of implanting a disease agent in a person is also called inoculation.

Although inoculation is based on the germ theory, it predates the alleged discoveries of Louis Pasteur (1849–1895) by hundreds of years. Indeed, both inoculation and the germ theory began their existence not as scientific discoveries but as religious superstitions. The Hindu superstition was transformed into "science" by Louis Pasteur through plagiarism and fraud.[16] Pasteur falsely took credit for the discoveries of Antoine Bechamp. He then twisted the science of Bechamp through fraud to conjure the myth of his germ theory as the cause of illness. Pasteur's germ theory for the cause of disease is the basis for the quackery and sin of the modern practice of vaccination. Bechamp's legitimate science-backed terrain theory for the cause of illness did not serve Satan's interest in killing, injuring, and enslaving mankind. And so Pastuer was promoted, and Bechamp was suppressed. Christians are called on to "keep that which is committed to thy trust, avoiding profane and vain babblings, and oppositions of science falsely so called: Which some professing have erred concerning the faith." 1 Timothy 6:20.

Burroughs Wellcome Pharmaceutical Company presented at the 17th International Congress of Medicine in London, England, in 1913, "The History of Inoculation and Vaccination for the Prevention of Disease."[17] In 2005, GlaxoSmithKline Pharmaceutical Company absorbed Burroughs Wellcome in a merger of the two companies. The 360-page International Congress of Medicine lecture memoranda from Burroughs Wellcome explain that inoculation against disease was started by Dhanwantari, the Vedic father of medicine, in 1500 B.C. In an account given in 1757 by one Howell, inoculation was practiced by itinerant Brahmins who went from house to house. Brahmin is the highest Varna in Vedic Hinduism. Brahmin came from the term Brahman, which is a magical force. The practice by the Brahmin required the recipients of the inoculation to "make a thanksgiving, Poojah, or offering to the goddess on their recovery."[18] Poojah is a Hindu word meaning worship, prayer, and offerings to a god or goddess.

The goddess to which an offering was to be made was Sitala, the goddess of smallpox, who "is the preeminent tutelary deity of villages in southwestern Bengal, and a goddess of the same name has a prominent role in Hindu pantheons throughout northern India."[19]

Pharmaceutical companies know full well that inoculation is a religious rite masquerading as a medical treatment. Below is a native drawing from India published in the Burroughs Wellcome lecture memoranda depicting a Malaba woman invoking the Hindu goddess of smallpox. The caption is as it appeared in the Wellcome Pharmaceutical Company lecture memoranda. Malabar is a region along the southwestern coast of India.

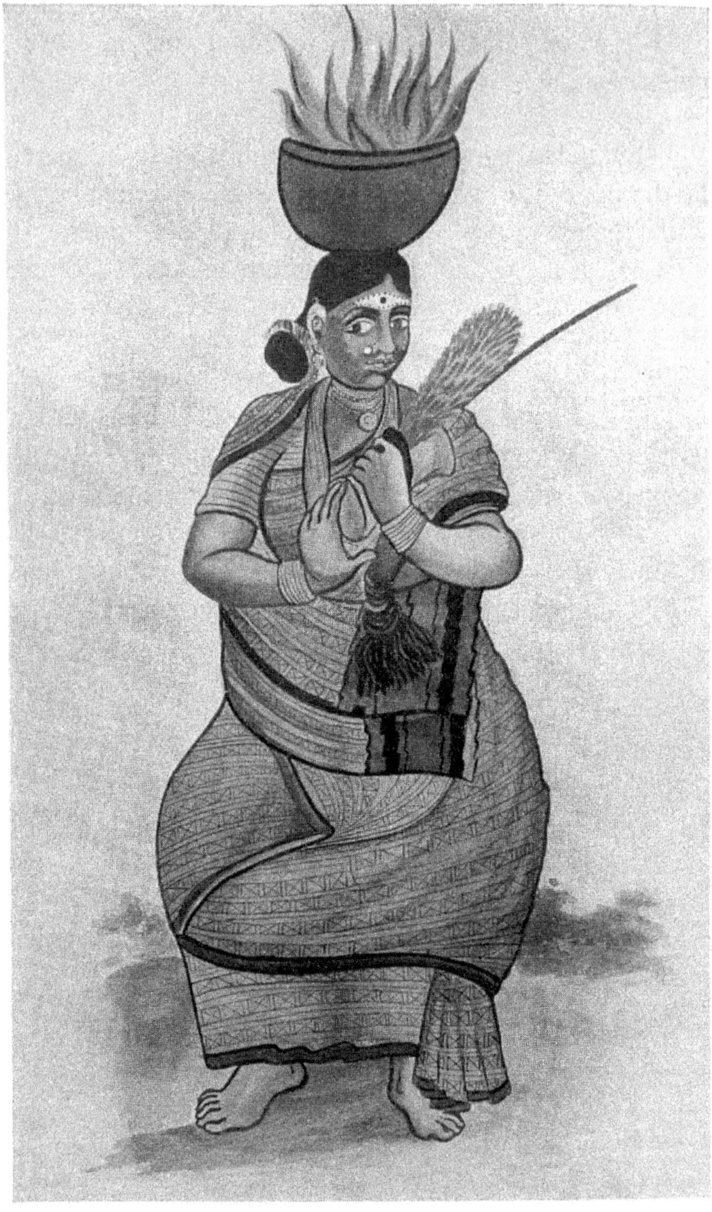

A MALABA WOMAN INVOKING THE GODDESS OF SMALLPOX AND CARRYING FIRE ON HER HEAD SYMBOLIC OF THE DISEASE

From a native drawing

Below is an ancient depiction of the Hindu veneration of the goddess of smallpox, which includes the practice of inoculation as part of the religious superstition. Burroughs Wellcome Pharmaceutical Company published the ancient drawing in its lecture memoranda at the International Congress of Medicine with a caption explaining:

> From an Antient Oriental Drawing. The goddess stands with two uplifted crooked daggers, threatening to strike on the right and left. Before her is a band of the executors of her vengeance. Two of them wear grinning red masks, carry black shields, and brandish naked scimitars. White lines, like, rays, issue from the bodies of the others, to indicate infection. On the left there is a group of men with spotted bodies, inflicted by the malady; bells are hung at their cinctures, and a few of them wave in their hands black feathers. They are preceded by musicians with drums, who are supplicating the pity of the furious deity. Behind the goddess, on the right, there advances a bevy of smiling young women, who are carrying gracefully on their heads baskets with thanksgiving offerings, in gratitude for their lives and their beauty having been spared. There is, besides, a little boy with a bell at his girdle, who seems to be conveying something from the right arm of the goddess. This action may probably be emblematic of inoculation. In a country where every thought, word and deed are mere repetitions of those of their progenitors, a composition like this bears the stamp of great antiquity.[20]

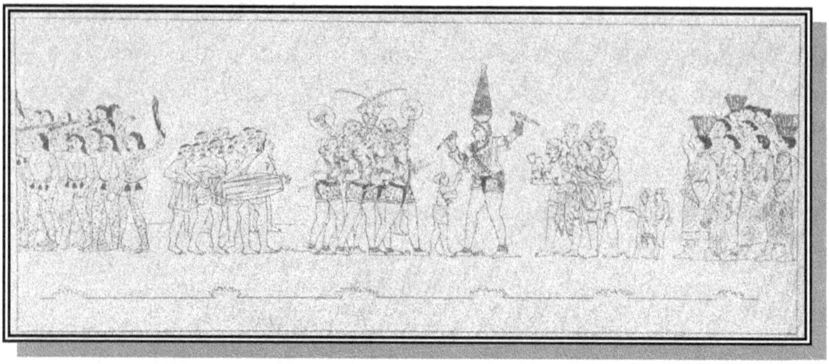

Ancient Depiction of Hindus Appeasing the Goddess of Smallpox Through the Superstitious Practice of Inoculation

Steve Halbrook confirmed that inoculation is founded on Hindu religious practices.

> James Martin Peebles, M.D., M.A., P.H.D., notes that "[s]mallpox inoculation was derived, not from scientific experimentation, but from a superstition practiced by the common people in India since the sixth century."[21] William H. York, in *Health and Wellness in Antiquity Through the Middle Ages*, elaborates:
>
> "Hindu mythology suggests that smallpox was likely present in India at roughly the same time as in Egypt. Religious texts make numerous allusions to the worship of Shitala, the goddess of smallpox, who was supposed to possess the body of individuals, thereby causing the disease. The Atharvaveda also describes a series of services and prayers that Brahmin priests would offer for the worship of Shitala, which included a ritual of inoculation in which people would breathe in dried scabs from smallpox lesions to induce a mild case of the disease. These unsystematic rituals likely led

> to the death of many and were probably not effective enough to have thwarted large-scale outbreaks of the disease, but they offer the earliest account of inoculation measures in the world."[22]

James Martin Peebles explains that the superstitious religious practice of inoculation was not limited to India:

> Mr. Porter, who was English ambassador at Constantinople in 1755, informs us, (Gentleman's Magazine, for October of that year): "It is the tradition and opinion of the inhabitants of the country that a certain angel presides over this disease. That it is to bespeak his favor and evince their confidence that the Georgians take a small portion of variolous matter, and, by means of scarification, introduce it between the thumb and the forefinger of a sound person. The operation is supposed to never miss its effect. To secure beyond all uncertainty the good will of the angel, they hang up scarlet cloths about the bed, that being the favorite colour of the Celestial inhabitants they wish to propitiate."[23]

Inoculation is a superstitious religious custom. Inoculation causes death and disease. Edward Jenner and Benjamin Jesty thought that by using cowpox puss as the antigen, they could induce an immune response to smallpox while reducing the risk of death because cowpox was much less deadly than smallpox. Today, the Jenner quackery continues on the theory that vaccination with something other than smallpox will give immunity to smallpox. The U.S. Food and Drug Administration (FDA) has licensed ACAM2000®, as a vaccine for smallpox.[24] The vaccine does not contain any smallpox (variola) virus. It contains a vaccinia virus in the genus Orthopoxvirus. While the virus is not cowpox, it is in the same genus (Orthopoxvirus) as cowpox. It is a variation of Jenner's cowpox vaccine. The consequences have proven to be the same, death and illness. The smallpox vaccine, ACAM2000®, is religious superstition masquerading as a medical treatment. It is based on the corrupt ethical judgment that the few should be sacrificed for the mythical hope that it will bring about a greater good. It justifies evil means by the hope of doing good. But the good that is hoped for is a phantom. It is quackery and sin.

The Wellcome memoranda reveal that the Hindus carried out the same process of vaccination using cowpox hundreds of years before Jenner and Jesty.[25] But Dominik Wujastyk, seeking to defend the legacy of Jenner and western medicine, disputes the claim that India was the first to use cowpox to vaccinate against smallpox.[26] Today, most use the terms vaccination and inoculation interchangeably to mean the same thing. But some, like Wujastyk, distinguish between vaccination, which Wujastyk limits to describing the use of a vaccinia (e.g., cowpox) virus and inoculation, which Wujastyk limits to describe the use of variola (smallpox) virus.

Wujastyk states that his research has uncovered that "no one disputed the fact that smallpox inoculation [using variola] was frequently practiced in India before the introduction of vaccination [using cowpox]."[27] But he claims that it was not true that the early Hindus used cowpox as the antigen for vaccination. That quibble leaves standing the fact that inoculation using variola from its beginning was based on a religious superstition complete with worship prayers and offerings to a Hindu smallpox goddess called Sitala. Modern-day vaccination finds its roots in that religious superstition and continues with the quackery of Jenner and Jesty.

Vaccination is a religious practice that has been proven to be medically ineffective and harmful.[28] In addition to the Hindus, other heathen tribes had practiced inoculation for centuries past.[29] The practice was usually abandoned once the superstitious treatment was found to be useless and harmful. But the enlightened medical doctors of today seem to be slow learners and are thus slow to abandon a practice that has been proven to be dangerous and ineffective.

The Hindu religion is a heathen religion. God commands us to have nothing to do with heathen practices. "And have no fellowship with the unfruitful works of darkness, but rather reprove them." Ephesians 5:11. We are called on to avoid such practices. "Beware lest any man spoil you through philosophy and vain deceit, after the tradition of men, after the rudiments of the world, and not after Christ." Colossians 2:8.

Christians have nothing religiously in common with Hindus. We are not to practice their heathen religion that masquerades under the guise of medicine. Christians are to separate themselves from the religious practices of heathens.

> Be ye not unequally yoked together with unbelievers: for what fellowship hath righteousness with unrighteousness? and what communion hath light with darkness? And what concord hath Christ with Belial? or what part hath he that believeth with an infidel? And what agreement hath the temple of God with idols? for ye are the temple of the living God; as God hath said, I will dwell in them, and walk in them; and I will be their God, and they shall be my people. Wherefore come out from among them, and be ye separate, saith the Lord, and touch not the unclean thing; and I will receive you, And will be a Father unto you, and ye shall be my sons and daughters, saith the Lord Almighty. (2 Corinthians 6:14-18)

Herbert M. Shelton describes vaccination as not merely quackery but "a criminal operation."[30] He elaborates:

> I would not go so far as to say that vaccination has never saved a single person from smallpox. It is a matter of record that thousands of the victims of this superstitious rite have been saved by the immunizing potency of death.[31]

Dr. Charles Creighton, M.A., M.D. (1847-1927) was a recognized authority in epidemiology. He had orthodox views of vaccination and believed them to be efficacious and safe. He was selected by the publishers of the Encyclopedia Britannica, Ninth Edition, to write the article on Vaccination. He did original and exhaustive research. His research opened his eyes to the reality that vaccines were ineffective and dangerous.[32] Dr. Creighton continued his research and wrote a book titled *Jenner and Vaccination: A Strange Chapter of Medical History*. Dr. Creighton explained that the book was written as he tried to find out **"how the medical profession in various countries could have come to fall under the enchantment of an illusion."**[33] One notable statistic that Dr. Creighton cited in his Encyclopedia Britannica article was that "in Bavaria in 1871 of 30,742 cases [of smallpox] 29,429 were in vaccinated persons, or 95.7 per cent, and 1,313 in the un-vaccinated, or 4.3 per cent."[34]

Upon reading Dr. Creighton's article in the Encyclopedia Britannica, Prof. Edgar M. Crookshank, who was the bacteriologist of King's College, did his own independent research on the efficacy and safety of vaccines in an attempt to assail the findings of Dr. Creighton. He was not able to refute Dr. Creighton's findings. He ended up writing two volumes titled, *The History and Pathology of Vaccination*, in which he presented unrefutable proof that vaccination was "uncertain, unscientific and dangerous."[35]

Herbert Spencer (1820-1903), biologist, could not understand how people could defend the "medical popery" of vaccination while condemning religious popery. Notice Dr.

Creighton reported that in Bavaria, 95.7% of the persons infected with smallpox were vaccinated against smallpox. That not only proves that the vaccines do not work, it shows that the vaccines cause the persons to be more suspetible to the illness they are supposed to prevent. The vaccination compromised their immune system, causing them to be more vulnerable to disease. There is no other explanation for the high percentage of vaccinated persons with smallpox. Dr. Viera Scheibner, Ph.D. principal research scientist and author of *Vaccination: 100 Years of Orthodox Research*, explains:

> The immunological research in the last 100 years has been demonstrating that vaccines actually do not immunize ... So, even the word immunize is incorrect, because that would imply that the vaccines actually immunize; they don't, they de-immunize, they suppress the immunize system, and all they cause is a harmful immune response.[36]

Dr. John Hodge concluded:

> That vaccination is not only useless, but positively injurious; That instead of protecting its subjects from the contagion of smallpox, it actually renders them more susceptible to it by depressing the vital powers and diminishing natural resistance.[37]

Dr. James Martin Peebles writes:

> The erudite Dr. A. Wilder, of New York, physician and author, assures us that if vaccination has any influence, it is that of changing the body from a natural and normal condition to an unnatural and diseased one; in which case, repeated vaccinating can be but an endeavor to make this unnatural and diseased condition permanent. The individual is

> thus rendered sickly, and placed in a state of chronic aptitude to contract other diseases.[38]

Dr. William Howard Hay in a 1937 address to the Medical Freedom Society explained how previously healthy children were struck with lifelong illness upon being vaccinated:

> It is now 30 years since I have been confining myself to the treatment of chronic diseases. During those 30 years I have run against so many histories of little children who had never seen a sick day until they were vaccinated and who, in the several years that have followed, have never seen a well day since. I couldn't put my finger on the disease they have. They just weren't strong. Their resistance was gone. They were perfectly well before they were vaccinated. They have never been well since.[39]

If vaccines are so clearly ineffective and dangerous, why are they falsely propagandized as safe and effective? Because the mantra of "safe and effective" is not based on science. It has become an unassailable religious maxim. It is a religious doctrine that cannot be questioned. All doctors who question the safety and effectiveness of vaccines will find themselves defrocked and relieved of their priestly duties. The so-called "science" of vaccines is a heathen religious practice. It is born of superstition and nurtured by money. The modern doctor administering vaccines is no different from a shaman priest who scares his victim into blindly following his edicts. Brett Wilcox, in his book, *Jabbed*, explains:

> Until fairly recently, traditional religion has provided the predominant paradigm that gives comfort in and purpose to pain, suffering, injustice, and death. Religion offered protection from bad

> weather, malignant spirits, vile people, and poor health. As the influence of religion decreased in modern society, the influence of the religion of Scientism took its place. Germs replaced evil spirits. Doctors replaced shaman. Pharmaceuticals replaced amulets and icons. And vaccines replaced prayers, ceremonies, and rites of passage.[40]

Brett Wilcox correctly characterizes the modern practice of Vaccinology as a religious rite dressed up as science.

> Framing government, medicine and pharma in a religious context may rankle those who have abandoned the confusion and chaos of religion for the perceived certainty of science, but science—as practiced in the modern profit and power-driven paradigm—is no less of a salvation-offering religion than is Christianity, Judaism or Islam. Pure science, on the other hand, is a method for uncovering facts and their interrelationship, but hardly worthy of worship. People of business have co-opted science and turned it into Scientism, the religion for the masses. Scientific bodies have displaced religious bodies just as scientific journals have displaced holy writ. The phrases "All scientists agree" and "The science is settled" have displaced phrases such as "God says" or "The Bible says."[41]

Attorney William Wagner explains in his book, *Vaccine Epidemic,* how the government has replaced God in the minds of the people, who do not question the edicts of government bureaucrats. The commands of the government to get vaccinated are not based on objective truth but rather on public policy dogma.

> The government … increasingly substitutes itself

> for God, as the source of our liberty. The paradigm shifts under this evolving legal philosophy. To evaluate state action that has an impact on parental decisions, the state replaces self-evident, unalienable standards with its own morally relative, utilitarian assessments. Thus the freedom of conscience and the sanctity behind parents directing the upbringing of their children no longer serve as moral benchmarks against which to measure whether government vaccination laws are right or wrong, good or bad, just or unjust. Instead, parents are told that questions regarding vaccination laws are public policy matters for the government to decide. Moreover, parents should not bother asking to participate in the debate if our view of the world is informed by religious principles since we are told we must only adopt public policy informed by secular dogma—without regard to any sacred, conscientious, or moral considerations. Beware. When the government eliminates a self-evident moral element from the law, it removes any moral reference point with which to measure whether laws are right or wrong, good or bad, just or unjust.[42]

People have lost sight of the truth that "the life of the flesh is in the blood." (Leviticus 17:11) They are thus easily tricked into polluting their blood with vaccines. They do not realize that vaccination is a religious ritual wherein the blood is contaminated.

The religion of Vaccinology ever so subtlety gains converts to its sacrament of vaccination by tricking people into thinking that the belief system of Vaccinology is different, it is superior, it is "science." The deluded masses do not perceive that they are being hoodwinked into turning from reliance on Almighty God in heaven to faith in science on earth. Brett Wilcox explains:

> Many people cite religious violence, intolerance, and hypocrisy as the motivation for their exodus from religious practice. However, when leaving their former faith, many of the same individuals fall to their knees in adoration of yet another object of devotion—the religion of Scientism. Despite having so plainly seen the flaws of their former churches, they often become blind to those of the white-coated ecclesiastics of their new secular faith. This peculiar phenomenon is never more evident than in the subsect of Scientism, The Church of Vaccinology.[43]

The disciples in this new religion of Vaccinology are kept ignorant of the cost to their bodies and souls. But the cost is real; they are being sacrificed by poisoning and, tragically, unwittingly sacrificing their children to the gods of Vaccinology. Brett Wilcox explains:

> The gods of Vaccinology are jealous, destructive, and vengeful. Their thirst for blood is not quenched with the sacrifice of a virgin or two. No, they demand the blood of virtually every human upon the planet. And the blood they crave most comes from the bodies of the faith-based community because it's harder to obtain.[44]

History testifies how heathen religions like Islam and Roman Catholicism use government force to gain converts and maintain adherents.[45] Historically, the synergy between religion and government has been close and mutually beneficial. The government-authorized heathen religion keeps the people docile and obedient to the oppressive government, while the government offers special protections to the religion. The force of government is used to eliminate religious competition. The primary target for government persecution is Christianity. That is because the kingdom of Jesus Christ is a spiritual kingdom that is not of this world. The Christian Church is outside the control of the government, and thus it is viewed as an enemy.

> Jesus answered, My kingdom is not of this world: if my kingdom were of this world, then would my servants fight, that I should not be delivered to the Jews: but now is my kingdom not from hence. Pilate therefore said unto him, Art thou a king then? Jesus answered, Thou sayest that I am a king. To this end was I born, and for this cause came I into the world, that I should bear witness unto the truth. Every one that is of the truth heareth my voice. (John 18:36-37)

A follower of Jesus Christ is called on to be unspotted by the heathen practices of vaccination. "Pure religion and undefiled before God and the Father is this, To visit the fatherless and widows in their affliction, and to keep himself unspotted from the world." James 1:27. We are not to take part in heathen religious practices like vaccination. *See* 2 Corinthians 6:14-18.

What is the religion of "scientism" to do when people object to their vaccine ritual? Simple, it uses its government partner to coerce people to get vaccinated. Laws and regulations mandate vaccinations before children can attend public or private schools. Similar regulations mandate vaccines for healthcare workers. The Center for Medicare and Medicaid Services stated: "Strategies that Work: Make the [flu] vaccinations mandatory for employees. Consequences of non-vaccination may result in termination or suspension of employment."[46] And, as has happened recently with the COVID-19 vaccines, the laws are being expanded to the entire population. Indeed, the government has mandated experimental (COVID-19) vaccines for whole swaths of the population.

Mandatory vaccinations violate the constitutional religious rights of the people. Vaccine requirements are driven by evil greed. Basic logic proves that fact. Robert F. Kennedy, Jr., used some basic grade school arithmetic to prove the point that the meningitis vaccine mandates only make sense for those who profit from the vaccine mandates:

> My opposition to new meningitis mandates for every New York State seventh and twelfth grader has nothing to do with autism and everything to do with arithmetic. … . Meningitis is a rare disease that [affected] only 390 people nationally last year. FDA and industry testing show the meningitis vaccine to be unusually low efficacy and high risk. The manufacturers' inserts predict that 1% to 1.3% of inoculated children will suffer "serious adverse effects." CDC's Pink Book forecasts that 0.3% of these will die from the vaccine. Of the 400,000 New York school children inoculated annually, some 4,000 will become [seriously] ill and nine will die in order to prevent around four people from contracting the disease. At between $84 and $117 per shot, and with the requirement for a two-shot series, the law is an $80 million annual windfall for vaccine manufacturers at taxpayer expense. This math makes sense only to the pharmaceutical companies and the Albany politicians who have taken their money.[47]

Vaccinology is a belligerent religion. It will seek to persecute those who are of a different faith. The heathen priests of Vaccinology are of the flesh. They will persecute those who have the Spirit of Jesus Christ. The Bible informs us "that was born after the flesh persecuted him that was born after the Spirit, even so it is now." Galatians 4:29.

The fact that most states allow for religious exemptions to vaccination testifies that vaccination is a religious practice. But the pharmaceutical industry, through its wholly controlled auxiliary, the American Medical Association (AMA), has been lobbying governments to disallow religious exemptions for vaccinations.

The AMA has stated that it will try to eliminate all religious exemptions for vaccinations. In its 2015 newsletter, the AMA said, "the AMA will seek more stringent state immunization requirements to allow exemptions only for medical reasons." The AMA bemoaned the fact that "only two states bar non-medical exemptions based on personal beliefs." The AMA states:

> New AMA policy recommends that states have in place an established decision mechanism that involves qualified public health physicians to determine which vaccines will be mandatory for admission to schools and other public venues. States should only grant exemptions to these mandated vaccines for medical reasons.[48]

The AMA has succeeded in its strategy, as evidenced by the passage of California Senate Bill 277 (SB 277) in 2015. That law removed personal or religious belief as a reason for obtaining an exemption from the vaccination requirements for entering private or public elementary or secondary schools in California. It also did not allow personal or religious belief exemptions for workers in daycare centers. That is just the beginning. That bill was followed by yet another California law (SB 792) signed by Governor Jerry Brown that requires parents who volunteer at public and private daycare and pre-schools to submit to the MMR, TDaP vaccines.[49] All who refuse are barred from volunteering at those facilities unless they have a medical exemption. Religious exemptions are not allowed, per SB 277.

The religion of Vaccinology, like all heathen religions, is

founded on a myth. The sacrament of vaccination is premised on the germ theory that disease is born by contagious viruses. For example, the modern medical myth is that smallpox is a contagious virus that is spread by the inhalation of airborne *variola virus.*[50] That is wrong. Dr. A.R. Campbell was a Texas doctor who discovered that smallpox was only spread by the bite of bedbugs (cimex Lectularius). Cimex is Latin for "bug" and Lectularius is Latin for "couch" or "bed."[51] Dr. Campbell proved that smallpox is not contagious and is not an airborne disease. In 1919 Dr. Campbell was nominated for the Nobel Prize in Medicine by the resolution of the legislature of the State of Texas for his work in eradicating mosquitoes assumed to cause malaria.[52] Dr. Campbell was the head bacteriologist for the city of San Antonio, Texas. Dr. Campbell constructed bat houses and colonized bats as you would bees. The bats would completely decimate the misquotes in the surrounding area.

Dr. Cambell regularly mingled with his smallpox patients, and he never contracted smallpox. But Dr. Campbell always found bed bugs in the homes of his patients who contracted smallpox. The medical myth is that vaccines have eradicated smallpox. Indeed, the CDC claims that "[t]hanks to the success of vaccination, the last natural outbreak of smallpox in the United States occurred in 1949."[53] The truth is that smallpox has been eradicated by modern sanitation and regular washing of bedding and clothing, which serve to eliminate bed bugs.[54]

Vaccination is justified on the same basis as sacrificing children to Molech. God calls it an abomination to sacrifice children to Molech. The heathen religious practice was to immolate the children to appease the pagan god, Molech. God states: "And thou shalt not let any of thy seed pass through the fire to Molech, neither shalt thou profane the name of thy God: I am the LORD." (Leviticus 18:21)

Parents would sacrifice their child to Molech to gain future protection against disease, famine, and war. There was tremendous pressure put on families to sacrifice their children for the greater good of the community. It was viewed as beneficial to sacrifice a few for the benefit of the many.

That is the same reasoning behind vaccination. It is understood that vaccines are inherently dangerous and will kill and injure some of those who are vaccinated. Indeed, the pharmaceutical companies and the government acknowledge that vaccines are inherently dangerous, which is the basis for the government granting pharmaceutical companies immunity from civil liability. The government thinks it is beneficial to sacrifice a few for the benefit of the many even when they know that there is no benefit to the many.

Vaccination is the shedding of innocent blood. One of the abominable sins of the Jews was the shedding of innocent blood through sacrificing their children to idols. "And shed innocent blood, even the blood of their sons and of their daughters, whom they sacrificed unto the idols of Canaan: and the land was polluted with blood." (Psalms 106:38)

In the case of the COVID-19 vaccines, Dr. Toby Rogers calculated that "[f]or every one child [allegedly] saved by the shot, another 117 would be killed by the shot."[55] But the CDC, has nonetheless placed the COVID-19 vaccine on the childhood vaccine schedule, with beginning doses starting at six months of age. The vaccine schedule is applied in whole or part by school districts nationwide as a prerequisite to entering school.

The concept of mandating vaccines is based on the theory of herd immunity. Under the herd immunity theory, there is indirect protection for the community from an infectious disease when a certain threshold of the population allegedly becomes immune to the disease through infection or vaccination. The World Health Organization advocates for developing so-called herd immunity through vaccination.[56] That same ethic drove parents to sacrifice their children to Molech. For the greater good of the herd, the child must be sacrificed. In the context of COVID-19, President Biden explained:

> The second reason to get vaccinated is to protect your community, your family, your friends, and your neighbors. Vaccines can save your own life, but they can also save your grandmother's life, your coworker's life, the grocery store clerk, or the delivery person helping you and your neighbors get through the crisis.[57]

Vaccination has much in common with the religion of Molech. It is the sacrifice of the few to protect the many. Doctors know that a certain percentage of children will die and be injured by vaccines. But as with the sacrifice of children to Molech, the medical community claims that "the benefits outweigh the risks and costs for many vaccines including polio, pertussis, measles, mumps and rubella. Thus, the use of these vaccines provides a net saving to society."[58] As with the worship of Molech, the few must be sacrificed for the benefit of society. Vaccination is the perverse ethic of doing evil that good may result. God calls such an ethic a damnable heresy. *See* Romans 3:8. God condemns it. The child sacrifices to Molech were ineffectual; it was based on mythology. In like manner, vaccination is ineffectual; it is also based on mythology. Just as Molech was no threat, so also viruses pose no threat. The sacrifice of the few to Molech did nothing to protect the many. In like manner, sacrificing the few to vaccination does nothing to protect the many. For example, it has been proven that the COVID-19 vaccine does not prevent the spread of the alleged virus known as SARS-CoV-2 and thus does not offer any immunity to the herd, as was alleged under the vaccine mandates.

There is scientific proof that the more vaccines administered to infants, the higher the infant death rate.[59] But vaccination is not based on science; it is based on religion. The religion of Molech. Parents obediently march their children to the pediatrician, who, like a priest of Molech, administers deadly poison to the children. The religious mantra is that vaccines are safe and effective; only a few will die. The few must die for the benefit of the many. Among the many surviving children, there will be those who will suffer lifelong ailments. And like Molech, the protection is a myth.

The First Amendment to the U.S. Constitution prohibits the government from establishing a religion or interfering with the people's God-given right to freely exercise religion. That means that the government is prohibited from requiring its citizens to engage in a religious ritual. The government cannot legally require anybody to engage in a religious rite, especially when it is known to cause death and disease. Vaccination is a heathen religious custom born from Satan's hatred of God and man. The First Amendment protects the people from religious tyranny, even when the religion is cloaked with the false patina of science. The constitutional protection should be at its zenith when the religious rite is premised on a degenerate philosophy that evil must be done so that some good may come about. God warns us about just such so-called science that would be used to deceive us.

> [K]eep that which is committed to thy trust, avoiding profane and vain babblings, and oppositions of **science falsely so called**: Which some professing have erred concerning the faith. Grace be with thee. Amen. 1 Timothy 6:20-21.

2 The Truth about the Polio Vaccine

The most often cited success story for vaccines is the alleged eradication of polio by the polio vaccines. Similar to the smallpox vaccine success myth, the polio vaccine success story is a medical tale more akin to a religious superstition than scientific fact.

Polio is short for Poliomyelitis. It is a combination of the Greek words for gray (polio) and marrow (mulos) and inflammation (itis). It denotes the inflammation of the gray matter of the spinal cord. The first great polio outbreak was the 1916 Northeastern United States polio outbreak. 25,000 people were stricken, and 5,000 died.

The 1916 polio outbreak began in Brooklyn, New York. Dan Olmstead reveals that a contagious virus did not cause the polio outbreak.[60] The first indication was that it was food-born. That is because it began with many who came down with polio after consuming ice cream at a particular ice cream shop in Brooklyn. But the illness struck adults as well. The ice cream shop owner was struck with the disease, but recovered. It turns out that the sugar that was used in making the ice cream was tainted with arsenic. How did that happen?

The tainted sugar was shipped to New York from Hawaii. There was a sugar plantation in Hawaii that was having a hard time financially and needed a solution to cutting labor costs. The problem was that weeds were choking out the sugar cane. In 1913 C.F. Eckart, head of the Hawaii Sugar Planters Association experiment station was hired by the plantation owners to solve the problem. Olmstead explains:

> The root of the problem at Olaa was the rainfall on the windward volcanic slope of the Big Island, which could reach 200 inches a year and allowed weeds to overtake the crop itself. The manpower required to keep ahead of them over the two-year growing season threatened whatever profit the plantation might eke out.[61]

Eckart's solution was to use arsenic to kill the weeds. The benefit of arsenic is that it killed the weeds but did not harm the sugar cane. But the problem was that the arsenic would absorb into the soil and then be taken up by the sugar cane. Thus, the arsenic ended up inside the sugar cane. The havested sugar cane was contaminated with the arsenic. After the sugar cane was refined and shipped to New York, it was introduced into ice cream and candy goods made by companies along the Northeastern United States. The people, primarily small children, who ate the sweets would then be stricken with polio caused by the ingestion of the arsenic.

The next great polio epidemic was after the widespread use of the pesticide DDT began in 1945. In the Mid- 1950's Physician Morton S. Biskind testified before Congress that polio resulted from central nervous system poison (CNS) and not a virus.[62] The principal poison being spread among the populace of the day was dichlorodiphenyltrichloroethane, commonly known as DDT. DDT was used during World War 2 to control mosquitoes. By 1945, DDT was available for public sale in the United States and began to be widely used.[63] The government and industry promoted it for use as an agricultural and household pesticide.

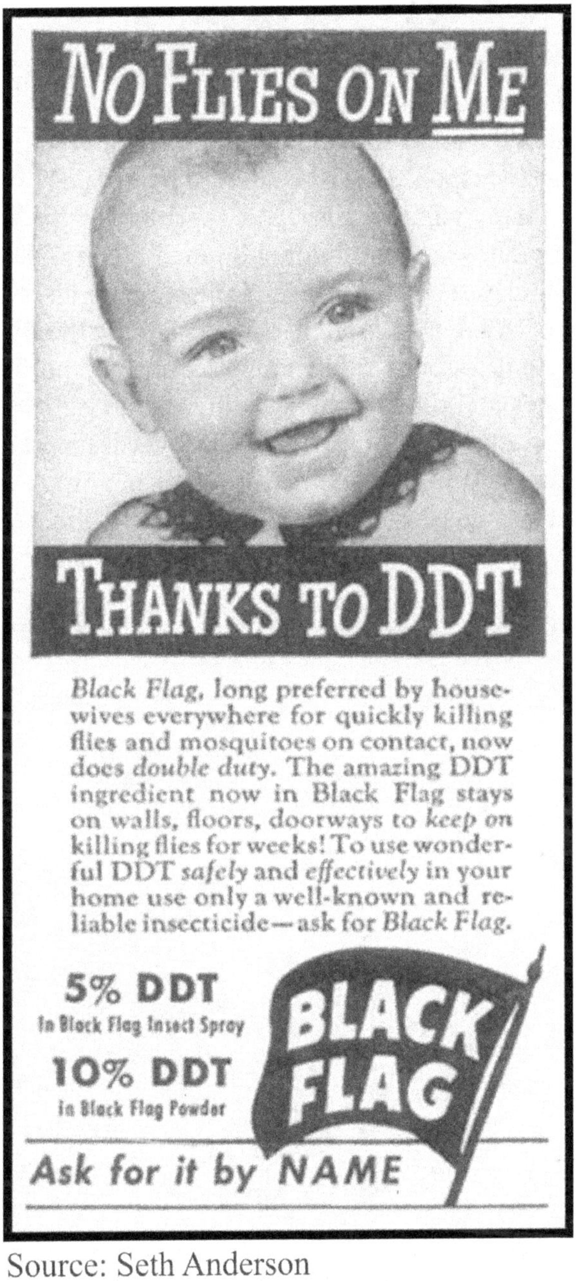

Source: Seth Anderson

Dr. Suzanne Humphries explains how in the 1940's and 50's DDT was thought to be safe:

> Insects were not just the bane of cattlemen and farmers throughout the world. Flies, in particular, were believed to spread polio outdoors and in the home. In response, fearful parents sprayed DDT on all their windowsills and sprinkled it on sandwiches in their children's lunch boxes. DDT in water was used to rinse clothes, bedding, and mattresses. It was thought to be a safe and effective insecticide—even safe enough to spray at public beaches and directly onto children in an effort to halt the spread of polio. [A DDT advertisement in the day said:] "Only a little fly you say? Yes ...but what a dangerous monster! He can carry polio, and many other horrible disease germs, right into your home!"[64]

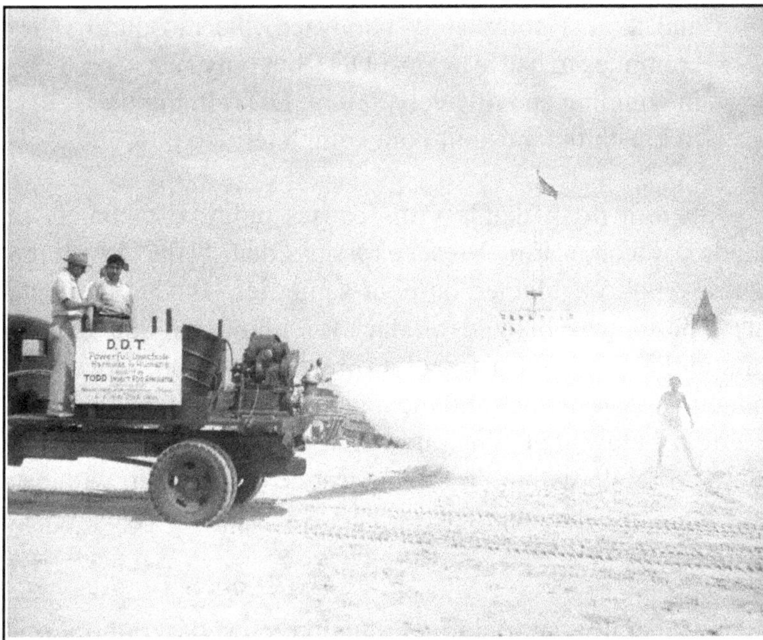

A beach on Long Island, New York is being sprayed with DDT on July 8, 1945. The new machine for spraying the insecticide is being tested for the first time. The beach goers have no fear of the DDT spray because they have been assured it is safe. The sign on the truck says: **"Powerful Insecticide Harmless to Humans."**

Dr. Humfrie's book, *Dissolving Illusions*, narrates the effects of DDT on a mosquito. The paralyzing effect on the mosquito is strikingly similar to that of a polio sufferer.

> [The]mosquito feels effects of DDT, gives frantic kick, leaps into air. As DDT enters nervous system and starts to paralyze muscles, mosquito seems to be trying to kick off paralyzing sensation. Paralysis of the nervous system affects the mosquito legs. The mosquito staggers, falls over, tries to push back onto its legs. It makes one last violent effort to rise but topples back onto its head. On its back

> and almost completely paralyzed, the mosquito continues to battle against DDT but only succeeds in wiggling convulsively. It took DDT 45 minutes to knock the mosquito out completely.[65]

It is a myth that a virus causes polio. But that is the orthodox theory. Jim West explains that "[i]n developing countries, polio is blamed on poor sanitation. But in the United States, polio was blamed on lack of immunity due to good sanitation!"[66] Jim West found a direct correlation between the production of pesticides and the incidence of polio. West created the graph below that illustrates that "[v]irtually all peaks and valleys correlate with a direct one-to-one relationship with each pesticide as it enters and leaves the US market."[67] West further explains:

> Generally, pesticide production precedes polio incidence by 1 to 2 years. I assume that this variation is due to variations in reporting methods and the time it takes to move pesticides from factory to warehouse, through distribution channels, onto the food crops and to the dinner table.[68]

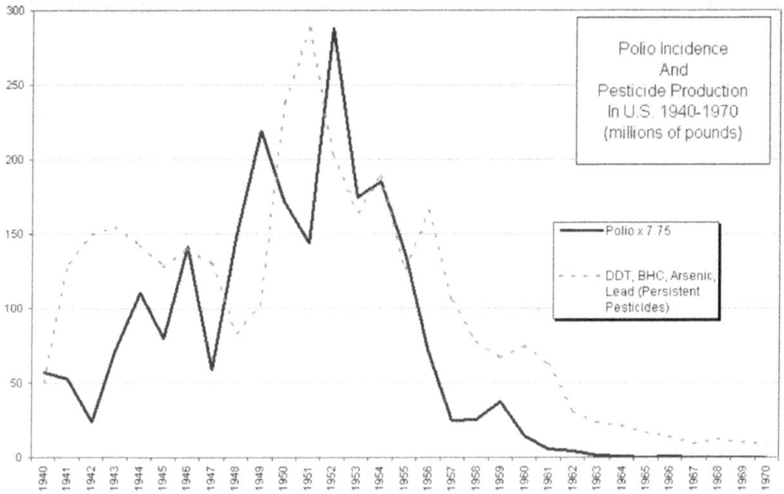

These pesticides represented in the graph are the major pesticides in use during the last major polio epidemic. West states:

> They persist in the environment as neurotoxins that cause polio-like symptoms, poliolike physiology, and were dumped onto and into human food at dosage levels far above that approved by the FDA. They directly correlate with the incidence of various neurological diseases called "polio" before 1965. They were utilized, according to Biskind, in the "most intensive campaign of mass poisoning in known human history."[69]

The graph shows that polio has no movement independent from pesticide movement. Yet, the virus theory for polio persists today. But one might argue that polio disappeared after the introduction of the polio vaccines. That is true, but the reduction in the incidence of polio after the introduction of the polio vaccines was not due to the effectiveness of the vaccines. Dr. Suzanne Humphries explains that there was a reduction in the use of dangerous pesticides like DDT at the time the polio vaccine was first introduced in 1955, and the criteria for reporting polio became more strict. [70]

The introduction of more strict criteria for reported polio upon the introduction of the polio vaccine had the effect of concealing vaccine-induced polio cases. After the polio vaccine was introduced, there were a significant number of vaccine-induced polio cases. But they were not reported as polio due to the strict requirements introduced for reporting a case of polio. Dr. Suzanne Humphries explains:

> In 1955, the year the Salk vaccine was released, the diagnostic criteria became much more stringent. If there was no residual paralysis 60 days after onset, the disease was not considered to be paralytic polio. This change made a huge difference in the documented prevalence of paralytic polio because most people who experience paralysis recover prior to 60 days.[71]

Recall the earlier outbreak of polio in 1916, which was caused by arsenic. Dr. Humprhies reveals that arsenic was a common ingredient in "therapeutic injections."

> After the removal of arsenic-containing pigments, arsenic poisoning resulted from medicines approved by the AMA in the form of supposedly therapeutic injections. Arsenic was used on fruits and vegetables in lead arsenate and calcium arsenate sprays, which resulted in human and animal ingestion. Washing or removing the outside contaminated layers of arsenic-treated produce was rarely recommended. Massive spray programs in the spring and at harvest are among the reasons why polio was once commonly referred to as summer diarrhea. Later, after cold storage for

> produce was used to extend the shelf life, the programs extended into the winter.[72]

Polio vaccines are unsafe and ineffective. Research reveals that polio is not caused by a virus.[73] If a virus does not cause polio, how does the polio vaccine that allegedly has a live virus cause polio?[74] In 1957, Eleanor McBean explained:

> R. B. Pearson made an exhaustive study of the data and experiments that have been made with polio vaccines and summed up his finding as follows: "Hence, I believe **there was no virus in the vaccine used. It was just a solution of the toxins and acid end-products of the decomposed proteins used that caused all the paralysis.** The acids generated by cooked meat in Dr. Pottenger's cats (experiment that caused polio in the cats) affected the nerves first, and the acids formed in the decomposed proteins used in the vaccines affected the nerves first. It is the same thing and, no so-called 'virus' is connected with it." (From Infantile Paralysis, by Pearson.)[75]

In India, approximately 491,000 children were struck down with polio due to the polio vaccine.[76] To conceal the causal link between the polio vaccine and resulting polio, officials renamed polio non-polio acute flaccid paralysis (NPAFP). Every sentient being familiar with the facts knows the children are being paralyzed by polio and that the polio vaccine causes it. Still, medical and government officials have decided to play the game of relabelling the disease to protect pharmaceutical companies. The polio vaccines causing polio was known at least since 2017. Yet, with that knowledge, pharmacuetical companies persist in pushing their live polio oral vaccines in third world countries.

On September 24, 2019, the Children's Health Defense

Team reported that despite knowing that the oral live polio vaccines cause polio, "the Gates Foundation is 'pushing hard[77] to get the [new oral] vaccine into the field as soon as possible,' speculating that it will have a lower risk of transmitting vaccine virus—however, the Foundation cautiously notes that 'the only way to know for sure will be to use the vaccine.'"[78]

Stop and reflect on the recklessness of the Gates Foundation. They are pushing new oral polio vaccines into the field on nothing but speculation that the vaccines will work and knowing full well that the downside is the vaccines will cause polio. The Gates Foundation is perfectly comfortable experimenting with the children by using the vaccines to see if they will work. All the while, they know that many of the children will contract polio from their vaccine and be paralyzed for life. They are experimenting with children. That is an outrage!

Two months later, on November 25, 2019, the Associated Press reported: "Four African countries have reported new cases of polio linked to the oral vaccine, as global health numbers show there are now more children being paralyzed by viruses originating in vaccines than in the wild."[79]

Brian Shilhavy, the editor of Heath Impact News, wrote an article titled, *Big Pharma and Corporate Media Finally Admit the Oral Polio Vaccine is a Failure – Causes Polio Instead of Preventing*.[80] Shilhavy also included another article after his post from the Children's Health Defense Team explaining the causal link between polio vaccines and polio.[81]

The most notable aspect of Shilhavy's story is the evident coercion imposed on mothers forced to have their children vaccinated. Notice in the picture below that there are four heavily armed officers standing guard to ensure no resistance to the vaccine. Please make no mistake about it. This is a forced vaccination program that the Pakistani government is administering not to benefit children but rather the pharmaceutical companies. The government is the customer who buys the vaccines. The government then forces the vaccines on the populace. The deal with the government grants pharmaceutical companies immunity from any injuries caused by their unsafe and ineffective vaccines. If children develop polio from the vaccine, the pharmaceutical company's attitude is that it's too bad, so sad, for them. There is simply no compensation for the lifelong disability.

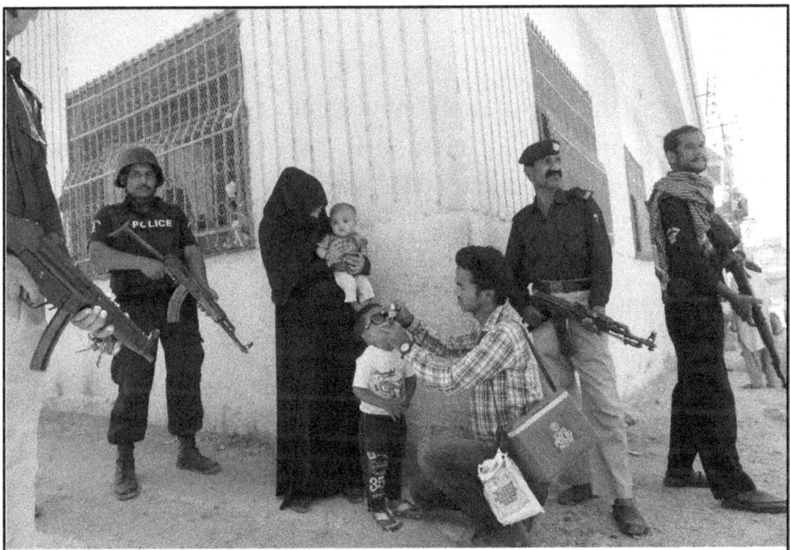

Photo by Asif Hassan/AFP taken during the 2016 Pakistan polio vaccine campaign. It shows the medical tyranny of forced vaccination under the protection of four heavily armed guards to ensure no resistance or interference.

3 Proof That the Measles Virus Does Not Exist

Children in the United States typically receive their mumps vaccination as part of the measles, mumps, and rubella (MMR) vaccine. The U.S. Centers for Disease Control and Prevention (CDC) advises children to receive their first dose between 12 and 15 months and their second between the ages of 4 and 6.[82] The CDC states that "[c]hildren can receive the second dose earlier as long as it is at least 28 days after the first dose."[83]

It has been proven in court that the alleged measles virus does not exist.[84] Dave Mihalovic, writing for Signs of the Times, reported:

> In a recent ruling, judges at the German Federal Supreme Court (BGH) confirmed that the measles virus does not exist. Furthermore, there is not a single scientific study in the world which could prove the existence of the virus in any scientific literature. This raises the question of what was actually injected into millions over the past few decades.

> Not a single scientist, immunologist, infectious disease specialist or medical doctor has ever been able to establish a scientific foundation, not only for the vaccination of measles but any vaccination for infants, pregnant women, the elderly and even many adult subgroups.[85]

The case stems from a reward offered by German biologist Dr. Stefan Lanka. He offered 100,000 euros to anyone who could provide scientific evidence that the measles virus existed. Doctor David Bardens attempted to claim the prize after providing six studies published in a medical journal that allegedly proved the existence of a measles virus.[86] Stefan rejected his proof, and Barden sued. Barden initially won in the regional court in Ravensburg, South Germany. But that decision was overturned by the German Federal Supreme Court.

The BBC reported when Dr. Stefan lost in the first hearing.[87] But, strangely, it did not report on Dr. Stefan's victory on appeal to the German Federal Supreme Court. The Supreme Court decision is significant. Dave Mihalovic explained:

> Five experts have been involved in the case and presented the results of scientific studies. All five experts, including Prof. Dr. Dr. Andreas Podbielski who had been appointed by the OLG Stuttgart as the preceding court, have consistently found that **none of the six publications which have been introduced to the trial, contains scientific proof of the existence of the alleged measles virus.**
>
> In the trial, the results of research into so-called genetic fingerprints of alleged measles virus have been introduced. Two recognised laboratories, including the world's largest and leading genetic Institute, arrived at exactly the same results

independently. **The results prove that the authors of the six publications in the measles virus case were wrong, and as a direct result all measles virologists are still wrong today: They have misinterpreted ordinary constituents of cells as part of the suspected measles virus.**

Because of this error, during decades of consensus building process, normal cell constituents were mentally assembled into a model of a measles virus. To this day, an actual structure that corresponds to this model has been found neither in a human, nor in an animal. With the results of the genetic tests, all thesis of existence of measles virus has been scientifically disproved.

The authors of the six publications and all other persons involved, did not realise the error because they violated the fundamental scientific duty, which is the need to work "lege artis", i.e. in accordance with internationally defined rules and best practice of science. **They did not carry out any control experiments.** Control experiments would have protected authors and mankind from this momentous error. This error became the basis of belief in the existence of any disease-causing viruses. The expert appointed by the court, Prof. Dr. Dr. Podbielski, answering to the relevant question by the court, as per page 7 of the protocol explicitly confirmed that the authors did not conduct any control experiments.[88]

That court finding thoroughly impeaches the scientific claims that there is such a thing as a measles virus. The six publications are the foundational proof for the supposed existence of a measles virus relied on by doctors and scientist worldwide.

The refutation of those studies, in turn, refutes the alleged theory that a virus causes measles. Dave Mihalovic explains:

> The six publications submitted in the trial are the main relevant publications on the subject of "measles virus." Since further to these six publications there not any other publications which would attempt by scientific methods to prove the existence of the measles virus, the Supreme Court judgment in the measles virus trial and the results of the genetic tests have consequences: **Any national and international statements on the alleged measles virus, the infectivity of measles, and on the benefit and safety of vaccination against measles, are since then of no scientific character and have thus been deprived of their legal basis.**[89]

That means that the measles vaccine is a complete fraud. Another significant outcome was the acknowledgment that the measles vaccine causes many severe allergies and autoimmune reactions. Dave Mihalovic explains:

> Upon enquiries which had been triggered by the measles virus contest, the head of the National Reference Institute for Measles at the Robert Koch Institute (RKI), Prof. Dr. Annette Mankertz, admitted an important fact. This admission may explain the increased rate of vaccination-induced disabilities, namely of vaccination against measles, and why and how specifically this kind of vaccination seems to increasingly trigger autism.
>
> **Prof. Mankertz has admitted that the "measles virus" contains [a] typical cell's natural components (ribosomes, the protein factories of**

> **the cell). Since the vaccination against measles contains [the] "whole measles virus," this vaccine contains cell's own structures. This explains why vaccination against measles causes frequent and more severe allergies and autoimmune reactions than other types of vaccination.** The court expert Prof. Podbielski stated on several occasions that by the assertion of the RKI with regard to ribosomes in the measles virus, the thesis of existence of measles virus has been falsified.[90]

What the court decision reveals is that vaccines are based on fraud. The viruses the vaccines are supposed to fight do not exist. Indeed, the MMR vaccine, of which measles is a constituent element, is a dangerous scam. Mike Adams, writing for *Natural News*, reports that Merck fraudulently spiked blood samples to falsely show the efficacy of its measles, mumps, and rubella vaccine (MMR).

> According to two Merck scientists who filed a False Claims Act complaint in 2010 -- a complaint which was unsealed three years ago -- vaccine manufacturer Merck knowingly falsified its mumps vaccine test data, spiked blood samples with animal antibodies, sold a vaccine that actually promoted mumps and measles outbreaks, and ripped off governments and consumers who bought the vaccine thinking it was "95% effective."[91]

That lawsuit was followed by a 2012 antitrust class action lawsuit against Merck filed by Chatom Primary Care, based in Alabama.[92] The complaint alleges that Merck engaged in fraud by artificially inflating MMR vaccine efficacy test results, destroying evidence of falsified data, lying to the FDA, and threatening a virologist in Merck's vaccine division with jail if he reported the fraud to the FDA.[93]

It is not surprising that the MMR has been ineffective in the real world. Dr. Joseph Mercola reveals that "[i]n 2009, more than 1,000 people in New Jersey and New York came down with mumps. At the time, questions arose about the effectiveness of the vaccine as 77 percent of those sickened were vaccinated."[94]

4 Injecting Disease

Vaccines are "usually administered through needle injections."[95] Vaccine active ingredients are allegedly viruses or bacteria.[96] They are commonly called antigens. An antigen is defined as "a substance that enters the body and starts a process that can cause disease."[97] The injected antigen is usually attenuated or inactivated to reduce the risk of disease. The theory behind vaccines promoted to the public is to "stimulate a person's immune system to produce immunity to a specific disease, protecting the person from that disease."[98] In addition to the antigens, vaccines contain an adjuvant, which is intended to stimulate the immune response of the person. Adjuvants are typically heavy metals like mercury or aluminum, which are neurotoxic.[99] Many contaminants find their way into the vaccines from the manufacturing process, including, but not limited to, antibiotics, formaldehyde, and aborted fetal tissue.[100]

Vaccination is a strange medical practice where instead of the doctor trying to cure a person of a disease to make him well again, the doctor purposely infects a well person with a disease in the hope that his reaction to the infection will be less than it would otherwise be if he had contracted the disease through the environment. Vaccination is not without risk. There can be dire consequences to the practice. There are side effects to vaccination that the medical community calls adverse events that can range from soreness in the injection site to fever, paralysis, and even death. The expectation, which is often not realized, is that the vaccinated person will develop an immunity to the disease and be thus protected from future infection. Unlike natural immunity from a disease contracted from the environment, which is typically lifelong, the immunity from vaccination, if it is present at all, is fleeting, requiring booster shots.

Vaccines are not given as therapeutic medicine to treat a person who is ill with a disease. Vaccines are given to people who are well. To get vaccinated is to take on a spirit of fear and reliance on man rather than God.

> But when Jesus heard that, he said unto them, They that be whole need not a physician, but they that are sick." (Matthew 9:12)

> For God has not given us a spirit of fear, but of power and of love and of a sound mind" (2 Timothy 1:7).

Christians are religiously bound to care for their bodies as they are the temple of the Holy Spirit. It is a sin to defile our bodies by injecting them with the polluting poisons of vaccines. The consequent death and illness that flow from vaccination fulfill God's promise to destroy those who would defile their bodies through vaccination.

> Know ye not that ye are the temple of God, and that the Spirit of God dwelleth in you? If any man defile the temple of God, him shall God destroy; for the temple of God is holy, which temple ye are. (1 Corinthians 3:16-17)

> What? know ye not that your body is the temple of

> the Holy Ghost which is in you, which ye have of God, and ye are not your own? For ye are bought with a price: therefore glorify God in your body, and in your spirit, which are God's. (1 Corinthians 6:19-20)

It is the wish of God that we prosper in our physical health. "Beloved, I wish above all things that thou mayest prosper and be in health, even as thy soul prospereth." 3 John 1:2. Vaccines are detrimental to health, and thus, it would violate God's command to be vaccinated. It is an established scientific fact that vaccines cause allergies and other ailments.

5 Poisonous Magic Potions

Merck is the largest vaccine manufacturer in the U.S. Merck claims to "make vaccines for 11 of the 17 diseases on the CDC's recommended immunization schedules."[101] Merck further claims it "distributed ~190M [vaccine] doses around the world in 2019."[102] Merck aspires "to be the premier research-intensive **biopharmaceutical** company."[103]

Another vaccine maker is Pfizer, which proclaims on its website that "[b]iotechnology is our foundation. Benefiting patients is our goal. Innovation, **pharmaceutical** development, and the most dedicated team of clinical researchers is how we do it."[104]

Jansen, a subdivision of Johnson & Johnson, is yet another U.S. pharmaceutical company that describes itself as making **pharmaceutical products**, including "vaccines to treat and cure infectious diseases."[105]

The most recent addition to the vaccine trade in the U.S. is Moderna, which considers itself a biotech company that it claims "has been named a top **biopharmaceutical** employer by Science for the past eight years."[106]

Notably, these companies all describe themselves as pharmaceutical companies. But when you read their websites, they claim to make medicines. Why do they not describe themselves as "medicine" companies? The reason is simple; they also make poisons, and poisons are not medicine.

Medicine means "Any substance, liquid or solid, that has the property of curing or mitigating disease."[107] It is derived from a Latin word "medicina, from medeor," meaning "to cure."[108]

Pharmaceutical, however, has a different, much more expansive definition. While pharmaceuticals can be medicines that cure, they can also be poisons that kill and injure.

Pharmaceutical is an adjective derived from the Greek word pharmacea, meaning "to practice witchcraft or use medicine; poison or medicine."[109] Indeed, the Greek word pharmakeia is translated in the English Bible as "witchcraft" and "sorcery." E.g., Galatians 5:20; Revelation 18:23. The Etymology Dictionary offers this: "from Late Latin pharmaceuticus 'of drugs,' from Greek pharmakeutikos, from pharmakeus 'preparer of drugs, poisoner.'"[110]

A supplier of a pharmaceutical is called a pharmacy. That noun is "directly from Medieval Latin pharmacia, from Greek pharmakeia 'a healing or harmful medicine, a healing or poisonous herb; a drug, poisonous potion; magic (potion), dye, raw material for physical or chemical processing.' This is from pharmakeus (fem. pharmakis) 'a preparer of drugs, a poisoner, a sorcerer' from pharmakon 'a drug, a poison, philter, charm, spell, enchantment.'"[111]

All of the pharmaceutical companies live up to their pharmaceutical billing by selling poisons that kill people. For example, Merck sold a product, Vioxx, to allegedly treat arthritis pain, knowing that it would kill many patients. Their studies showed that Vioxx caused patients to suffer heart attacks and die. Their studies showed that it increased heart attacks by 400% over the control group. Despite that danger, Merck pushed the poison for approval by the FDA. The New Atlantean reports Merck's efforts to get Vioxx approved by the FDA despite the studies showing that the drug killed people.

> Merck resorted to a public relations campaign that aggressively marketed the drug with the help of celebrity endorsements from the likes of Bruce Jenner before it was even approved, a standard of scientific review that revolved around obfuscating the intent of its studies, funding ghostwritten studies that painted the drug in a positive light, creating fake medical journals to laud the drug, and even working in tandem with the FDA to suppress scientific dissent by intimidating doctors who questioned the safety of the drug. Ultimately, the nefarious campaign behind getting Vioxx approved by the FDA would succeed.[112]

Merck falsely promoted Vioxx as safe and effective, knowing it would kill people. Predictably, Vioxx ended up causing 88,000 heart attacks and killing 38,000 people.[113] That is a death toll equivalent to fifteen (15) Pearl Harbors. The New England Journal of Medicine caught Merck altering its testing data by removing evidence in the data that Vioxx kills people.[114] As the body count mounted, the lawsuits followed, and Merck ended up paying $4.85 billion into a settlement fund, ending thousands of lawsuits.[115] Merck pled guilty to criminal charges for their "false statements about the drug's cardiovascular safety." Merck ended up paying $950 million to settle the criminal and civil charges brought against it by the U.S. Department of Justice.[116]

Pfizer acts more like a criminal enterprise. It has been described as "a rogue pharmaceutical corporation[] knowingly and deliberately put[ing] patients' lives at risk."[117] Pfizer's criminality in selling poisons to the public under the guise that they are safe medicines is breathtaking. For example, Pfizer peddled a dangerous antipsychotic drug, Geodon. Pfizer knew Geodon had a life-threatening side effect of altering the heart's rhythm, which posed the risk of sudden death.

Knowing this, Pfizer nonetheless mobilized an army of more than 250 psychiatrists nationwide to whom Pfizer paid handsome speaking fees to promote the deadly drug by convincing other doctors to employ Geodon for off-label use and switch their patients from other, safer drugs.[118] Geodon was just one of four poisonous drugs that in 2009 led to Pfizer paying the largest health care fraud fine in history, $2.3 billion.[119] That case uncovered evidence that Pfizer paid kickbacks to healthcare providers to induce them to prescribe their dangerous drugs. That is just the tip of the iceberg. Over the past 30 years, Pfizer has paid more than $4.7 billion to settle 34 civil and criminal settlements with the federal and state governments.[120]

Johnson & Johnson and its subsidiary Jansen have been sued repeatedly for injury and death caused by their pharmaceutical poisons. For example, it marketed off-label the antipsychotic drug Risperdal. The side effects of the drug included gynecomastia (abnormal breast tissue growth in males), type 2 diabetes, stroke, cardiac arrest, and death. The harm caused by that drug gave rise to 14,000 lawsuits against Johnson & Johnson and its subsidiary Jansen.[121] The U.S. Department of Justice prosecuted Johnson & Johnson and Jansen for their criminality in marketing Risperdal. Incidentally, Risperdal was only one of three drugs for which the DOJ was prosecuting Johnson & Johnson. The companies jointly pled guilty to criminal charges and paid $2.2 billion to settle the criminal and civil claims brought by the DOJ. The Justice Department stated that "the conduct at issue in this case jeopardized the health and safety of patients."The Justice Department stated the obvious in its press release about the criminal case settlement: the companies "put profit over patients' health."[122] That seems to be a pattern with all of the pharmaceutical companies.

On or about August 26, 2019, Johnson & Johnson was ordered to pay $572 million to the State of Oklahoma for fueling the opioid addiction crisis in that state.[123] The judge ruled that Johnson & Johnson engaged in deceptive marketing of its opioid drugs, Duragesic and Nucynta sold through its subsidiary Jansen Pharmaceuticals. Jack Fortier and Brian Mann reported for NPR that "Johnson & Johnson also profited by manufacturing raw ingredients for opioids and then selling them to other companies, including Purdue, which makes Oxycontin."[124] Purdue Pharmaceuticals was a co-defendant in the case. Purdue settled with the State of Oklahoma for $272 million.

Incidentally, Perdue Pharmaceuticals was shut down in 2020 and ordered to pay $8 billion in criminal penalties, forfeiture, and civil fines for fraud in its marketing of Oxycontin.[125] Purdue engaged in a scheme where it marketed its opioid products to more than 100 health care providers that Purdue knew were diverting opioids to addicts. Purdue used the traditional scheme of pharmaceutical companies to pay doctors through a doctor-speaker program to induce those doctors to write more prescriptions for Purdue's opioid products. The opioid crisis, fueled by the greed of pharmaceutical companies, reportedly killed 400,000 people from opioid overdoses.[126] According to the CDC, about half of those deaths were from Perdue Pharmacuetical's Oxycontin. Perdue is owned by the Billionaire Sackler family, who are supporters of Israel and large donors to Tel Aviv University. The Sackler School of Medicine in Tel Aviv is resisting a call to have the Sackler name removed from its school.[127]

Although it was clear early on that Oxycontin was addictive and dangerous, Purdue Pharmaceuticals continued to fraudulently market Oxycontin as a non-addictive pain killer knowing full well that the drug would kill people. "Purdue and three executives pleaded guilty in 2007 to federal charges of misbranding drugs and were ordered to pay $635 million."[128] As Purdue saw their profits drop in the U.S. as their criminal drug scheme was being exposed, they decided to move to Latin America, Asia, the Middle East, Africa and other regions. The Los Angeles Times reported in 2016:

> Prescriptions for OxyContin have fallen nearly 40% since 2010, meaning billions in lost revenue for its Connecticut manufacturer, Purdue Pharma. So the company's owners, the Sackler family, are pursuing a new strategy: Put the painkiller that set off the U.S. opioid crisis into medicine cabinets around the world. A network of international companies owned by the family is moving rapidly into Latin America, Asia, the Middle East, Africa and other regions, and pushing for broad use of painkillers in places ill-prepared to deal with the ravages of opioid abuse and addiction.[129]

Purdue Pharmaceuticals marketed its Oxycontin internationally through subsidiary companies and used the same deceptive marketing campaigns claiming it was safe and not habit-forming. The marketing was designed to overcome the deep-seated resistance of doctors who did not want to load up their patients on opioids because of the fear of addiction. The marketing campaign was designed to overcome the doctors' resistance it labeled "opiophobia." Purdue Pharmaceuticals was focused on making money no matter whom they destroyed. "The love of money is the root of all evil." 1 Timothy 6:10.

Moderna is the new pharmaceutical company on the block. The only product to make it to market in the history of that company as of 2023 has been its COVID-19 vaccine. As documented in this book, that product has caused extensive death and injury. That is what pharmaceutical companies do best.

The pharmaceutical companies only care about making money; they do not care whom they injure and kill. Brett Wilcox reveals the sociopathic behavior of pharmaceutical companies. For example, in 1979, a series of sudden infant deaths could be attributed to DTP vaccines from Wyeth Pharmaceutical Company.[130] You would think the company would then recall the batch causing the deaths. But Wyeth did no such thing. Instead, Wyeth "senior management" instituted a policy memorialized in an August 27, 1979, memo that thereafter there would be a practice of "limiting distribution of a large number of vials from a single lot to a single state, county, or city health department."[131] Doing that ensured that the death from "hot lots" of DTP vaccines would be spread nationwide, the hope being that the deaths being less concentrated would thus be less noticeable. Wyeth understood that their DTP vaccines were killing children; their objective once the deadliness of their vaccine became known to the public was to ensure that the deaths were less noticeable so they would be less likely to be attributed to the DTP vaccine.

Brett Wilcox compares the behavior of Wyeth to drug dealers. "Drug dealers routinely kill for profit. Vaccine sociopaths have knowingly put at risk virtually every person on the planet to protect and increase their profits. Wyeth provided a disturbing example of sociopathy."[132]

Even scarier is that it is the policy of the U.S. Government to cooperate with the pharmaceutical companies in covering up any dangers posed by vaccines so that the population will not think that vaccines are unsafe or ineffective. This policy includes injecting dangerous vaccines into people's arms even though the pharmaceutical companies and the government know the vaccines will kill and injure the population. Below is a direct quote from the 1972 Executive Reorganization and Government Research of the Committee on Government Operations United States Senate:

> [E]ven when the contaminating virus was found to be oncogenic [cancer causing] in hamsters, the DBS [Division of Biologics Standards] and its expert advisory committee decided to leave existing stocks on the market rather than risk eroding public confidence by a recall. ... There has been a tendency on the part of certain higher government circles to play down any open discussion of problems associated with vaccines.[133]

Congress found that the pharmaceutical companies, with the cooperation of the Federal Government, intentionally allowed vaccines known to be contaminated with carcinogenic viruses to be left on the market and injected into people "rather than risk eroding public confidence by a recall" of the dangerous vaccines. That shocking finding was not isolated; it is part of a confidence game (a.k.a., a con game) designed to deceive the public into having confidence that vaccines are safe and effective when they are, in reality, dangerous and ineffectual. That is the behavior of sociopathic religious zealots. They will kill and harm people to keep the con game going and money rolling in.

For example, Congressman Percy Priest chaired a full investigation in 1956 of polio vaccine malfeasance by the pharmaceutical companies, including an instance where Cutter Pharmaceutical Company was making dangerous polio vaccines due to unsanitary and incompetent manufacturing practices that resulted in live polio viruses contaminating what was supposed to be an inactivated polio vaccine. Federal regulators knew the issue, but nothing was done to stop it. The Cutter vaccines caused children to be paralyzed with polio. Congressman Priest decided that the malfeasance should be covered up. The public should not be informed about the dangers of contaminated and dangerous polio vaccines that federal regulators allowed to be administered to children.

> [M]any responsible persons had felt that the public should be spared the ordeal of "knowledge about controversy." If word ever got out that the Public Health Service had actually done something damaging to the health of the American people, the consequences would be terrible. ... We felt that no lasting good could come to science or the public if the Public Health Services were discredited.[134]

The public is being conned into believing that vaccines are safe and effective when they are poisons that kill and injure. Brett Wilcox explains that the vaccine industry is nestled in a deceptive premise that vaccines are presumed safe and effective.

> How does the Unholy Trinity—the vaccine industry, medical establishment, and government—get away with calling vaccines "safe and effective" when the US Supreme Court has ruled that vaccines are "unavoidably unsafe?" The short answer is: it lies.[135]

So we see that these companies have chosen a word, pharmaceutical, to describe their businesses to include potions and poisons that are part of the curious dark arts of witchcraft. Indeed, vaccination is a practice embraced by those who worship Satan. For example, the Satanic Temple requires all attendees at their 2023 Satan Conference to be vaccinated and masked.[136] Satanists do not conform to the norms of society. But the vaccine requirement is not the Satanic Temple conforming to society; it is proof that society has conformed to the sorcery of Satanism by injecting poisons into their bodies. Those poisonous potions are made for them by pharmaceutical companies. And that is why pharmaceutical companies are not called medicine companies.

6 The American Medical Association

The pharmaceutical industry launched the American Medical Association (AMA) in 1847 to crush competition from non-patent medicinal therapies.[137] Gathering funding from the Rockefeller and Carnegie foundations the AMA moved to shut down all homeopathic schools of medicine. "Establishments and research which were were not drug based were refused funding and soon dissolved in favor of the lucrative pharmaceutical industry."[138] In 1900 there were 22 homeopathic medical schools in the U.S. But through a well-planned Machiavellian scheme, they were all closed by 1950. If a person did not graduate from an approved medical school, it was impossible to find a job as a doctor.

And, of course, grabbing the reigns of government to serve its ends was one of the key means to destroying the competition. Homeopathy, naturopathy, vitamin therapy, and alternative cancer and arthritis treatments were vilified as quackery, and the government went to work for the pharmaceutical companies to stop the "quackery." The Center for Media and Democracy explains:

> The birth of the AMA in 1847 launched an organized push for a "totalitarian medical

> pharmaceutical police state".Funded by the drug industry, a single, medical monopoly was established using the insurance industry, the U.S. Department of Justice, the Federal Trade Commission (FTC), the Internal Revenue Service (IRC), the U.S. Postal Service and other state and federal agencies. From the onset, the AMA is characterized as a greed motivated trade union, eliminating competitors to its own financial and political interests. Funded by the Carnegie Foundation, Abraham Flexner was ostensibly empowered to investigate the quality of medical education in all 161 medical schools that existed in 1910. In league with Rockefeller billions, Flexner helped destroy the credibility and funding sources for nearly all schools using non-drug based medicine.[139]

The pharmaceutical companies and their AMA have gained control over words as though they are trademarks that cannot be used except when referring to a pharmaceutical drug. Dr. Richard Shulze, N.D., M.H. explains:

> Unfortunately the word "cure" is the sole property of the drug companies. If a nutritional supplement company uses this term they are attacked judiciously. This often leads to bankruptcy. As a result, many natural cures are buried.
>
> Today in the US, only a medical doctor can diagnose a disease, prescribe something, and cure you. Nobody else can say "diagnose", "prescribe" and "cure". That means that nobody can cure you but a medical doctor....I can't say "Chaparral is the cure for a tumour". I can't say garlic is the cure for cholestrol or high blood pressure. They have made

the laws. So that makes me look stupid, impotent, and it makes the herbs look weak and wimpy.

I can't as a herbalist, say that an herb will cure, even though a lot of prescription drugs are made from herbs.

This was a tactic by organised medicine to wipe out the opposition, by making them look silly and impotent…they have the words…they control the high ground. They can walk out and say, "Yes, if you take this drug, you will cure yourself." But they hired lawyers and got the government behind them. If I say that I go to jail. It isn't because the herbs don't work and the drugs are better, it's just because they have more money, they lobbied more and got the law passed in their favour. That is why people get this idea that herbs don't cure you.[140]

7 Dangerous Placebos

The gold standard for a scientific study is a randomized controlled trial (RCT). In an RCT, the study participants are selected from the targeted population and randomly assigned to either a trial or control group. In a vaccine study, the trial group receives the vaccine being tested for efficacy and safety. The control group is supposed to receive a placebo injection, which should be an inert liquid like saline. The study participants and administrators should be kept blind as to which persons are in each group.

The control group is supposed to give the background base for determining adverse events. The adverse events in the trial group are compared to the adverse events in the control group to determine if the vaccine is safe. But pharmaceutical companies have a problem. They know their vaccines are unsafe and could never pass muster as safe and effective in a properly conducted RCT. They could fudge the data, but the problem with doing that is it's a crime and they don't want to go to jail.

The pharmaceutical companies have figured out a way to rig their vaccine studies to conceal the health dangers of their vaccines and, at the same time, avoid jail. Pharmaceutical companies use a trick to make their dangerous vaccines appear safe. They use a bioactive ingredient, which they falsely call a "placebo," to administer to the control group. The bioactive injections cause adverse events in the control group. This raises the background adverse events so that when the vaccine group is compared to the control group receiving the "placebo," the vaccine group's adverse events do not look so bad by comparison.

That is what Merck did when it tested Gardasil. Gardasil® is a quadrivalent human papillomavirus recombinant vaccine (qHPV) made by Merck, The 2006 Gardasil package insert describes two placebos used in its testing.[141] One placebo was a inert saline injection given to 320 members of the control group and another was an injection containing amorphous aluminum hydroxyphosphate sulfate (AAHS) given to another 3,470 members of the control group. The total number of persons in the control group was 3,790 (3,470+320=3,790). When the total control group of 3,790 participants was listed they were described as receiving a "placebo." But AAHS cannot be truly described as a placebo. It is a bioactive ingredient that is formulated to cause the body to have an immune response.

A placebo is an innocuous, inactive substance that does not have a physiological effect on the body.[142] Some prefer to call such inert substances dummies.[143] Indeed, Merck acknowledges that a placebo is supposed to be inert and inactive. "On its website, qHPV vaccine's sponsor [Merck] defines a placebo as 'an inactive pill, liquid, or powder that has no treatment value'. This definition is consistent with the decades old notion of placebos as pharmacologically inert substances used to obtain unbiased assessments in experimental research."[144]

But when Merck sought FDA approval for Gardasil in 2006, it administered AAHS to the control group, while misleadingly calling it a placebo. Furthermore, Merck concealed the independent reporting of the systemic effect of the actual placebo (saline solution) on the control group. This was purposeful because Merck specifically broke out the different localized reactions to the injections site for the “"Aluminum-Containing Placebo" and the saline “placebo.” That is because it was expected that there would likely be some reaction to the injection site for anything injected into the body. But systemic reactions, like fever and nausea, are a whole other matter. Merck lumped the AAHS control group and the saline placebo control group together when reporting systemic reactions. This had the effect of elevating the systemic adverse events caused by the “placebo” injections. Merck reported the combined 3,790 members of the AAHS and saline control group as a single “placebo” group. It made it appear that the systemic adverse event rate of approximately 38.6% for the Gardasil test group was not so bad because the combined 3,790 members of the control group had 35.1% systemic adverse events. Merck purposely obscured that 92% of the control group received AAHS.

Even though 92% of the control group received a bioactive AAHS injection, Merck described the control group throughout the 15-page package insert as receiving a “placebo.” The first mention of an “Aluminum-Containing Placebo” appeared on page 6. But it was only in a chart heading. AAHS is not mentioned again until pages 10 and 12, where it is again listed as an "Aluminum-Containing Placebo," and only in a chart heading. But there was no explanation.

Interestingly, the insert explains: “Each 0.5-mL dose of the [Gardasil] vaccine contains approximately 225 mcg of aluminum (as amorphous aluminum hydroxyphosphate sulfate adjuvant) [AAHS]” among other ingredients. Thus, the test subjects and 92% of the control group were injected with AAHS. When you realize that the purpose of AAHS is to stimulate the immune response and that immune response is the catalyst for adverse events, you get an idea of the trick Merck was pulling. They wanted the control group’s immune system ramped up to have as many adverse events as possible to make the expected adverse events from Gardasil not look so bad by comparison to the "placebo" injected control group.

Once Merck received its 2006 FDA approval for Gardasil it slithered back and rewrote its package insert to explicitly describe the use of AAHS as the "placebo" in the control group.[145] In September 2008, Merck published a new Gardasil package insert that made 68 references to AAHS use in the control group. Suddenly the group of 3,790 people in the control group that was labeled in 2006 as receiving a "Placebo" was now listed as receiving "AAHS control or Saline Placebo." Merck then explains in the package insert that "AAHS Control = Amorphous Aluminum Hydroxyphosphate Sulfate." Once they obtained FDA approval and the coast was clear, Merck decided to go back and tidy up its package insert to reflect what was really happening in the trials.

Peter Doshi, Ph.D., is an Associate Professor of Practice, Sciences, and Health Outcomes Research at the University of Maryland School of Pharmacy. He wrote an article with other scientists exposing the fraud of vaccine researchers using bioactive placebos. In particular, he cited the example of the Merck Gardasil study using AAHS with Merck misleadingly calling it a "placebo." Dr. Doshi correctly identifies that practice as an ethical issue. Dr. Doshi describes the problem:

> [T]he efficacy and safety analyses of these five qHPV [Guaradasil] vaccine trials were conducted as if the trials were controlled with inert placebo when they were not. None of the key publications for these trials, which have been used to inform regulatory and health decision making, appear to discuss how AAHS-containing control could affect the interpretation of results.[146]

Doshi was troubled that Merck lied to the trial participants by telling them they would receive an inactive placebo. When in fact they were receiving a bioactive AAHS injection.

> We also consider that the use of the term 'placebo' to describe an active comparator like AAHS inaccurately describes the formulation that the control arm participants received, and constitutes an important error that requires correction. If trial participants were told they could receive 'placebo' (widely defined as referring to an 'inactive' or 'inert' substance) without being informed of all non-inert contents of the control arm injection, this raises ethical questions about trial conduct as well.[147]

Using a bioactive ingredient that is actually one of the adjuvants used in the Gardasil injection renders the study results almost useless. Dr. Doshi explains:

> With respect to adjuvants in vaccines, the FDA has noted that 'adjuvants have their own pharmacologic activity, which may affect both the immunogenicity and the safety of vaccines. Adverse reactions may include local reactions such as pain, swelling, injection site necrosis, and granulomas. Systemic reactions may include nausea, fever, arthritis, as well as potential immunotoxic reactions. Unexpected, rare events may also occur'.[148]

Dr. Doshi opined that the reasons given by Merck for using AAHS in the control arm were not credible. Merck claimed that it wanted to test only the HPV virus-like particles and therefore used the AAHS in the control group. But that appears to be a deceptive cover story that makes no sense. If that was Merck's objective, it could not accomplish it by only using AAHS. Merck should have included all other excipients that were in the Gardasil vaccine to inject in the control group. Dr. Doshi explains:

> According to qHPV vaccine's prescribing information, each dose of vaccine contains '9.56 mg of sodium chloride, 0.78 mg of L-histidine, 50 mcg of polysorbate 80, 35 mcg of sodium borate, <7 mcg yeast protein/dose and water', in addition to AAHS and HPV virus-like particles. To test HPV virus-like particles, as the manufacturer stated was its intention in using an AAHS control, the control would logically have also included these other ingredients in addition to AAHS.[149]

Finally, Dr. Doshi explains that the study would be irrelevant even if Merck included all other ingredients in the control group injection. To conduct such a study would be scientifically irrational. A vaccine trial aims to assess the safety and efficacy of the vaccine as manufactured and not just one component of the vaccine. That is because there is a synergism between the ingredients in the vaccine, and people are injected with all those ingredients, not just the antigen in the HPV virus-like particles.

> [T]he stated rationale of using AAHS control, to characterise the safety of the HPV virus-like particles, lacks clinical relevance. The clinically relevant question is what are the effects (benefits and harms) of qHPV vaccine—the whole product, not one of its components.[150]

Clearly, the real reason that Merck used AAHS and misleadingly labeled it as a "placebo" in its control group was to ramp up the adverse events in the control group to then show that the Gardasil vaccine was safe compared to the control group receiving a "placebo." Those reading the study will not realize that the "placebo" was not a placebo at all but an injection of a bioactive substance made up of amorphous aluminum hydroxyphosphate sulfate (AAHS).

Merck is not alone. All pharmaceutical companies making childhood vaccines use the same deceptive trick. An author of a book titled *Turtles All the Way Down* needed to remain anonymous to protect himself from backlash in the medical community. The anonymous author explains how the pharmaceutical companies rig the trials while staying out of jail:

> Vaccine trials in general, and childhood vaccine trials specifically, are purposely designed to obscure the true incidence of adverse events of the vaccine being tested. How do they do this? By using a two-step scheme: First, a new vaccine (one which does not have a predecessor), is always tested in a Phase 3 RCT in which the control group receives another vaccine (or a compound very similar to the experimental vaccine, see explanation below). A new pediatric vaccine is never tested during its formal approval process against a neutral solution (placebo). Comparing a trial group to a control group that was given a compound that is likely to cause a similar rate of adverse events facilitates the formation of a false safety profile.[151]

The pharmaceutical companies use the word "placebo" to describe the injection given to the control groups in their studies of childhood vaccines. But the "placebos" always contain bioactive ingredients that cause adverse events. Those adverse events in the control group are then used as the supposed background rate of adverse events to compare the tested vaccine's safety. The tested vaccine may be quite dangerous, but because it is often being compared to an equally dangerous bioactive "placebo" the pharmaceutical companies can announce that the vaccine is safe because it does not significantly increase the rate of adverse events as compared to the control group receiving a "placebo." Shocking as it may sound, it is a historical, scientific fact that no vaccine on the CDC childhood vaccine schedule was ever tested in a randomized controlled trial using an inert placebo for the control group.

The CDC has described the hepatitis A vaccine as "very safe." The CDC recommends that children get a two-shot administration beginning as early as 12 months old.[152] Merck, in 1996, tested its hepatitis A vaccine (VAQTA®) against a control group that was given a "placebo" containing an aluminum diluent. Aluminum is a bioactive ingredient that not only stimulates the immune system but it is also neurotoxic. There are significant side effects to being injected with such a heavy metal. Merck described the placebo as (alum diluent). That means that the aluminum was a diluent. A diluent is a substance used to dilute other ingredients. That suggests the "placebo" carried other unspecified ingredients diluted in the aluminum carrier.

It is not surprising then to find that the 1996 Merck VAQTA® hepatitis A study showed systemic side effects for the control group receiving the 'placebo" that in most instances were equal to or greater than those in the test group getting the VAQTA® vaccine. With that trick, Merck was able to say in their VAQTA® package insert that "[t]here were no significant differences in the rates of any adverse events or adverse reactions between vaccine and placebo recipients after Dose 1."[153]

Another example of the "placebo" scam run by pharmaceutical companies is a 2002 safety trial study for a new DTaP (diphtheria, tetanus, and pertussis) vaccine. The CDC has concluded that "DTaP and Tdap vaccine [*sic*] are safe and effective at preventing diphtheria, tetanus, and pertussis."[154] The CDC based its conclusion that the DTaP vaccine was safe on a rigged study.

In the DTaP study, the "control group" received the older DTP vaccine.[155] In that study, 1 in every 22 subjects in the experimental group became so ill that they were admitted to the hospital.[156] But a similar rate of hospitalization was also reported in the control group. The study thus reported that the "rates of vomiting, convulsions and hospitalizations ... were not significantly different between the two groups."[157] The study showed that the new DTaP vaccine and the older DTP vaccine both have a high rate of adverse events, which caused many children to be hospitalized. But the point of the study was to measure the safety of the new vaccine against the older vaccine and not to measure the vaccine's safety in absolute terms. With the rigged criteria of relative safety, the FDA and the vaccine maker were able to announce a finding that the new vaccine was just as safe as the older vaccine because the rate of hospitalization was the same for both. But no rational person would ever say that a vaccine is safe that causes 1 out of every 22 children to be hospitalized. The trial showed that both the old and new vaccines were unsafe. But because the vaccine maker did not use an actual placebo there was no comparison to an inert (saline solution) the danger of the new DtaP was obscured.

The scam artists at the Pharmaceutical companies argue that when they have a childhood vaccine that has been proven effective, it is unethical not to administer that established vaccine to the control group. That is their cover story, but it is a provable lie. The testing of Prevnar® proves the lie. Prevnar® is supposed to guard against pneumococcus bacterium. Before Prevnar® there was no established childhood vaccine against pneumococcus bacterium. And so, no ethical claim could be made not to use an inert saline solution for the control study group. Nonetheless, Pfizer chose not to test Prevnar® against a true control group using a saline solution. Instead, Pfizer used a bioactive meningococol bacterium "placebo."

It gets worse; the control "placebo" was an investigational vaccine. An investigational vaccine is an experimental vaccine that has only been tested in a laboratory and is approved by the FDA for use on persons for testing purposes only.[158] An investigational vaccine has not been shown to be safe or effective. That means the "placebo" vaccine given to the control group was an unproven and possibly unsafe vaccine that could cause unknown adverse events. The testers introduced an unknown variable into their test.

Pfizer went a step further in contaminating the test. Pfizer gave both the control group and the test group the DTaP vaccine. The Pfizer Prevnar® insert states:

> Efficacy was assessed in a randomized, double-blinded clinical trial in a multiethnic population at Northern California Kaiser Permanente (NCKP) from October 1995 through August 20, 1998, in which 37,816 infants were randomized to receive either Prevnar® or a control vaccine (an investigational meningococcal group C conjugate vaccine [MnCC]) at 2, 4, 6, and 12-15 months of age. Prevnar® was administered to 18,906 children and the control vaccine to 18,910 children. Routinely recommended vaccines were also administered which changed during the trial to reflect changing AAP and Advisory Committee on Immunization Practices (ACIP) recommendations.[159]

Pfizer did all it could to obscure the dangerousness of Prevnar. It was as though they knew that Prevnar would be shown in the study to be dangerous to children. The test did not disappoint. Sure enough, the study resulted in about 1,000 infants being hospitalized; that amounted to one out of every 35 infants in the study being hospitalized.[160] One out of every 16 children in the trial needed to be taken to the emergency room within 30 days of being vaccinated.

The study reported 5 cases of sudden infant death syndrome (SIDS) among the Prevnar test group and 8 cases of sudden infant death syndrome among the control group receiving the "placebo." Prevnar was shown to kill children, yet because they rigged the study to ramp up the control group's deaths by giving the control an experimental vaccine, they concluded that Prevnar was safe. Furthermore, the study authors stated: "The number of SIDS deaths in the efficacy study from October 1995 until April 20, 1999, was similar to or lower than the age and season-adjusted expected rate from the California State data from 1995-1997."[161] The study authors compared the SIDS data in the study to the SIDS data from a state that mandates childhood vaccinations and does not allow religious exemptions.

It is interesting that many of the childhood vaccine studies report SIDS data. But when people try to link SIDS to vaccines, they are considered conspiracy theorists or anti-vax wackos.

But Pfizer was not done. They must keep the poisons coming. Prevnar was purported to work against 7 strains of pneumococcus bacteria. In 2010, it updated its Prevnar vaccine to cover 13 pneumococcus bacterial strains. The new vaccine was branded Prevnar 13. How did they study the new vaccine for efficacy and safety? Well, they were not about to use an inert saline solution for the control group. So, they tested Prevnar 13 against the control group receiving the previously approved predecessor Prevnar vaccine.[162] What was the result? The Prevnar 13 package insert reveals:

> **Serious adverse events** reported following vaccination in infants and toddlers occurred in **8.2%** among Prevnar 13 recipients and **7.2%** among Prevnar recipients.[163]

You read that correctly. The FDA approved Prevnar 13 as safe even when **8.2% (one out of every 12 children) suffered a "serious adverse event"** from the vaccine. But because Prevnar 13 was compared to an equally dangerous predecessor vaccine, it was deemed by the FDA to be safe. There was a lot of money at stake with Prevnar and its successor vaccine, Prevnar 13. Reuters reported in 2014 that Prevnar and Prevnar 13 combined annual sales of almost $4.5 billion made them Pfizer's second-biggest franchise.[164]

This same scam is being run for adult vaccines. For example, Jeremy Howick revealed that "in the COVID-19 vaccine developed by the University of Oxford, the control group receives a meningitis and septicaemia vaccine as a placebo." [165] The Oxford COVID-19 vaccine is made by AstraZeneca and sold under the brand names Covishield and Vaxzevria.

On April 29, 2020, Pfizer-BioNTech announced the phases 1-2 studies (NCT04368728) of its COVID-19 vaccine.[166] The trial was described as "a Phase 1/2, randomized, **placebo-controlled**, observer-blind, dose-finding, and vaccine candidate-selection study in healthy adults."[167] One would naturally think that Pfizer-BioNTech would conduct the study using an inert saline solution. But you would be wrong.

The Informed Consent Action Network (ICAN) filed a Freedom of Information Act request with the FDA asking for the ingredients of the "placebo" used in the Pfizer-BioNTech studies. The FDA responded by denying the request. The FDA stated in pertinent part that information was a "trade secret" and thus "confidential commercial information."[168]

Dear reader, think about that. The placebo used in the control groups for the Pfizer-BioNTech COVID-19 vaccine trials is considered a confidential trade secret. We know from that alone that the placebo was not an inert substance like saline because saline is not and cannot be a trade secret. Thus, we know that the ingredients for the "placebo" were very likely bioactive. Pfizer-BioNTech likely used their usual procedure of administering a bioactive ingredient to the control group to set a very high level of adverse events against with which to measure the mRNA COVID-19 vaccine to make the mRNA COVID-19 falsely appear safe. We now know that their scheme worked because the Pfizer-BioNTech COVID-19 vaccine won emergency use authorization and immediately began injuring and killing people.

8 Food Allergies

Vinu Arumugham, in an article written for the Journal of Developing Drugs, reveals that "Nobel Laureate Charles Richet demonstrated over a hundred years ago that injecting a protein into animals or humans causes immune system sensitization to that protein."[169] What does that mean for the person receiving the vaccine? Arumugham explains that "[s]ubsequent exposure to the protein can result in allergic reactions or anaphylaxis."[170] Thus, food proteins injected into a person through a vaccine can have the effect of causing a subsequent allergic reaction by that person who subsequently eats food that contains the food proteins in the vaccine.

Vaccines are the source of the explosion in food allergies in the United States. Indeed, there are more than 15 million Americans who suffer from life-threatening food allergies. Arumugham reveals how this happens.

> Vaccines contain adjuvants such as pertussis toxins and aluminum compounds that also bias towards allergy. Adjuvants also increase the immunogenicity of injected food proteins. This combination of atopic children and food protein injection along with adjuvants contributes to

millions developing life-threatening food allergies.

That means that vaccines can cause food allergies. Arumugham reveals that this scientific fact of vaccine-induced allergies "has since been demonstrated over and over again in humans and animal models."[171] Vaccines contain food proteins derived from chicken eggs, casein, gelatin, soy, agar, peanut oil, etc. Those ingredients sound innocent enough. And if they were eaten they would not be harmful and, indeed, would be nutritious. But when those same ingredients are injected into a human body, in a significant number of cases, a person develops an allergic reaction or even anaphylaxis to that food protein.

The allergic reaction is caused because accompanying the food protein is an adjuvant whose purpose is to stimulate the body's immune response to the antigen. The problem is that the stimulated immune response is not limited to the antigen. The body also develops an immune response to the food proteins in the vaccine. The stimulated immune response to the food protein causes an allergic reaction to the food when consumed.

For example, casein is a phosphoprotein derived from milk. Trace amounts of casein are often found in vaccines. Indeed, the DTaP children's vaccine is cultured using bovine casein as a medium. There has been an explosion of people who have developed allergies to milk. According to the American College of Allergy, Asthma, and Immunology, "cow's milk is the most common food allergy in children under the age of 5."[172] It is probable that milk allergies in young children are a direct result of the stimulated immune response to the bovine casein in the DTaP vaccine.

Anaphylaxis caused by peanuts is the leading cause of death among food allergies. Brett Wilcox, in his book, *Jabbed*, reveals that "[a]ccording to Heather Fraser, author of *The Peanut Allergy Epidemic*, the explosion of peanut and many other allergies in recent years is linked to the use of peanut oil in vaccines."[173]

Robyn Charron scrutinized the evidence gathered in Heather Fraser's book, *The Peanut Allergy Epidemic*. She concluded that Fraser was correct. The explosion in peanut allergies directly results from vaccinations. Charon states:

> A lot of people might be surprised to know that there are food oils in injectable vaccines. In the 1930s there was cottonseed oil in vaccines, followed by a short-lived spate of cottonseed oil allergies of about a decade that quietly went away with a change in formula. In the 1960s and 1970s a flu vaccine used peanut oil as an adjuvant to make a smaller amount of influenza antigen elicit a bigger antibody response from the immune system. From 1950-1980 an injectable penicillin was suspended in peanut oil to allow for a slow release of penicillin while the body metabolized the oil. The occasional anaphylactic death from subsequently eating peanuts made headlines.[174]

Charron explains how the oil used in a vaccine doesn't need to be peanut oil to cause a peanut allergy. Oils in vaccines that are closely related to peanut oil cause peanut allergies. Charron identifies the use of castor oil in the original formula of the Vitamin K shot given to newborns as causing peanut allergies because castor oil is known to cross-sensitize immune systems to peanut oil. When the Vitamin K injection was reformulated in 2006 to replace castor oil with lecithin derived from soybean and egg that only exacerbated the resulting food allergies because soybean and peanuts have molecular weights that cause cross-reactivity. The soybean oil in the vaccine is sensitizing some babies to peanuts. Charron further explains how the bacterial Hib vaccine causes peanut allergies:

> It is now known that the structure and weight of the Hib bacteria proteins are very similar to the structure and weight of the peanut protein, which leads to cross reactivity to peanuts and tree nuts. We are, essentially, creating anaphylactic babies in the same manner researchers create anaphylactic mice: administering a peanut-like protein fused to adjuvant bacterial toxin.[175]

Shockingly, that fact regarding vaccine-induced allergies has been known by the scientific community for more than one hundred years, but the pharmaceutical companies, which largely fund the medical schools, keep physicians, most notably pediatricians, in the dark about it. Indeed, medical doctors are only given a few hours of instruction on vaccines during medical school. Physicians are ill-equipped by their medical training to assess the safety of vaccines. That ignorance is by design.

9 Vaccines Cause Autism

Autism has exploded from a rate of 1 in 10,000 children in 1970 to 1 in 54 children by 2020.[176] That explosion in autism has correlated with the increase in childhood vaccinations. The correlation is unmistakable. The conclusion is ineluctable; childhood vaccinations cause autism. With each new vaccine comes an increased incidence of autism. In the United States, children have gone from receiving only the DTP and smallpox vaccines in 1940 to receiving the MMR, polio, and DTP shots in 1980, to now receiving 11 vaccines, involving 29 separate shots before the child reaches the age of 15 months old, according to the 2023 CDC childhood vaccine schedule.[177] The poor children have their immune systems bombarded with 19 shots before they reach six months old.[178]

Synaptogenesis is the formation of synapses in the brain, which are the contact points where information is transmitted between neurons. Intense synaptogenesis occurs in children as they grow during the first 18 months. Vaccines produce immune activation, which disrupts synaptogenesis in a child's brain. There is likely a synergistic effect caused by neurotoxic ingredients in the vaccines, like aluminum or mercury, at the very time the brain is developing. This adverse effect on the child's brain causes autism.

A medical researcher explains:

> The science reviewed here tells a consistent and compelling story: that vaccines may cause autism by stimulating immune activation and elevated cytokines in the brain. Al [aluminum] adjuvants are implicated as a cause of autism because they can be transported into the brain, because they cause microglial activation at vaccine-relevant dosages, and because aluminum induces IL-6 in the brain.[179]

Aluminum is used as an adjuvant in vaccines given to children. Vaccine advocates claim that an aluminum adjuvant dissolves in the blood and is removed by the kidneys. But that claim is based on the assumption that the aluminum is ingested by drinking it. That is not the case when aluminum is contained in a vaccine injected into the body. Research has shown that aluminum travels from the injection site throughout the body to the brain.[180] The aluminum remains in the organs of the body, wreaking havoc. Aluminum causes inflammation in the brain. A single vaccine shot contains more than enough aluminum to inflame an infant's brain.[181]

Researchers using fluorescence microscopy have found high levels of aluminum in the brain tissue of those who have autism.[182] That is significant because, as explained by Dr Chris Shaw, Neuroscientist and aluminum researcher at University of British Columbia, "the existing evidence on the toxicology and pharmacokinetics of Al [aluminum] adjuvants...altogether strongly implicate these compounds as contributors to the rising prevalence of neurobehavioural disorders in children."[183]

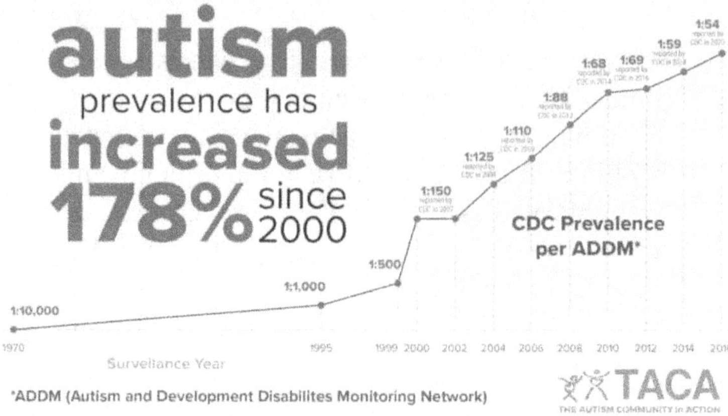

A study of newborn boys showed that those who were vaccinated with Hepatitis B had threefold greater odds for autism compared to boys who were not vaccinated.[184] Another study involving 666 children that compared 405 vaccinated children with 261 unvaccinated children revealed that vaccinated children had 4.7 times greater diagnoses of autism.[185]

That study raised a furor among the powerful pharmaceutical companies and allied interests. They took immediate action to force the Frontiers in Public Health Journal to retract publication of the study. It was republished in the Journal of Translational Science, but similar pressure was brought on that journal and it subsequently also retracted publication of the study. It is interesting to note that those who denigrate that study never discuss the details of the study. They limit their discussion to general allegations of bias, with no specifics. Indeed, they cannot allow the information in the study to be generally known.[186] The study can be downloaded from the link provided at the endnote at the end of this sentence.[187] See also the study by Dr. Andrew Wakefield that linked vaccines to autism that *The Lancet* retracted.[188]

You will never hear of a study alleging no connection between vaccination and autism suddenly withdrawn from publication. Indeed, when you look at the studies closely, they studiously limit their study to only the MMR vaccine. Often they are comparing groups where the unvaccinated group has actually received other vaccines, it is just that they did not receive the MMR vaccine. And so the results are announced that the study shows that the MMR vaccine does not cause autism because the rates of autism are the same as for the non-MMR group.

To keep the vaccine wagon rolling, the pharmaceutical companies and their minions must have some studies to establish the safety of their unsafe vaccines. Since their vaccines are dangerous, and they most certainly cause autism, the only way a study can show they are safe is if they rig the study.

In a 2019 Denmark study, the largest study of its kind, researchers in Denmark compared 625,842 vaccinated children with 31,619 unvaccinated children.[189] The unvaccinated children were those that had not received the MMR vaccination. Whereas the vaccinated children had received the MMR vaccination. They concluded that the MMR vaccine did not cause any appreciable difference in the rate of autism between the groups. That is how it was portrayed to the public. But let us look at that study a little closer.

The Novo Nordisk Foundation funded the study.[190] Furthermore, the two principal researchers both received additional financial grants from the Novo Nordisk Foundation during their work on the autism/MMR research.[191] The Novo Nordisk Foundation is a Danish charitable trust with significant corporate pharmaceutical interests.[192] Its wholly owned subsidiary, Novo Holdings, is the holding company for the pharmaceutical companies Novo Nordisk A/S and Novozymes. Novo Nordisk Foundation's assets were estimated in 2021 to be worth approximately US$93.73 billion, making it one of the largest charitable foundations in the world.[193] They have interlocking interests with other giant philanthropic foundations like the Bill and Malinda Gates Foundation.[194] The Gates and Novo Nordisk foundations use their charitable trusts to push agendas that enhance corporate profits.

Pharmaceutical companies, like Novo Nordisk, have an interest in seeing the vaccines continue to be given to children. That is because they make a lot of money on pharmaceuticals that are subsequently needed to address the injuries caused by the vaccines.

Novo Nordisk also profits directly from vaccine manufacturing. Novo Nordisk makes Cetyl Trimethyl Ammonium Bromide (CTAB), which is a germicide that is a powerful cationic surfactant "used in vaccine downstream processing in both bacterial and viral vaccines."[195] Novo Nordisk explains that "CTAB (Cetrimonium Bromide) is recommended by the WHO in bacterial vaccine manufacturing as a purification agent for polysaccharide vaccines."[196] Notably, "[p]olysaccharide vaccines are commonly found in standard children vaccination programs."[197] If a vaccine (like the MMR vaccine) is shown to be unsafe or ineffective, that will hurt the profits of Novo Nordisk.

The Danish research study was also funded by the Danish Ministry of Health.[198] The Danish Health Authority is interested in seeing a study outcome favorable to childhood vaccines. After all, their official stance is that "All young children are vaccinated against the following diseases: Diphtheria, tetanus, whooping cough, polio, ... Meningitis ... Measles, mumps and German measles [rubella] [a.k.a. MMR]."[199]

He who pays the piper calls the tune. The researchers understood that if their research found that the MMR caused autism, the government and Novo Nordisk would be very unhappy with them. Their research grants from the Novo Nordisk

Foundation and the government would end if they found a causal link between the MMR vaccine and autism. It is no big surprise that the researchers concluded what they were paid to conclude. It is interesting to study how they rigged their study to find that MMR vaccines do not cause autism.

The study is rather suspicious because at the outset it cites to Dr. Wakefield's study that was retracted by *The Lancet* that showed a direct correlation between childhood vaccines and autism. That suggests that their research was designed to rebut Dr. Wakefield's study. Indeed, in an email to NPR, the lead researcher, Anders Hvid suggested that the research was prompted by the fact that "the idea that vaccines cause autism is still around despite our original and other well-conducted studies."[200] Hvid was concerned that "[p]arents still encounter these claims [that vaccines cause autism] on social media, by politicians, by celebrities, etc."[201] Although he did not come out and say so, his comments suggested that his research was to refute the MMR-autism causation argument. He had an agenda.

Hvid states that he was concerned about the argument that "vaccines" cause autism. But that is not what he researched. To answer that question he raised about vaccines causing autism, one must compare vaccinated and unvaccinated children. But Hvid did not do that. He compared two groups of vaccinated children. He compared a group that received a single vaccine against five diseases against another group that received that same vaccine plus another vaccine against three diseases. In Denmark, that single vaccine against five diseases is given four times at intervals of 3 months of age, 5 months of age, 12 months of age, and 5 years of age.[202] The second vaccine is given twice, at 15 months old and again at 4 years old.[203] The single vaccine group received the diphtheria, acellular pertussis, tetanus, inactivated poliovirus, and Haemophilus influenza type b (a.k.a., DtaP-IPV/Hib) vaccine. The double vaccine group received the additional vaccine against measles, mumps, and rubella (MMR).

The researchers were careful to label the unvaccinated group "MMR-unvacciated" and the vaccinated group "MMR-vaccinated." The reason for that nomenclature was that the MMR-unvaccinated group was only not vaccinated with the MMR vaccine. The unvaccinated group was not truly unvaccinated. 26,890 of the 31,619 children in the "MMR-unvaccinated" group received other vaccinations. Thus, more than 85% of the children labeled as "MMR-unvaccinated" received vaccinations. They received diphtheria, acellular pertussis, tetanus, inactivated poliovirus, and Haemophilus influenza type b vaccines (a.k.a., DtaP-IPV/Hib). Any one of those vaccines could cause an increase in autism in the "MMR-unvaccinated" group. And certainly, the cumulative effect of those seriatim vaccinations on a young child could be devastating to a child's undeveloped immune system. The only vaccine missed by the unvaccinated group was the MMR vaccine. The high numbers of autism sufferers in the MMR-unvaccinated group would then be compared to the MMR-vaccinated group and allow the researchers to claim that the MMR vaccine does not cause autism because the rate of autism would be similar. The Denmark study authors concluded:

> The study strongly supports that MMR vaccination does not increase the risk for autism, does not trigger autism in susceptible children, and is not associated with clustering of autism cases after vaccination.[204]

That conclusion in the Denmark study can be likened to a study of the intoxicating properties of rum. In our hypothetical rum study, we will have 10 persons consume a shot of vodka, a shot of whiskey, a shot of gin, a shot of tequila, and a shot of rum, and another 10 persons will consume all of those shots of alcoholic beverages but not the shot of rum. Both groups of persons (all 20) end up drunk. Thus, just as do the vaccine researchers, we can conclude that rum could not have caused the drunkenness because both the 10 persons who drank rum and the

10 persons who did not drink rum got drunk. We can then publicly announce that our study proves that rum is not an intoxicating liquor. Those are the kinds of shenanigans being pulled by "scientists" portraying dangerous vaccines as safe to the public.

And so the non-MMR group, being not truly an unvaccinated group, is presenting a higher autism number than would be the case for a truly unvaccinated group. When looking at a study that truly compares a vaccinated group vs. an unvaccinated group, the results are significant. A recent study that compared truly unvaccinated children with vaccinated children revealed that vaccinated children had 4.7 times greater diagnoses of autism.

Notably, the Danish researchers acknowledged the elephant in the room. "A general criticism of observational vaccine effect studies is that they do not include a completely unvaccinated group of children."

They should have compared a purely unvaccinated group against a vaccinated group. But they did not do that. The mainstream media misinforms the public that "[t]here's strong new evidence that a common childhood vaccine is safe."[205] They trumpet statements of the co-author of the Denmark study, Anders Hviid, stated that he hopes the findings will reassure parents. He further stated, "[p]arents should not avoid vaccinating their children for fear of autism."[206] Does that sound like an objective researcher? He is showing his bias by reassuring parents that they should not be afraid that vaccines cause autism. But how would he know that? His study compared two vaccinated groups. And his study was limited to the MMR vaccine. But he went further in his comment to cover all vaccines. That sounds like a promoter of vaccines, not an objective researcher. And it seems that he had an agenda. Mission accomplished.

Pedro Alcantara of the Asociacion Espanola de Pediatria

posted the following public comment alleging that the study came to a misleading conclusion.

> Both the control group and the study have previously received a cocktail of vaccines: DTaP-IPV/Hib by 12 months of age. Obviously, if some or all of the vaccines in the cocktail caused autism in susceptible kids, by the time the MMR is administered all the susceptible kids would already be autistic and the extra MMR wouldn't affect much the incidence in the study group relative to the control group. Therefore the correct conclusion would be that "Later MMR vaccination does not increase the risk in comparison to a cocktail of previously administered vaccines". By omitting this last point from the conclusion the reader is misled into believing that the MMR vaccine has been proven safe in absolute terms, that is, compared to lack of vaccination. By making a grand universal statement that "MMR vaccination does not increase the risk for autism, does not trigger autism in susceptible children, and is not associated with clustering of autism cases after vaccination" the authors unduly extrapolate their observations to unvaccinated subjects. Lawmakers maybe mislead into taking wrong decisions affecting public health.[207]

Anthony R. Mawson, Department of Epidemiology and Biostatistics, School of Public Health, Jackson State University, posted a public comment to the authors of the study that said in pertinent part:

> The effect of these analyses was therefore to compare autism rates in two highly vaccinated groups, thereby obliterating the potential impact of

> vaccines in general. Comparisons should instead be between fully vaccinated and completely unvaccinated groups of children, or between MMR-only vaccinated and completely unvaccinated children in terms of autism.[208]

While the authors of the study responded to comments made by other researchers, they did not respond to the remarks of Anthony Mawson or Pedro Alcantara. It seems that they had no good explanation for what they did. The researchers rigged the study to falsely show that MMR vaccines do not cause autism by ensuring that both the MMR-vaccinated and the MMR-unvaccinated groups were vaccinated.

Such fraudulent studies are planned in advance for the purpose of coming out with a predetermined result. Brett Wilcox, in his book, *Jabbed*, explains:

> When research emerges demonstrating the risks associated with vaccines and vaccine ingredients, the government often responds by conducting fraudulent studies to shore up the faith of vaccine believers. Dr. Gordon Douglas, director of strategic planning for vaccine research at the National Institutes of Health, explained as much in a 2001 presentation at Princeton University when he said,
>
> "Four current studies are taking place to rule out the proposed link between autism and thimcrosal. In order to undo the harmful effects of research claiming to link the [measles] vaccine to an elevated risk of autism, we need to conduct and publicize additional studies to assure parents of safety."[209]

The Director of Strategic Planning for the NIH, who is

supposed to be a public servant looking out for children's safety, is concerned that the studies linking the measles vaccine to autism might be believed. He does not care that the studies are accurate and the prove a real risk of autism. His only concern is that the study may undermine the security that parents have in the safety of the vaccine. He does not warn the parents based on scientific research that the MMR vaccine is dangerous. Instead, he plans out four studies that he announces before they are concluded will "undo the harmful effects of research" that proves that the vaccine is causing autism. How can he be so sure that the four studies he cites will show that the vaccines do not cause autism? Because the studies are rigged.

Brett Wilcox reveals the entities that are really pulling the strings on the puppet known as Dr. Gordan Douglas.

> Robert F. Kennedy Jr. pointed out that when Douglas spoke at Princeton, he was also employed by Aventis, a company that manufactures thimerosal containing vaccines. In addition, Douglas had formerly served as president of Merck's vaccination program. While serving in that capacity in 1991— the beginning of the thimerosal generation and the autism epidemic.[210]

Dr. Douglas knows full well that the mercury-laden thimerosol is neurotoxic. He knew that using mercury in childhood vaccines would cause brain damage (i.e., autism). Brett Wilcox exlpains:

> Robert F. Kennedy [Jr.] asserts that Dr. Maurice Hilleman, one of the fathers of Merck's vaccination programs, warned Dr. Gordon Douglas ... that six-month-old children administered the shots on schedule would suffer mercury exposures 87 times the existing safety standards. He

> recommended that thimerosal use be discontinued, "especially where use in infants and young children is anticipated."[211]

Dr. Douglas knew from the beginning that the MMR vaccine from Merck caused autism. Yet, right up until 2001, when thimerosal was finally removed, Dr. Douglas was trying to rig fraudulent studies to prove that the MMR vaccine was safe.

The American Academy of Pediatrics (AAP) "calls for the on-time, routine immunization of all children and adolescents" and further "reminds pediatricians that every visit is an opportunity to vaccinate."[212] The AAP further recommends "COVID-19 vaccination for all infants, children, and adolescents 6 months of age and older."[213] That is an appalling recommendation in light of the VAERS data showing that the COVID-19 vaccines are associated with 35,347 deaths, 27,113 cases of myocarditis and pericarditis, and 66,462 permanent disabilities as of June 2, 2023.[214] That dangerous recommendation can be explained by the fact that the AAP receives funds from COVID-19 vaccine maker Pfizer.[215] Indeed, the AAP is almost entirely funded by pharmaceutical companies. Among its top ten donors are pharmaceutical giants Johnson & Johnson, Merck, and Sanofi, all vaccine makers.[216] He who pays the piper calls the tune.

Furthermore, the AAP argues against religious liberties by calling for eliminating religious exemptions to vaccinations. "The AAP views nonmedical exemptions to school-required immunizations as inappropriate for individual, public health, and ethical reasons and advocates for their elimination."[217]

The AAP falsely states that vaccines are not associated with autism.[218] The AAP makes that statement even though the AAP knows that vaccines cause permanent brain damage. The AAP has posted a 1998 paper written by CDC researchers that showed the measles vaccine causes permanent brain damage.[219]

Autism is brain damage caused by vaccines. That 1998 study does not stand alone. There are 214 peer-reviewed studies linking vaccines and autism.[220] Several studies have shown that a vaccinated child is more than four times more likely to be stricken with autism than an unvaccinated child.[221]

Steve Kirsch reports that a "large clinical pediatric practice I am personally very familiar with has eschewed the use of all vaccines and acetaminophen and achieved a zero autism rate over the past 25 years even though autism rates were skyrocketing in adjacent clinics."[222] Another pediatric clinic, Homefirst Medical Services, which has treated more than 30,000 children over a 47-year period, found not a single case of autism among the unvaccinated children.[223] Compare that to the shockingly high rate of 1 in 54 autistic children (as of 2020) reported by the CDC. Incidently, Steve Kirsch conducted a study and found that the rate of autism is closer to 1 out of 3 children.[224]

Dr. Lyons Weiler, Ph.D., is the Scientific Director of the Bioinformatics Analysis Core and a Senior Research Scientist at the University of Pittsburgh. Dr. Weiler got a call from one of the top autism experts in the world, who told Dr. Weiler: "We [autism experts] all know vaccines cause autism. We just aren't allowed to talk about it."[225] Steve Kirsch explains that if autism researchers publically admitted that vaccines cause autism, "they would lose their funding, their job, their license to practice medicine, their hospital privileges, their board certifications, etc."[226]

10 Kangaroo Court

Thus far, the federal government and the pharmaceutical companies have not admitted what is obvious, that vaccines cause autism. Research has shown that thimerosal in vaccines is neurotoxic and the proximate cause of autism. While the FDA's decision to remove mercury-laden thimerosal from childhood vaccines was a step in the right direction, autism has continued because other excipients, such as aluminum, are almost as neurotoxic and continue to cause autism. Oddly, although the CDC removed thimerosal from childhood vaccines, it still maintains that it is safe. The CDC has the following information on its website about thimerosal.

> **Is thimerosal safe?**
>
> Yes. Thimerosal has been used safely in vaccines for a long time (since the 1930s).
>
> Scientists have been studying the use of thimerosal in vaccines for many years. They haven't found any evidence that thimerosal causes harm.
>
> **Is thimerosal still used in vaccines for children?**

> No. Thimerosal hasn't been used in vaccines for children since 2001.
>
> However, thimerosal is still used in some flu vaccines. Yearly flu vaccines are recommended for all children. If you are worried about thimerosal, you can ask for a flu vaccine without it.
>
> **Does thimerosal cause autism?**
>
> No. Research does not show any link between thimerosal and autism.[227]

The CDC further states, without equivocation, that childhood vaccines do not cause autism. The CDC says on its website that "there is no link between receiving vaccines and developing [autism spectrum disorder] ASD."[228]

That deception is typical of the CDC. The CDC knows that childhood vaccines are the cause of autism. Furthermore, the CDC knows that the mercury in thimerosal is dangerous and causes autism. They know that because in 1999, Thomas M. Verstraeten, M.D., who works for the CDC in the NIP, Division of Epidemiology and Surveillance Vaccine Safety and Development Branch, prepared a report based on a study he did that showed that those who received vaccines containing thimerosal were 7.6 times more likely to suffer from autism.[229] Furthermore, more than 165 studies have determined that thimerosal is harmful.[230]

Actions speak louder than words. In 2001, the FDA ordered that thimerosal be taken out of childhood vaccines in the U.S. because the FDA determined that the mercury contained in thimerosal was dangerous to children.[231] How could the FDA now claim that thimerosal is safe when it removed thimerosal from the childhood vaccines because they determined it was unsafe? The FDA is double minded. "A double minded man is unstable in all his ways." (James 1:8)

It has been a religious mantra of federal health agencies that vaccines do not cause autism. They and their pharmaceutical company partners know that if it was officially acknowledged that vaccines were the cause of the explosion in autism, it would expose the claim that vaccines are safe as a complete fraud. The government will not budge from its irrational position and will do all it can to create the illusion that vaccines are safe in its written edicts. But the actions of government agencies reveal the truth, that they genuinely know vaccines are dangerous. For example, the Vaccine Injury Compensation Program (VICP) has paid millions of dollars to compensate children for the autism caused to them by their childhood vaccines.[232] At the same time, the VICP has posted in the internet a statement that "HHS has never concluded in any case that autism was caused by vaccination."[233]

Under the 1986 National Childhood Vaccine Injury Act (NCVIA), Congress created an administrative forum that gave Vaccine Injury Compensation Program (VICP) original jurisdiction for all vaccine injury claims.[234] The VICP protects vaccine manufacturers from liability by requiring those injured by vaccines bring their claims for injuries against HHS.[235] They are prohibited from suing manufacturers or healthcare practitioners until they exhaust the administrative process under the VICP.[236] Under the NCVIA, the vaccine makers are immune from liability for failing to disclose known risks to parents or guardians of those being vaccinated.[237]

Mary Holland led a team of researchers from Pace University Law School that found 39 cases of vaccine injury where there was confirmation of autism or autism spectrum disorder where the VICP awarded damages for the autism caused by vaccines.[238] But the offical position of HHS is that they have never awarded any damages to those claiming autism was caused by a vaccine. On February 20, 2009, David Bowman, from the

Office of Communications Health Resources and Services Administration (HRSA) sent an email giving the HRSA official position regarding compensation for autism caused by vaccines.

> In response to your most recent inquiry, HRSA has the following statement:
>
> The government has never compensated, nor has it ever been ordered to compensate, any case based on a determination that autism was actually caused by vaccines. We have compensated cases in which children exhibited an encephalopathy, or general brain disease. Encephalopathy may be accompanied by a medical progression of an array of symptoms including autistic behavior, autism, or seizures.
>
> Some children who have been compensated for vaccine injuries may have shown signs of autism before the decision to compensate, or may ultimately end up with autism or autistic symptoms, but we do not track cases on this basis.[239]

Ginger Taylor summarizes what Bowman said. "What Bowman is saying is that 'vaccines don't really cause autism, they cause brain damage that may cause autism. And we don't pay attention if it does.'"[240] Taylor lampooned the idiocy of the schizophrenic official position of HRSA by writing a parallel satire.

Vaccines Do Not Cause Autism

The government has never compensated, nor has it ever been ordered to compensate, any case based on a determination that autism was actually caused by vaccines. We have compensated cases in which children exhibited an encephalopathy, or general brain disease. Encephalopathy may be accompanied by a medical progression of an array of symptoms including autistic behavior, autism, or seizures.

Some children who have been compensated for vaccine injuries may have shown signs of autism before the decision to compensate, or may ultimately end up with autism or autistic symptoms, but we do not track cases on this basis.

Gunshots Do Not Cause Death

The government has never compensated, nor has it ever been ordered to compensate, any case based on a determination that death was actually caused by gunshot. We have compensated cases in which people exhibited a perforation, or general hole in the body. Perforation may be accompanied by a medical progression of an array of symptoms including bleeding, organ damage, or death.

Some people who have been compensated for gunshot injuries may have shown signs of dying before the decision to compensate, or may ultimately end up dead or with fatal symptoms, but we do not track cases on this basis.

What the government has done in the VICP is award damages for what they call encephalopathy. What they are actually doing is awarding damages for autism, but they have changed the terminology for the award from autism to encephalopathy. It is all a word game. If a parent claims damages alleging that vaccines caused autism, their claim will almost certainly be denied. But if they steer clear of the word autism and claim, instead, that the vaccines caused encephalopathy, their claim could be approved. We have now entered the psychopathic world of Alice's Wonderland. "When I use a word,' Humpty Dumpty said in rather a scornful tone, 'it means just what I choose it to mean — neither more nor less.'"

On February 12, 2009, the VICP special masters ruled in a unique series of test cases that decided the fate of more than 5,000 claims for vaccine-induced autism injuries. The special masters decided that the evidence that vaccines caused autism was unpersuasive. One of the masters could not help but demean the parents and expert doctors who testified that vaccines caused autism in the children. The special master, George Hastings Jr., wrote that the physicians "are guilty, in my view, of gross medical misjudgment."[241]

The VICP test case hearings were a sham, a show trial, complete with fraudulent reports. One doctor, Andrew Zimmerman, had reported in a separate case (Hannah Poling), that vaccines caused Hannah Poling's autism. Yet, the attorneys for the government used a separate report written by Dr. Zimmerman wherein he contradicted himself by saying: "There is no scientific basis for a connection between measles, mumps, and rubella (MMR) vaccine or mercury (Hg) intoxication and autism."[242]

A government attorney had Dr. Zimmerman's report in the Poling case in his possession when he argued to an appeals court that "we are not even at a stage where [a link between vaccines and autism] is medically or scientifically possible."[243] The lawyer knew that was false because his expert, Dr. Zimmerman, had made that link in his Poling report.

Dan Olmstead explains how Rolf Hazlehurst has rock-solid proof of fraud in the VICP test hearings that ended any chance of compensation for more than 5,000 autistic children.

> [H]e has the goods on the sleazy, corrupt and in fact criminal behavior engaged in by HHS attorneys to hide the evidence that his son and so many others were vaccine-injured and now face a lifetime of the neurological catastrophe called autism.[244]

Rolf Hazlehurst is an Assistant District Attorney General for the State of Tennessee, and the father of Yates Hazlehurst, one of the six test cases that were thrown out in the VICP decision. Hazlehurst is an attorney. His legal opinion is that the government committed criminal fraud in the VICP proceedings.

> Well, the government's expert witness in neurology put in writing, yes, vaccines cause autism. Here's how vaccines cause autism. And the Department of Justice and HHS concealed it.
>
> The bottom line is that during the autism omnibus proceedings, the United States Department of Justice, representing the United States Department of Health and Human Services, willfully and intentionally concealed critical material evidence about how vaccines cause autism. ...
>
> Let me put that in perspective for you. If I did to a criminal, in a United States court of law, what the Department of Justice did to vaccine-injured children in the so-called vaccine court, I would be disbarred and I would be facing criminal charges.[245]

Below are the answers to questionnaires sent by Mary Holland and her research team to parents of autistic children who won their cases in the VICP court.[246] How could they win when the federal government's official position is that vaccines do not cause autism, and the government has never compensated any child based on a determination that a vaccine caused his autism? The claims were won because the vaccines caused encephalopathy, not autism. It is a deceitful word game. Don't be fooled. These cases litigated and won in the VICP court prove that vaccines cause autism. The accounts below are hard to read. They give a window into the heart-breaking devastation caused by vaccines. Please pray for these and all families damaged by vaccines.

Question: How is your child's life today?

(A) A. is profoundly autistic. She is non-verbal, has major behavioral issues, is self-injurious. . .classic and very severe autism. . ..She cannot be left alone ever. . ..A. was a beautiful baby, who was developing normally, but who had obvious reactions to her first two DPT vaccines. One left her leg swollen and red, and she developed a high fever and screamed after the other. But the doctors did not hesitate to give A. her third DPT shot when she was 5 months old, and she went over the edge. She had the shot at 4:00 p.m., and by 6:00 p.m. she had a fever of 105 to 106 degrees. . ..After that day, she was gone. Over the years, we have lost many friends and are distant from many family members because A. is so hard to love and be around. It is very heartbreaking to see people reject her, and to have them suggest that we should have institutionalized her.

(B) B. (aged 44) has no speech, no functional use of his hands, and will no longer stand He has a couple of seizures every day. . ..B.'s teeth had to be pulled because he would not allow anyone near his mouth to brush them. He is not potty trained. He is very sensory defensive, flaps his hands, and makes moaning noises.

(C) C. is a "giant baby" because although she is an overweight 18- year-old, she functions at the level of a 2-year old. She has no life really, compared to her peers. She has very little functional communication, and can only say a few words, like "eat" or short phrases that she repeats incessantly. . ..She is still in diapers, with no probability that she will ever be potty trained C. now has frequent periods (every 4 to 6 months) of frustration, extreme rage, and self-injurious behavior.

Question: What was the impact of the vaccine injury on your family?

Devastating.

Question: Was your child's claim resolved fairly?

(A) No, it was a war.

(B) DOJ attorneys were disrespectful and combative. ... The Compensation Program should be about compensation and not about defense of the vaccine program.

(C) The attorney for the government was absolutely horrible. She was cold, insulting, and did whatever she could to keep us from being compensated. She pushed for C. to be put in a group home because it would be cheaper than allowing her to live with her family, and she argued against very basic home safety devices, like latches on cupboards, a fence for the yard, and a special swing where C. would not fall out when a seizure hit.

11 Toxic Excipients

Vaccines contain excipients that are added to the antigen. According to the CDC, only the antigen is considered the "active ingredient."[247] But that does not mean that the excipients do not serve an active function. And it does not mean that the exipients do not actively affect the injected patient. Excipients are often toxic and cause long-term adverse health effects, including severe immunological and brain disorders. The excipients fall into three basic categories: 1) adjuvants, 2) preservatives, and 3) stabilizers.[248] Adjuvants are designed to stimulate the immune response to the antigen in the vaccine. Preservatives prevent degradation and contamination. Stabilizers help keep the vaccines potent during storage.

There are also trace chemicals and materials found in the vaccines. For example, vaccines often contain antibiotics that are used to prevent contamination of bacteria during manufacturing. Vaccines contain cell culture materials used to grow the antigen, such as egg protein and aborted fetal tissue. The trace chemicals are often dangerous, although they may be listed as "inactive ingredients." For instance, the CDC describes toxins found in vaccines, such as formaldehyde, which is used to inactivate viruses, "inactive ingredients."[249] Formaldehyde is a dangerous toxic chemical that disrupts cellular functions and is cytotoxic (causes cell death).[250] Please understand that the CDC does not test the vaccines to determine what ingredients are in them. The CDC simply takes the vaccine manufacturers at their word and republishes the ingredients found in the vaccine package insert.

Vinu Arumugham discovered that "there are no specifications limiting allergen content in vaccines approved for use in the United States." What does that mean for vaccine patients? It means that no safe level has been established for any allergens contained in vaccines. Those who make vaccine excipients such as sorbitol and Polysorbate 80 are not limited in any way by government regulations as to the residual allergens contained in their injectable grade products. Arumugham made the disturbing discovery that "[s]ince there are no limits, suppliers do not test for allergens in production. Further, residual allergens that may be present in the excipients are not even listed in the vaccine package inserts." Thus, there is no way for a doctor to know all of the excipient ingredients in the vaccine being injected into his patient. The doctor (and the patient) are literally flying blind. Each new vaccine injection poses a risk of the patient developing food or other allergies.

Aluminum

A common adjuvant is aluminum.[251] Indeed, the CDC lists aluminum, aluminum hydroxide, aluminum phosphate, aluminum sulfate, or aluminum hydroxyphosphate sulfate as ingredients in 27 vaccines.[252] Aluminum is a dangerous neurotoxin and carcinogen. Research has established that "[t]he adverse neurologic, hematopoietic, skeletal, respiratory, immunologic, and other effects associated with excessive aluminum (Al) exposures are well known."[253]

Research has proven that the neurological effects of aluminum include "impairment on neurobehavioral tests for psychomotor and cognitive performance and an increased incidence of subjective neurological symptoms."[254] Indeed, "studies clearly identify the nervous system as the most sensitive target of aluminum toxicity."[255] In studies involving "intramuscular administration of aluminum hydroxide or aluminum phosphate vaccine adjuvants in rabbits, increased levels of aluminum were found in the kidney, spleen, liver, heart, lymph nodes, and brain (in decreasing order of aluminum concentration)."[256]

Pediatrician Dr. Paul Thomas explains:

> Aluminum, the adjuvant in most vaccines, is the largest and most powerful trigger of autoimmunity. There's an entire book about it called, *Vaccines and Autoimmunity*, edited by Schoenfeld. There are hundreds of articles pointing to this issue. That's just a small piece. ... [Y]our baby's born, and the first thing they do is give your baby a hepatitis B vaccine with a huge dose, 250 mcg. of aluminum, TEN TIMES THE MAXIMUM TOXIC DOSE, according to the FDA. [The FDA] has had an active policy up since 2000 stating not to exceed 5 micrograms/Kg/day of parenteral aluminum. ... And this is also where mandatory vaccine laws are just harmful.[257] (emphasis in original)

Mercury

In 1999, the U.S. Food and Drug Administration (FDA) determined that mercury in childhood vaccines, in the form of thimerosal, exceeded FDA guidelines for mercury exposure. But it was not taken out of childhood vaccines in the U.S. until 2001.[258] Mercury is a known neurotoxin. The mercury safety standards were determined by measuring methylmercury. But the mercury in thimerosal metabolizes in the body as ethylmercury.

The FDA had no safety guidelines for ethylmercury. The FDA did not know what to do, so they correctly required vaccine companies to reduce or eliminate the use of thimerosal in vaccines. The CDC identifies thimerosal as a preservative. Mercury is an effective preservative because it kills bacteria; indeed, it is a heavy metal poison that kills all cells on contact, including the brain cells of infants, as it courses through their fragile bodies. It is still being used in vaccines. While thimerosal has been removed from childhood vaccines, according to the CDC, it remains an ingredient in influenza, tetanus, and Diptheria vaccines.[259]

Eli Lilly, the thimerosal patent holder, contracted for a safety study on thimerosal. The study was determined later to be fraudulent. Researchers H.M. Powell and W.A. Jamieson, both Lilly employees, published the fraudulent study, which the FDA still cites on its website today as proof that thimerosal is safe. The FDA speaks with a forked tongue. It removed thimerosal from childhood vaccines because of mercury toxicity, but it still claims it is safe. That is because thimerosal remains in other vaccines, some of which have since ended up on the childhood vaccine schedule (e.g., the influenza vaccine). The FDA presently states:

> Prior to introduction of thimerosal in the 1930's, data were available in several animal species and humans providing evidence for its safety and effectiveness as a preservative (Powell and Jamieson 1931). Since then, thimerosal has been the subject of numerous studies ... and has a long record of safe and effective use preventing bacterial and fungal contamination of vaccines, with no ill effects established other than minor local reactions at the site of injection.[260]

That is a lie. Thimerosal has devastated children's lives, causing lifelong autism and digestive disorders. But the FDA does not stop there. As of 2016, the FDA had posted on its website the following details about the Powell and Jamieson study:

> The earliest published report of thimerosal use in humans was published in 1931 (Powell and Jamieson 1931). In this report, 22 individuals received 1% solution of thimerosal intravenously for unspecified therapeutic reasons. Subjects received up to 26 milligrams thimerosal/kg (1 milligrams equals 1,000 micrograms) with no reported toxic effects, although 2 subjects demonstrated phlebitis or sloughing of skin after local infiltration. Of note, this study was not specifically designed to examine toxicity; 7 of 22 subjects were observed for only one day, the specific clinical assessments were not described, and no laboratory studies were reported.[261]

That statement was removed from the FDA website some time after 2016. Technically what the FDA says about the Powell and Jamieson study is true. But what is not explained is why "7 of 22 subjects were observed for only one day." 7 of the 22 subjects were observed for only one day because they died that day![262] You read that correctly. 7 out of the 22 subjects died the day they were injected with thimerosal. But the table for the study did not reflect that the study subjects had died. Most of the remaining study patients died by the end of the second day.[263] Those facts were not revealed until 2002. Powell and Jamieson knew before the human studies that thimerosal was toxic because they had done animal studies. A significant number of the animals died from mercury poisoning.[264]

What is reprehensible is that the FDA has known since at least 2002 that the Powell and Jamieson 1931 study was fraudulent. In 2002 an Eli Lilly whistleblower revealed the fraud.[265] But the FDA still cites that scam study as proof that injecting toxic mercury into people is safe.

The FDA knows that the mercury in thimerosal causes autism because in 1999 Thomas M. Verstraeten, M.D., from the CDC, NIP, Division of Epidemiology and Surveillance Vaccine Safety and Development Branch, did a retrospective study involving 400,000 children and determined that those who received vaccines containing thimerosal were 7.6 times more likely to suffer from autism.[266] More than 165 studies have focused on thimerosal, which found it to be harmful. Dr. Brian Hooker, M.D., reports:

> 16 [of those 165 studies] were conducted to specifically examine the effects of Thimerosal on human infants or children with reported outcomes of death; acrodynia; poisoning; allergic reaction; malformations; auto-immune reaction; Well's syndrome; developmental delay; and neurodevelopmental disorders, including tics, speech delay, language delay, attention deficit disorder, and autism.[267]

Polyethylene Glycol

Both the Moderna and the Pfizer/BionTech COVID-19 mRNA vaccines contain lipids, which have polyethylene glycol (PEG) as part of the lipid ingredients.[268] While PEG is not strictly an adjuvant, it allegedly enhances the effect of mRNA vaccines by helping the mRNA access cells. PEG has been proven to cause hypersensitivity reactions.[269] A hypersensitivity reaction is an exaggerated or inappropriate immune response that can include anaphylaxis.[270] "The Anaphylaxis is a medical emergency because it can lead to an acute, life-threatening respiratory failure."[271] Indeed, as of March 5, 2021, "at least 1,689 recipients of the Pfizer and Moderna injections have reported anaphylactic or serious allergic reactions."[272] The anaphylaxis was predictable. Prior research documented the detrimental effects of PEG on drug delivery. On September 25, 2020, Robert Kennedy, Jr., warned the

FDA and NIH about the dangers of PEG in the (at that time) proposed mRNA vaccines.[273] No action was taken by the FDA, NIH, Moderna, or Pfizer to mitigate the risk inherent in the mRNA vaccine PEG excipients.

Polysorbate 80

Polysorbate 80 is an excipient contained in the Johnson & Johnson (aka Janssen) COVID-19 vaccine.[274] It is also an ingredient in the following vaccines: DtaP-IPV, Hep B influenza Meningaogoccal, Pneumococcal, Rotavirus, Tdap, Shingles.[275] Polysorbate 80 is used in vaccines as a surfactant that allows the antigen to evenly dissolve in the excipient vaccine ingredients. Polysorbate 80 is manufactured from food sources such as coconut, palm, sunflower, tapioca, wheat, corn, etc. That sounds safe enough, but Vinue Arumugham explains that it is impossible to guarantee that these products from which the polysorbate 80 is derived do not contain residual allergen proteins. Polysorbate 80 has been proven to cause hypersensitivity reactions.[276] A hypersensitivity reaction is a type of exaggerated or inappropriate immune response that can include anaphylaxis.[277] "The Anaphylaxis is a medical emergency because it can lead to an acute, life-threatening respiratory failure."[278] Indeed, CNBC reported that "[t]wo trial participants suffered severe allergic reactions shortly after getting Johnson & Johnson's Covid-19 vaccine."[279]

Brett Wilcox, in his book, *Jabbed*, deconstructs the FDA's argument that the ingredients in vaccines are safe.

> "Vaccine Ingredients," [is] a subject of utmost importance, because vaccines are chemical concoctions produced by pharmaceutical companies and the simple truth is that nature did not arrange for the ingredients in vaccines to be injected into the blood streams of humans or any

other creature. So what exactly does the FDA have to say about vaccine ingredients?

“A vaccine is made-up of various ingredients and each ingredient present in a vaccine is there for a specific reason. Different ingredients have different roles in a vaccine, and vaccines licensed for use in the United States are demonstrated to be safe and effective before they are used by the public.”

But enough said. The FDA has decreed that vaccines include "various ingredients" and each ingredient is there "for a specific reason" accomplishing "different roles." And, since the FDA pronounces vaccines "to be safe and effective," any sane parent or patient would be a fool not to conclude that all of those unnamed ingredients are also "safe and effective."

Let’s test that theory using FDA’s logic. Formaldehyde, ethylmercury, aluminum, 2-phenoxyethanol, MRC-5 cells, peanut oil, polysorbate 80, and potassium chloride, are a few of the dozens of ingredients found in vaccines. Formaldehyde—embalming fluid—is defined as a carcinogen, but when placed in vaccines, it miraculously becomes safe and effective. Ethylmercury and aluminum are neurotoxins and are synergistically neurotoxic when ingested, but when injected they change into something that’s “safe and effective.” 2-phenoxyethanol is an insecticide. Humans are not insects, but somehow injecting humans with this insecticide is “safe and effective.” Potassium chloride is used in lethal injections to shut down the heart and stop

> breathing, but when injected into babies it's "safe and effective." Of course, the dosage in vaccines is a small fraction of a lethal dosage, but less of a poison does not equal safe, it equals less toxic. MRC-5 cells are cells from aborted human fetuses. Foreign proteins—human or otherwise—can result in a host of medical problems including autoimmune disorders when ingested, but when injected, they're "safe and effective."[280]

Foreign Proteins

Anaphylaxis has been a known side effect of vaccines since 1913. Indeed, the less severe anaphylaxis, an allergic reaction, is so predictable and prevalent that it should be considered a design feature of vaccines. Eleanor McBean explains the debilitating effects of injecting foreign proteins into the bloodstream through vaccination.

> All vaccines and serums are foreign proteins and therefore a virulent poison. If any protein enters the body illegitimately, through any channel other than the digestive tract, it becomes a strong poison. Proteins in themselves cannot be used by the body—they first require to be broken up by the various processes of digestion into Amino Acids before they become useful as a nutrient to the organism and can be taken into the blood stream to be used as building materials. Injections of therapeutic serums in human beings and animals result in impairment and great injury to some of the most vital organs—heart, lungs, liver, kidneys, nerves etc.[281]
>
> ANAPHYLAXIS or SERUM POISONING or DISEASE, sometimes called SERUM SHOCK, are

> the terms being used to indicate the harmful after-effects of vaccination. We cannot tell in advance of the inoculation the amount of damage which will be done in any particular individual, whether he will die of anaphylaxis, be severely damaged for life or throw it off with a minimum amount of harm to himself. The degree of injury done to the organism may have no immediate noticeable effect but will find expression eventually, especially if the harmful practice is continued. It may result in constitutional debility, degeneration, chronic disease, and death. Some of the symptoms following vaccination and resulting in Serum Sickness are: Fever, Glandular Enlargement, Urticaria, Leucopenia, Leukotaxis, Sciatica, Phlebitis, Pain and Tenderness of the Joints, Paralysis, Heart Failure, Collapse and Death.[282]

Eleanor McBean wrote that in 1957. She was revealing what scientists, government agencies, and pharmaceutical companies have known with certainty since 1913; injecting protein into the bloodstream acts as a poison that causes anaphylaxis (i.e., serum poisoning). A less severe anaphylaxis is typically called an allergic reaction.

Sasha Latypova is a former pharmaceutical executive with 25 years of experience in clinical trials, clinical technologies, and regulatory approvals. She owned and managed several contract research organizations doing work for more than 60 pharmaceutical companies worldwide, including, but not limited to, Pfizer, Johnson and Johnson, Novartis, AstraZeneca, and GSK. Latypova reveals that vaccines work in the exact opposite way as we're told they do. She states that it's impossible to make a vaccine that does anything but poison somebody.[283] She states that "vaccines prime our bodies to react badly to anything that's injected into us, including benign substances like milk or egg proteins. Hence the proliferation of allergies, such as allergies to milk, eggs, wheat, peanuts, etc."[284]

Latypova explains that "this has been known since 1913, when Charles Richet—a French physiologist and self-proclaimed eugenicist—won a Nobel Prize for figuring out that injecting animals with toxins primes them for harmful or deadly reactions if they encounter the same toxins in the environment, even in small amounts. He called these reactions 'anaphylactic' reactions, but said that these reactions also included allergies."[285] Latypova explains that, "[i]t's impossible to vaccinate for anything. And Richet has demonstrated it conclusively and was given Nobel Prize for it ... because he figured out how to poison everyone by sensitizing them to the most commonly occurring things in their environment."[286] Vinu Arumugham confirms Latypova's findings; he explains in a research paper:

> Nobel Laureate Charles Richet demonstrated over a hundred years ago that injecting a protein into animals or humans causes immune system sensitization to that protein. Subsequent exposure to the protein can result in allergic reactions or anaphylaxis. This fact has since been demonstrated over and over again in humans and animal models. The Institute of Medicine (IOM) confirmed that food proteins in vaccines cause food allergy, in its 2011 report on vaccine adverse events. The IOM's confirmation is the latest and most authoritative since Dr. Richet's discovery. Many vaccines and injections contain food proteins. Many studies since 1940 have demonstrated that food proteins in vaccines cause sensitization in humans. ... Vaccines contain adjuvants such as pertussis toxins and aluminum compounds that also bias towards allergy. Adjuvants also increase the

> immunogenicity of injected food proteins. This combination of atopic children and food protein injection along with adjuvants, contributes to millions developing lifethreatening food allergies.[287]

The Nobel Prize Foundation describes the standard view of the theory behind vaccination.

> Our immune system protects us from attacks by microorganisms and poisonous substances. After experiencing an attack, the immune system learns to defend itself against new attacks—we become immune. One of the ways this is used is with vaccinations, when a low dosage of an infectious substance provides immunity.[288]

That is the standard theory of vaccination. But the Nobel Prize Foundation explains that Charles Richet discovered that vaccines have the opposite effect. Vaccination actually makes one sicker.

> Through studies involving dogs, Charles Richet demonstrated an opposite effect in 1902. After an initial low dose of a substance, a new dose some weeks later could produce a severe reaction. He called the phenomenon anaphylaxis. The result had important implications for our understanding of allergies.[289]

Charles Richet was a eugenicist. He was part of the same eugenics philosophy shared by Bill Gates. Eugenicists think that the earth is overpopulated, and thus it is proper to poison people through vaccination to keep the population in check. Vaccination is the most ingenious way of poisoning because it is slow-acting and brings on death over a long time through a series of disabling diseases that are difficult to trace to their source–vaccines. The government agencies propped up seemingly to protect the public in actuality act as gatekeepers for the pharmaceutical companies to conceal the dangerousness of vaccines and their causal link to life-shortening diseases.

The medical profession and governments know that vaccines contain harmful poisons. Their protestations to the contrary are simply lies. Indeed, adverse reactions to vaccines are listed in the ICD-CM as "poisoning." **Poison is "a substance that through its chemical action usually kills, injures, or impairs an organism."**[290] As we have seen, the vaccine ingredients contain excipients like aluminum, formaldehyde, antibiotics, Polyethylene Glycol, and polysorbate 80 that are neurotoxic and carcinogenic. The adverse events from vaccines sometimes result in death. Most survive the vaccinations only to have a lifetime of health issues. But the poisons in the vaccines are so slow-acting that most do not realize that their allergies, heart conditions, autism, infertility, cancer, and neuromuscular diseases are caused by vaccines. The medical establishment knows the vaccine ingredients are poisonous, and they say so in their billing codes, known as the International Classification of Diseases Clinical Modification (ICD-CM).

The CDC explains:

> [ICD-9-CM and] ICD-10-CM—the International Classification of Diseases, [Ninth and] Tenth Revision[s], Clinical Modification—[...are] based to code and classify medical diagnoses. [ICD-9-CM and] ICD-10-CM [...are] based on [ICD-9 and] ICD-10, the system[s] used to code and classify mortality data from death certificates.[291]

The modern trend in the ICD-CM is away from specifying the specific vaccine that caused the poisoning instead to identifying the vaccine under a generic category of vaccines. For example, "poisoning by tetanus vaccine" under the ICD-9-CM has been swept into the generic category of "Poisoning by other bacterial vaccines" under the ICD-10-CM. "Poisoning by measles vaccine" under the ICD-9-CM has been swept into the generic category of "Poisoning by other viral vaccines" under the ICD-10-CM. The ICDM-9-CM has specific code listings for poisoning by tetanus, diphtheria, measles, poliomyelitis, tuberculosis, typhoid, paratyphoid, cholera, pertussis, smallpox, typhus, yellow fever, and rabies vaccines. Many of those specific ICD-9-CM listings have been recategorized into general categories under the ICD-10-CM. Below are a few examples:

> ICD-9-CM Diagnosis Code 978.4: **Poisoning by tetanus vaccine.**[292]
> ICD-9-CM Diagnosis Code 978.4 converts approximately to 2025 ICD-10-CM T50.A92A **Poisoning by other bacterial vaccines**, intentional self-harm, initial encounter.[293]
>
> ICD-9-CM Diagnosis Code 978.5: **Poisoning by diphtheria vaccine.**[294]
> ICD-9-CM Diagnosis Code 978.5 converts approximately to 2025 ICD-10-CM T50.A92A **Poisoning by other bacterial vaccines**, intentional self-harm, initial encounter.[295]
>
> ICD-9-CM Diagnosis Code 979.4: **Poisoning by measles vaccine.**[296]
> ICD-9-CM 979.4 converts approximately to: 2025 ICD-10-CM Diagnosis Code T50.B91A (effective October 1, 2024): **Poisoning by other viral vaccines**, accidental (unintentional), initial encounter.[297]
>
> ICD-9-CM Diagnosis Code 979.5: **Poisoning by**

poliomyelitis vaccine.
ICD-9-CM Diagnosis Code 979.5 converts to approximately 025 ICD-10-CM T50.B91A **Poisoning by other viral vaccines**, accidental (unintentional), initial encounter.[298]

Aborted Fetal Tissue Used in Making Vaccines

Vaccines often contain aborted fetal tissue, and those that do not contain aborted fetal tissue are often developed using aborted fetal tissues. The Vaccine Education Center for the Children's Hospital of Philadelphia explains:

> Vaccines for varicella (chickenpox), rubella (the "R" in the MMR vaccine), hepatitis A, rabies (one version, called Imovax®) and COVID-19 (one U.S.-approved version, Johnson & Johnson (J&J)/Janssen) are all made by growing the viruses in fetal cells. All of these, except the COVID-19 vaccine, are made using fibroblast cells. The COVID-19 vaccine (J&J/Janssen) is made using fetal retinal cells.[299]

The CDC states that there are "[n]o tissues such as aborted fetal cells, gelatin, or any materials from any animal"[300] in the COVID-19 vaccines. But that is misleading because the CDC does not reveal that aborted fetal cells are used in the manufacturing of the COVID-19 vaccines. Furthermore, the CDC is basing its statement that there are no materials from any animals or aborted fetal cells on the fact that the process of making vaccines includes a filtering step that is supposed to remove the animal and fetal cells. That filtering step, though, is not 100% successful. There remain in the vaccines trace amounts of human fetal and animal cells. The British Columbia (BC) immunization information website, run by the BC Ministry of Health, the BC Centre for Disease Control (an agency of the BC Provincial Health Services

Authority), the BC Pharmacy Association, and other government and industry organizations, explains that vaccines contain trace amounts of animal and human cells used in production.

> Animal and human cell cultures may be used in the process of making mRNA or viral vector COVID-19 vaccines, but the vaccines do not contain animal or human cells or tissue. The purification process removes nearly all of the cell components so that only **trace amounts of DNA and protein may be present in the vaccine.**[301]

Dr. Brianne Barker, associate professor of biology at Drew University, explains that "in order to make the [Johnson and Johnson COVID-19] vaccine, the scientists give PerC6 [fetal] cells DNA so that they can make the parts of the virus and build that molecular machine—basically the PerC6 [fetal] cells are the factories that make the vaccine for us."[302] The PERC6 fetal cells are allegedly later filtered out of the J&J COVID-19 vaccine before it is put into vials for injection.[303] Pfizer/BioNTech and Moderna used the HEK293 fetal cell lines in their testing stages for their COVID-19 vaccines.[304]

The HEK293 fetal line derived from an elective abortion in the 1970s is routinely used to produce proteins and cultivate viruses.[305] HEK is an acronym for human embryonic kidney cells.

The WI-38 fetal line was derived from fetal tissues harvested from an elective abortion in the 1960s to generate attenuated viruses.[306]

The MRC-5 fetal line was derived from fetal lung tissues harvested from an elective abortion in 1966. The abortion records indicate that it was taken from a 14-week male fetus removed for psychiatric reasons from a 27-year-old woman with a genetically normal family history. MRC-5 is used to generate attenuated viruses.[307]

The origin of PERC6 fetal line is documented through direct testimony before the Food and Drug Administration's Vaccines and Related Biological Products Advisory Committee from Dr. Alex Van Der Eb, who stated: "So I isolated retina [cells] from a fetus, from a healthy fetus as far as could be seen, of 18 weeks old. There was nothing special in the family history, or the pregnancy was completely normal up to 18 weeks, and it turned out to be a socially indicated abortus, abortus provocatus, and that was simply because the woman wanted to get rid of the fetus."[308] The PERC6 fetal line is currently used in the research and development of vaccines.

Novavax has publicly proclaimed: "No human fetal-derived cell lines or tissue, including HEK293 cells, are used in the development, manufacture or production of the Novavax COVID-19 vaccine candidate, NVX-CoV2373."[309]

The HEK293 fetal line mentioned by Novavax refers to the human embryonic kidney (HEK) cells of the victim of an elective abortion in the 1970s.[310]

HEK293 is not the only human fetal cell line. It is rather suspicious that Novavax would specifically cite that particular cell line and claim that it was not used in the "development, manufacture or production" of its COVID-19 vaccine when it turns out that Novavax, indeed, used that very cell line when "testing" the efficacy of its vaccine. Is not testing part of the development of the vaccine? Absolutely!

It seems that Novavax has been caught in a subtle deception. It is more properly described as a bald-faced lie. Novavax funded research that studied the efficacy and safety of their COVID-19 vaccine. That study expressly states that it involved the use of "human embryonic kidney (HEK) 293F cells."[311] Novavax cannot distance itself from the testing because researchers who worked on the study were identified as being employed by or affiliated with Novavax, Jing-Hui Tian, Alyse D. Portnoff, Nita Patel, Michael J. Massare, Greg Glenn, and Gale Smith.[312]

When presented with that damning evidence, Novavax claimed that it "did not use HEK293 cells in the testing of NVX-CoV2373."[313] Novavax, apparently, understood that testing was part of the development of its COVID-19 vaccine and decided to deny that it used the aborted fetal cell line of HEK293 in its testing, although the published paper was, in part, a "testing" study. Thus, rendering Novavax's denial untrue.

Furthermore, the statement from Novavax denying that it used aborted fetal cells in testing its COVID-19 vaccine was later impeached by a letter sent by Novavax to the Charlotte Lozier Institute, wherein Novavax officially admitted:

> Testing was conducted to compare the structural integrity of the SARS-CoV-2 spike protein produced in the Sf9 insect cells versus the spike protein produced in the mammalian human embryonic kidney HEK 293F cells. The comparison determined the Sf9 cell technology produced spike proteins were comparable in structural integrity as the spike proteins produced in the HEK 293F cell.[314]

It seems that Novavax is pathological in its deception. In the same letter sent by Novavax to the Charlotte Lozier Institute, where it admitted that its vaccine was tested on aborted fetal tissue, Novavax stated that "fetal-derived cell lines were not used in the manufacture, testing, or production of the Novavax COVID-19 vaccine."[315]

"Oh what a tangled web we weave when first we practice to deceive."

The Inova Hospital System is spreading the Novavax lie. Indeed, the Inova imprimatur of the Novavaz vaccine includes the provably false statement that "the Novavax vaccine has no linkage to cell lines from aborted fetuses." Inova prefaces its conclusion with an official statement from Novavax that "no human fetal-derived cell lines or tissues are contained in the Novavax COVID-19 vaccine, adjuvanted, or used in the development, manufacture, or release testing."

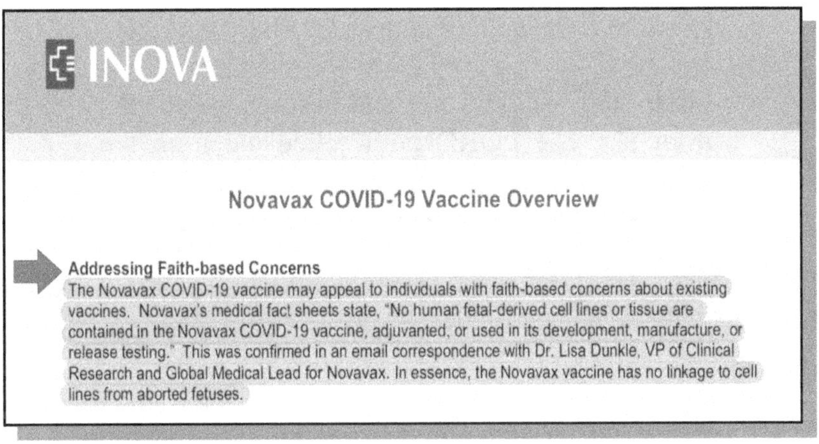
INOVA

Novavax COVID-19 Vaccine Overview

Addressing Faith-based Concerns
The Novavax COVID-19 vaccine may appeal to individuals with faith-based concerns about existing vaccines. Novavax's medical fact sheets state, "No human fetal-derived cell lines or tissue are contained in the Novavax COVID-19 vaccine, adjuvanted, or used in its development, manufacture, or release testing." This was confirmed in an email correspondence with Dr. Lisa Dunkle, VP of Clinical Research and Global Medical Lead for Novavax. In essence, the Novavax vaccine has no linkage to cell lines from aborted fetuses.

Release testing is something that is done after the release of a product. Apparently, Novavax is now quibbling that they did not test their product on aborted fetal cells after the product was released. I guess they hope that will be enough to pull the wool over the eyes of most who will not realize that Novavax, in fact, tested their COVID-19 vaccine on aborted fetal cells before releasing it. Proof that the equivocation is simply an effort by Novavax to obfuscate their guilt in using aborted fetal tissue is found in the statement by INOVA that "[i]n essence, the Novavax vaccine has no linkage to cell lines from aborted fetuses." Read that again. INOVA interprets Novavax's claim that there was no release testing using fetal tissue, as meaning that the vaccine has no linkage to aborted fetuses. That is what Novavax wants people to believe. But it is a deception; it is not true.

Abortion is the sin of unjustifiable homicide. God states that we are living souls from the moment of conception in the womb.

> For thou hast possessed my reins: thou hast covered me in my mother's womb. I will praise thee; for I am fearfully and wonderfully made: marvellous are thy works; and that my soul knoweth right well. (Psalms 139:13-14)

> Listen, O isles, unto me; and hearken, ye people, from far; The LORD hath called me from the womb; from the bowels of my mother hath he made mention of my name. (Isaiah 49:1)

Indeed, we are ordained to be living souls by God before our conception in our mothers' wombs. God forms us in the womb.

> Before I formed thee in the belly I knew thee; and before thou camest forth out of the womb I sanctified thee, and I ordained thee a prophet unto the nations. (Jeremiah 1:5)

God is the creator of all things, including the creator of each man in his mother's womb.

> As thou knowest not what is the way of the spirit, nor how the bones do grow in the womb of her that is with child: even so thou knowest not the works of God who maketh all. (Ecclesiastes 11:5)

God of the Lord of all, both born and unborn.

> I was cast upon thee from the womb: thou *art* my God from my mother's belly. (Psalms 22:10)

Fetuses in the womb are sentient. We see that in Luke when, Elizabeth was greeted by Mary, who was pregnant with Jesus. John the Babtist, who was unborn and in Elizabeth's womb jumped for joy upon hearing the Mary's greeting.

> And it came to pass, that, when Elisabeth heard the salutation of Mary, the babe leaped in her womb; and Elisabeth was filled with the Holy Ghost: (Luke 1:41)

God hates the shedding of innocent blood.

> These six things doth the LORD hate: yea, seven are an abomination unto him: A proud look, a lying tongue, and **hands that shed innocent blood**, An heart that deviseth wicked imaginations, feet that be swift in running to mischief, A false witness that speaketh lies, and he that soweth discord among brethren. (Proverbs 6:16-19)

The Holy Bible states that God elected Jacob as the heir to the promise. God elected Jacob before he was born.

> That is, They which are the children of the flesh, these are not the children of God: but the children of the promise are counted for the seed. For this is the word of promise, At this time will I come, and Sara shall have a son. And not only this; but when Rebecca also had conceived by one, even by our father Isaac; (For the children being not yet born, neither having done any good or evil, that the

> purpose of God according to election might stand, not of works, but of him that calleth;) It was said unto her, The elder shall serve the younger. As it is written, Jacob have I loved, but Esau have I hated. (Romans 9:8-13)

Notice also what God states about Jacob and Esau. God elected Jacob before they were born and before either he or Esau had done any good or evil. That means that children who are aborted have not done any evil. There is no justification for their death; they are innocent. The killers are culpable, and those who encourage and abet them in their deadly scheme are accomplices in that sin. Unless they repent and turn in faith to Jesus Christ, they will be punished by God accordingly. *See* Matthew 25:31-46; Romans 2:3-9; 2 Corinthians 5:10; Revelation 20:11-15.

Abortion is homicide. God has commanded that we shall not kill one another. "Thou shalt not kill." (Exodus 20:13)

12 Moral Hazard

The COVID-19 vaccine is killing exponentially more than needed for the regulatory agencies to rise up and take it off the market. But, suspiciously, the COVID-19 vaccines are getting a pass. Why, with the carnage from the COIVD-19 vaccines so clearly apparent, is there still a push to vaccinate the population? The answer is simple. When the Swine Flu vaccine caused death and illness, the vaccine makers were liable for the damages. But now it is different. The drug companies now have immunity from civil liability for the injuries they cause through their vaccines.

The dangers of vaccines are inherent in the practice and cannot be avoided. Vaccines have been acknowledged by the U.S. Supreme Court and the U.S. Congress to be unavoidably unsafe. Congress passed the National Vaccine Injury Act (NVIA) of 1986, granting pharmaceutical companies immunity for injuries caused by the vaccines they manufactured. As explained by the U.S. Supreme Court in *Bruesewitz v. Wyeth*[316], the reason for that protection is that Congress deemed vaccines to be unavoidably unsafe;[317] thus no manufacturer would make a vaccine if they had to suffer the liability for injuries they would unavoidably cause.[318]

Mary S. Holland explains the issue: "The success of the

national vaccine program has come at a cost. Some children are permanently disabled or die from their vaccine exposures. … Between 1980 and 1986, people who claimed vaccine injury brought over three billion dollars of damages claims to U.S. civil courts against vaccine manufacturers."[319]

In response to the litigation that held them accountable for the injuries caused by their vaccines, the vaccine manufacturers lobbied Congress, and in 1986 they were able to get the NVIA law passed. That law protected them from civil liability for injuries caused by vaccines that they manufactured.

The underlying legal reasoning of Congress for the 1986 NVIA law was a concept borrowed from the Restatement of Torts law that vaccines were "unavoidably unsafe." Holland explains that "[t]he Restatement describes all vaccines as 'unavoidably unsafe' products and implicitly recommended that manufacturers not be liable for injuries if doctors administered them properly."[320]

The NVIA set up a system of government compensation for vaccine injuries that has, in practice, served more to prevent compensation than anything else. Robert F. Kennedy explains:

> Parents, legal guardians and legal representatives can file on behalf of children, disabled adults, and individuals who are deceased. According to the vaccine-injured and their loved ones, the program has failed miserably as a litigious, broken system where the injured are up against a government vaccine program, government owned vaccine patents, government health officials who administer the program and government paid attorneys from the Department of Justice. There is no judge, no jury of your peers and no discovery. Claimants feel the system is set up for their claims to fail.[321]

The U.S. Supreme Court in *Bruesewitz*, supra, ruled that language in the statute categorically preempts even design defect claims against vaccine manufacturers. Holland explains that U.S. Supreme Court ruling "removed incentives for pharmaceutical corporations to conduct the extensive research and development necessary to ensure that FDA-approved vaccines remain as safe and effective as possible after licensure. FDA approval alone has not been a sufficient guarantee of drug safety, owing in part to the FDA's limited authority to compel further safety research after final approval."[322]

Holland reveals the real-world consequences of the NIVA for vaccine recipients:

> [Gayle] DeLong showed that the proportion of people that reported a serious complication from a vaccine after [enactment of the NVIA in] 1986 is more than double the proportion of people who experienced a serious complication from a disease before a vaccine for it was available. The difference is statistically significant and is likely greater because of underreporting.
>
> DeLong's analysis suggests that the Vaccine Act "gave firms greater incentives to capture the regulator: If consumers cannot sue firms for product liability, the only barrier to sales is regulatory approval."[323]

The NVIA protects vaccine makers from liability for "unavoidable" injuries caused by vaccines. The NVIA states in pertinent part:

> No vaccine manufacturer shall be liable in a civil action for damages arising from a vaccine-related injury or death associated with the administration

> of a vaccine after October 1, 1988, if **the injury or death resulted from side effects that were unavoidable** even though the vaccine was properly prepared and was accompanied by proper directions and warnings.[324]

In order to make sure the immunity from liability pill goes down easier for the public, the NVIA mandated that the Secretary of HHS "promote the development of childhood vaccines that result in fewer and less serious adverse reactions than those vaccines [presently] on the market."[325]

That requirement was supposed to be performed by a task force made up of the "Director of the National Institutes of Health [NIH], the Commissioner of the Food and Drug Administration [FDA], and the Director of the Centers for Disease Control [CDC]."[326]

The NVIA statute required that "within 2 years after December 22, 1987, and periodically thereafter, the Secretary [of HHS] shall prepare and transmit to the Committee on Energy and Commerce of the House of Representatives and the Committee on Labor and Human Resources of the Senate a report describing the actions taken pursuant to subsection (a) during the preceding 2-year period."[327]

The NIH, FDA, and CDC scoundrels thumbed their noses at Congress. They violated the law by not filing the required reports with the U.S. Congress. Why did they not file the required reports? The only logical reason is that they did not meet as required, and they did not "promote the development of childhood vaccines that result in fewer and less serious adverse reactions than those vaccines [presently] on the market"[328] as required by the statute.

That is clear evidence that the component agencies of HHS

(CDC, NIH, and FDA) have no interest in the development of safe vaccines for children.

Robert F. Kennedy Jr. discovered the scofflaws at HHS when he filed a Freedom of Information Act request with HHS requesting the reports prepared and transmitted to Congress as required by the NVIA. HHS refused to comply with the request. He sued HHS.[329] After being served with the lawsuit, HHS admitted that they never filed any required reports with Congress.[330] That means that the component agencies of HHS (CDC, NIH, and FDA) never formed the required task force and made no effort to see that vaccines were made safer.

The CDC, NIH, and FDA never met to develop a plan for safe vaccines for children. Why? Because CDC, NIH, and FDA know that the pharmaceutical companies have no interest making vaccines safe for children! Vaccines are unavoidably unsafe and the vaccine makers like it that way. Pharmaceutical companies get rich when people are made sick. It is a racket where they cause injury via their vaccines and then make the patent medicines to address the symptoms of the injuries they have caused. There was a fly in their ointment, and that was civil liability for the injuries they caused. The immunity granted by the NVIA solved that problem. Since the NVIA, the pharmaceutical companies have been off to the races creating one ineffective and unsafe vaccine after another.

As explained by Texans for Vaccine Choice, "[t]he [NVIA] removed all liability from vaccine manufacturers when their products injure or kill. Realizing that removing consumer accountability would eliminate any motivation for manufacturers to ensure their products are as safe and effective as they can possibly be, the Mandate for Safer Childhood Vaccines clause was added to the the Act as a check-and-balance." But we now know that there is no check-and-balance. Robert F. Kennedy Jr. explains:

> This speaks volumes to the lack of seriousness by which vaccine safety is treated at HHS and heightens the concern that HHS doesn't have a clue as to the actual safety profile of the now 29 doses, and growing, of vaccines given by one year of age.[331]

The CDC, when asked, was unable to provide any evidence that any childhood vaccine has ever been tested for safety using a placebo control. Indeed, Robert F. Kennedy Jr. points out that "not one of the 72 vaccines on the schedule mandated for our children, have been tested with a placebo." There is a reason. No vaccine could ever survive being tested for safety and effectiveness against a placebo. The pharmaceutical companies know that their vaccines are not only ineffective, they are injurious. Research has shown that childhood vaccines cause injuries.[332] And that is by design. A design for which the U.S. Supreme Court has ruled the drug companies have immunity from civil liability.

The CDC, NIH, and FDA know it is a fool's errand to try to convince the drug companies to manufacture something safe when to do so would undermine the drug companies' pecuniary interests. The surreptitious goal of the drug companies is to make people sick through vaccines. That is why the CDC, NIH, and FDA had nothing to report to Congress regarding their efforts to develop vaccines with "fewer and less serious adverse reactions." The goal of the vaccine makers is to cause injury. The pharmaceutical companies, CDC, NIH, and FDA all know that vaccines will unavoidably cause injuries. They have no interest in mitigating the damage caused by vaccines because those injuries make the pharmaceutical companies rich through the patent medicines they sell to address the injuries caused by the vaccines.

For example, on December 13, 2021, Pfizer announced:

> Pfizer will acquire Arena, a clinical stage company

> developing innovative potential therapies for the treatment of **several immuno-inflammatory diseases**. Under the terms of the agreement, Pfizer will acquire all the outstanding shares of Arena for $100 per share in an all-cash transaction for a total equity value of approximately $6.7 billion. The boards of directors of both companies have unanimously approved the transaction.[333]

Pfizer is acquiring a company that makes drugs that treat the very immuno-inflammatory injuries caused by Pfizer's COVID-19 vaccine. Arena has drugs in the pipeline to treat cardio inflammatory diseases like myocarditis; the Pfizer COVID-19 vaccine has become notorious for causing myocarditis.[334] Also notable is Arena's development of a drug (Termanogrel) to address microvascular obstructions, which several doctors have identified as the root cause of many illnesses resulting from Pfizer's COVID-19 vaccine.[335] For example, Dr. Charles Hoffe, MD — who practices in British Columbia, Canada — explained in very simple terms how the mRNA COVID vaccines create the spike proteins which cause widespread microscopic blood clotting that will eventually kill many people within three years of taking the shots.[336] Pfizer now wants to get in on the action of offering overpriced patent medicines to give to desperate patients suffering from the deadly side-effects of their vaccine. How much more Machiavelian can you get?

Pharmaceutical companies, like Pfizer, act much like a firefighter who is also an arsonist. That sounds strange, but firefighter arson is a real phenomenon. In 1998, Glendale, CA, Fire Department Captain and Arson Investigator John Orr was convicted of four counts of murder and twenty counts of arson for fires he started dating back to 1984.[337] Orr, like Pfizer, showed no remorse and did not much care who he killed. Orr is not alone. There are many historical accounts of arson fires perpetrated by firefighters. The U.S. Fire Administration reported:

> Slowly, the fire service is shedding light on a situation that occurs rarely but which is nevertheless serious: some firefighters intentionally start fires. A very small percentage of otherwise trustworthy firefighters cause the very flames they are dispatched to put out.[338]

Indeed, the U.S. Fire Administration reported that the South Carolina Forestry Commission (SCFC) said that 47 firefighters had been charged with arson in South Carolina alone. The U.S. Fire Administration report explained that the motives behind firefighter-perpetrated arsons varied. But one of the potential motives is financial. The arsonist firefighter may be seeking increased overtime pay, or he may be fighting fires for a paid-on-call fire service.

Pfizer acts like a firefighter who causes fires for financial gain, but instead of setting a house ablaze, it destroys the health of the vaccinated patient. Like the firefighter who enters the scene to put out the fire he started, Pfizer enters the scene to provide pharmaceutical drugs to treat the ailment caused by its vaccines. Pfizer then profits by supplying the drugs to treat the harm caused by its vaccines.

Pfizer is hell-bent on profiting from the injuries its vaccines cause. On October 5, 2022, Pfizer announced that it acquired Global Blood Therapeutics, Inc. (GBT), a biopharmaceutical company.[339] The primary money-making drug from GBT is nOxbryta®, which treats sickle-cell anemia. But the company researches and develops drugs for all blood and hemolytic disorders. It is the ideal company for Pfizer to acquire because Pfizer's COVID-19 vaccine causes all manner of blood and hemolytic disorders.[340]

On March 13, 2023, Pfizer announced that it had acquired one of the world's leading oncology companies, Seagen, for $43 billion. It has now been established that COVID-19 vaccines cause cancer.[341] Indeed, as Eustace Mullins explains in his book, *Murder by Injection*, all vaccines cause cancer.[342] Cancer was practically unknown before the scheme of compulsory vaccinations.[343] Pfizer is "flush with windfall cash from its hugely successful BioNTech-partnered COVID-19 vaccine."[344] Pfizer is deploying the billions of dollars in profits from its COVID-19 vaccine to acquire companies that address cancer caused by its COVID-19 vaccine. With the acceleration of new vaccines, Pfizer sees cancer treatments to address the cancers caused by vaccines as a growth industry. The acquisition of Seagan is all about making money. Pfizer states that cancer is a growing disease, and they want to profit from it:

> Oncology continues to be the largest growth driver in global medicine, and this acquisition will enhance Pfizer's position in this important space and contribute meaningfully to the achievement of Pfizer's near- and long-term financial goals.[345]

Believe it or not, the COVID-19 vaccine manufacturers are protected from civil liability beyond the NVIA. The Food and Drug Administration granted emergency use authorization (EAU) for the COVID-19 vaccines. Because the COVID-19 vaccines administered in the U.S. under an EUA are not FDA-approved. The COVID-19 vaccines, being EUA vaccines, fall under the blanket civil liability protection provided by the PREP Act, which is an almost insurmountable barrier to just compensation for injuries caused by EUA vaccines.[346] While certain of the COVID-19 vaccines have been approved by the FDA (Moderna's SPIKEVAX and Pfizer-BioNTech's Comirnaty), suspiciously, those approved branded vaccines are not available in the United States.[347]

A "declared public health emergency" as described in the PREP Act is the legal landscape under which the COVID-19 vaccine is being developed. Under the PREP Act, there is a moral hazard where manufactures of the COVID-19 vaccines will be protected from any liability for injuries caused by their COVID-19 vaccines. They have no financial incentive to make a vaccine that is safe or effective. They can sit back and count their billions in profits as they injure the public with impunity. The demand for the product is guaranteed by a marketplace that is rigged by the U.S. and state governments, which will pay for the vaccine and then mandate that the public consume that vaccine. The attitude of the vaccine manufacturers toward the consumer who is injured is "oh well, too bad, so sad, it sucks to be you."

"For the love of money is the root of all evil: which while some coveted after, they have erred from the faith, and pierced themselves through with many sorrows." 1 Timothy 6:10.

The vaccine manufacturers are virtually immune from liability for their negligence in manufacturing vaccines.[348] This creates a moral hazard where there is no financial incentive for the vaccine manufacturers to make their vaccines safe.

Mary S. Holland has written an excellent law review article in the Emory Law Journal that explains the moral hazard created by Congress in enacting the 1986 U.S. National Childhood Vaccine Injury Act, which established the National Vaccine Injury Compensation Program (NVICP). There is also the subsequent 2005 PREP Act which established the Countermeasure Injury Compensation Program.[349]

The NVICP had the effect of protecting vaccine manufacturers from civil liability for injuries caused by vaccines that they manufactured. A plaintiff must first pass through the rigorous legal labyrinth of a special vaccine court to obtain compensation from the government. There are a few who push their cases and are able to win in that court.

The vaccine court wears down the plaintiffs. Thus, there are many thousands of vaccine injury victims who suffer in silence. You can expect the same with the COVID-19 vaccine. Indeed it will be even worse. In 2005, Congress passed a tort shield law, the PREP Act, to protect manufacturers of drugs and other "covered countermeasure[s]," including vaccines, from the risk of damages in the event of a declared public health emergency. The standards for recovery for injuries due to the COVID-19 vaccine under the PREP Act are even more onerous than those under the NVICP. "The Countermeasures Injury Compensation Program (CICP) is a Federal government program that administers the compensation Program specified by the Public Readiness and Emergency Preparedness Act (PREP Act)."[350] There is a strict one year statute of limitations under the PREP Act. Except under rare exceptions, an injured person must file suit within one year of receiving the vaccine alleged to have caused the injury.[351] Of the thousands of injuries suffered by people from vaccines, the CICP program has only compensated 29 claimants since 2005, paying out a total of $6 million.[352]

Vaccine Manufacturers have little concern about the safety of the vaccines because when you are injured by their experimental vaccine, they will be immune from liability.

The vaccine manufacturers are cheering on vaccine mandates. That is why the vaccine manufacturers work so closely with the ultimate force, governments. The governments of the world are their real customers. The governments pay for the vaccines. And the governments will then force those overpriced, ineffective, and unsafe vaccines on their people. On July 22, 2020, the Wall Street Journal Editorial Board pointed out that "[l]ife probably won't return to normal until we have a widely distributed Covid-19 vaccine."[353]

13 Edmund Massey's Sermon Against Vaccination

In his 1722 pamphlet, "A Sermon Against the Dangerous and Sinful Practice of Inoculation," Edmund Massey explains that vaccination is a sin. Notice that Massey's sermon was in 1722. That was 27 years before Edward Jenner was born. That is proof that the practice of administering disease into the blood of healthy persons did not start with Edward Jenner. The word vaccine had not yet been coined in the medical community when Massey gave his 1722 sermon. Massey called the practice of contaminating the blood of healthy people with disease

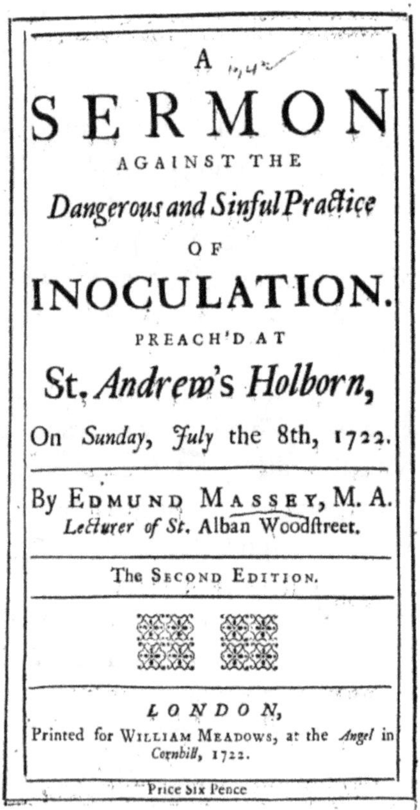

A
SERMON
AGAINST THE
Dangerous and Sinful Practice
OF
INOCULATION.
PREACH'D AT
St. *Andrew's Holborn,*
On *Sunday, July* the 8th, 1722.

By EDMUND MASSEY, M. A.
Lecturer of St. Alban Woodſtreet.

The SECOND EDITION.

LONDON,
Printed for WILLIAM MEADOWS, at the *Angel* in *Cornhill,* 1722.

Price Six Pence

inoculation. It was not until 1798 that Jenner published his fraudulent report and coined the term *variolae vaccinae* from which we get the word, vaccine. Massey's sermon reveals that inoculation (i.e., vaccination) is a heathen religious practice masquerading as a medical procedure. Massey explains that the Holy Bible reveals that all diseases are under the sovereign control of God. Disease is brought upon men for one of two reasons: 1) to try our faith, and 2) to punish our sin. Indeed, God explains his sovereignty over all good and evil. "I form the light, and create darkness: I make peace, and create evil: I the LORD do all these things." (Isaiah 45:7) God uses disease and hardship to correct his elect.

> Behold, happy is the man whom God correcteth: therefore despise not thou the chastening of the Almighty: For he maketh sore, and bindeth up: he woundeth, and his hands make whole." (Job 5:17-18)

The Bible reveals that God sometimes delegates his power to bring disease in rare occasions. For example, in Job, God permitted Satan to strike Job with a noisome disease that caused boils from head to toe. Job 2:4-7. Notice how God gave Satan permission to strike Job with disease.

> And Satan answered the LORD, and said, Skin for skin, yea, all that a man hath will he give for his life. But put forth thine hand now, and touch his bone and his flesh, and he will curse thee to thy face. And the LORD said unto Satan, Behold, he is in thine hand; but save his life. So went Satan forth from the presence of the LORD, and smote Job with sore boils from the sole of his foot unto his crown. (Job 2:4-7)

Edmund Massey opines that Job's disease was brought

about by some form of infusion of a toxin similar to the practice of vaccination.

> The silence of scripture hath given interpreters occasion of guessing at the distemper, which the Devil here inflicted upon Job. But among them all, it appears not certainly what it was. I will therefore desire to give an opinion, equally I think true, with any that hath yet been taken notice of. It is this, That the Devil by some venomous Infusion into the Body of Job, might raise his blood to such a ferment, as threw out a confluence of inflammatory pustules all over him, from head to Foot. That is, his distemper might be what is now incident to most men, and perhaps conveyed to him by some such way as that of inoculation.[354]

Massey explains the motive of Satan in striking Job with the terrible disease.

> The tempter's aim was still the same as before; to make his patient let go his Integrity, throw off his dependance upon Almighty God, and renounce that allegiance which is justly due to him, as creator and governor of the world.[355]

The attack on Job was unusual because God delegated his power over disease to Satan. That disease was not to punish Job for sin but to test (and prove) Job's faithfulness to God. Massey explains:

> Our Text indeed ascribes Job's distemper to the power of the Devil; but the foregoing verse shows that power to have been delegated to him, and limited by Almighty God, who alone being omnipotent, the powers that be, whether natural or

> Political, must all be derived from him [God]. 'Tis true, he has communicated several parts of his sovereignty to the sons of men, but still the exercise of it will ultimately be resolved into his permission. And it is as true, that there are several branches of authority, which he [God] has reserved to himself, in displaying of which, he acts upon prerogative, and without human intervention. I choose to instance in the infliction of diseases, which I will attempt to prove are utterly unlawful to be inflicted, by any who profess themselves Christians.[356]

God allowed Satan to strike Job with disease to test Job's faith. By God's grace, Job made it through the disease; God ultimately restored Job to health. Now godless and greedy men, under the auspices of Satan, are injuring people for money by the hundreds of millions. Satan's objective, as it was with Job, is to drive men to curse God. "There is no new thing under the sun." Ecclesiastes 1:9. Vaccination is an evil, devil-inspired enterprise.

The usual course is that disease is brought on directly from God. Paul offers us another example where God sent "the messenger of Satan to buffet" him by striking Paul with thorn of pain of some kind in his side. God did this to keep Paul humble. Paul explained that it was part of God's plan to make him weak in the flesh so that he would be strong in the spirit.

> And lest I should be exalted above measure through the abundance of the revelations, there was given to me a thorn in the flesh, the messenger of Satan to buffet me, lest I should be exalted above measure. For this thing I besought the Lord thrice, that it might depart from me. And he said unto me, My grace is sufficient for thee: for my strength is made perfect in weakness. Most gladly therefore

> will I rather glory in my infirmities, that the power of Christ may rest upon me. Therefore I take pleasure in infirmities, in reproaches, in necessities, in persecutions, in distresses for Christ's sake: for when I am weak, then am I strong. (2 Corinthians 12:7-10)

Another reason for God to bring disease is to punish a person for his sin. The malady is thought to flow from the actions of the natural laws set in place by God.

> For he that eateth and drinketh unworthily, eateth and drinketh damnation to himself, not discerning the Lord's body. **For this cause many are weak and sickly among you, and many sleep.** (1 Corinthians 11:29-30)

> And likewise also the men, leaving the natural use of the woman, burned in their lust one toward another; men with men working that which is unseemly, and **receiving in themselves that recompence of their error which was meet**. (Romans 1:27)

> Be not deceived; God is not mocked: **for whatsoever a man soweth, that shall he also reap. For he that soweth to his flesh shall of the flesh reap corruption**; but he that soweth to the Spirit shall of the Spirit reap life everlasting. Galatians 6:7-8

All elect Christians are the spiritual seed of Jesus Christ. Galatians 3:16, 29. Nonetheless, if we transgress his commandments, he will correct us. One of the means of correction is through disease. But his correction of us does not affect the eternal promise of salvation.

> Also I will make him my firstborn, higher than the kings of the earth. My mercy will I keep for him for evermore, and my covenant shall stand fast with him. **His seed also will I make to endure for ever, and his throne as the days of heaven. If his children forsake my law, and walk not in my judgments; If they break my statutes, and keep not my commandments; Then will I visit their transgression with the rod, and their iniquity with stripes.** Nevertheless my lovingkindness will I not utterly take from him, nor suffer my faithfulness to fail. My covenant will I not break, nor alter the thing that is gone out of my lips. (Psalms 89:27-34)

But if we make the Lord our refuge and fortress, he will deliver us from disease. We are not to fear the pestilence by night.

> I will say of the LORD, He is my refuge and my fortress: my God; in him will I trust. **Surely he shall deliver thee from the snare of the fowler, and from the noisome pestilence.** He shall cover thee with his feathers, and under his wings shalt thou trust: his truth shall be thy shield and buckler. Thou shalt not be afraid for the terror by night; nor for the arrow that flieth by day; **Nor for the pestilence that walketh in darkness;** nor for the destruction that wasteth at noonday. (Psalms 91:2-6)

If we keep his commandments and take refuge in the Lord, no evil plague of disease will come near us.

> Because thou hast made the LORD, which is my refuge, even the most High, thy habitation; **There shall no evil befall thee, neither shall any plague**

> **come nigh thy dwelling.** For he shall give his angels charge over thee, to keep thee in all thy ways. (Psalms 91:9-11)

To take a vaccine is to eschew the promises of God and put trust in man. Vaccination implicitly encourages sin by promising that there will be no consequential disease. People are beguiled by the devil's promise of immunity from future diseases. But the disease comes anyway because vaccines come with a promise that cannot be delivered. Often the disease comes from the vaccine itself. Vaccination is a sin. Those suffering from vaccine-induced disease should repent, humble themselves before God, and call on his mercy.

Massey calls vaccination a diabolical practice that promotes vice and immorality by giving people the false hope of sin without consequences by assuring them that through injection with an antigen, they will be protected from future illness. Rather than live a clean and moral life, they can now throw caution to the wind and live it up since they are immune from the consequences of their sin.

> Remembering then our text, I shall not scruple to call that a diabolical operation, which usurps an authority founded neither in the laws of nature or religion, which tends in this case to anticipate and banish providence out of the world, and promotes the increase of vice and immorality.[357]

With that in mind, it is clear that we should not purposely cause disease through vaccination. Disease is an evil that is under the control of God, and for man to usurp that power is a sin. It is a sin to do what is solely in the province of God. It is a sin to cause disease. Disease brings death, and making someone ill that could lead to his death is a violation of the commandment of God. "Thou shalt not kill." Exodus 20:13.

Sincere Christian beliefs are founded on the Holy Bible. The Bible says:"For the life of the flesh is in the blood..." Leviticus 17:11, and "... the life of all flesh; the blood of it is for the life thereof." Leviticus 17:14. Therefore, in order to preserve the life of one's flesh, one must keep one's blood unpolluted from foreign proteins, antigens, adjuvants, and other pollutants typically found in vaccines. It is a sin to do evil that some imagined good may come. Romans 3.8.

14 Vaccines Cause Diseases

Eustace Mullins reveals in his book, *Murder by Injection*, that Dr. W. B. Clarke wrote that "Cancer was practically unknown until compulsory vaccination with cowpox vaccine began to be introduced. I have had to deal with a least two hundred cases of cancer, and I never saw a case of cancer in an unvaccinated person."[358] In a speech elaborating on Dr. Clarke's statement Mullins stated:

> Other doctors have said the same thing, that vaccination is really a time bomb within the human system that can go off five years, ten years, 40 years after you have the vaccinatin you could have the time bomb go off, you could have a stroke, a heart attack because it's always there in your system, you never get rid of it. And, apparently, it's always an alien force in your physique.[359]

The process of death begins with poisoning through vaccination. For example, the explosion in deadly cancers is primarily caused by vaccination. All one needs to hear is that he has been diagnosed with cancer to understand that death is near. With some cancers, the death rate is 90%.[360] The barbarous practices of surgery, chemotherapy, and radiation offer little succor other than the hope of delaying the fast-approaching date of death. Certainly, there are persons who have "beat cancer," but there is a significant plurality who succumb to the disease. Dr. Dennis Turnbull, who had studied cancer for 30 years declared: "I have no hesitation in stating that in my judgement the most frequent disposing condition for cancerous development is infused into the blood by vaccination and re-vaccination."[361] Dr. Forbes Laurie, late Medical Director of the Metropolitan Cancer Hospital (London), said: "I am thoroughly convinced that the increase of cancer is due to vaccination."[362] Dr. Robert Bell, the famous cancer specialist of the British Cancer Hospital, stated: "The chief, if not the sole cause of the monstrous increase in cancer has been vaccination."[363]

Dr. Herbert Snow, Surgeon of the London Cancer Hospital, had this to say: "I am convinced that some 80 per cent of these cancer deaths are caused by the inoculations or vaccinations they have undergone. These are well-known to cause grave and permanent disease of the heart also."[364] Regarding the heart, in the book, *Murder by Injection*, Eustace Mullins reveals that Dr. Snow stated: "In recent years many men and women in the prime of life have dropped dead suddenly, often after attending a feast or a banquet. I am convinced that some eighty per cent of these deaths are caused by the inoculation or vaccination they have undergone. They are well known to cause grave and permanent disease to the heart."[365]

If some in the medical community know vaccinations cause grave and permanent disease to the heart, why does the public not rise up against vaccination? Dr. Snow explained that the public is kept ignorant of the dangers because "[t]he coroner always hushes it up as 'natural causes.'"[366] The medical community has a cult of secrecy regarding the causal link between vaccination and deadly diseases.

It seems that Dr. Snow's 80% vaccine causal rate for heart

disease and cancer might be an understatement. A recent study points the needle of causation closer to 100%. That study compared the health of a group of 1,482 unvaccinated persons to the national statistics on the health of vaccinated persons.[367] The study revealed that 48% of vaccinated adults had some form of heart disease, compared to zero percent (0%) of unvaccinated adults.[368] Six percent (6%) of vaccinated adults had cancer compared to zero percent (0%) of unvaccinated adults.[369] That study is not widely publicized, and most do not know about it. The secrecy cult in the medical establishment will ensure that it stays that way. In his book, *Cancer and Vaccination*, Esculapius says:

> No candid and scientific inquirer who has read the works of such authorities as Doctors Creighton, Crookshank and Scott Tebb, can be surprised that an alarming increase in cancer is now evident. Those who adopt the brutal practice of calf-lymph vaccination are but too surely sowing the wind which they must inevitably reap as the whirlwind, a whirlwind of corruption, disease and national deterioration. Where the so-called, human lymph is employed, syphilis, leprosy and tuberculosis follow in its train; and wherever calf-lymph is used, tuberculosis and cancer spread like a conflagration.[370]

Sir Thomas Paget (M.D.), tells us that "the progress of vaccine infection in the blood shows us that a permanent morbid condition is established; in the tissues themselves, it is also established by this specific poison."[371] Dr. Benchetrit states that serums and vaccines "are principally responsible for the increase of those two really dangerous diseases, cancer and heart disease."[372] Dr. F. P. Millard, prominent Osteopath of Toronto and President of the National League for Prevention of Spinal Curvature says: "Abolish vaccination, and you will cut the cancer death-rate in half."[373]

Cancer is just one of the many diseases spread by vaccination. Eleanor McBean states that "[w]herever an honest survey is made after a vaccination campaign it is noticed that there is always a marked increase in disease."[374] Thomas Morgan, in his *Medical Delusions* reports a survey that was made of the city of Youngstown, Ohio, after a general vaccination order of school children. "It was found that nearly all the cases of scarlet fever, measles and diphtheria had been recently vaccinated. What is true of this city is true everywhere, and any close observer can satisfy himself in this direction."[375] In or about 1955, Eleanor McBean took up Morgan's challenge and checked the Los Angeles Health Index for 1954. She found that the total number of cases of 48 diseases recorded in the index, including but not limited to chickenpox, scarlet fever, measles, mumps, and syphilis, more than doubled after the annual June 1954 vaccine campaign.[376] Dr. Peebles, (world renowned researcher and authority on vaccination) stated in his book on Compulsory Vaccination:

> We shall never stamp out smallpox, cancer, consumption, or leprosy, so long as we continue to STAMP THEM IN through the idiotic and vicious practice of vaccination. The Germans endeavored to stamp out syphilis by stamping it in with syphilized vaccine. They have abandoned that practice now and in time they will abandon vaccination altogether.[377] (emphasis in original)

A 2018 human research study of the efficacy and safety of influenza vaccines "did not observe that influenza vaccination significantly reduced overall hazard of influenza."[378] In addition, the study found that the hazard of acute respiratory illness (ARI) caused by non-influenza respiratory pathogens was higher in vaccinated individuals compared to unvaccinated individuals.[379]

A 2013 animal research study found that the influenza vaccine caused vaccine-associated enhanced respiratory disease

(VAERD), wherein the animals ended up with enhanced influenza (pH1N1) infection.[380] "Vaccinating pigs with whole inactivated H1N2 (human-like) virus vaccine (WIV-H1N2) resulted in enhanced pneumonia and disease after pH1N1 infection."[381]

15 Unsafe and Ineffective Flu Vaccines

People are injected with more influenza vaccines than all other shots combined.[382] Lies drive the marketing to get the flu vaccine. The CDC falsely represents the number of people who die each year from the flu to scare the elderly into getting the flu shot. The CDC adds deaths from pneumonia to flu deaths to come up with a combined figure for flu and pneumonia deaths. For example, on April 6, 2023, the CDC reported on its "Influenza" page the mortality for 2021 as "Number of deaths: 41,917."[383] Even though it was on the "Influenza" page, the figure was reported under the heading "Influenza and pneumonia deaths." Interestingly, the CDC reveals that the total number of influenza-only deaths was reported to be 608. Thus, 99% of the deaths being reported as "influenza and pneumonia deaths" in 2021 were from pneumonia.

It is misleading to report the combined deaths from flu and pneumonia. That is because, as explained by Dr. David Rosenthal, director of Harvard University Health Service, the relationship between pneumonia and the flu is not unique.[384] Many other diseases can cause pneumonia.[385] People can die from pneumonia without ever having the flu. But because people typically do not die from influenza, the CDC has decided to hook the alleged flu deaths to pneumonia to scare the public into getting flu shots. Jon

Rappaport reported:

> In December of 2005, the British Medical Journal (online) published a shocking report by Peter Doshi, which spelled out the delusion and created tremors throughout the halls of the CDC. Here is a quote from Doshi's report:
>
> "[According to CDC statistics], 'influenza and pneumonia' took 62,034 lives in 2001—61,777 of which were attributable to pneumonia and 257 to flu, and in only 18 cases was the flu virus positively identified."[386]

The CDC used that sleight of hand until 2008, to announce that "every year ... about 36,000 people die from flu."[387] But that is twisting the truth because very few of those deaths are from the flu. The CDC had been doing that for years. On or about 2004, pediatrician Kenneth Stoller on behalf of the International Hyperbaric Medical Association, admonished the CDC about this deception and asked them to stop doing it.[388] On or before 2010, the CDC decided to change from saying that "every year ... about 36,000 people die from flu" to saying that "[e]ach year ... 36,000 people die from flu-related causes."[389] But, again, that is a lie. The 36,000 figure is coming from combining flu and pneumonia deaths. There is nothing unique about the relationship between the flu and pneumonia. It is misleading to call pneumonia a "flu-related cause" of death. People can die from pneumonia without ever having the flu. This is all done to fan the flames of fear to convince the uninformed masses to get a flu shot.

Glen Nowak, Ph.D., the Associate Director for Communications National Immunization Program in the CDC, gave a presentation in 2004 before the American Medical Association where he explained how the CDC uses the media to drum up demand for influenza vaccines.[390] His slide presentation is posted on the AMA website. In the presentation, he listed the media message that "Flu kills 36,000 per year" as the #2 predominant message pumped out from the CDC to the media during the week of September 21-28, 2003. That message, we now know, was a lie.

Dr. Novak's presentation states that his goal was "to broaden understanding and thinking about influenza vaccination communication– especially when it comes to greatly increasing coverage." He explained how the CDC will insert particular messages in the media to increase the uptake of the influenza vaccines for 2004-2005. One of his slides presents: "'Recipe' that Fosters Influenza Vaccine Interest and Demand." The recipe is a seven-step plan for "Generating Interest in, and Demand for, Flu (or any other) Vaccination." Dr. Novak's slide show was in 2004. The CDC has since evolved to now reporting the statistic for flu deaths under the heading: "influenza and pneumonia deaths." The CDC does not break out a separate report that only lists flu deaths because that puny number would not scare people into getting a flu vaccine.

Some of the pertinent slides that indicate the kind of messages that the CDC planned on feeding to the media are cut and pasted below:

> Medical experts and public health authorities publicly (e.g., via media) state concern and alarm (and predict dire outcomes)– and urge influenza vaccination.
>
> Framing of the flu season in terms that motivate behavior (e.g., as "very severe," "more severe than last or past years," "deadly")
>
> Continued reports (e.g., from health officials and media) that influenza is causing severe illness

> and/or affecting lots of people– helping foster the perception that many people are susceptible to a bad case of influenza.
>
> Visible/tangible examples of the seriousness of the illness (e.g., pictures of children, families of those affected coming forward) and people getting vaccinated (the first to motivate, the latter to reinforce)
>
> References to, and discussions, of pandemic influenza–along with continued reference to the importance of vaccination.[391]

Below are the text in slides where Dr. Novak addresses some of the expected issues during the vaccine campaign.

> Vaccination demand, particularly among people who don't routinely receive an annual influenza vaccination, is related to heightened concern, anxiety, and worry.
>
> Effectively addressing parent concerns about a) the number and timing of vaccinations and b) thimerosal[392]
>
> Some component of success (i.e., higher demand for influenza vaccine) stems from media stories and information that create motivating (i.e., high) levels of concern and anxiety about influenza.

The CDC is marketing to scare the public into getting an unsafe and ineffective flu shot. The CDC knows that the shot is almost worthless in protecting people from the flu. Yet, the CDC states:

> Everyone 6 months and older in the United States should get an influenza (flu) vaccine every season with rare exception. CDC's Advisory Committee on Immunization Practices has made this "universal" recommendation since the 2010-2011 flu season.[393]

In his book, *Jabbed*, Brett Wilcox explains the worthlessness of the influenza vaccines.

> GSK tested Fluarix in 2 European countries during the 2006-2007 influenza season and found that 3.2 percent of the unvaxxed subjects came down with the flu or an "influenza-like illness" (ILI) while 1.2 percent of the subjects in the Fluarix group contracted the flu or an influenza-like illness. This equates to a 62.5% efficacy rate.
>
> The math used to obtain 62.5% is as follows: Divide 3.2 into 1.2 to get .375 or a 37.5% reduced incidence of flu in the treatment group. Subtract 37.5 from 100 to get an efficacy rate of 62.5%. This figure is not technically a lie, but it is absolutely deceptive. It gives the impression that Fluarix prevents the flu in 62.5% of people who get the jab. GSK knows full well that according to its own efficacy test that for every 100 people who are vaccinated with Fluarix, only 2 people derive any benefit (3.2 minus 1.2 equals 2). 2 out of 100 equals an absolute risk reduction or vaccine efficacy rate of 2% with a corresponding vaccine worthless rate of 98%.
>
> According to the 2015 meta-analysis conducted by the Cochrane Collaboration, the 98% worthless rate is fairly consistent among flu vaccine

> recipients. The Collaboration reviewed 90 reports and found that on average flu jabs prevent 2.5% of people from coming down with an influenza-like illness and only 1.4% of people from contracting the flu. In other words, the flu jab is from 97.5% to 98.6% worthless.[394]

Wilcox points out that the above figures do not account for those who get sick because of the flu vaccine. The CDC adamantly states that "Flu vaccines CANNOT cause the flu"[395](emphasis in original). That is just another government lie. The inserts for Novartis' flu vaccine, FLUARIX, states that 16% of participants in its trial suffered flu-like symptoms within seven days of getting vaccinated.[396] So, how can the CDC and Novartis claim that the flu vaccine does not give one the flu? Simple, they do not count what happens within the first seven days of getting the shot. Novartis monitored the study subjects immediately after the vaccination. But they did not consider what happened in the first two weeks when calculating the efficacy of the vaccine. That two-week cut-out ensured that inconvenient evidence that showed that the vaccine was making people sick would not affect the efficacy statistics. The Novartis excluded the first two weeks of data after vaccination when calculating the vaccine efficacy because the first seven days showed a spike in flu-like symptoms among the test subjects. The study's raw data showed that for every two people helped by the vaccine, 16 were made sick from it. The vaccine is 8 times more likely to harm than help. Novartis did not count the 16% who came down with flu-like symptoms within the first week of the shot when reporting the vaccine's efficacy.

Adding insult to injury, almost half of the flu vaccines contain dangerous mercury. Congressman Bill Posey made the following statement on the floor of the House of Representatives in 2013.

> Some believe that toxins like thimerosal, which is

> 50% ethylmercury, have played a role in the rise in autism and neurodevelopmental disabilities. In 2000 there was near universal agreement that mercury should be removed as a preservative for vaccines. Yet, today, nearly half of all annual flu vaccines, which are recommended for children and pregnant women, still contain mercury as a preservative—not simply trace amounts of mercury. It's 2013! Why are we still injecting ethylmercury into babies and pregnant women?[397]

Congressman Dan Burton submitted a report in the House of Representatives after a three-year investigation initiated by the Committee on Government Reform. Below is an excerpt from that report:

> The research is explicit that fetal brains are more sensitive than the adult brains to the adverse effects of methylmercury, which include:
>
> Severe brain damage
>
> Delayed achievement of developmental milestones
>
> Neurological abnormalities such as brisk tendon reflexes
>
> Widespread damage to all areas of the fetal brain, as opposed to focal lesions seen in adult tissue
>
> Microcephaly
>
> Purkinje [neuron] cells failed to migrate to the cerebellum
>
> Inhibition of both cell division and migration,

> affecting the most basic process in brain development[398]

Knowing the dangers of mercury to an unborn child and that half of the flu vaccines contain mercury, the CDC still recommends that "[p]regnant women should receive a seasonal flu shot."[399] Russell Blaylock, M.D., a (retired) board-certified neurosurgeon, highly respected authority, and expert on brain damage caused by vaccines, stated: "I cannot think of anything more insane than vaccinating pregnant women."[400]

Lest you think that the mercury-free flu vaccine is safe, think again. The Medical Director and Chief Operating Officer of the Cleveland Clinic Wellness Institute, Daniel Neides, M.D., warns that the mercury-free flu vaccine is also dangerous. Dr. Neides posted the following article on January 6, 2017, on the Cleveland Clinic website.

> I am tired of all the nonsense we as American citizens are being fed while big business - and the government - continue to ignore the health and well-being of the fine people in this country. Why am I all fired up, you ask?
>
> I, like everyone else, took the advice of the Centers for Disease Control (CDC) - the government - and received a flu shot. I chose to receive the preservative free vaccine, thinking I did not want any thimerasol (i.e. mercury) that the "regular" flu vaccine contains.
>
> Makes sense, right? Why would any of us want to be injected with mercury if it can potentially cause harm? However, what I did not realize is that the preservative-free vaccine contains formaldehyde.

WHAT? How can you call it preservative-free, yet still put a preservative in it? And worse yet, formaldehyde is a known carcinogen. Yet, here we are, being lined up like cattle and injected with an unsafe product. Within 12 hours of receiving the vaccine, I was in bed feeling miserable and missed two days of work with a terrible cough and body aches.

My anger actually stems from a constant toxic burden that is contributing to the chronic disease epidemic. And yet the government continues to talk out of both sides of its mouth. We want our citizens to be healthy and take full advantage of the best healthcare system in the world (so we think), yet we don't treat our bodies with the love and attention they deserve.

***

Link to autism?

***

Slight detour. Why do I mention autism now twice in this article. Because we have to wake up out of our trance and stop following bad advice. Does the vaccine burden - as has been debated for years - cause autism? I don't know and will not debate that here. What I will stand up and scream is that newborns without intact immune systems and detoxification systems are being over-burdened with PRESERVATIVES AND ADJUVANTS IN THE VACCINES.

The adjuvants, like aluminum - used to stimulate

the immune system to create antibodies - can be incredibly harmful to the developing nervous system. Some of the vaccines have helped reduce the incidence of childhood communicable diseases, like meningitis and pneumonia. That is great news. But not at the expense of neurologic diseases like autism and ADHD increasing at alarming rates.

When I was in medical school in the late 1980s, the rate of autism was 1 in 1,000 children. For those born in the 1950's and 60's, do you recall a single student in your grade with an Individualized Education Program (IEP) for ADHD or someone with a diagnosis of autism? I do not.

As of 2010, the rate of autism in the U.S. escalated to 1 in 68 children. The deniers will simply state that we do a better job of diagnosing this "disorder". Really? Something (s) are over-burdening our ability to detoxify, and that is when the problems begin.

***

For those who want to dive in further, help me understand why we vaccinate newborns for hepatitis B - a sexually transmitted disease. Any exposure to this virus is unlikely to happen before our second decade of life, but we expose our precious newborns to toxic aluminum (an adjuvant in the vaccine) at one day of life.

And when they actually need the protection, many who have received this three-shot series in the first year of life will lack antibody protection--as immunity may not last.[401]

Two days after Dr. Neides posted that article, the Cleveland Clinic posted this response.

> Cleveland Clinic is fully committed to evidence-based medicine. Harmful myths and untruths about vaccinations have been scientifically debunked in rigorous ways. We completely support vaccinations to protect people, especially children who are particularly vulnerable. Our physician published his statement without authorization from Cleveland Clinic. His views do not reflect the position of Cleveland Clinic and appropriate disciplinary action will be taken.[402]

Did you notice the threat of disciplinary action? Well, the Cleveland Clinic acted and summarily fired Dr. Neides. There are many doctors who agree with Dr. Neides, but they keep their mouths shut because they know it will mean the end for their medical careers to criticize the safety or efficacy of vaccines.

In 2016, Dr. Nick Delgado made the astounding statement that he had spoken to some 500 doctors in the previous three years. He asked them privately if they would be willing to share their views on vaccinations. They told him, "No, I can't talk about it." Their response to his "Why not?" was "Because my license is at risk."[403]

Brett Wilcox recounts, "Andrew Wakefield, said that doctors tell him all the time that they'd like to speak up but are afraid of what it would do to their careers. Wakefield says he has little patience or tolerance for such people anymore. They took an oath to 'First Do No Harm,' and in remaining silent, they violate that oath and what it means to be a doctor."[404]

Del Bigtree, the producer of Vaxxed, described the situation of doctors being scared to speak out about the dangers of vaccines in an interview with ABC:

> The real sad thing is the [number] of doctors I've spoken to that say, "Del, I know that vaccines are causing autism, but I won't say it on camera because the pharmaceutical industry will destroy my career just like they did to Andy Wakefield." And that's where we find ourselves: being bullied by an industry that doesn't really care about our children.[405]

So, it is not just mercury that is dangerous to the mother and her unborn child. The other excipients in the flu vaccines cause severe adverse effects. Alexander Langmuir, former head of the CDC, was fired when he refused to say that people should get the flu vaccine. Langmuir said:

> I would not take the flu vaccine. My wife does not take the flu vaccine. No one should take the flu vaccine. And in fact when I was head of CDC, I wanted to make that as a public statement and I refused to say that you should take the flu vaccine. That's why I'm now professor at Harvard.[406]

FLUARIX is a flu vaccine that does NOT contain thimerosal.[407] Yet, the FLUARIX package insert lists the following adverse events experienced by people injected with the vaccine:

> Lymphadenopathy, tachycardia, vertigo, conjunctivitis, eye irritation, eye pain, eye redness, eye swelling, eyelid swelling, abdominal pain or discomfort, swelling of the mouth, throat, and/or tongue, asthenia, chest pain, feeling hot, injection site mass, injection site reaction, injection site warmth, body aches, anaphylactic reaction including shock, anaphylactoid reaction,

hypersensitivity, serum sickness, injection site abscess, injection site cellulitis, pharyngitis, rhinitis, tonsillitis, convulsion, encephalomyelitis, facial palsy, facial paresis, Guillain-Barré syndrome, hypoesthesia, myelitis, neuritis, neuropathy, paresthesia, syncope, asthma, bronchospasm, dyspnea, respiratory distress, stridor, angioedema, erythema, erythema multiforme, facial swelling, pruritus, Stevens-Johnson syndrome, sweating, urticarial, Henoch-Schönlein purpura, and vasculitis.[408]

16 The Ends Do Not Justify the Means

Causing disease in someone violates the great commandment that "as ye would that men should do to you, do ye also to them likewise." Luke 6:31. Edmund Massey explains:

> The Holy Scriptures give us frequent instances of God's giving power unto men to heal diseases; and by his blessing a power is still continued. But that one was ever granted to inflict diseases, will I think hardly appear; unless in the case of Moses with the Egyptians, and Elisha with his servant Gehazi. But both these cases were miraculous, and of God's own immediate appointment, to vindicate the honour of his servants the prophets, and for the punishment of sacrilege and idolatry, and cannot be drawn into precedent by any not invested with the same character and authority. Men may, and have invented racks and tortures for each other, but no man, let his Crimes be what they will, was ever yet condemned to an immediate sickness, or sentenced to lie languishing in a fever, for want of a sufficient authority, which no body but a present set of adventurous practitioners have of late

pretended to assume.[409]

It is a sin for man to kill another man. Matthew 19:18. But it is not a sin for God to kill a man. In like manner, it is a sin for a man to bring about disease in another through vaccination, but it is not sin for God to bring about disease in another.

> See now that I, even I, am he, and there is no god with me: **I kill, and I make alive; I wound, and I heal**: neither is there any that can deliver out of my hand. Deuteronomy 32:39.

Indeed, God sent disease among the Egyptians and killed the firstborn of each Egyptian household.

> He [God] made a way to his anger; he spared not their soul from death, but gave their life over to the **pestilence**; And **smote all the firstborn in Egypt**; the chief of their strength in the tabernacles of Ham. (Psalms 78:50-51)

Massey explains that disease is within the sovereign authority of God. It is not for man to usurp that authority and inject antigens to cause disease through vaccination in the hope that later the person will develop an immunity to the pathogen.

> It will easily be granted, therefore, that such a procedure, for want of a competent authority, is unlawful. That if diseases, as beforementioned, are sent unto us for the trial of our faith, or the punishment of our sins; He alone to whom our faith must approve itself, and our sins are manifest, has properly the power of inflicting them.[410]

God is sovereign. "All things were made by him; and without him was not any thing made that was made." John 1:3

"And he is before all things, and by him all things consist." (Colossians 1:17) Indeed, God knows the end from the beginning.

> According as he hath chosen us in him before the foundation of the world, that we should be holy and without blame before him in love: Having predestinated us unto the adoption of children by Jesus Christ to himself, according to the good pleasure of his will. (Ephesians 1:4-5)

Indeed, God can use evil for good ends. But don't get it twisted. What is permissible for God is not permissible for man. God is omnipotent; he knows the end from the beginning. Man is not omnipotent; man has no way of being sure that a good end will result from his evil means. While with God, good ends justify evil means, with man, good ends can never justify evil means. Man cannot commit the evil sin of injecting a vaccine containing harmful antigens, toxic adjuvants, and noxious contaminants to infect a person with a disease to accomplish the supposed good end of creating a theoretical future immunity from that disease. Indeed, the death and disease from vaccines testify to the error of man working to have the ends justify the means.

The example of Asa, King of Judah, reveals how God is displeased with evil means to accomplish good ends. In the case of Asa, he used greed and deception to trick the King of Syria into attacking Asa's enemy, the King of Israel. This displeased God because Asa relied on his own evil means to conquer his enemy, Israel. God wanted Asa to depend on him and not on his own evil devices.

> And at that time Hanani the seer came to Asa king of Judah, and said unto him, **Because thou hast relied on the king of Syria, and not relied on the LORD thy God, therefore is the host of the king of Syria escaped out of thine hand.** Were not the

> Ethiopians and the Lubims a huge host, with very many chariots and horsemen? yet, because thou didst rely on the LORD, he delivered them into thine hand. For the eyes of the LORD run to and fro throughout the whole earth, to shew himself strong in the behalf of them whose heart is perfect toward him. Herein thou hast done foolishly: therefore from henceforth thou shalt have wars. (2 Chronicles 16:7-9)

Asa started his reign as king by relying on God, but as God gave him success, he ended up relying on himself and not trusting God. As his health failed and he was struck with a disease, he acted on fear and turned to his physicians instead of turning to God. Consequently, he died of the illness. Fear is the opposite of faith.

> And Asa in the thirty and ninth year of his reign was diseased in his feet, until his disease was exceeding great: yet in his disease **he sought not to the LORD, but to the physicians.** And Asa slept with his fathers, and died in the one and fortieth year of his reign." (2 Chronicles 16:12-13)

Nationally renowned Dr. Paul Offit, M.D. condones the concept of the means justifying the ends. "Paul Offit, is a pediatrician specializing in infectious diseases and an expert on vaccines, immunology, and virology. He is the co-inventor of a rotavirus vaccine that has been credited with saving hundreds of lives every day. Offit is the Maurice R. Hilleman professor of vaccinology, professor of pediatrics at the Perelman School of Medicine at the University of Pennsylvania and director of The Vaccine Education Center at Children's Hospital of Philadelphia (CHOP). Offit is currently a member of National Institutes of Health (NIH) working group on vaccines, a subgroup of the 'Accelerating COVID-19 Therapeutic Interventions and Vaccines'

(ACTIV) comprised of experts to combat COVID-19. He is also a member of the FDA's Vaccines and Related Biological Products Advisory Committee (VRBPAC). Previously, he was a member of the Centers for Disease Control and Prevention's (CDC) Advisory Committee on Immunization Practices."[411] Dr. Offit invokes the authority of the Pope of the Roman Catholic Church as he tries to advocate for the use of evil means of using aborted fetal tissue to justify the alleged good ends of preventing disease by vaccination.

> Now, the Catholic Church, through the Pontifical Academy of Life have weighed in on this issue because obviously for the Catholic Church, abortion is a sin, a sin worthy of excommunication, a sin that causes one to lose, frankly, the ability to participate in the sacraments of the church or Catholic life. So, I think Catholics have reasonably asked the question, "Can we get these vaccines?" And the Pontifical Academy of Life, at the time headed by Joseph Ratzinger who became Pope Benedict XVI, has ruled that "yes" it is OK to get it. In fact it's important to get these vaccines because vaccines save lives; vaccines prevent suffering; vaccines prevent hospitalization and occasionally death. And the Catholic Church, like any major religion, cares deeply about the health and well-being of children.[412]

The Roman Catholic Church is the classic religious cult that justifies compromising religious principles to conform with the ways of the world. Indeed, the Roman Catholic Church is a Machievlian organization whose evil aims are hidden behind pomp and circumstance of elaborate liturgical ceremony and costumes. The Vatican is truly the habitation of seducing spirits "speaking lies in hypocrisy." See 1 Timothy 4:1-3.

The papacy presents a public facade of righteousness. That

pubic facade, however, is a smokescreen that conceals an anti-Christian agenda. The papacy is the progeny of the hypocritical scribes and Pharisees, condemned by Jesus. Matthew 23:13-15. The Roman Catholic Church funds organizations that work to undermine biblical standards, all the while claiming to uphold those very standards.

For example, the Catholic Campaign for Human Development (CCHD) gives millions of dollars in grants to numerous radical left organizations. CCHD was founded in 1970 as the Catholic bishops' anti-poverty program. In 1997 CCHD funded the following organizations, all of which endorsed the National Organization for Women's (NOW) 1996 "Fight for the Right" [to abortion] march in San Francisco: Association of Community Organizations for Reform Now (ACORN) ($310,000 grant from CCHD), Asian Immigrant Women Advocates ($20,000 grant from CCHD), the Center for Third World Organizing (CTWO) ($25,000 grant from CCHD), the Chinese Progressive Association ($30,000 grant from CCHD), and the Santa Clara Center for Occupational Safety and Health ($30,000 grant from CCHD).[413] ACORN was a co-sponsor of the February 1996 conference of the Feminist Majority Foundation which advocates abortion rights. The CTWO advocates homosexual marriage laws. CTWO in turn sponsors WAGE (Winning Action for Gender Equality), which is harshly critical of those such as Christians who support the traditional nuclear family and Christian values.

CCHD funds many radical left and communist front organizations indirectly by funding coalitions of allegedly charitable groups.[414] For example, in 1997 CCHD awarded a grant to Greater Birmingham Ministries, which in turn sponsored another coalition, Alabama Arise. Members of Alabama Arise included the AFL-CIO and the American Civil Liberties Union (ACLU).[415] CCHD also awarded a grant to the Philadelphia Unemployment Project Coalition for JOBS; that coalition included AFSCME locals, the Pennsylvania AFL-CIO, the state chapter of

NOW, and the Woman's Law Project (WLP).[416] NOW is an aggressive proponent of abortion and special sodomite rights. NOW supports partial birth abortions and opposes any restriction on abortion, including parental notification. The WLP is a legal services provider in Philadelphia that advocates lesbian and homosexual parenting rights and abortion rights. AFSME and the AFL-CIO both contribute to groups that advocate abortion rights and homosexual "marriage." The ACLU is the leading opponent of religious freedom in schools and opposes restrictions on abortions.

Some might argue that the Catholic bishops just made some errors. The evidence, however, suggests that the leftist anti-American slant to the CCHD grants is knowing and purposeful. For the past ten years the Capital Research Center has publicized to all who would listen the radical left slant to the CCHD grants, but the CCHD has done little to nothing to curtail the support of the radical anti-Christian left.[417]

The CCHD responded in 1998 to criticism by proposing changes to its guidelines. The new guidelines were adopted, and they specifically forbade the CCHD from awarding grants to organizations which "promote or support abortion, euthanasia, the death penalty, or any other affront to human life and dignity."[418] Apparently the new guidelines were merely lip service, designed to appease conservative Catholics. There, in fact, has been no significant change in the grants by the CCHD. The CCHD is still funneling money to radical left, communist, and pro abortion organizations.

For Example, not only did the CCHD not cut off its funding of ACORN in 1999-2000, they increased the funding for 17 state and local chapters of ACORN by 18%, to a total of \$517,000.[419] The CCHD also continued to fund the Philadelphia Unemployment Project during 1999-2000. The project's "Jobs Campaign" coalition includes a branch of ACORN, AFSCME locals, the Pennsylvania and Philadelphia AFL-CIO, the state chapter of NOW, and the Women's Law Project, all of which support abortion rights.[420] In addition, the CCHD continues its perennial financial support to affiliates of the Industrial Areas Foundation (IAF). IAF was founded by Saul Alinsky, who was author of *Rules for Radicals*, which is a bible for left-wing political protest groups.[421] The CCHD is carrying out the official, but covert, un-American and anti-Christian policies of the Roman Catholic Church. Suzanne Belongia, CCHD director in Winona, Minnesota, in an attempt to defend CCHD pointed out that Pope John Paul II, officially endorsed CCHD when he visited Washington, D.C., early in his pontificate.[422]

The information about the CCHD grants gives us a little peak at the wolf under the sheep's clothing. Politician Huey Long once said, "if you have a reputation as an early riser, you can sleep until noon."[423] Publicly the Catholic Church is against abortion and for traditional family values; while behind the scenes the Roman church is financially supporting pro abortion and anti-Christian groups. The CCHD reveals the Roman Catholic Church as the consummate Machiavellian political organization.

A hypocrite is a person who pretends to have religious beliefs or morals that are the opposite of his behavior. The Roman Catholic hierarchy are the same as the hypocrites that Jesus criticized.

> Ye hypocrites, well did Esaias prophesy of you, saying, This people draweth nigh unto me with their mouth, and honoureth me with their lips; but their heart is far from me. But in vain they do worship me, teaching for doctrines the commandments of men. (Matthew 15:7-9)

But God is not like man. God's crucifixion of Jesus Christ illustrates how, with God, the ends justify the means. God used evil means for good ends. The crucifixion of Jesus Christ was a torturous death, but God used that evil for good; it is the means through which Jesus Christ atoned for the sins of his elect. And it was all orchestrated by God.

Judas betrayed Jesus as prophesied by God hundreds of years earlier. Jesus stated, while praying to God the Father: "While I was with them in the world, I kept them in thy name: those that thou gavest me I have kept, and **none of them is lost, but the son of perdition; that the scripture might be fulfilled."** (John 17:12)

The betrayal of Jesus by Judas was planned by God. In Jeremiah we read a prophecy written approximately 600 years before the betrayal of Jesus by Judas: "Yea, mine own familiar friend, in whom I trusted, which did eat of my bread, hath lifted up his heel against me." (Psalms 41:9 AV) Jesus, referring to the prophecy in Jeremiah, told the apostles: "I speak not of you all: I know whom I have chosen: but that the scripture may be fulfilled, He that eateth bread with me hath lifted up his heel against me." (John 13:18)

Jesus knew Judas would betray him: "For he knew who should betray him; therefore said he, Ye are not all clean." (John 13:11) Judas had no more a free will in the matter than a pencil has a free will to write. Judas, like the pencil, was an instrument completely under God's control.

God did not leave our salvation to the chance that Judas might not betray Jesus. God is love. 1 John 4:8. It would be the very antithesis of love to leave our salvation to chance. God is not a gambler.

Judas was preordained by God to betray Jesus. Judas had no choice in the matter. God predicted what Judas would do hundreds of years before he did it and then predicted it to his apostles moments before it happened. Jesus then personally gave Judas orders to hurry up and betray him. Judas could not resist the will of God.

> Jesus answered, He it is, to whom I shall give a sop, when I have dipped it. And when he had dipped the sop, he gave *it* to Judas Iscariot, the son of Simon. And after the sop Satan entered into him. Then said Jesus unto him, That thou doest, do quickly. (John 13:26-27)

Not only did Judas not have a free will to choose whether to betray Jesus, but every single act of Herod, Pontius Pilate, the Jews, and the Romans was preordained and orchestrated by the sovereign God of Heaven. "For of a truth against thy holy child Jesus, whom thou hast anointed, both Herod, and Pontius Pilate, with the Gentiles, and the people of Israel, were gathered together, **For to do whatsoever thy hand and thy counsel determined before to be done."** (Acts 4:27-28) In fact, God orders the steps of all men and controls their very tongue. "The preparations of the heart in man, and the answer of the tongue are from the Lord." Prov. 16:1.

While God may do evil so that good may come of it, man my not do that same thing. Man cannot do evil (cause disease) in order that some good may come of it. That is the theory of vaccination. The ends cannot justify the means. We are forbidden to do evil in order to obtain some good end. Bad means corrupt the intended good. "And not rather, (as we be slanderously reported, and as some affirm that we say,) Let us do evil, that good may come? whose damnation is just." (Romans 3:8) Indeed, "whatsoever is not of faith is sin." (Romans 14:23)

A person is injected with a pathogen on the theory that the recipient's body will become immune to the disease. Even if that theory were correct, it would be a sin to inject a person with an antigen to cause an immune response. That is to "do evil that good may come." That is a sin. See Romans 14:23. But the good that is expected is a phantom; the medical theory of vaccination is fallacious. Job explains: "But ye are forgers of lies, ye are all physicians of no value." (Job 13:4)

The gospel message is that those who have saving faith and are thus justified will live by that faith. Their faith is a living faith, not a dead faith. "For therein is the righteousness of God revealed from faith to faith: as it is written, The just shall live by faith." Romans 1:17. See also Galatians 3:11. Indeed, God has a warning for those who purport to believe but who do not live by faith. "Now the just shall live by faith: but if any man draw back, my soul shall have no pleasure in him." (Hebrews 10:38) "Not every one that saith unto me, Lord, Lord, shall enter into the kingdom of heaven; but he that doeth the will of my Father which is in heaven." (Matthew 7:21) Faith brings obedience. It is special obedience wrought by God through faith that God imparts in the believer. "But now is made manifest, and by the scriptures of the prophets, according to the commandment of the everlasting God, made known to all nations for the obedience of faith." (Romans 16:26) We are called on to have nothing to do with evil. We are to avoid even the appearance of evil. We are to "abstain from all appearance of evil." 1 Thessalonians 5:22. Indeed, we are to reprove evil. "And have no fellowship with the unfruitful works of darkness, but rather reprove them." (Ephesians 5:11) Vaccination is an unfruitful work of darkness forged by lies. Christians are duty-bound to reprove the evil practice.

17 The Sacrament of Vaccination

Doctors who have practiced for years and have seen the ineffectiveness of and damage done by vaccines are at a loss to explain the practice. They realize that it is not based on science. When considering why such a practice would continue in the face of such damning evidence against it, they come to the only logical conclusion left; vaccination is a superstitious religious practice.

Robert S. Mendelsohn, M.D., (1926-1988) was a practicing pediatrician for 30 years and a professor of pediatrics at the University of Illinois College of Medicine. He wrote a syndicated newspaper column and appeared on over 500 television and radio shows. In his book *Confessions of a Medical Heretic*, he characterized the medical profession as akin to a religious cult. Dr. Mendelsohn criticized the flu shot as a "farce." Dr. Mendelsohn called the alleged swine flu epidemic of 1976 a "fiasco." He portrayed doctors as powerful priests of a primitive and mysterious religion with arcane doctrines that the laity cannot understand. The central ethic of the religion is dishonesty. Dr. Mendelsohn states that "[t]he doctor is taught in his seminary, which he calls a medical school, to never tell the truth to patients."[424] Dr. Mendelsohn viewed vaccination as akin to religious superstition, where the cult member is left in a worse state after the "sacrament" is injected into the arm.

> If you follow the sounds of medical-governmental drum-beating in favor of a "preventive" procedure, you'll more often than not find yourself in the midst of one of the Church's least safe and effective sacraments. For instance, with some immunizations the danger in taking the shot may outweigh that of not taking it![425]

The only way to properly understand the dangers of vaccination is to realize that it is the product of a so-called science that runs on lies and disinformation. The practice of vaccination is the product of a medical practice based on superstition and greed. Dr. Mendelsohn stated:

> Once you understand Modern Medicine as a religion, you can fight it and defend yourself much more effectively than when you think you're fighting an art or a science.[426]

Dr. Richard Moskowitz, M. D. reflected on the ineffectiveness and dangers of vaccines and could not come up with a rational explanation for the practice. How can one justify vaccinating the population with a vaccine only to find that most of those vaccinated become ill with the disease for which they were vaccinated? Add to that the often debilitating side effects of the vaccines, and you are left with no scientific justification for the practice. Dr. Moskowitz concluded that vaccination could only be explained by a mindset in the medical community that has been taken over by religious superstition where each vaccination is a sacrament. Vaccines are administered without regard to the fact that they have been proven ineffective and unsafe because the reason for the administration is not medical science but rather religious dogma.

> The fact is that we have been taught to accept vaccination as a kind of involuntary Communion, a sacrament of our participation in the unrestricted growth of scientific and industrial technology, utterly heedless of the long-term consequences to the health of our own species, let alone to the balance of Nature as a whole. For that reason alone, the other side of the case urgently needs to be heard.
>
> ***
>
> [W]ith all due respect, I cannot have faith in the miracles or accept the sacraments of Merck, Sharp, and Dohme and the Centers for Disease Control. I prefer to stay with the miracle of life itself, which has given us illness and disease, to be sure, but also the arts of medicine and healing, through which we can acknowledge and experience our pain and vulnerability, and sometimes, with the grace of God and the help of our friends and neighbors, an awareness of health and well-being that knows no boundaries. That is my religion; and while I would willingly share it, I would not force it on anyone.[427]

Olivier Clerc states in his book, *The New World Religion: How Beliefs Secretly Influence Medical Dogmas and Practices*:

> [P]hysicians have taken the place of priests; vaccination plays the same role as baptism; the search for health has replaced the quest for salvation; the fight against disease has replaced the fight against sin; eradication of viruses has taken the place of exorcising demons; the hope of physical immortality (cloning, genetic engineering)

takes priority over eternal life.[428]

Clerc observes the replacement of actual science with false science driven by the desire for riches. The Bible warns that the love of money is the root of all evil. 1 Timothy 6:10. Christians are called on to be wary of false religious doctrines like vaccination that are cloaked in so-called science. "[K]eep that which is committed to thy trust, avoiding profane and vain babblings, and oppositions of science falsely so called. Which some professing have erred concerning the faith." 1 Timothy 6:20-21. Christians are marching their children into the pediatrician's office to take part in a dangerous ritual of vaccination without realizing they are engaging in a heathen religious practice that is cloaked in the garb of medical science.

Clerc traces the substitution of Christian values with heathen superstition to the adoption of Louis Pasteur's mythological germ theory that has given rise to the dangerous practice of vaccination.

> We traditionally associate the birth of modern medicine with the publication of the work of French biologist Louis Pasteur (1822-1895), the father of vaccines. This choice fits perfectly with my thesis, as it was with Pasteur that the progressive and systematic transference of Christian symbolism to medicine began.[429]

Brett Wilcox, in his book, *Jabbed*,[430] argues that vaccines are a ritual of religion and not a medical treatment based on science. It is easy to accept Wicox's premise once one understands the fraud, corruption, and superstition surrounding vaccination. The practice of injecting poisons into the body to prevent disease can only be understood as a superstitious religious practice because the science that supports it only appears to do so because the studies have been designed to conceal vaccine dangers. At the same time, the studies are conducted to falsely portray benefit where there is none. Wilcox explains:

> Vaccines, on the other hand, are infallible in the sect practiced by vaccine believers and sociopaths. Their infallibility is proclaimed in the primary vaccine creed: "Vaccines are safe and effective." Questioning the creed is verboten as is legal redress against vaccine manufacturers. The creed is an essential part of the vaccine paradigm because, unlike other pharmaceuticals, vaccines are administered to healthy individuals. Parents wouldn't let medical professionals jab their healthy kids if they didn't have faith in the creed. Vaccines—the sacred cow of public health—are a golden calf to the sociopaths who manufacture and manipulate the faith of the human herd. And with over 250 vaccines in development, that calf is growing ever more golden. By 2020, profits from the global vaccine market are expected to swell from nearly $24 billion to $61 billion. Referring to vaccines as a sacred cow and a golden calf is apropos from both religious and etymological perspectives. "Vacc" in the word "vaccine" is from the Latin word "cow." The original "vaccine" was a preparation of the cowpox virus taken from infected cows and inoculated in humans with the belief that it would provide immunity to smallpox.[431]

Those who question the legitimacy of vaccination are treated like religious heretics. They are vilified and shunned. Doctors are defrocked from the medical priesthood by the medical boards. The believers are indoctrinated to fear the invisible contagion such that anyone who does not receive the sacrament of vaccination is excommunicated as posing a threat to the entire community. Few ever stop to consider that if the vaccines were effective, those vaccinated should have nothing to fear. But the fact that the vaccinated believers still fear infection from the unvaccinated (i.e., the unclean; untouchables) is an implicit acknowledgment that they understand that the vaccines do not work. Wilcox explains:

> The Unholy Trinity—the pharmaceutical industry, the medical establishment and government—has successfully convinced the faithful that abstaining from vaccinations puts the entire flock at risk of damnation in the form of lethal disease outbreaks. Under the bonds of such indoctrination, people who otherwise respect legal and religious freedom heartily endorse the use of scorn, shame, hostility, name calling, discrimination, loss of the right of public education, loss of parental rights, fines, and even imprisonment for those who refuse to inject any and all vaccines the indoctrinated impose upon the rest of the flock. Former pharmaceutical representative Brandy Vaughan, now an industry whistleblower, relates the following: "I've being called a murderer, told that I should be in jail, burned at the stake, that my child will kill other children on the playground, that he should be taken away from me." Such accusations protect believers against the uncomfortable realization that the sanctuary in which they worship may not be what it claims to be, that the data supporting their beliefs is more smoke and mirrors than it is science. Leaving the Church is not for the faint of heart. Just as churches often hide, falsify, or erase faith-destroying information from their congregants, the sociopaths who run The Church of Vaccinology routinely hide, falsify or erase faith-destroying information from the public. Thus,

> the spotlight of truth must not only shine on vaccines, it must also shine on the people who profit from the deliberate spread of vaccine-related propaganda and misinformation.[432]

Dr. Paul Offit is the co-inventor of the rotovirus vaccine. He is an expert in vaccines and immunology and the Chief of Infectious Diseases at Children's Hospital of Philadelphia. Offit is also the Maurice R. Hilleman Professor of Vaccinology at the Perelman School of Medicine at the University of Pennsylvania. Dr. Offit gives an example of the kind of nonsense being preached by the priesthood of vaccinologists. When trying to justify injecting vaccines containing heavy metals like mercury and aluminum and other dangerous adjuvants and excipients into tiny babies, Offit stated that it was not the ingredient that is dangerous but the dosing of that ingredient. Offit stated that "you can overdose on water. People who drink large quantities of water during a short period of time have occasionally suffered seizures as they've exceeded their bodies ability to hold onto sodium. As Paracelsus, a chemist, once said, 'The dose makes the poison.'"[433]

While it is technically accurate that one can drink too much water, it is a strange and deceptive argument to make when discussing vaccine toxicology. Marco Cáceres was beside himself to understand how Offit could use such reasoning to justify injecting vaccines containing known poisons into babies.

> You can overdose on drinking too much water? We are supposed to take this as a scientific comparison of the effect of highly toxic chemicals and metals being injected into fatty tissue, and ultimately the bloodstream and brain? Repeatedly injected, without much pause, over the course of our lifetime, from the time we are a fetus in our mother's womb, through our infancy, teenage and adult years, and finally until we are elderly and in

> the twilight of our years?
>
> The first inclination is to chuckle and say, "He's kidding, right?" But no, Dr. Offit doesn't give the impression he's joking around. The quote from Paracelsus is one of his favorites, which he often uses in interviews. The man really believes it's solely about the dose, and that whether it's mercury or water (… or applesauce, for that matter), it all comes down to how much you consume or inject.[434]

It gets worse. Offit is on record saying that a baby's immune system could handle as many as 100,000 vaccine shots.[435] This is the same man who said that dosing was everything and that one can overdose on too much water. Like all snake oil salesmen, he changes his tune depending on the audience. According to Offit, you should be more concerned with your child drinking too much water than allowing a doctor to inject 100,000 vaccines containing toxic chemicals into your child. But when you understand that Offit is the co-patent holder for a vaccine against rotavirus, it is clear that he is being paid handsomely to say such strange things.

This was not an off-the-cuff statement by Dr. Offit. He posted the statement in an official newsletter sent out from the Children's Hospital of Philadelphia (CHOP), where he is the director of the CHOP Vaccine Education Center. Under the heading: "Myth 1: Getting so many vaccines will overwhelm my child's immune system" is found the following statement:

> Compared to what they typically encounter and manage during the day, vaccines are literally a drop in the ocean." In fact, Dr. Offit's studies show that in theory, healthy infants could safely get up to 100,000 vaccines at once.[436]

When he was confronted with that statement, Dr. Offit reaffirmed that he genuinely believed it to be true that a child could safely get 100,000 vaccines injected into him at once. Dr. Offit said:

> "The 100,000 number makes me sound like a madman. Because that's the image: 100,000 shots sticking out of you. It's an awful image," Offit says. "Many people — including people who are on my side — have criticized me for that. But I was naive. In that article, I was being asked the question and **that is the answer to the question."**[437]

Offit reaffirmed, **"that is the answer to the question."** He said he understood that he sounded like a madman. But he did not say he was exaggerating or using hyperbole. Instead, he explained that was the answer to the question and truly believed what he said. He is correct that saying such a thing makes him sound like a madman; but believing it makes him a madman.

J.B. Handley, Co-Founder of Generation Rescue, comments:

> Not only is Offit's comment insane, it's also wildly dangerous and untrue. 100,000 vaccines given to a baby would cause immediate death, every single time. How profoundly disrespectful to the THOUSANDS of parents for whom ONE vaccine caused death for their child. ONE!!
>
> Let's look at the Vaccine Injury Compensation Program website for a moment, just to further highlight how crazy Offit's comments really are. What does it tells us? It shows 11,970 claims of injury and 1,006 claims of death, in every case from ONE vaccine. Offit is saying a baby can

> handle 100,000 of something that has killed, at a bare minimum, more than 1,000 Americans,[438]

Assuming a vaccine dose range between 0.5 ml and 2.0 ml we find that at the lowest dosage volume, 100,000 vaccines will equal a total of 50 liters or 13.2 gallons of vaccine solution, and at the upper range, it would be 200 liters or 52.8 gallons injected into a child. Please be mindful that those gallons of vaccines would contain such excipient ingredients including, but not limited to, formaldehyde (a carcinogenic embalming fluid), ethylmercury (neurotoxin), aluminum (neurotoxin), 2-phenoxyethanol (insecticide), MRC-5 cells (aborted fetal tissue causing autoimmune disorders), polysorbate 80 (causing an immune response that can include anaphylaxis) and polyethylene glycol (PEG) (can cause hypersensitivity including anaphylaxis).

But according to the high priest of vaccinology, Paul Offit, there would be no problem injecting gallons of vaccines containing such chemicals into an infant. He wears the white clerical garment and is called a doctor. He is part of the medical priesthood whom you are expected to believe without question, regardless of how inane is his opinion. You must have faith; most of all, you must be obedient. The man is a religious zealot dressed up as a doctor, he is a quack, as are all priests in the cult of vaccinology. Brett Wilcox probably says it best:

> Prepare to enter the Inner Sanctum of The Church of Vaccinology. Prepare to drink from the Holy Grail. Prepare to kiss the hand of the Patron Saint of The Church, the Reverend Doctor Paul Offit. One proclamation echoes within the sacred chambers far more than any other. It embodies the religion's central tenet, the core doctrine, the cosmic creed:
>
> "Vaccines are safe and effective."

So it is, so it has ever been, and so it will ever be. Amen and amen.

The Unholy Trinity—pharma, the medical establishment, and government—has uttered, published, and broadcast this statement with such repetition that merely thinking or hearing it induces society into a hypnotic response, effectively shutting down critical thought processes while turning on faith-based magical thinking. "Vaccines are safe and effective." In a religious context, this proclamation is a creed. In organizational terms, it's policy. In marketing, it's the hook. In social psychology, it's propaganda. In literary parlance, it's myth. In legal vernacular, it's fraud. In the art of mind control, it's described as conversational hypnosis or "sleight of mouth." Under oath, it's perjury. In short, it's bunk.[439]

18 Government Fraud

Medical quackery is the ignorant, misinformed, or dishonest practice of medicine. Certainly, medical fraud would fall within the ambit of quackery. The FDA defines health fraud drug products as follows:

> In general, health fraud drug products are articles of unproven effectiveness that claim to treat disease or improve health.[440]

The FDA elaborates on that definition and considers the deceptive promotion or distribution of a product that has not been scientifically proven safe and effective to constitute health fraud.

> The FDA defines health fraud as the deceptive promotion, advertising, distribution, or sale of a product represented as being effective to prevent, diagnose, treat, cure or lessen an illness or condition, or provide another beneficial effect on health, but that has not been scientifically proven safe and effective for such purposes.[441]

By that definition, all emergency use authorized (EUA) products constitute health fraud and, at the very least, quackery.

That is because EUA products, like the COVID-19 vaccines, have not been proven safe and effective. The standard for an EUA product is simply that "the known and potential benefits of the product, when used to diagnose, prevent, or treat such disease or condition, outweigh the known and potential risks of the product."[442] It is a balancing of the risk to the benefits. The danger from the vaccine could be pretty serious. And indeed, the vaccine could be ineffective. But a determination has been made that the benefits outweigh the risks of the vaccine. That is not the same as determining that the vaccine is safe and effective.

But then we have vaccines that the FDA has approved on the promise that they are safe and effective. But, almost always, those vaccines later turn out to be either unsafe, ineffective, or both. For example, the FDA-approved influenza vaccines have been repeatedly proven ineffective. And yet these ineffective vaccines are nonetheless promoted by the CDC. Promoting an ineffective vaccine is medical fraud; the CDC is engaging in quackery.

In an October 20, 2022 presentation by the CDC National Center for Immunization & Respiratory Diseases, members of the Advisory Committee on Immunization Practices revealed that the "2021–2022 influenza vaccination provided low to non-significant protection against predominant influenza A/H3N2 illness of varying severity."[443] The committee further stated that the ineffectiveness of the influenza vaccine was not a surprise because all of the vaccines in prior years have also been ineffective. "Protection was similar to pre-pandemic A/H3N2-dominant seasons."[444]

With that in mind, you would think that CDC Director Rochelle Walensky would step in and stop vaccinations for the flu. You would be wrong. Instead, Walensky promoted ineffective flu vaccines. On November 11, 2022, Walensky tweeted:

> Influenza like illness continues to increase across the United States. Flu vaccine uptake has lagged compared to prior seasons. It is time to get your flu vaccine as well as your updated #COVID19 vaccine if you have not yet done so.[445]

CDC Director is promoting a vaccine that her agency has said offers "low to non-significant protection." The data shows that for the elderly, the vaccine was detrimental. An elderly person who had been vaccinated against the flu was more likely to get the flu. Walensky is engaging in what the FDA defines as health fraud by promoting a vaccine that has not been scientifically proven safe and effective. Walensky is a quack. Walensky adds insult to injury by promoting the unsafe and ineffective COVID-19 vaccine. This is the same Rochelle Walensky who had fallen ill with COVID-19 just a few weeks before her tweet promoting the flu vaccine and a month after receiving her bivalent COVID-19 booster.[446] She has personal knowledge that the COVID-19 vaccines do not work, yet she continues to promote them. Walensky is promoting "health fraud drug product[s]," which are defined by the FDA as "articles of unproven effectiveness that claim to treat disease or improve health."[447]

Igor Chudov considers the influenza vaccines as the perfect example of medical quackery.

> Non-working, non-proven (flu vaccines are NEVER tested with randomized trials prior to rollouts) treatments are called medical quackery, and the quacks promoting such treatments should be called charlatans.
>
> You would think that the CDC, upon hearing news of the utter ineffectiveness of flu vaccines, would withdraw them from circulation, right? Would you suppose that our authorities care about us, so they

> would never promote treatments with negative effectiveness?
>
> Actually, promoting non-working flu vaccines is prioritized almost as highly as promoting harmful Covid vaccines![448]

The approval of the drug Aduhelm is another example of government medical fraud and quackery. The FDA is a component agency of HHS. HHS announced a 14.5 % increase in the Medicare premium for 2022. One-half of the increase was for the purpose of paying for a drug called Aduhelm.[449] The FDA approved Aduhelm to treat Alzheimer's disease.[450] Aduhelm is made by Biogen of Cambridge, Massachusetts. A one-year treatment for the drug is $28,200. Medicare estimated that Aduhelm would cost it $30 billion in one year.

Here is the rub. Adulhelm does not work; it is a complete fraud; it is unsafe and ineffective. The FDA states that "health fraud drug products are articles of unproven effectiveness that claim to treat disease or improve health."[451] By its own definition, the FDA is an accomplice to health fraud. You might think that I am engaging in hyperbole. You might think that certainly the safety and effectiveness of Aduhelm are supported by scientific studies. Well, the safety and effectiveness of Aduhelm were studied, but the drug was found to be both ineffective and unsafe. Indeed, during its 2019 medical trials, Aduhelm was found so clearly unsafe and ineffective that the clinical trials were suspended.

Despite the fact that the Aduhelm was shown to be unsafe and ineffective in trials, Biogen sought FDA approval for the drug anyway. The 11-member FDA panel of expert scientists voted not to approve the drug. The vote was 10 voting no and one voting not certain. Thus, none of the members of the FDA's own advisory panel voted to approve Aduhelm. How could they approve it? The studies were clear; it does not work. Yet, the FDA approved it anyway. Three FDA panel members resigned in protest of the FDA decision.

One FDA panel member who resigned, Dr. Aaron Kesselheim, a professor of medicine at Harvard Medical School and Brigham and Women's Hospital, stated that "[t]his might be the worst approval decision that the FDA has made that I can remember."[452] The New York Times reported:

> He said the agency's approval of the drug, aducanumab, which is being marketed as Aduhelm, a monthly intravenous infusion that Biogen has priced at $56,000 per year, was wrong "because of so many different factors, starting from the fact that there's no good evidence that the drug works."

Incidentally, Biogen later dropped the price to $28,200 after all the bad press. The New York Time article further reveals:

> Two other members of the committee resigned earlier this week, expressing dismay at the approval of the drug despite the committee's overwhelming rejection of it after reviewing clinical trial data in November.
>
> The committee had found that the evidence did not convincingly show that Aduhelm could slow cognitive decline in people in the early stages of the disease — and that the drug could cause potentially serious side effects of brain swelling and brain bleeding. None of the 11 members of the committee considered the drug ready for approval: Ten voted against and one was uncertain.

***

> Beyond the steep price tag of the drug, additional costs to screen patients before treatment and for regular MRIs required to monitor their brains for problems could add tens of thousands of dollars to the tab. Medicare is expected to shoulder much of the bill.
>
> "Giving patients a drug that doesn't work and of course has important risks that are going to require multiple MRIs at a price of $56,000 a year is putting patients in a really challenging position and putting doctors in a difficult position as well," Dr. Kesselheim said.[453]

So, there you have it. The FDA has approved an ineffective and dangerous drug to enrich a company to the tune of $30 billion per year at taxpayers' and medicare participants' expense. The FDA is a captured agency engaging in criminal fraud. The FDA cannot be trusted.

"For the love of money is the root of all evil: which while some coveted after, they have erred from the faith, and pierced themselves through with many sorrows." 1 Timothy 6:10.

19 Vaccines Are Dangerous Medical Quackery

The COVID-19 vaccine is not an anomaly. It is just the most recent vaccine atrocity. Vaccination is medical quackery.[454] But because vaccinations fulfill the perverted ends of Satan and his minions, the practice flourishes. Vaccines are unsafe and ineffective. James Howenstine, M.D., in his book, *A Physicians Guide to Natural Health Products*, revealed that "[a] New Zealand study disclosed that 23% of vaccinated children develop asthma compared to zero in unvaccinated children."[455] One suppressed study proves that "vaccinated children appear to be significantly less healthy than the unvaccinated."[456]

In that study funded by The Institute for Pure and Applied Knowledge (IPAK) and published in the International Journal of Environmental Research and Public Health it was determined that unvaccinated children are significantly healthier than vaccinated children.[457] The conclusion from the study is that vaccinating children causes them to suffer a "significant" increase in asthma, allergies, breathing issues, behavioral issues, ADHD, respiratory infections, otitis media (ear infections), ear pain, infections, conjunctivitis (eye infections), eye disorders, eczema, dermatitis, urticaria (hives), and anemia.

The study made a notable finding. "Remarkably, zero of the 561 unvaccinated patients in the study had attention deficit hyperactivity disorder (ADHD) compared to 0.063% of the (partially and fully) vaccinated."

The chart below shows the "[c]umulative office visits in the vaccinated (orange) vs. unvaccinated (blue) patients born into [Dr. Paul Thomas' pediatric] practice: the clarity of the age-specific differences in the health fates of individuals who are vaccinated (2763) compared to the 561 unvaccinated in patients born into the practice over ten years is most strikingly clear in this comparison of the cumulative numbers of diagnoses in the two patient groups. The number of office visits for the unvaccinated is adjusted by a sample size multiplier factor (4.9) to the expected value as if the number of unvaccinated in the study was the same as the number of vaccinated."[458]

The study reported: "The visual impact of the cumulative office visit plots is striking; more so than other plots, the time element (day of life) provides an index by which to compare the accumulation of human pain and suffering from potential vaccine side effects ... [chart below]. These results are worth studying closely and noticing the variation among the cumulative office visits per condition and the stark differences between the rates of billed office visits in the most and unvaccinated patients born into the practice." Below are charts that graphically illustrate the difference in the number of office visits for various diagnosed ailments between vaccinated children ([upper light gray] orange line) and unvaccinated ([lower dark gray] blue line) children. The stark difference illustrates the significantly better health of unvaccinated children.

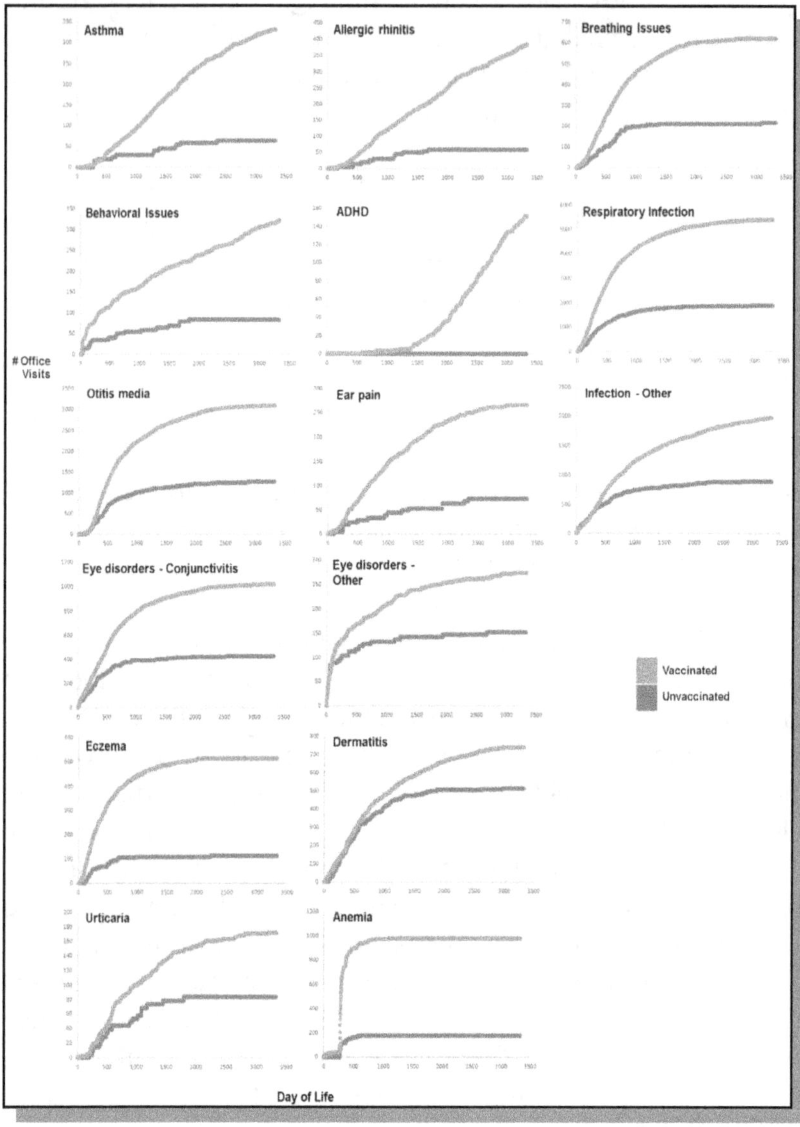

The above study was later retracted based on the unsubstantiated complaint from an anonymous source.[459] The study's authors revisited the data to address the claim by the complainant and found that the complaint was without merit.

Their confirmation study was published and has not been refuted or retracted. Their revisit of the study confirmed their initial conclusions that vaccinated children are significantly less healthy than unvaccinated children.

> Studies finding associations between vaccines and adverse conditions have been targeted for retraction. Here, we revisit data from one such study, comparing the increase in office visits for conditions independent of the routine "well-child" visits (hereafter, Health Care Visits; HCVs).The retraction occurred after >1/4 of a million people had read the peer-reviewed study. It was targeted by one anonymous reader who complained he did not believe the published results. His complaint hinged on the supposition —unsupported by any data —that vaccinated children made their scheduled HCVs more regularly than unvaccinated, implying that those unkept appointments led to fewer diagnoses. We show, here, new data from the same practice that the opposite is true. When the data for vaccinated versus unvaccinated children are examined, the critic's claim is exactly reversed.[460]

Steve Kirsch explains the motive behind the skulduggery in retracting Dr. Thomas' study.

> The [Thomas] study was unethically retracted by the journal over the objection of the authors, i.e., the journal didn't follow the COPE guidelines. They said that "the conclusions were not supported by strong scientific data" which is NOT a valid reason to retract a study once it is published. The journal retracted the paper after an anonymous person claimed (without any evidence) that the

> results could be due to fewer office visits by the unvaxxed. The author provided evidence that this was not the case, but the journal ignored the evidence. Why? Because the paper got 250,000 views, it had to be retracted because it was counter-narrative and too popular. Later, a new paper showed proof that the reason the journal gave for retracting the paper was clearly false. The journal decided not to admit they were wrong and did not reverse the retraction of the Thomas paper. This is corruption of the highest magnitude.[461]

Please notice the chart below relating to ADHD (Attention-Deficit/Hyperactivity Disorder). ADHD begins to manifest as soon as the vaccinated children begin going to school and their ADHD behavior becomes noticeable relative to their classmates. What the study chart does not break out from ADHD are the children who are also suffering from autism. Autism falls within a spectrum and is often referred to as Autism spectrum disorder (ASD). Children and Adults with Attention-Deficit/Hyperactivity Disorder (CHADD) is an organization that provides support, education and encouragement to parents, educators and professionals regarding ADHD issues on a grassroots level. CHADD explains the relationship between ADHD and ASD:

> More than half of all individuals who have been diagnosed with ASD also have signs of ADHD. In fact, ADHD is the most common coexisting condition in children with ASD. On the flip side, up to a quarter of children with ADHD have low-level signs of ASD, which might include having difficulty with social skills or being very sensitive to clothing textures, for example.
>
> Both ADHD and ASD are neurodevelopmental

> disorders (brain development has been affected in some way). That means both conditions/disorders affect the central nervous system, which is responsible for movement, language, memory, and social and focusing skills. A number of scientific studies have shown that the two conditions often coexist, but researchers have not yet figured out why they do.

Objective research has established a direct link between vaccination and ASD. The chart below tells a clear story that vaccines cause ADHD. CHADD says that researchers have not yet figured out why ASD and ADHD often coincide with one another. That is not true. All one need to do is look at the chart below and realize that ADHD and ASD are both neurodevelopmental disorders to understand that they are both caused by vaccine poisoning.

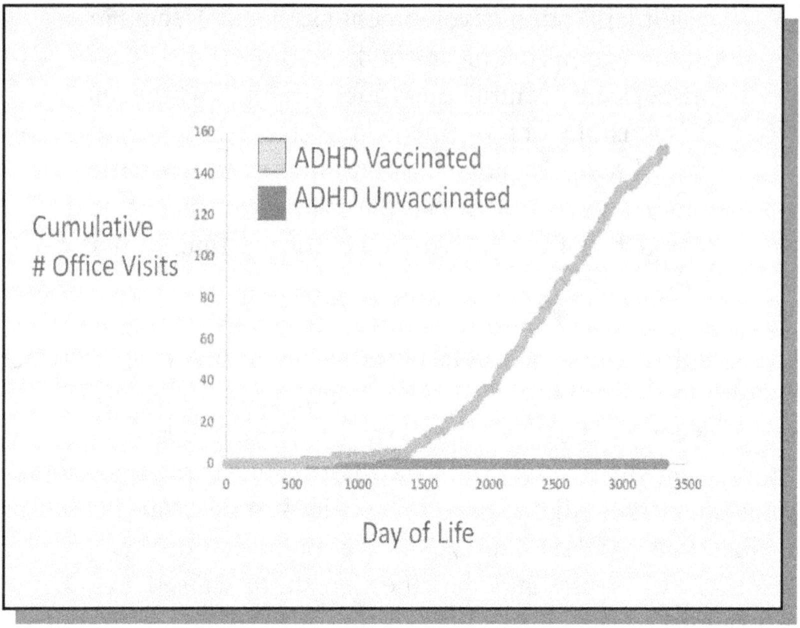

The two researchers who conducted the study, Dr. James Lyons-Weiler and Dr. Paul Thomas are not anti-vaccination doctors. But publishing data that refutes the vaccine paradigm comes with a cost. As a direct result of this study, the state medical board suspended the medical license of one of the researchers, Dr. Paul Thomas, within a week of the publication of the article. The suspension was in retaliation for having published the study showing the harmful effects of childhood vaccinations. The suspension was an unprecedented action because it was done summarily prior to any adversarial hearing. He is being punished as an object lesson for anyone who would have the temerity to publish the truth about vaccinations being harmful to the health of patients. Jeremy Hammond explains:

> On December 3, 2020, the Oregon Medical Board issued an emergency suspension order to prevent renowned pediatrician Paul Thomas, MD, from

seeing his patients by stripping him of his license.

The ostensible reason given by the board for this action against Thomas, who is affectionately known as "Dr. Paul" by his patients and peers, is that his "continued practice constitutes an immediate danger to public health".

Thomas is perhaps most well known as coauthor, along with Dr. Jennifer Margulis, of the book The Vaccine-Friendly Plan, which provides guidance to parents who want to protect their children from infectious diseases but have concerns about vaccines. The book is a bestseller currently showing a five-star rating from over 1,800 customer reviews at Amazon.com.

Since 2008, Thomas has practiced pediatrics out of his clinic, Integrative Pediatrics, which is in Beaverton, Oregon, within the metropolitan area of Portland.

The main accusation leveled at Thomas by the state medical board is that he has "breached the standard of care" in his practice by having many patients who are not vaccinated strictly according to the routine childhood schedule recommended by the Centers for Disease Control and Prevention (CDC).

The story the medical board tells is one of a reckless and "bullying" doctor who coerces his pediatric patients' parents not to follow the CDC's recommendations and whose gross negligence in this regard has caused harm to children and negatively impacted the health of the community.[462]

But that's not the true story.

The *true* story is that parents have flocked to Integrative Pediatrics precisely because they've been bullied, with the state's approval, by pediatricians in other practices who choose to dutifully serve the bureaucrats in government by compelling parents to strictly comply with the CDC's schedule.

Parents who *did* comply and then witnessed their children suffer harm as a result are mocked and derisively labeled "anti-vaxxers" for learning hard lessons from their firstborn children that they then apply to younger siblings by making different parenting choices. (Often, such parents respond to the derogatory label by insisting on being described as "ex-vaxxers", but government officials and the major media institutions refuse to hear them.)

Parents who *do* vaccinate their children, but not strictly according to the CDC's schedule, are also lumped into the group monolithically labeled "the anti-vaccine movement" by apologists for the one-size-fits-all approach of public vaccine policy.

These parents have all been told a million times that vaccines are "safe and effective". They are well aware of the arguments in favor of vaccinations that we all hear incessantly from government officials, medical professionals, and the mainstream media.

They are also perfectly familiar with the tale of how, in 1998, public enemy number one, Dr. Andrew Wakefield, published a fraudulent study in The Lancet, later retracted, claiming to have found an association between the measles, mumps, and rubella (MMR) vaccine and autism. In my own case, our son's pediatrician told us during an early well-child visit that Wakefield was serving time in prison for what he'd done, which I knew was untrue. This attempt to persuade us into compliance consequently served only to reaffirm our conviction that we shouldn't assume doctors are trustworthy and should rather do our own research, think for ourselves, and trust our own judgment. These parents know that numerous studies have since been published that failed to find an association.

They know that, by choosing to dissent from or criticize public vaccine policy, they are placing a target on their back. They know they will be met with disapproval by other members of their own family, accused of being irresponsible parents, scolded, and scorned. They know that they will be viciously attacked by government officials and policy advocates masquerading as journalists, as well as by doctors and other members of their community. (I, too, have experienced rifts within my family over this issue, and, naturally, as someone who has for years been publicly criticizing public vaccine policy, I have experienced countless personal attacks on my character.) (parenthetical originally in endnote)

And yet, despite the bullying and intimidation, they remain unmoved. There is one simple reason for this: they see it as their duty as responsible parents to act in their children's best interest no matter what societal pressures are placed on them to conform with expected behavior. Consequently, they do their own research, think for themselves, draw their own conclusions, and take a stand to protect their children.

In many cases in Portland, parents who face the scornful intimidation of a routine well-child visit at their pediatrician's office and still insist on exercising their right to make an informed choice not to vaccinate are told that they must either comply with the CDC's recommendations or find another pediatrician. (Just since publishing this article, my family has also experienced this kind of bullying due to a policy change at our son's pediatric practice. On May 5, 2021, we were given an ultimatum by one of the doctors there to either vaccinate him according to the AAP's recommendations (synonymous with the CDC's recommendations) or never come back. We declined the unnecessary and risk-carrying pharmaceutical products and so were expelled. [...]) (parenthetical originally in endnote)

And, so, they go to Dr. Paul.

With respect to the medical board's suspension order, Paul Thomas says that he knew the moment The Vaccine-Friendly Plan was published that this day was coming. He knew at the time that, because he was challenging the CDC's schedule and therefore the "standard of care" of the medical establishment, he would be placing a target on his back and risking his career.

But he did it anyway.

Why?

The Oregon Medical Board wants us to believe it's because he's a villain who demonstrates reckless disregard and poses a danger to public health. The media have run with that story.

But what the results of the study do demonstrate to a reasonable degree of certainty is that his unvaccinated patients are healthier than vaccinated children and place less of a burden on the health care system.

However, what neither the board's order nor the media have disclosed is that the board's suspension order was issued just eleven days after Thomas published a study in a peer-reviewed medical journal showing that, among the children born into his practice, those who remained completely unvaccinated were diagnosed at significantly lower rates than vaccinated children for a broad range of chronic health conditions and developmental disorders.

The difference in health outcomes was even more dramatic when Thomas and his coauthor, research scientist Dr. James Lyons-Weiler, looked at cumulative incidence of office visits for given diagnoses rather than incidence of diagnoses alone. This result strongly suggests that his vaccinated patients not only suffer from a higher rate of chronic health conditions, but also that their conditions are more severe, therefore requiring more frequent visits to his clinic.

The study is titled "Relative Incidence of Office Visits and Cumulative Rates of Billed Diagnoses Along the Axis of Vaccination." It was published in the International Journal of Environmental Research and Public Health on November 22, 2020.

As Thomas and Lyons-Weiler emphasize in the study, they do not show that vaccinations are the cause of the evidently worse health outcomes among vaccinated children. But what the results of the study do demonstrate to a reasonable degree of certainty is that his unvaccinated patients are healthier than vaccinated children and place less of a burden on the health care system.[463]

Importantly, this was data that the medical board had asked Thomas to produce to support his practice of vaccinating patients according to the principles of his "Vaccine-Friendly Plan".

Yet, when Thomas surmounted this challenge by obtaining Institutional Review Board (IRB) approval and publishing the deidentified data comparing health outcomes between vaccinated and unvaccinated children, the board's emergent response was to suspend his license until further notice "while this case remains under investigation"—and on grounds that are completely belied by the publicly available evidence. (endnote deleted)

The real story here isn't one of a rogue doctor dismissing science and recklessly endangering his pediatric patients by bullying their parents into accepting "alternative" care. The real story is one of a rogue medical board dismissing science and recklessly endangering public health by encouraging pediatricians to bully their parents into strict compliance with the CDC's schedule and selecting Paul Thomas, MD, to set an example to other physicians of what their punishment will be if they instead choose to respect parents' right to informed consent.

But that story doesn't begin in December of 2020. To tell the true story and fully appreciate its significance, we need to go back and review the sequence of events that led Paul Thomas to this pivotal moment in his life's journey.

On 16 July 2021, the MDPI retracted the article with the following cryptic notice. "The journal retracts the article 'Relative Incidence of Office Visits and Cumulative Rates of Billed Diagnoses along the Axis of Vaccination' cited above. Following publication, concerns were brought to the attention of the editorial office regarding the validity of the conclusions of the published research. Adhering to our complaints procedure, an investigation was conducted that raised several methodological issues and confirmed that the conclusions were not supported by strong scientific data. The article is therefore retracted. This retraction is approved by the Editor in Chief of the journal. The authors did not agree to this retraction."[464] The MDPI did not indicate what were the "methodological issues" or specify how the conclusions "were not supported by strong scientific data." That lack of specificity for such an extraordinary action suggests the retraction of the article by the MDPI was not due to methodological

> issues or that it was not supported by strong scientific data but was rather due to financial and political pressure put on MDPI.

The following report was posted on the Institute for Pure and Applied Knowledge (IPAK) website:

> Independent journalist Jeremy Hammond has authored a definitive and thorough report[465] that reveals that the Oregon Medical Board is guilty of wrong-doing because they tried to coerce Dr. Thomas into changing his lawful pediatric practice into an unlawful medical practice under Oregon's state law.

The IPAK report explains that the real story isn't a negligent doctor dismissing science and recklessly endangering his pediatric patients by hoodwinking parents into not vaccinating their children. The real story is one of a villainous medical board endangering public health by encouraging pediatricians to scare parents into strict compliance with the CDC's schedule. The rogue medical board selected Dr. Thomas, MD, to set an example to other physicians of what would happen to them if they choose to accede to the parents' right to informed consent.

> Under Oregon state law, phyisicians, including pediatricians, must provide for fully informed consent and respect vaccine refusal. The board had tried to sanction Dr. Thomas for allowing patients to use antibody titre-testing as evidence of immunity. It [the Hammond report[466]] found that the board's actions were "ludicrous given the fact that Oregon law only requires one dose of mumps vaccine, and it specifically allows for the use of antibody testing as evidence of immunity in lieu of evidence of vaccination."

> The report also completely rebuts all eight of the allegations of medical misconduct alleged by the Oregon Medical Board. Under current Oregon law, The Board answers to the Governor of the State of Oregon.[467]

Rhoda Wilson reveals in the April 11, 2022, edition of The Expose a groundbreaking study comparing the health of a group of 1,482 unvaccinated adults and children to the national statistics on the health of vaccinated adults.[468] The study conducted by an organization called *The Control Group* reveals that unvaccinated adults are significantly healthier than vaccinated adults.[469]

The Control Group filed a complaint in federal court seeking a declaratory judgment and injunctive relief against the federal government alleging its vaccine laws, regulations, and policies are unscientific and violate the constitutional rights of the people.[470] But their complaint was dismissed and "on October 3, 2022, the US Supreme Court denied The Control Group's petition for writ of certiorari. So this health freedom case is now closed."[471]

Despite the failure of the Control Group in court, the facts that they established in their study will have a long-term benefit to all who seek justice in the future. The study is robust and unimpeachable. Dr. Stephen Malthouse states:

> Every so often a study comes along that shakes the bedrock of medicine. The Control Group compared unvaccinated adults to vaccinated adults in the US and what they discovered is incredible. Perhaps one of the most surprising findings is that vit K shots, containing aluminum in most cases (although not always disclosed on the list of ingredients), played a significant role in adult (and childhood) chronic disease. If you get rid of vit K shots and all vaccinations, the incidence of heart

> disease, asthma, autism, and other severe disorders goes practically to zero.[472]

Below is a sample of some of the charts that were filed as exhibits in the litigation by the Control Group.

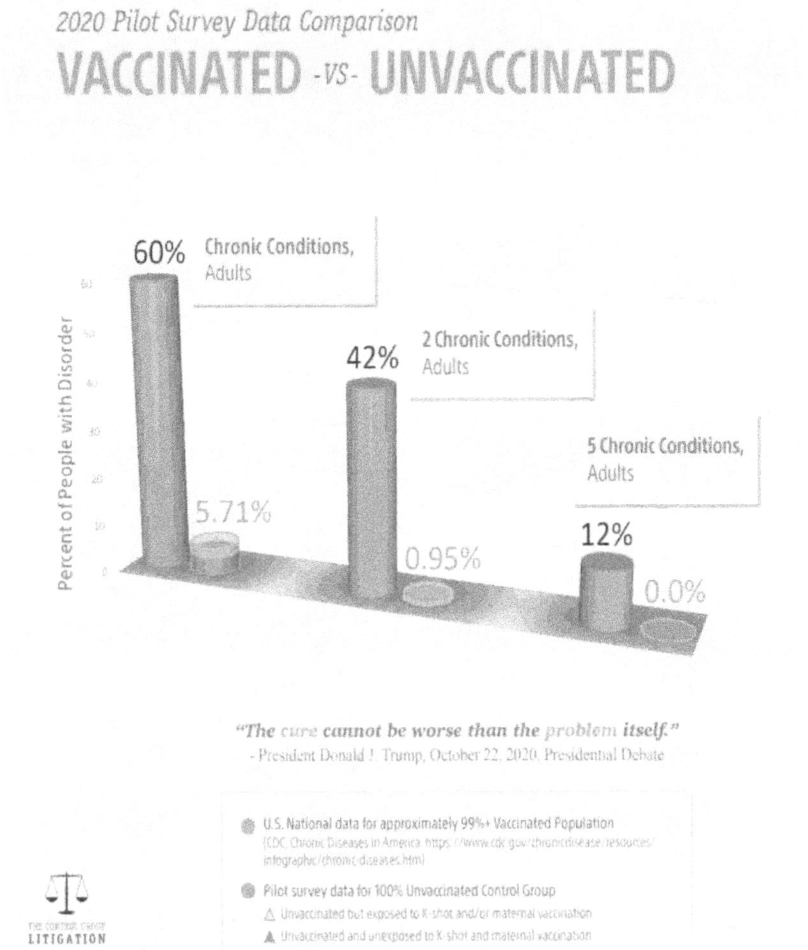

60% of adults in the vaccinated population had chronic health conditions, while **5.71%** of adults in the unvaccinated group had chronic health conditions. **42%** of adults in the vaccinated population had 2 chronic health conditions, while **0.95%%** of adults in the unvaccinated group had 2 chronic health conditions. **12%** of adults in the vaccinated population had 5 chronic health conditions, while **0.0%%** of adults in the unvaccinated group had 5 chronic health conditions.

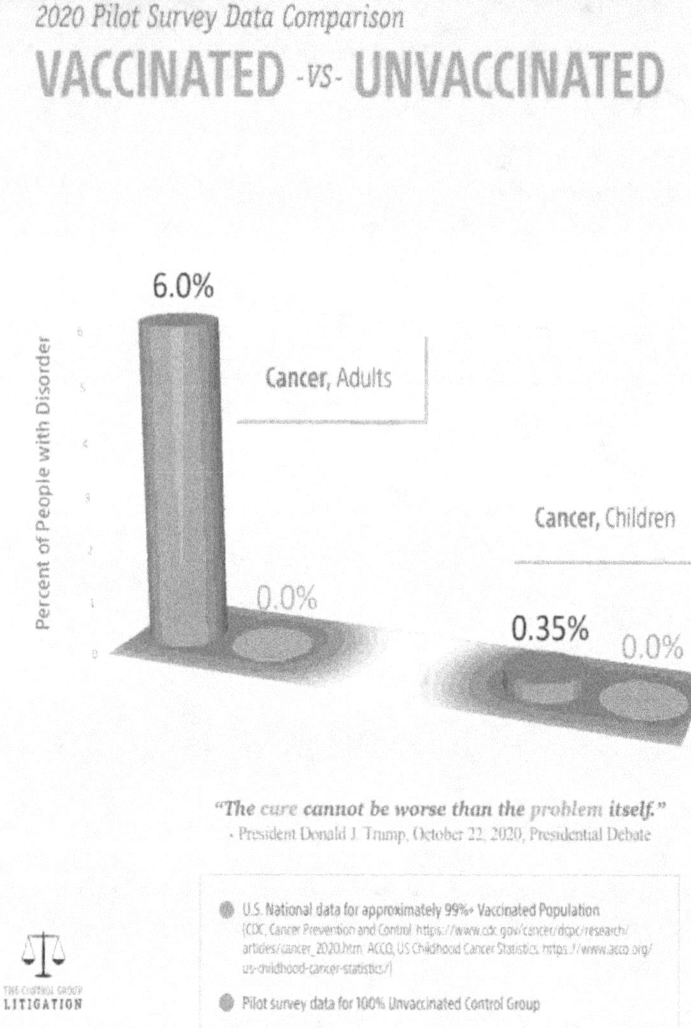

6% of adults in the vaccinated population had cancer, while **0%** of adults in the unvaccinated group had cancer. **0.35%** of children in the vaccinated population had cancer, while **0.0%** of children in the unvaccinated group had cancer.

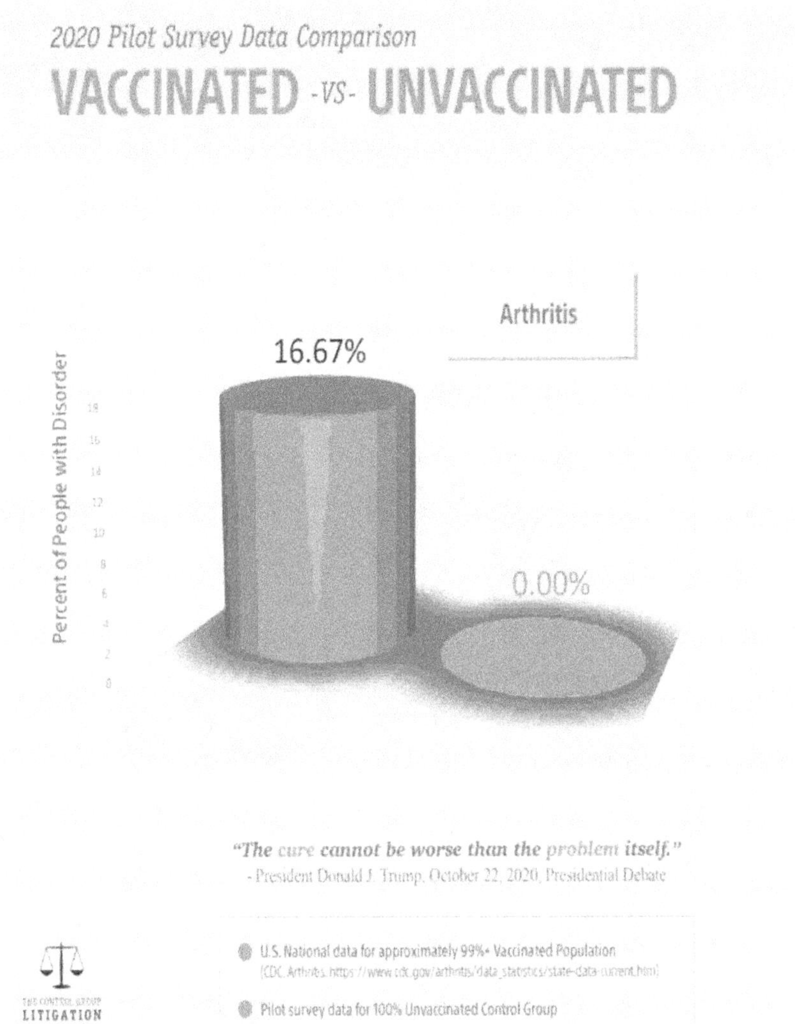

16.67% of adults in the vaccinated population had arthritis, while **0.0%** of adults in the unvaccinated group had arthritis.

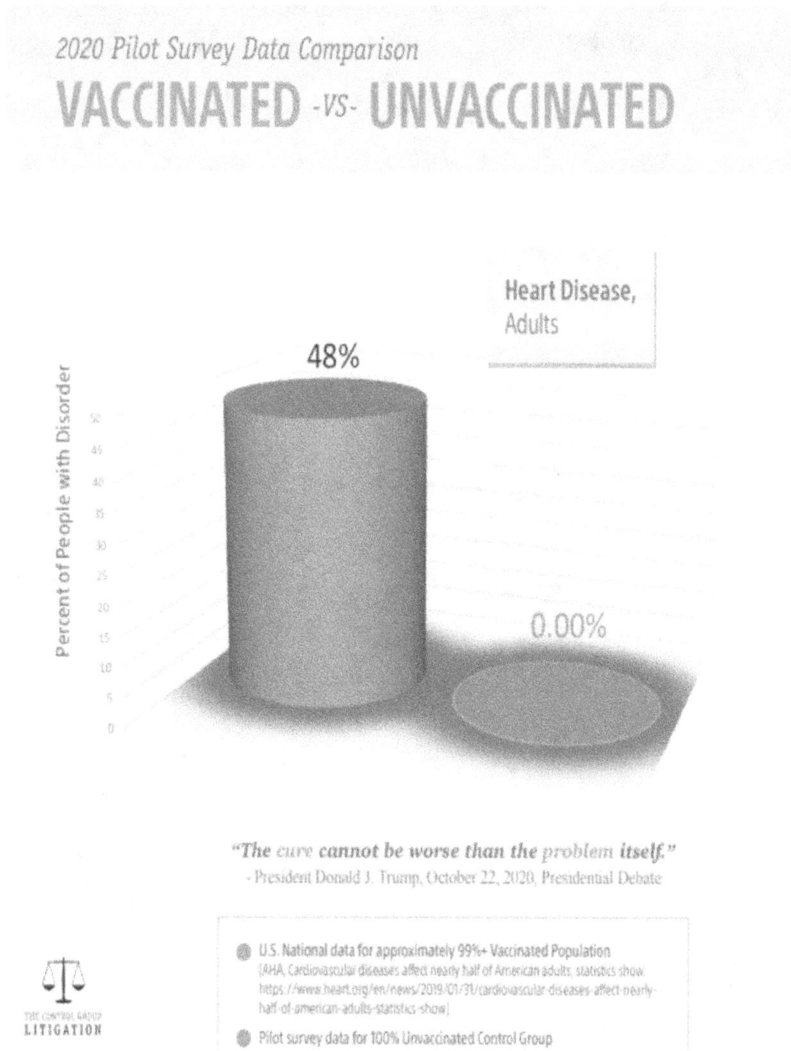

48% of adults in the vaccinated population had heart disease, while **0%** of adults in the unvaccinated group had heart disease.

Yet another study in 2020 came up with the same results. The study found that vaccinated children were much sicker than unvaccinated children. The researchers concluded:

> In this study, based on a convenience sample of children born into one of three distinct pediatric medical practices, higher ORs [odds ratios] were observed within the vaccinated versus unvaccinated group for developmental delays, asthma and ear infections.[473]

The 2017 Mawson study comparing the health of vaccinated children to the health of unvaccinated children concluded that the vaccinated children were much less healthy than the unvaccinated children.[474] Indeed, the study showed that vaccinated children were 2.4 times more likely to have chronic illnesses, 2.9 times more likely to develop eczema, 3.7 times more likely to incur a neurodevelopmental disorder, 4.2 times more likely to develop autism, 4.2 times more likely to develop ADHD, 5.2 times more likely to develop learning disabilities, and 30.1 times more likely to develop allergic rhinitis.

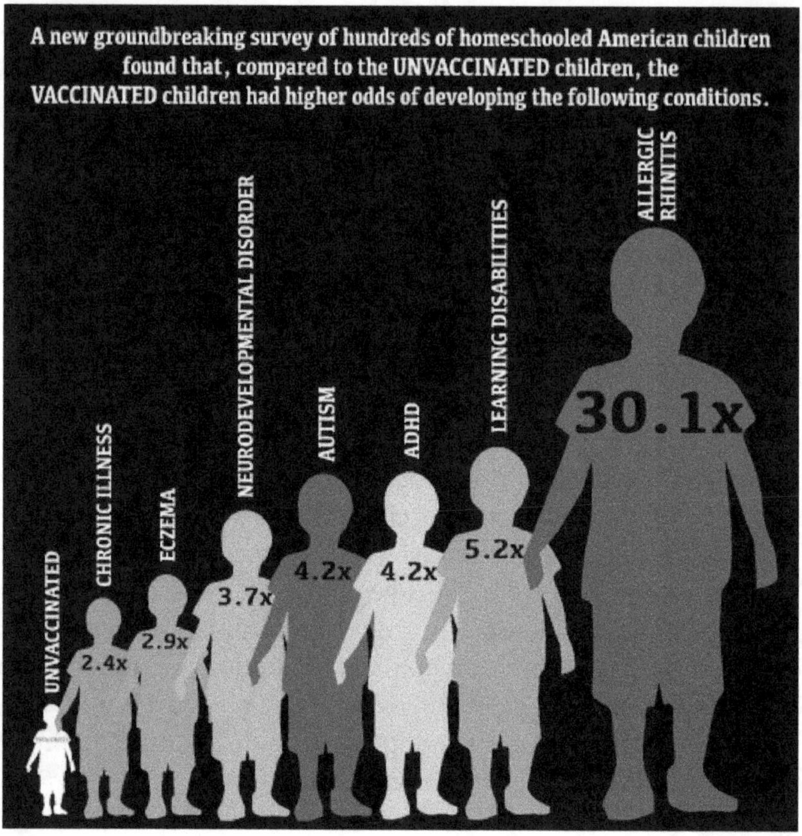

Other studies have confirmed the Mawson results.[475] For example, Steve Kirsch surveyed the parents of 10,000 children and found a 5-fold increase in autism for vaccinated children compared to unvaccinated children.[476] A study of 9,000 boys in California and Oregon found that "vaccinated boys had a 155% greater chance of having a neurological disorder like ADHD or autism than unvaccinated boys."[477] It seems that sinus issues are endemic with vaccines. The Mawson study showed a 30.1-fold greater incidence of allergic rhinitis among the vaccinated children compared to the unvaccinated children; Kirsch found that vaccinated children showed a 33-fold greater incidence in sinusitis compared to the unvaccinated children.

In November 2012, Dr. Coleen Boyle, the CDC's Director of the National Center on Birth Defects and Developmental Disabilities, testified under oath before the House Committee on Oversight and Government Reform that "we have not studied vaccinated versus unvaccinated [children]." Robert F. Kennedy Jr. states, "that was perjury."[478] Kennedy, through Freedom of Information requests, found out that, indeed, the CDC has done vaccinated vs. unvaccinated comparative health studies.

Kennedy discovered that in 1999, the CDC employed an in-house researcher, Thomas Verstraeten, to conduct a vaccinated vs. unvaccinated study using CDC's giant Vaccine Safety Datalink (VSD). The study evaluated whether cumulative ethylmercury exposure from thimerosal-containing vaccines after one month of life increased "the subsequent risk of degenerative and developmental neurologic disorders and renal disorders before the age of six."[479] The study results proved that vaccines were dangerous to the health of children. The study concluded that "high exposure to ethylmercury from thimerosal-containing vaccines in the first month of life increases the risk of subsequent development of neurologic development impairment."[480]

In particular, the study found that the relative risk of autism for vaccinated children was 7.6 times greater than the unvaccinated children. The study also found that the relative risk of sleep disorders for vaccinated children was 5 times greater than unvaccinated children. The study further found that the relative risk of speech disorders for vaccinated children was 2.1 times greater than unvaccinated children. The study found that the relative risk for neurological development disorders for vaccinated children was 1.8 times greater than unvaccinated children.

The CDC could not allow that information to get out. So they instituted a plan to coverup the results of the study. Robert F. Kennedy Jr. explains:

> The world's largest vaccine maker GSK whisked Verstraeten off to a sinecure in Brussels and CDC handed his raw data to his CDC boss Frank DeStefano and another researcher, Robert Davis who served as a vaccine industry consultant. Those two men tortured the data for 4 years, removing all unvaccinated children, to bury the autism signal before publishing a sanitized version purporting to exculpate the vaccine. The CDC then cut off public access to the VSD and to this day aggressively blocks any attempts by researchers to study health outcomes in vaccinated vs. unvaccinated populations.[481]

The fraudulently altered study that ended up being published changed the actual conclusion in the original study from showing that "high exposure to ethylmercury from thimerosal-containing vaccines in the first month of life increases the risk of subsequent development of neurologic development impairment"[482] to, instead, say that "[n]o consistent significant associations were found between TCVs [thimerosal-containing vaccines] and neurodevelopmental outcomes."[483]

Kennedy caught government health officials red-handed lying to Congress and engaging in fraud to conceal the dangers of childhood vaccines. This is not merely negligence or dereliction of duty; it is part of a well-funded conspiracy to injure and kill children. This is the behavior of sociopathic criminals. The childhood vaccine scheme constitutes organized crime that is more sophisticated and more dangerous than any mafia syndicate.

The pharmaceutical companies and the governments of the world know that vaccines cause harm. All published vaccine studies funded by pharmaceutical companies and governments are scams. Steve Kirsch explains how pharmaceutical company and government funded researchers accomplish the deception.

> When you read the peer-review literature carefully, you'll find that they always consider the "unvaccinated" group to have kids without the particular vaccine under study. So when they compare the MMR vaccine, they compare it to the kids who didn't get the MMR vaccine. So it's like comparing the autism rates of kids who got 28 vaccines with the rates of kids who got 27 vaccines. This is how they hide the signal. They design studies which are designed to fail. Just because they don't find a signal, it doesn't mean that it isn't there. It just means their study design didn't find the signal. They will NEVER compare the chronic disease rates in kids who got all recommended vaccines (well over 50 shots, many with multiple vaccines) vs. completely unvaccinated kids. It simply has never happened. The excuse that unvaccinated kids are too hard to find is ridiculous. The Amish have thousands of such kids and there are hundreds of such kids that can be located in a heartbeat. All they have to do is call me and I'll be happy to help.[484]

Steve Kirsch challenged the seminal government-funded research study from Denmark that allegedly showed no causation between the MMR vaccine and autism.[485] Kirsh alleged that the researchers purposely "chose a study design that was designed to look credible but obscure any signal."[486] In essence, the study was a scam. Kirsch challenged one of the study's principal authors, Professor Anders Hviid, to provide the underlying data and defend his study. Kirsch even offered him $25,000 if Professor Hviid could successfully defend his study. Professor Hviid refused the offer and took steps to block Kirsch. Kirsch sent Professor Hviid an article he wrote detailing his challenge of the research and asked him for comments; Hviid did not respond and instead immediately made his tweets only viewable by followers;

Professor Hviid then did not allow Kirsch to follow him on Twitter. Professor Hviid refuses to address the errors in his study. As Kirsch points out, truth does not mind being questioned; a lie does not like being challenged.

There is convincing evidence that the Denmark autism study was part of a coordinated plan to mislead the public about the dangers of vaccines.[487] Fraud is woven through the warp and woof of the study. Notably, one of the study's co-authors, Dr. Paul Thorsen, is presently a fugitive from justice; he is charged with wire fraud and money laundering for stealing infant disability and autism study grant money.[488]

A randomized study published in 2018 by the highly respected Dr. Peter Aaby found that the Diphtheria–Tetanus–Pertussis (DTP) vaccine caused children to die at a higher rate than unvaccinated children.[489] By the way, Dr. Aaby is not against vaccinations. Indeed, he promotes vaccinations. Yet he concluded that the DTP vaccine is killing children. Aaron Siri explains that Dr. Aaby is a long-time promoter of vaccines:

> Dr. Aaby is renowned for studying and promoting vaccines in Africa with over 300 published studies. ... Among his accolades, in 2000, Dr. Aaby was awarded the Novo Nordisk Prize, the most important Danish award within health research, and in 2009, the Danish Ministry of Foreign Affairs selected Dr. Aaby as a leader in the fight against global poverty.[490]

The conclusion of Dr. Aaby's study was that "[a]lthough having better nutritional status and being protected against three infections, 6–35 months old DTP-vaccinated children tended to have higher mortality than DTP-unvaccinated children. All studies of the introduction of DTP have found increased overall mortality."

Other studies have shown that the mortality rate for DTP-vaccinated children is two (2) times greater than for unvaccinated children. Dr. Aaby explains that "[a]ll studies that documented vaccination status and followed children prospectively indicate that DTP has negative effects; a meta-analysis of the eight studies found 2-fold higher mortality for DTP-vaccinated compared with DTP-unvaccinated."

Doubling the mortality rate is bad enough, but that is not the whole story. The studies referenced by Dr. Aaby were biased in favor of the vaccinated group because the vaccinated groups were healthier babies. Dr. Aaby explains that "the 'unvaccinated' control children in previous studies having been a frail subgroup, too frail to get vaccinated." Thus, the unvaccinated babies did not receive the DTP vaccine because the doctors determined they were too frail and unhealthy to tolerate a vaccination. But when the study measured babies of similar health, the detrimental effect of the DTP vaccine is revealed in all its horror. Dr. Aaby explains that "DTP [vaccination] was associated with 5-fold higher mortality than being unvaccinated."[491]

That is bad enough, but it gets worse. You see, the unvaccinated group cited by Dr. Aaby in his conclusion simply means unvaccinated with DTP. The "unvaccinated" babies in that group had, in fact, been vaccinated with the oral polio vaccine (OPV). When the children that received the OPV are excluded from the unvaccinated group, the mortality rate for children receiving a DTP vaccine skyrockets to ten (10) times that for children receiving no vaccination. That suggests that there is also an increase in mortality due to the OPV.

When isolating only the DTP-vaccinated children and comparing them to the truly unvaccinated children, the simple conclusion is that vaccinating a child with the DTP vaccination increases his chances of dying in the first 6 months of his life by ten (10) fold.

Dr. Aaby concluded that "[a]ll currently available evidence suggests that DTP vaccine may kill more children from other causes than it saves from diphtheria, tetanus or pertussis. Though a vaccine protects children against the target disease, it may simultaneously increase susceptibility to unrelated infections." Many countries, including the U.S., replaced The DTP vaccine with the DTaP vaccine long ago.[492] The 'a' stands for 'acellular' pertussis.

The newer DTaP vaccine is alleged to be somewhat safer than the DTP vaccine, but it is just as ineffective as the DTP vaccine. A 2014 study proved that the DTaP vaccine is ineffective. The study examined the effectiveness of the DTaP vaccine in preventing the 2012 Wisconsin pertussis outbreak.[493] Researchers determined that the efficacy of the vaccine quickly waned. For example, only 11.9% of the children who had received the DTaP vaccine in 2008 and 2009 were protected from getting pertussis during the 2012 Wisconsin pertussis outbreak. Mathematician Igor Chudov reviewed the statistics in the study and concluded that the protection afforded by the DTaP vaccine was effectively zero four years after vaccination.[494] The DTaP vaccine is worthless. Yet, governments and doctors falsely promote the DTaP vaccine as safe and effective.

The DTP vaccine is still being administered in about 40 countries worldwide. What informed parent would agree to vaccinate their child with the DTP vaccine? Indeed, why would any informed parent allow their child to be inoculated with any vaccine?

The above 2018 study by Dr. Aaby confirmed the results of a prior 2017 study he did showing the deadliness of the DTP vaccine. In 2017, the Informed Consent Action Network (ICAN) and the Vaccine Science Foundation (VSF) informed the UN about Dr. Aaby's 2017 study showing the deadliness of the DTP vaccines. Yet, with that knowledge, the UN continued to fund and promote the DTP vaccines. ICAN again implored the UN to stop the DTP program after Dr. Aaby's 2018 study was published. Yet the UN continued to promote and fund DTP vaccinations, knowing that the vaccine was killing children.

Attorney Aaron Siri sent a letter on January 28, 2021, on behalf of the ICAN to the United Nations Special Rapporteur on Torture and Other Cruel, Inhuman or Degrading Treatment or Punishment. In that letter, Siri called out UNICEF for funding and promoting the DTP vaccine while knowing that the vaccine is killing children. It seems that the UNICEF vaccine program killing children is quite profitable. Siri reveals in his letter that "in 2019 alone, UNICEF purchased over $1.656 billions of vaccine products from these companies and spent an equally significant sum paying companies for their distribution, in total amounting to over a third of UNICEF's budget."[495] As shocking as it may sound to read, it is a fact that high officials are knowingly killing children for profit through vaccination. Siri challenged the UN to stop killing children through the DTP vaccine program.

> The seminal study regarding DTP and mortality found that children receiving this product during the first six months of life died at 10 times the rate when compared to children that did not receive this product. Despite this, and many similar studies, the United Nations Children's Fund ("UNICEF"), continues to purchase, promote, and distribute DTP to developing and underdeveloped countries, and pushes its use on every newborn child long after knowing that the clear dangers it poses caused developed nations to stop using DTP decades ago. ... UNICEF has and continues to be instrumental and the central worldwide actor in the purchase,

> promotion and distribution of DTP in many developing countries. UNICEF has continued this conduct despite the clear evidence that it increases mortality and despite the fact that DTP has not been subjected to a single randomized placebo-controlled trial to prove its safety.[496]

One thing the medical system has done to conceal that vaccines are causing infant deaths is to label the deaths as being a "syndrome." Hence, we find that what used to be called crib death is now called sudden infant death syndrome (SIDS). Thus, the focus is on the death, leaving the medical community to conjure up some mythical cause to steer the public away from vaccines.

The medical community refuses to acknowledge that vaccines cause SIDS. Instead, they falsely claim that "[r]esearchers do not know exactly what causes SIDS."[497] They claim that they do not know what causes SIDS, but from that alleged position of ignorance, they recommend a way to prevent it by having babies sleep on their backs. A campaign was instituted to do that called "Back To Sleep." When back-sleeping was found not to stop SIDS, the medical community changed the program's name in 2022 to "Safe To Sleep."[498] The medical community maintained the back-sleeping recommendation but added a bunch of other precautions to the mix. It does not matter to the medical community that its recommendations are ineffective. Effectiveness is not the point; concealing vaccines as the cause of SIDS is the goal of "Safe To Sleep."

The Safe To Sleep program is propaganda for the public. Knowledgeable doctors know full well that vaccines cause SIDS. The incidence of SIDS has increased in tandem with rising vaccination rates.[499] The unmistakable correlation cannot be missed. It is being covered up by medical sociopaths who act as protectors of the pharmaceutical companies making the deadly vaccines.

Furthermore, anecdotal proof is abounding. Often anecdotal cases can be dismissed as "idiopathic." But when cases of sudden infant deaths happen to identical twins immediately following vaccination, the inference of causation is compelling. Indeed, one doctor explains that "cases of identical twins developing a condition immediately following an intervention are often considered a gold standard in proving causality.[500] That doctor tracked down 10 cases of twin SIDS, each happening shortly after receiving vaccines, including, but not limited to, DTP, hepatitis B, and oral polio. The vaccines killed the twins. Any other cause is almost impossible. Such evidence is being concealed because it would end the profitable practice of infant vaccinations.

Mathematician Igor Chudov made a significant discovery. He uncovered evidence of a correlation between infant vaccinations and infant deaths.[501] The correlation is that children who do not receive vaccines are less likely to die as infants. Of course, correlation does not necessarily mean causation, but one can make reasonable inferences when there is no other probable cause. Indeed, the correlation of decreased infant deaths with decreased vaccinations without any other causal link establishes probable cause that the vaccines are causing infant deaths.

Chudov looked at Florida statistics reflecting a drop in childhood vaccinations in 2021.[502] He found that the reduction in childhood vaccinations correlated with a concomitant decline in infant deaths.[503] Keep in mind that Chudov was not examining COVID-19 vaccines. The vaccines under consideration were the routine vaccines received in accordance with the childhood vaccine schedule.

Infant vaccination decreased by 14.1% in 2021, which correlated directly with a drop in 2021 in all-cause infant mortality of 8.93% in 2021. Notably, the the decrease in infant mortality happened as deaths of other age groups increased significantly.

That 8.93% drop in infant mortality happened at the same time that there was a 14% drop in childhood vaccinations. Carina Blackmore, the Director of the Division of Disease Control and Health Protection Coverage For the State of Florida, stated that in 2021 there was a decrease in childhood vaccinations in Florida by "an alarming 14.1 percentage points since 2020, from 93.4 to 79.3 percent statewide."[504]

Chudov concluded that the "14 percent decrease in vaccination coverage is associated with 9 percent decrease in infant mortality."[505] That significant finding should be of concern for all parents and doctors. That kind of evidence has been known for years. But governments and social scientists have kept it hidden from the public. The medical community is also aware of the evidence revealing the dangers of vaccines, but doctors and scientists have shown a suspicious lack of curiosity about the damning evidence. There is a good reason the medical community has disregarded this incriminating evidence - "money." For the love of money is the root of all evil." 1 Timothy 6:10. Pharmaceutical companies massively fund virtually every medical school. He who pays the piper calls the tune.

In addition, pediatricians do not want to hear about or explore any evidence about the dangers of vaccines because they make large amounts of money by administering those vaccines. Indeed, most pediatricians refuse to treat unvaccinated children because they are paid a bounty for every fully vaccinated child in their practice above a certain threshold.[506]

Furthermore, in 2021, the American Medical Association (AMA) amended its Code of Medical Ethics Section 8.7 to include an ethical responsibility to encourage patients to get vaccinated.[507] With that, the AMA (being under the thumb of the pharmaceutical industry) has determined that it is an ethical violation for a physician not to encourage patients to accept immunization.[508] A physician cannot be neutral on the issue of vaccination; he must "encourage" vaccination or be subject to license suspension by their state medical board for violating the AMA code of ethics.[509]

Mark Blaxill and Amy Becker studied mortality rates during the COVID-19 lock-downs.[510] They discovered a startling fact. Infant mortality actually went down during the COVID-19 lockdowns. There was a significant decrease in the number of infant deaths. Blaxill and Becker attributed that drop to the inability of parents to do well-baby doctor checkups with the obligatory vaccinations. Fewer vaccines = fewer infant deaths. Blaxill and Becker stated:

> Starting in early March, expected deaths [for children under 18 years old] began a sharp decline, from an expected level of around 700 deaths per week to well under 500 by mid-April and throughout May. The Centers for Disease Control and Prevention. National Center for Health Statistics Mortality Surveillance System.
>
> As untimely deaths spiked among the elderly in Manhattan nursing homes and in similar settings all over the country, something mysterious was saving the lives of children. As springtime in America came along with massive disruptions in family life amid near-universal lockdowns, roughly 30% fewer children died.
>
> ***
>
> Was this a protective effect of school closures? Were teenagers getting themselves into risky situations at a lower rate? No. There was very little effect among school age children or adolescents.[511]

Incidentally, since the publication of Blaxill and Becker's

article, the CDC has removed the page that memorialized the fact that almost all of the reduction in childhood deaths came from infants. Blaxill and Becker explain that the CDC statistics showed:

> **Virtually the entire change came from infants.** Somehow, the changing pattern of American life during the lockdowns has been saving the lives of hundreds of infants, over 200 per week.
>
> ***
>
> What has changed during this period that might have such an effect?
>
> ***
>
> One very clear change that has received publicity is that public health officials are bemoaning the sharp decline in infant vaccinations as parents are not taking their infants into pediatric offices for their regular well-baby checks. In the May 15 [2020] issue of the CDC Morbidity and Mortality Weekly Report (MMWR), a group of authors from the CDC and Kaiser Permanente reported **a sharp decline in provider orders for vaccines as well as a decline in pediatric vaccine doses administered.** Santoli, Jeanne M et al. Effects of the COVID-19 Pandemic on Routine Pediatric Vaccine Ordering and Administration — United States, 2020. cdc.gov.[512] [Online] May 15, 2020. These declines began in early March, around the time infant deaths began declining.[513]

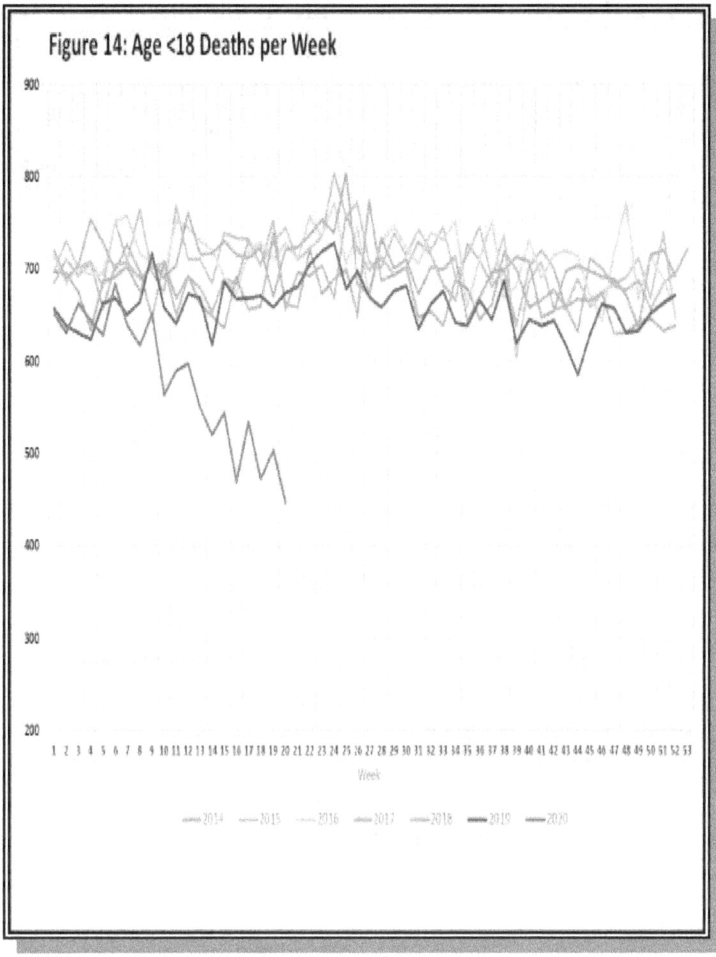

Figure 18: Chart showing a precipitous drop in child deaths early in 2020 that correlated directly with the COVID-19 lookdowns. Virtually the entire drop in deaths among children under 18 years old came from infants. The COVID-19 lockdowns prevented parents from taking infants for well-baby checkups and getting vaccinated. The reduction in infant deaths also correlated directly with a sharp decline in provider orders for vaccines and a decline in pediatric vaccine doses administered.

A 2011 study compared the infant mortality rate (IMR) of 34 countries to the number of vaccines required by their 2009 national vaccine schedule within the first year of infancy.[514] If vaccines were safe and effective, as the pharmaceutical companies and the CDC claim, the greater the number of childhood vaccines would mean a lower infant mortality rate. But the opposite was found. The study revealed a direct correlation between the number of childhood vaccines and the mortality rate. The more vaccines administered to infants, the higher the infant death rate.

In 2009, the U.S. vaccine schedule called for 26 vaccine doses within the first year after birth, and the infant mortality rate in the U.S. was 6.22 per 1,000. The U.S. had the highest number of infant vaccines of all 34 countries in the study. The report also found that the U.S. had the highest infant mortality rate among all 34 countries. The researchers explained:

> Despite the United States spending more per capita on health care than any other country, 33 nations have better IMRs. Some countries have IMRs that are less than half the US rate: Singapore, Sweden, and Japan are below 2.80. According to the Centers for Disease Control and Prevention (CDC), "The relative position of the United States in comparison to countries with the lowest infant mortality rates appears to be worsening."
>
> ***
>
> The infant mortality rate is expressed as the number of infant deaths per 1000 live births. According to the US Central Intelligence Agency (CIA), which keeps accurate, up-to-date infant mortality statistics throughout the world, in 2009 there were 33 nations with better infant mortality rates than the United States. The US infant

mortality rate of 6.22 infant deaths per 1000 live births ranked 34th.

The researchers broke the countries into five categories based on the number of vaccines routinely given to the children in each country. The researchers then charted the number of vaccines in each quintile against the average mortality rate for those countries. The chart revealed a direct correlation between the number of vaccines and the average infant death rate. The more vaccines administered to infants, the higher the infant death rate.

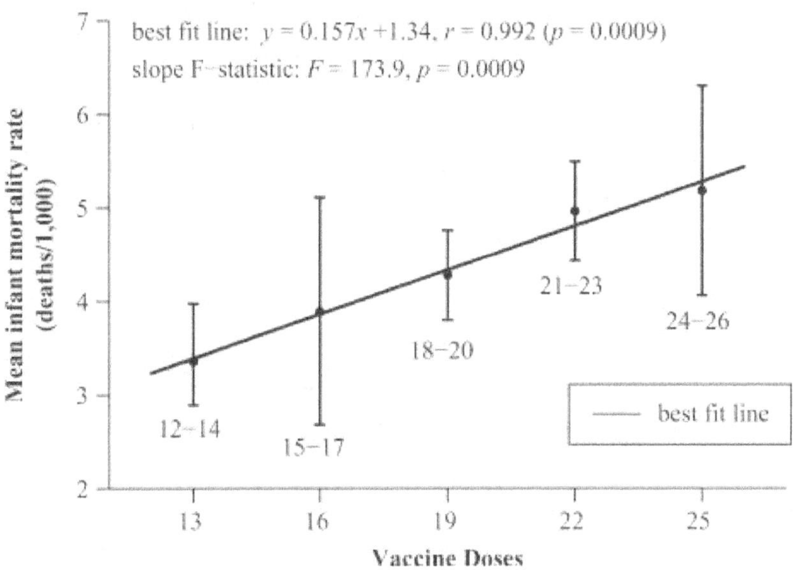

The *r*-value between the number of infant vaccines and infant deaths was 0.992. The lowest *r*-value possible is 0.0, and the highest positive *r*-value is 1.0. An *r*-value of 1.0 means a perfect one-to-one positive linear correlation between two variables. Generally, an *r*-value greater than 0.7 indicates a strong correlation between variables. In this case, an *r*-value of 0.992 indicates a very strong correlation that more infant vaccines will result in more infant deaths. The r^2 for the statistics was 0.983.

That means an increase in infant vaccinations explains 98.3% of infant deaths. The *p*-value for the statistics was 0.0009. That means that the probability of the outcome happening by chance was 0.09%. Thus, it can be said with a high degree of scientific certainty that as more vaccines are given to infants, those vaccines will cause more infant deaths. That is scientific proof that vaccines kill infants.

Lest you think that the above quoted doctors and their studies are anomalies, please understand that doctors and scientists through the centuries have witnessed first-hand the injuries caused by vaccines and have been speaking out against that superstitious practice.

Dr. Archie Kalokerinos was a vaccine believer when he first worked as a medical doctor among Australia's aboriginal people in the 1950s. But he soon realized that the children were becoming sick and dying after getting vaccinated. He wrote a book about his experience titled *Every Second Child*. Brett Wilcox explains:

> *Every Second Child* was so named because up to half of the vaccinated Aboriginal infants died following vaccination, which Kalokerinos attributed to an acute vitamin C deficiency. Kalokerinos learned independently what professionals had come to learn in Africa and India and what vaccine manufacturers had known all along: vaccines injure and sometimes kill immunocompromised children.[515]

Dr. Kalokerinos reveals in his book the devastation wrought by the vaccine programs in the aboriginal populations of Australia:

> A health team would sweep into an area, line up all

the Aboriginal babies and infants and immunise them. There would be no examination, no taking of case histories, no checking on dietary deficiencies. Most infants would have colds. No wonder they died. Some would die within hours from acute vitamin C deficiency precipitated by the immunisation. Others would suffer immunological insults and die later from 'pneumonia', 'gastroenteritis' or 'malnutrition'. If some babies and infants survived, they would be lined up again within a month for another immunisation. If some managed to survive even this, they would be lined up again. Then there would be booster shots, shots for measles, polio and even T.B. Little wonder they died. The wonder is that any survived. The excitement of this realisation is difficult to describe. On one hand, I was enthralled by the simplicity of it all, the 'beautiful' way by which the pattern fitted everything I had been doing. On the other hand, I almost shook in horror at the thought of what had been, and still was going on. We were actually killing infants through lack of understanding.[516]

20 The AMA Cracks Down

The medical establishment cannot allow doctors to inform their patients about the dangers of vaccines. They certainly do not want studies like the one conducted by Dr. Thomas, supra, to be undertaken that reveal that vaccines are unsafe and ineffective. So, in 2021, the American Medical Association (AMA) amended its Code of Medical Ethics Section 8.7 to include this requirement: "As professionals committed to promoting the welfare of individual patients and the health of the public and to safeguarding their own and their colleagues' well-being, physicians have an ethical responsibility to encourage patients to accept immunization when the patient can do so safely."[517]

With that, the AMA has determined that it is an ethical violation for a physician to not encourage patients to accept immunization. A physician cannot be neutral on the issue of vaccination; he must "encourage" vaccination or be subject to license suspension by their state medical board for violating the AMA code of ethics.

Ethical Opinion 8.7 seems obviously intended to persuade doctors to encourage vaccinations. But, in my opinion, there is a giant loophole in EO 8.7. Notice that EO 8.7 uses the word immunization and not vaccination. That is a notable difference.

The AMA seems to use vaccination and immunization interchangeably, they are related and often viewed as synonymous, but they are not identical concepts. One can gain natural immunity without a vaccine and thus be viewed as “immunized.” But recall that the CDC defines immunization as only obtained “through vaccination.”[518] That implies no natural immune protection from a disease once a person recovers. Under that CDC rubric, the AMA can narrow the definition of immunization to only vaccination.

The CDC definition of immunization limits a doctor to an AMA ethical obligation to recommend a vaccine for an illness. Under the AMA Ethical Opinion 8.7, doctors are encouraged to recommend “immunization,” not “vaccination.” Although scientifically a doctor could recommend a course of homeopathic steps to obtain natural “immunity” instead of recommending vaccine immunity, doing so would violate the AMA Ethical Opinion 8.7 if the AMA adopts the CDC definition of immunization, which is limited to vaccination.

There is another loophole. Assuming that the AMA adopts the CDC's definition of immunization as only vaccination, a physician only has an ethical responsibility to encourage a patient to accept vaccination "when the patient can do so safely." But the pharmaceutical companies have admitted, and the U.S. Supreme Court has ruled that vaccines are "unavoidably unsafe." Thus, a physician could argue that no patient can be vaccinated safely.

The problem with that argument is that it assumes that words have meaning and we are working in a field of honest science. In reality, vaccinology is founded on a religious dogma that all vaccines are safe and effective. If a doctor contradicts that sacred maxim, he could find himself "excommunicated" from his "medical" practice even though he can prove that the sacred dogma is wrong.

The AMA Ethical Opinion 8.7 means that doctors are ethically bound by the AMA to subvert their oath to do no harm and instead encourage their patients to submit to injections of harmful vaccines. Indeed, even vaccines that have a proven track record of harm must be recommended. The America's Frontline Doctors (AFLD), in a complaint filed against the federal government explains the problem the new AMA ethical opinion presents.

> In this updated opinion, the astonishing position was taken that not only do physicians have an ethical and moral obligation to inject themselves with the experimental COVID-19 vaccination, but they also have **an ethical duty to encourage their patients to get injected with the experimental COVID-19 vaccination.** The ethics opinion repeatedly uses the phrase "safe and effective" as a descriptor for the experimental COVID-19 vaccination. The AMA's ethics opinion goes on to state that institutions may have a responsibility to require immunization of all staff![519]

Indeed, the AMA even recommends a script for doctors' offices answering machines and websites recommending the dangerous and ineffective COVID-19 vaccines. The AMA calls it a script for inquiries. But it is not in response to any question from the patient. The proposed script is propaganda from doctors' offices, which locks all the doctors into a position as a member of the office advocating an unsafe and ineffective vaccine. The AFLD complaint explains:

> The AMA even offers a "COVID-19 vaccine script for patient inquiries". Despite being styled as a script for inquiries, the script clearly intends for phone messages and office websites to lead with the following message for every caller, not simply

> those who wish to inquire about vaccines. The proposed script reads: "We are encouraging our patients to receive the COVID-19 vaccine when it is available and offered to them."[520]

The AFLD explains that the AMA ethical opinion creates an untenable conflict for physicians. A physician now must recommend a dangerous vaccine or risk losing his career. The AFLD reveals that the massive power of pharmaceutical companies is driving this.

> To illustrate just how unresolvable these conflicts are, it is necessary to consider the massive power of big pharmaceutical companies over the institutions who employ the physicians and the ease with which a physician's career can be destroyed through widely unregulated reporting which opens an investigation that can and often does render the physician virtually unemployable. Not only do physicians have to choose between their ethical obligations to their patient to do no harm and their current job; the reality is that many of them will be choosing between their patients and their medical career.[521]

The AMA Ethical Opinion 8.7 requires that physicians have an "ethical responsibility to encourage patients to accept immunization when the patient can do so safely." That proviso for safety seems to be an adoption of the American Medical Association (AMA) Council on Ethical and Judicial Affairs recommendation. In a report dated November 20, 2020, the AMA council stated on page 3, line 31, that "[v]accines are medically contraindicated for individuals who have histories of severe allergic reactions from prior doses of vaccine."[522] It further stated on page 4, line 1: "It is not ethically problematic to exempt from vaccination an individual with medical contraindications."[523]

But the AMA policy recommendation takes an Orwellian turn. On page 2, line 48, of that policy recommendation it states: "Policy also opposes non-medical exemptions, including non-medical exemptions from mandated pediatric immunizations."[524] That statement was an affirmation of the AMA policy opposing all non-medical, exemptions. The AMA Policy statement H-440.970 provides:

> 1. Our AMA believes that nonmedical (religious, philosophic, or personal belief) exemptions from immunizations endanger the health of the unvaccinated individual and the health of those in his or her group and the community at large.
>
> Therefore, our AMA (a) supports the immunization recommendations of the Advisory Committee on Immunization Practices (ACIP) for all individuals without medical contraindications; **(b) supports legislation eliminating nonmedical exemptions from immunization; (c) encourages state medical associations to seek removal of nonmedical exemptions in statutes requiring mandatory immunizations, including for childcare and school attendance;** (d) encourages physicians to grant vaccine exemption requests only when medical contraindications are present; (e) encourages state and local medical associations to work with public health officials to develop contingency plans for controlling outbreaks in medically-exempt populations and to intensify efforts to achieve high immunization rates in communities where nonmedical exemptions are common; and (f) recommends that states have in place: (i) an established mechanism, which includes the involvement of qualified public health physicians, of determining which vaccines will be

> mandatory for admission to school and other identified public venues (based upon the recommendations of the ACIP); and (ii) **policies that permit immunization exemptions for medical reasons only.**
>
> 2. **Our AMA will actively advocate for legislation, regulations, programs, and policies that incentivize states to eliminate non-medical exemptions from mandated pediatric immunizations.**[525]

The AMA is the avowed enemy of religious and bodily freedom. The AMA actively lobbies to thwart the freedom of every American to choose whether or not to be vaccinated. They require doctors to become shills for the pharmaceutical companies by opining that it is medically unethical for a physician not to affirmatively "encourage patients to accept immunization."

Please understand that reality the next time you speak with a doctor about vaccination. He is NOT giving you his unbiased opinion. He will be in Jeopardy of being disciplined by the state medical board if he recommends against vaccination. Oddly, the doctor would be subject to discipline even if he is neutral on vaccinations. The doctor is under an "ethical" obligation to "encourage" vaccination. He can only be assured of not violating Ethical Opninon 8.7 by affirmatively encouraging his patients to be vaccinated.

21 Pediatricians Are Paid Bounties

This author talked to a couple with a newborn baby who had to leave their pediatrician's office because the pediatricians would not allow them to forgo getting their child vaccinated. The pediatricians continually pushed to allow the nurse to vaccinate their newborn baby. When the parents requested that the nurses and doctors please stop continually pestering them to have their child vaccinated, she was told that their office would allow a delay in the vaccination schedule but they would eventually have to get their child fully vaccinated.

The pediatric office has posted on its website a notice that it follows "the national standards of care set forth by the Centers for Disease Control and Prevention (CDC) and the American Academy of Pediatrics (AAP)."[526] According to the CDC vaccination schedule, their child would need to receive more than 47 total doses of vaccines (including boosters) that covered 17 different diseases before the child reached 15 months old. That pediatric practice of 15 doctors stated that if the parents persisted in not allowing them to vaccinate their child they would need to abide by their written policy, which required them to "find another pediatrician who agrees with your beliefs."[527]

The parents called pediatricians to find another doctor for their newborn child. The first four offices that the parents called refused to treat their child unless they agreed to have him vaccinated. A fifth office finally agreed to see their child without him being vaccinated, but only if they submitted a religious exemption.

The American Academy of Pediatrics (AAP) is a corporate and government mouthpiece that touts the wares of drug and vaccine manufacturers. Most Pediatricians mindlessly follow the recommendations of the AAP. The AAP advocates strong-arm tactics to coerce parents to vaccinate their children; it advises pediatricians that it is an "acceptable option to pediatric care clinicians to dismiss families who refuse vaccines."[528]

Moral degenerates run the AAP. For example, the AAP has issued an official policy statement supporting transitioning prepubescent children from male to female and vice versa.[529] The AAP thinks that prepubescent children should be allowed to change their gender despite objections from parents. The AAP approves transgenderism and states that it is outdated thinking to opine that a prepubescent child is not mature enough to change his or her gender. The AAP says that parents and doctors should affirm a child's decision to transition from one gender to another and not try to dissuade the child from that course. The AAP calls efforts to stop a child from identifying as or transitioning to a sex other than his or her biological sex "inappropriate," "deleterious," "unfair," "deceptive," and "outside the mainstream of traditional medical practice." The AAP states that it approves children undergoing cross-sex hormone therapy and irreversible transexual "gender affirming" surgeries. The AAP thinks that Pediatric primary care providers should be "a reliable source of validation, support, and reassurance" to prepubescent children seeking to transition from one gender to another. The AAP undermines the authority of parents over their children. In cases where the family objects to their child transitioning from one sex to another, the

AAP recommends that pediatricians seek legal help to ensure that they do not violate the local consent laws in their efforts to help the child transition over the objection of the parents.

It seems that there is a medical phalanx set up to push parents into vaccinating their children. The Immunization Action Coalition (IAC) provides doctors with a "Sample Vaccine Policy Statement: Ready for you to adapt for your practice."[530] That policy statement template states, in pertinent part that "if you should absolutely refuse to vaccinate your child despite all our efforts, we will ask you to find another healthcare provider who shares your views. We do not keep a list of such providers, nor would we recommend any such physician."[531]

The Immunization Action Coalition is funded "in partnership with the Centers for Disease Control and Prevention (CDC)" which "provided financial support to IAC."[532] The Children's Health Defense revealed that the CDC has acted as a captured government agency that is under the control of the vaccine industry.

> The latest data and science show that specific vaccines are unequivocally not safe. Yet government officials – with well-documented conflicts of interest with the $50 billion vaccine industry – systematically obscure the risks while exaggerating the benefits of vaccines.
>
> The government has quietly admitted culpability by paying out over $4 billion for thousands of injuries and deaths caused by vaccines underscoring that vaccine injuries can and do happen, including autism. And, an HHS-funded study concluded that fewer than 1% of vaccine injuries are even reported.

> Big Pharma is exerting influence over WHO, FDA and CDC to fast track and short cut safety studies in order to gain more profits faster. Big Pharma has zero financial risk when children get vaccine injured because the government prevents victims from suing big pharma – resulting in big pharma not being concerned about child vaccine safety.
>
> ***
>
> And CDC, frankly, is a vaccine company; it owns 56 vaccine patents and buys and distributes $4.6 billion in vaccines annually through the Vaccines for Children program, which is over 40% of its total budget. Further, Pharma directly funds, populates and controls dozens of CDC programs through the CDC foundation. A British Medical Journal editorial excoriates CDC's sweetheart relationship with pharma quotes UCLA Professor of Medicine Jerome R. Hoffman "most of us were shocked to learn the CDC takes funding from industry… It is outrageous that industry is apparently allowed to punish the CDC if the agency conducts research that has potential to cut into profits."[533]

The parents of the above mentioned child have come up against a massive syndicate funded by vaccine manufacturers. The couple's ordeal in finding a pediatrician who will treat their unvaccinated child is not unusual. Alex Pietroski, a reporter for Waking Times, alleged that "it is now very difficult to find a pediatrician who will accept a family who doesn't vaccinate. Even parents who partially vaccinate or follow a different schedule have a hard time finding a doctor. Here's why: doctors have to vaccinate a certain percentage of their patients or they don't get their bonus. BCBS [Blue Cros Blue Shield] says doctors need to vaccinate 63% of their patients to get the payout [of $400 per vaccinated child]."[534]

This author researched Pietroski's allegation. Indeed, many pediatricians refuse to see child patients whose parents have decided not to have their children receive vaccines.[535] Doctors are increasingly encouraged to refuse service to the unvaccinated child patients based on a policy published in 2016 by the American Academy of Pediatrics (AAP) that allows pediatricians to dismiss the child patients of parents who refuse vaccines.[536] The Greenville News reported that "[a] two-month-old baby was recently denied care at a Carolina Forest pediatrician's office due to his parents' stance on vaccines."[537] The report reveals:

> That decision stems from a policy adopted by recommendation of the American Academy of Pediatrics, according to Brian Argo, chief financial officer of Conway Medical Center, which operates CPG Pediatrics.[538]

You will notice that the spokesman for the pediatric office was the "chief financial officer." Why would the chief financial officer be the one who is giving the reasons for the policy of refusing service to unvaccinated children? Brian Argo has an MBA[539], not an MD; he is a financial expert; he is not a medical expert. You would think that there would be a medical reason for the policy. You would think that the pediatrics office would appoint a medical doctor to give a medical reason for the policy. Instead, the pediatric office appoints a financial officer to present the rationale for refusing service to unvaccinated children. But he does not give a financial reason, nor does he give a medical reason; he gives as the reason a recommendation by the AAP. Unsurprisingly, he did not say that the pediatric office makes a lot of money by vaccinating children, and every unvaccinated child in its medical practice threatens that money stream.

Pietroski, however, alleges that there is a financial motive at the core of pediatricians not allowing unvaccinated children in their practice. Pietroski made a fantastic allegation that many pediatricians will not treat unvaccinated children because they need a certain threshold of patients in their medical practice to be vaccinated to be paid a bounty from insurance companies for each vaccinated child. It seems that the stick of medical licensure suspension for violating the AMA and AAP regulations if the pediatrician fails to vaccinate children is matched by the carrot of financial reward for doctors who push vaccines on the uninformed parents of children.

I researched Pietroski's allegation. What I found was surprising. The evidence establishes that his allegation is true. One example of this is under the Blue Cross Blue Shield *Childhood Immunizations- Combo 10* program. Under that program, if a pediatrician can convince 63% of the parents of children in their practice to receive the full schedule of the ten listed vaccines before the child's second birthday, the pediatrician will receive a $400 bounty per vaccinated child from Blue Cross Blue Shield.[540] That program presents a perverse monetary incentive for pediatricians to push for childhood vaccines. By the way, this is only one of the incentive programs being run by one insurance company in Michigan. There are, no doubt, many others. Below is a screenshot from page 15 of the 2016 Blue Cross Blue Shield "Performance Recognition Program, Provider Incentive Program," outlining the details of its *Childhood Immunizations- Combo 10 program*.

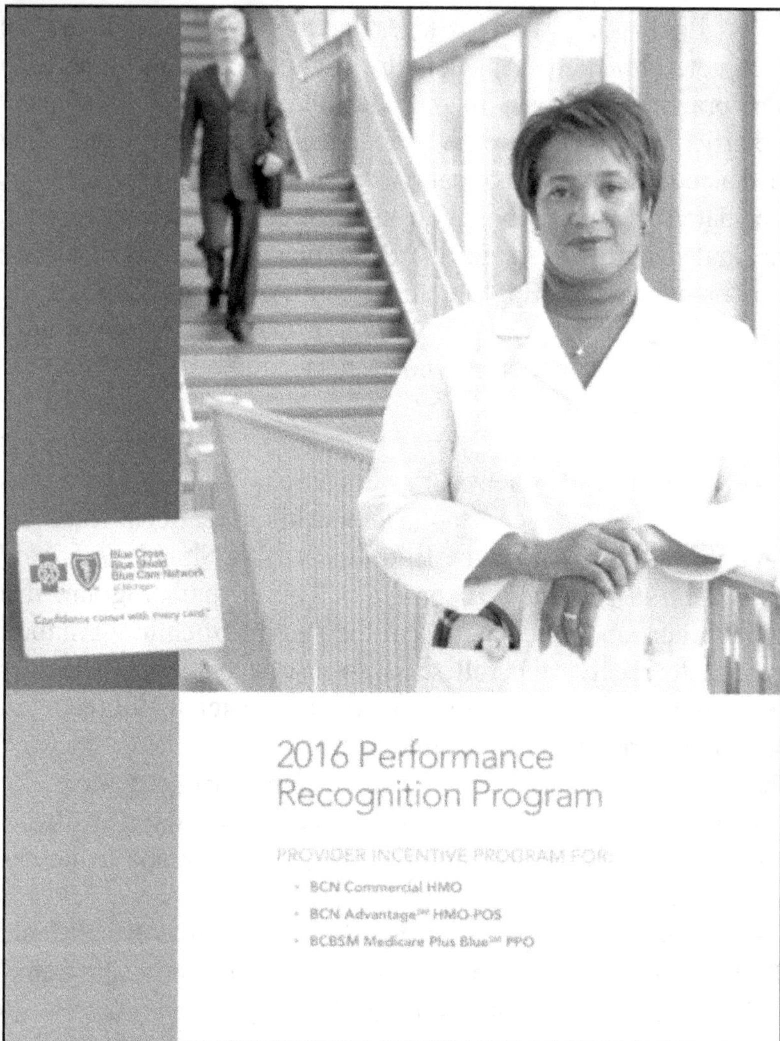
2016 Performance Recognition Program

PROVIDER INCENTIVE PROGRAM FOR:

- BCN Commercial HMO
- BCN Advantage℠ HMO-POS
- BCBSM Medicare Plus Blue℠ PPO

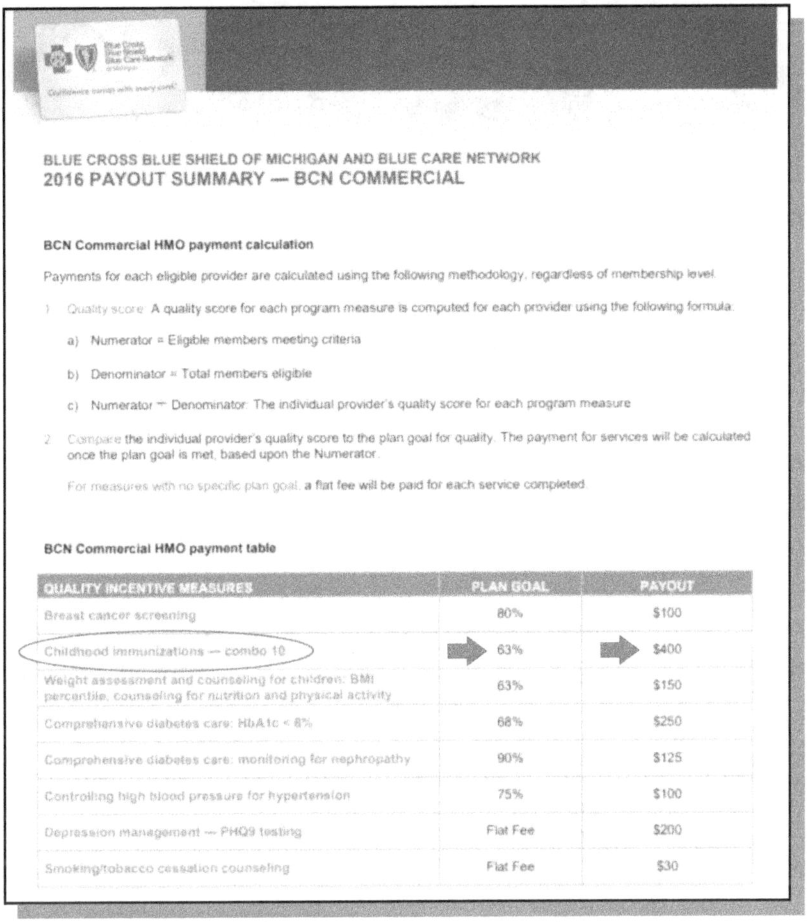

BLUE CROSS BLUE SHIELD OF MICHIGAN AND BLUE CARE NETWORK

2016 PAYOUT SUMMARY — BCN COMMERCIAL

BCN Commercial HMO payment calculation

Payments for each eligible provider are calculated using the following methodology, regardless of membership level.

1. Quality score: A quality score for each program measure is computed for each provider using the following formula:
   a) Numerator = Eligible members meeting criteria
   b) Denominator = Total members eligible
   c) Numerator ÷ Denominator: The individual provider's quality score for each program measure
2. Compare the individual provider's quality score to the plan goal for quality. The payment for services will be calculated once the plan goal is met, based upon the Numerator.

   For measures with no specific plan goal, a flat fee will be paid for each service completed.

BCN Commercial HMO payment table

QUALITY INCENTIVE MEASURES	PLAN GOAL	PAYOUT
Breast cancer screening	80%	$100
Childhood immunizations — combo 10	63%	$400
Weight assessment and counseling for children: BMI percentile, counseling for nutrition and physical activity	63%	$150
Comprehensive diabetes care: HbA1c < 8%	68%	$250
Comprehensive diabetes care: monitoring for nephropathy	90%	$125
Controlling high blood pressure for hypertension	75%	$100
Depression management — PHQ9 testing	Flat Fee	$200
Smoking/tobacco cessation counseling	Flat Fee	$30

Figure 21: Chart (annotated) with instructions appearing on page 4 of the Blue Cross Blue Shield 2016 Performance Recognition Program.

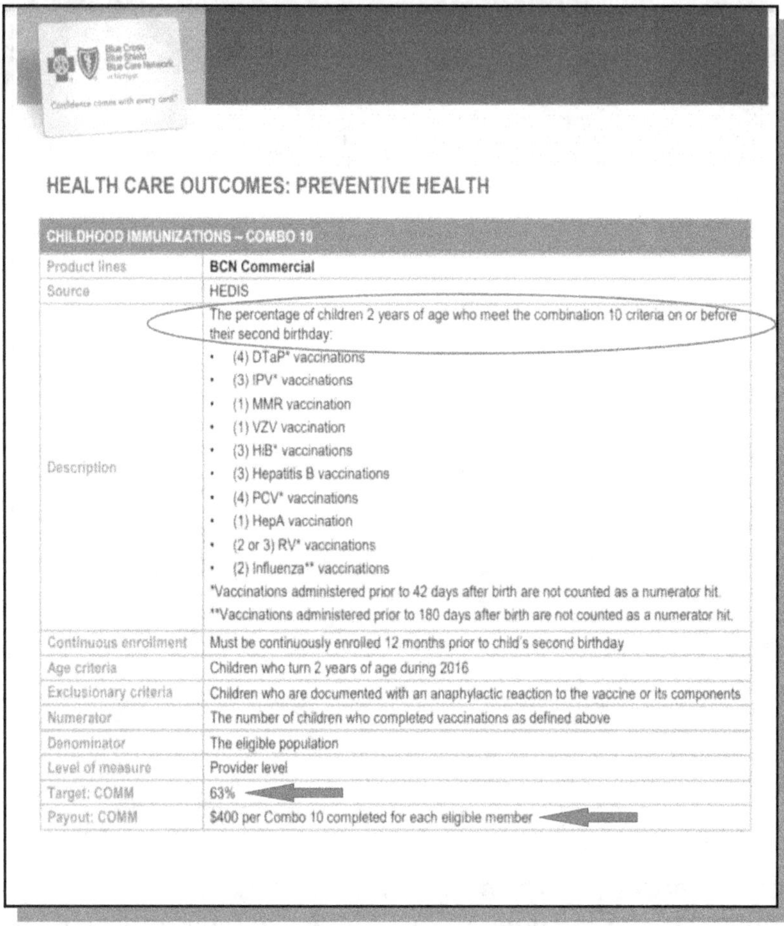

HEALTH CARE OUTCOMES: PREVENTIVE HEALTH

CHILDHOOD IMMUNIZATIONS – COMBO 10	
Product lines	**BCN Commercial**
Source	HEDIS
Description	The percentage of children 2 years of age who meet the combination 10 criteria on or before their second birthday: • (4) DTaP* vaccinations • (3) IPV* vaccinations • (1) MMR vaccination • (1) VZV vaccination • (3) HiB* vaccinations • (3) Hepatitis B vaccinations • (4) PCV* vaccinations • (1) HepA vaccination • (2 or 3) RV* vaccinations • (2) Influenza** vaccinations *Vaccinations administered prior to 42 days after birth are not counted as a numerator hit. **Vaccinations administered prior to 180 days after birth are not counted as a numerator hit.
Continuous enrollment	Must be continuously enrolled 12 months prior to child's second birthday
Age criteria	Children who turn 2 years of age during 2016
Exclusionary criteria	Children who are documented with an anaphylactic reaction to the vaccine or its components
Numerator	The number of children who completed vaccinations as defined above
Denominator	The eligible population
Level of measure	Provider level
Target: COMM	63%
Payout: COMM	$400 per Combo 10 completed for each eligible member

Figure 22: Chart (annotated) appearing on page 15 of the Blue Cross Blue Shield 2016 Performance Recognition Program.

The Blue Cross Blue Shield *Childhood Immunizations-Combo 10* program pays a bounty of $400 per child. But the pediatrician must have at least 63% of his patients vaccinated to receive any money. If the vaccinated population of children in his practice drops below 63%, the pediatrician receives nothing. To meet the plan goal, the eligible children receiving the required ten vaccines (numerator) is divided by the total eligible children in the practice (denominator). If that figure is 63% or more, then the doctor receives his bounty based on the number of children in the numerator. The Blue Cross Provider Incentive Program states: "The payment for services will be calculated once the plan goal is met [63%], based upon the Numerator."[541] If the fraction is less than 63% the doctor receives nothing.

It would not be unusual for a pediatrician to make approximately $53,000 yearly from Blue Cross Blue Shield's childhood vaccine incentive program. In 1999, a research study published in the Journal of the American Medical Association examined eighty-nine pediatric practices in 31 states involving 373 individual pediatric practitioners.[542] The study found that "each practitioner cared for an average of 1546 patients" over a two-year period. That is an average of 773 patients each year. The study was not a measure of office visits; it was a measure of individual patients treated regardless of the number of office visits. Thus, one patient visiting the office three times over the two-year period would be counted as a single patient. The study found that 27.4% of all pediatric patients were 2 years old or younger. On average, each pediatrician treated 211.8 (773 x 0.274 = 211.8) patients that were two years old or younger per year. That means that the average pediatrician can count on a bounty payout of approximately $84,720 per year from the Blue Cross Blue Shield Childhood Immunizations- Combo 10 program.

The $84,720 figure assumes that the doctor is able to convince 100% of his parents to vaccinate their children. If he is only able to convince 63% of parents, which is the bare minimum to qualify for the bounty, he would stand to make $53,374. Thus, the average pediatrician can make between $53,374 and $84,720 per year in vaccine bounty payments. The critical driver for him to push vaccinations on every parent is that if his rate of child vaccinations drops below 63% he will make nothing under that program.

This financial incentive to have a certain threshold (63%) of fully vaccinated children in their practice explains perfectly why some pediatricians will not allow unvaccinated children in their practice. Every child in their practice who is not fully vaccinated will bring them closer to their minimum threshold and threaten their $400 bounty for each vaccinated child. The Pediatrician, who you think should be looking out for your child's best interest, has a monetary incentive to ignore the mountain of evidence that vaccines are both ineffective and dangerous to children. Now you know why there has been no push-back from pediatricians about the acceleration of vaccines being injected into infants. They are financially incentivized to be willfully ignorant doctors.

The avarice of doctors has reached such a level that some will risk the lives of their patients for a buck. In a 2016 post on *Wellness and Equality*, the writer reveals how one pediatrician was willing to inject a vaccine into a child even after the child had a prior severe life-altering vaccine reaction. The pediatrician did not care about the harm the vaccine could cause to the child.

> When my friend's child suffered a life-threatening reaction to a vaccine a week after her first birthday, my friend assumed her pediatrician would write her a medical exemption from future vaccines. Shortly after receiving a routine set of vaccines, the happy, vibrant one-year-old spiked a 106 degree fever, began having seizures, and was hospitalized. When the unexplained "illness" passed after a week in the hospital, the little girl had lost her ability to walk. My friend describes how her daughter, who had learned to walk several months earlier at 9 months, suddenly "stumbled around like a drunk person" for weeks following the vaccines. My friend met with a team of pediatricians, neurologists, and naturopathic doctors, and they agreed: Her daughter had

suffered a brain injury caused by a reaction to one of the vaccines. Hoping the injury would be temporary and that she might recover and ease her brain inflammation if they could help her small body quickly eliminate the vaccine additives that caused the reaction, my friend's daughter underwent an intensive detoxification program overseen by a nutritionalist. Slowly, her daughter relearned to walk.

My friend is a practicing attorney who graduated from a Top 10 college. The evidence was overwhelming that her daughter's reaction had been caused by vaccines, she told me.

But a few months later, when she took her daughter back into the pediatrician for a visit, he wanted to vaccinate her daughter again. She was baffled. Why?

After a reader sent us a link to a PDF file of Blue Cross Blue Shield's Physician Incentive Program available online, *Wellness & Equality* learned that insurance companies pay pediatricians massive bonuses based on the percentage of children who are fully vaccinated by age 2.[543]

Some pediatricians are money-grubbers who care nothing about the well-being of the children they treat.

For the love of money is the root of all evil: which while some coveted after, they have erred from the faith, and pierced themselves through with many sorrows. (1 Timothy 6:10)

Once Blue Cross and Blue Shield realized their scheme

was being publicized, it took steps to prevent further revelations.

> After *Wellness & Equality* published [the] article, Blue Cross Blue Shield locked online access to their incentive program and then removed the page altogether.[544]

J.B. Handley, the co-founder of Generation Rescue, revealed the dark secret of how much money pediatricians make by administering vaccines to children.

> [W]henever I meet a pediatrician I ask them a simple question: what percentage of your revenue come from vaccine administration? The number always astounds me. The answers I get are that anywhere from 50-80% of their revenue comes from giving vaccines. Imagine that.[545]

In his book, Jabbed, Brett Wilcox revealed that "a pediatrician told a Minnesota audience in 2016 that he loses $700,000 a year because he doesn't push vaccines according to the U.S. vaccine schedule."[546]

COVID-19 Vaccine Bounties

On April 13, 2023, U.S. Congressman Thomas Massie reported on Twitter that Anthem Medicaid paid a bounty to push COVID-19 vaccines under its "COVID-19 Vaccine Provider Incentive Program."[547] The bounty gave progressively increased payments for each vaccinated patient based on the percentage of Anthem vaccinated members. For example, if the doctor provided at least one dose of a COVID-19 vaccine before September 1, 2021, to a patient, the doctor would receive a $20 bonus per vaccine administered if at least 30% of his Anthem patients were vaccinated. However, the payment increased to $125 per vaccinated patient if 75% of the Anthem members were vaccinated. The amount increased substantially if the patient was vaccinated between September 21, 2021, and December 31, 2021. If the doctor provided at least one dose of a COVID-19 vaccine to a patient before December 31, 2021, the doctor would receive a $100 bonus per vaccine if at least 30% of his Anthem patients were vaccinated. However, the payment per COVID-19 vaccine increased to $250 per vaccinated patient if 75% of the Anthem members were vaccinated before December 31, 2021. Below is the official schedule of bounties provided to doctors by Anthem, which Rep. Massie obtained. Other insurance companies almost certainly have similar incentive programs. You have reason to question your doctor's objectivity when he recommends you take the COVID-19 vaccine. He likely has a pecuniary interest in convincing you to take the vaccine.

Anthem Medicaid

Anthem Blue Cross and Blue Shield Medicaid

COVID-19 Vaccine Provider Incentive program

Getting vaccinated against COVID-19 is one of the best and safest ways people can protect themselves and their families against the virus. As a participating practice in the COVID-19 Provider Vaccine Incentive program, we recognize your hard work by offering incentives for helping patients make the choice to become vaccinated.

Eligibility

The COVID-19 Vaccine Provider Incentive program is open to you if you are a participating Kentucky primary care provider with an Anthem Blue Cross and Blue Shield Medicaid (Anthem) panel size of 25 or more members. All Anthem members identified as receiving COVID-19 vaccination services are included in the methodology. Vaccine results will be determined by a COVID-19 vaccine claim or by confirmation from the Kentucky Vaccine Registry.

The results will be calculated for two time periods:

- September 1, 2021 – Initial incentive payment
- December 31, 2021 – Final incentive payment

How you can qualify for a bonus

If your practice meets the below thresholds for vaccination with at least one dose by September 1, 2021, you will receive the initial incentive payment based on the following rates:

- 30% Anthem members vaccinated – $20 bonus per vaccinated member
- 40% Anthem members vaccinated – $45 bonus per vaccinated member
- 50% Anthem members vaccinated – $70 bonus per vaccinated member
- 60% Anthem members vaccinated – $100 bonus per vaccinated member
- 75% Anthem members vaccinated – $125 bonus per vaccinated member

The final incentive payment is calculated based on members who are newly vaccinated between September 1, 2021 and December 31, 2021 (see the *Appendix* for calculation examples). If your practice meets the below thresholds for vaccination with at least one dose by December 1, 2021, you will receive the final incentive payment based on the following rates:

- 30%Anthem members vaccinated – $100 bonus per newly vaccinated member
- 40% Anthem members vaccinated – $150 bonus per newly vaccinated member
- 50% Anthem members vaccinated – $175 bonus per newly vaccinated member
- 60% Anthem members vaccinated – $200 bonus per newly vaccinated member
- 75% Anthem members vaccinated – $250 bonus per newly vaccinated member

https://providers.anthem.com/ky

22 Buying Influence to Injure and Kill

The strange phenomenon of colleges nationwide issuing vaccine mandates in virtual lockstep is explainable. They were not making independent judgments about the safety and efficacy of the COVID-19 vaccines. They mandated the COVID-19 vaccines because the federal government paid them to do it. The federal government created a financial incentive for universities to mandate COVID-19 vaccines.

College administrators don't care about the well-being of the students; they care about money. The universities are staffed with highly qualified scientific researchers with worldwide data and studies at their fingertips. College administrators know with certainty that the COVID-19 vaccines are unsafe and ineffective. But they have been paid off. The universities mandating the COVID-19 vaccines are run by sociopaths who are perfectly okay with injuring the students and staff because they get money from the federal government to do it.

U.S. colleges and universities are being paid billions of dollars from the federal government Coronavirus Aid, Relief, and Economic Security (CARES) Act to mandate student and staff COVID-19 vaccinations. The precondition for receiving the

CARES money is that the universities comply with COVID-19 vaccine mandates.

The universities do not serve the students. They are more beholden to their paymaster, the federal government. **For example, Yale University made more money from the CARES Act in 2022 ($607 million) than from student tuition ($475 million).**[548] Dr. Michael Nevradakis, Ph.D., and Lynn Comerford, Ph.D., revealed that "since 1998, Yale has received $9 billion from HHS — $1 billion of which has been disbursed since 2020."[549] It is no surprise then to find that Yale's "COVID-19 Vaccination Policy" includes an oppressive COVID-19 vaccine mandate.

> The university requires all students, faculty, staff, and postdoctoral/postgraduate trainees — other than those with approved medical or religious exemptions — to receive a primary COVID-19 vaccine series and to obtain a booster shot within 14 days of eligibility. Additionally, students — other than those with approved medical or religious exemptions —must receive an updated, bivalent booster by the start of the spring semester (in any event, no later than January 31, 2023), regardless of how many previous monovalent boosters they received.[550]

On April 1, 2021, HHS announced that it was establishing a nationwide network of "trusted voices" to encourage people to get COVID-19 vaccinations. The trusted voices were labeled "The COVID-19 Community Corps." Among the founding members of this Orwellian campaign to poison the populace through deceptive marketing were the nation's premier medical and health associations, including, but not limited to, the American Medical Association (AMA), American Academy of Pediatrics (AAP), American College of Obstetricians and Gynecologists (ACOG), American College of Physicians (ACP), and American

Association of Nurse Practitioners (AANP).[551]

Why would these medical organizations agree to work with HHS to encourage people to get COVID-19 vaccines? The answer is as old as time; they are being paid very handsomely to prostitute themselves and act as shills and huxters for the government. For example, the ACOG alone received $11 million from HHS.[552] Attorney Maggie Thorp, and her OBGYN husband Jim Thorp, M.D., revealed that receipt of the money was contingent on "ACOG's full compliance with CDC guidance on COVID-19 infection and control."[553] The ACOG is not just a professional organization; it holds great sway over its members. Maggie and Jim Thorp explain:

> Meet the American College of Obstetricians and Gynecologists (ACOG). Founded in 1951, ACOG holds itself out as the "premier professional membership organization for obstetricians and gynecologists" and is the leading organization representing physicians and specialists in obstetrical care. ACOG is entrenched across two continents – it has more than 60,000 members and is composed of 12 geographic districts made up of 98 sections spanning North, South, and Central America.[554]

The ACOG had initially taken the position that "[i]n the interest of patient autonomy, ACOG recommends that pregnant individuals be free to make their own decision regarding COVID-19 vaccination."[555] But after HHS made its $11 million payoff to ACOG, on July 30, 2021, the ACOG changed its position on the COVID-19 vaccine from one of deference to the mother's decision to one of strongly recommending the COVID-19 vaccine for pregnant women. That recommendation was made in the face of no evidence of the vaccines' safety or efficacy for pregnant women; indeed, the COVID-19 vaccine clinical trials failed to include pregnant women. There was no science to support ACOG's change in position, but the payment of $11 million certainly explains it.

Flush with its windfall of $11 million from HHS, ACOG obediently whipped its doctors into line by publishing "key recommendations," including:

> The American College of Obstetricians and Gynecologists (ACOG) strongly recommends that pregnant individuals be vaccinated against COVID-19. Given the potential for severe illness and death during pregnancy, completion of the initial COVID-19 vaccination series is a priority for this population.
>
> ***
>
> ACOG recommends that pregnant and recently pregnant people up to 6 weeks postpartum receive a bivalent mRNA COVID-19 vaccine booster dose following the completion of their last COVID-19 primary vaccine dose or monovalent booster.[556]

All patients who refuse to get the COVID-19 vaccine must have their medical record reflect their refusal. Notably, one of the ACOG "key recommendations" is for the doctor to convince the patient who refused previous vaccination efforts to get vaccinated at the next office visit.

> For patients who do not receive any COVID-19 vaccine, the discussion should be documented in the patient's medical record. During subsequent office visits, obstetrician–gynecologists should address ongoing questions and concerns and offer vaccination again.[557]

This hard-sell strategy clearly deviates from ACOG's previous position that "pregnant individuals be free to make their own decision regarding COVID-19 vaccination." A little known fact is that under the "Cooperative Agreement" between HHS and the ACOG that was part of the arrangement to get the millions of dollars from HHS, "the recipient is expected to provide to CDC copies of and/or access to COVID-19 data collected with these funds."[558] That means the patient's decision whether to get a COVID-19 vaccine will likely be reported to the CDC. The CDC is a component agency of HHS.

The $11 million payoff from the HHS turned the ACOG into liars. One of the "Key Messages" about COVID-19 from the ACOG is the claim that the COVID-19 vaccines do not cause infertility, spontaneous abortion, or fetal defects. That assurance is false. Evidence from Pfizer's studies reported in January 2021 (and publically revealed under an FOIA order on April 28, 2023) showed that rats who had taken the COVID-19 vaccine were twice as likely to suffer pregnancy loss.[559] Furthermore, the Pfizer studies showed a 14-fold increase in birth abnormalities among the COVID-19 vaccinated rats compared to the control group.[560]

On April 29, 2023, it was revealed that in human trials, the Pfizer COVID-19 vaccine was shown to cause spontaneous abortions in 21% of women receiving the COVID-19 vaccine.[561] Babies born to mothers who had been vaccinated suffered damages ranging from pneumothorax to death.[562] Indeed, 19% of the infants exposed to the COVID mRNA vaccine via their mothers' milk suffered from 48 different adverse events ranging from diarrhea to vomiting.[563] Amy Kelly, who is the Program Director of the War Room/DailyClout Pfizer Documents Analysis Project, explains:

> Despite Pfizer and the FDA knowing by April 20, 2021, the extent of damage to fetuses and babies, including the fact that fetuses and newborns had

> died, on April 23, 2021, inexplicably [CDC Director] Dr. Rochelle Walensky held a White House press briefing where she recommended pregnant women get vaccinated.[564]

ACOG is as culpable as the CDC. While the ACOG had no scientific or medical reasons, they had eleven million other reasons to "strongly recommend[] that pregnant individuals be vaccinated against COVID-19." The ACOG doctors have literally been given a script to follow to deceive and badger their patients into getting vaccinated. The script did not allow for any consideration of each patient's unique health needs or condition. It is a one size fits all recommendation to get vaccinated. There is no proviso in the script for informed consent. It is a script to push, prod, and cajole compliance. The ACOG script prodding pregnant women to get vaccinated remains unchanged despite the mountain of evidence that the COVID-19 vaccines are ineffective and dangerous. It is a violation of the Hippocratic oath to first do no harm. It is not the practice of medicine; it is more the administration of a superstitious religious sacrament.

You realize who is behind this effort to poison and kill mothers and infants when you follow the money. The "CDC Foundation" was created by Congress.[565] It is a public charity that has been given statutory authority to fund the CDC. The CDC accepts funds from the CDC Foundation. Of course, the CDC Foundation wields tremendous control over the CDC. The funds the CDC Foundation provides are then funneled to medical associations such as the ACOG to push doctors into administering vaccines. Take a wild guess who funds the CDC Foundation? The CDC Foundation is funded by all the usual suspects: pharmaceutical companies that make vaccines like Pfizer, Merck, Johns & Johnson, and organizations that profit from vaccines or are funded by those who so profit, like the Bill & Malinda Gates Foundation, the GAVI Alliance, and the World Health Organization.[566] He who pays the piper calls the tune. The powerful pharmaceutical interests use their funding control over the CDC to, in turn, see that those funds are used to control what the doctor tells his patients about the safety and efficacy of vaccines. This is a new spin on trickle-down economics. Any doctor who kicks against the pricks and does not follow orders soon finds himself out of a job.

23 The Blind Leading the Blind

Both patients and doctors are kept in the dark about the ineffectiveness and dangers of vaccines. Doctors act as blind guides leading their blind patients into a ditch. Suzanne Humphries, M.D., board-certified in nephrology and family medicine, has this to say regarding how little doctors know about vaccines.

> Do you know how much doctors learn about vaccines in medical school? When we participate in pediatrics training, we learn that vaccines need to be given on schedule. ... We are indoctrinated with the mantra that 'vaccines are safe and effective'—neither of which is true. ... Doctors today are given extensive training on how to talk to 'hesitant' parents—how to frighten them by vastly inflating the risks during natural infection. They are trained on the necessity of twisting parents' arms to conform, or fire them from their practices. Doctors are trained that nothing bad should be said about any vaccine, period.[567]

Bob Sears, M.D., a board-certified pediatrician who authored the book, *The Vaccine Book: Making the Right Decision for Your Child*, said this about the woeful vaccine training of doctors:

> Doctors, myself included, learn a lot about diseases in medical school, but we learn very little about vaccines, other than the fact that the FDA and pharmaceutical companies do extensive research on vaccines to make sure they are safe and effective. We don't review the research ourselves. We never learn what goes into making vaccines or how their safety is studied. We trust and take it for granted that the proper researchers are doing their job. So, when patients want a little more information about shots, all we can really say as doctors is that the diseases are bad and the shots are good. But we don't know enough to answer all of your detailed questions about vaccines, nor do we have the time during a regular health check up to thoroughly discuss and debate the pros and cons of vaccines.[568]

TV's *The Doctors* co-host Rachael Ross, M.D. in 2016 said the following after screening the movie *Vaxxed*:

> They don't teach us about the ingredients; they don't teach us about the studies behind it. … what they teach us is that they've always been given and that they cure diseases and that you just do it. And honestly from the outside looking in now and in saying this to all you people, I almost feel like an ass. ... I am just blindly following like a robot following through with this with no real data, no real information, didn't know what was in them. … that's part of what makes us all feel real bad, and it's part of why physicians are very resistant to this information. … You have to sit at home and

> re-digest everything that you've learned and come to terms with the damage that you've potentially caused over the years.[569]

Kathryn A. Hale, M.D., MPH, FACOG, who is an OB/GYN, published a blog titled, "I saw VAXXED and I was shattered!" She states that "[a]fter watching VAXXED, one thing is clear, there is a definite link between the MMR vaccine and autism. Children are being damaged and something needs to be done."[570] She further explained how she and other doctors simply trust and follow the edicts of the CDC. She did not realize that the CDC is not trustworthy.

> For many in public health and medicine in general, the individuals that work at CDC are placed on a pedestal. We view them and their research as the epitome of scientific excellence. We regard their findings and recommendations as the gospel. We trust them to pursue hard science and trust that when they publish data, they are not being influenced by anything more that the pursuit of truth. I was shattered when I saw VAXXED because this movie told the story of a situation where something other than truth motivated certain professionals involved in safety research involving the MMR vaccine. I learned for the first time about the whistle-blower Dr. William Thompson. The truth he exposed, revealed in black and white an instance where life-saving information was withheld. Information that could have saved countless lives.
>
> My heart broke for the parents of children with autism. There was story after story of beautiful babies who were developing perfectly and engaged with their families up until they received the MMR

> vaccine. I fought back tears as Polly Tomey shared how she defended her choice to follow the pediatrician's advice to give her child the MMR vaccine despite concerns expressed by her mom and a good friend. Our patient's place such trust in us as physicians. As physicians, we place our trust in organizations such as the CDC to give us the information we need to keep our patients safe. It changes you when you find that those you thought you could trust could not be trusted.[571]

Now you know the sad truth that most doctors are ignorant about the ingredients, safety, and efficacy of vaccines. When doctors recommend vaccines, they do it from a position of ignorance. They are not competent to advise you about something they know little or nothing about. Open your eyes so that you are not led into a ditch by blind doctors. "[T]hey be blind leaders of the blind. And if the blind lead the blind, both shall fall into the ditch." Matthew 15:14.

But what about doctors who are not blind? What about doctors who are aware of the high probability that vaccines are damaging children but go out of their way to remain ignorant? Their blindness enters a stage known as willful blindness, where they purposely avoid taking steps to confirm or allay their suspicions. Such willful ignorance is not different from actual knowledge.

In controlled substance prosecutions for illegal dispensing, willful ignorance is sufficient to prove actual knowledge to support a conviction. The *en banc* U.S. Court of Appeals for the Ninth Circuit explains: "As our cases have recognized, deliberate ignorance, otherwise known as willful blindness, is categorically different from negligence or recklessness. A willfully blind defendant is one who took deliberate actions to avoid confirming suspicions of criminality."[572] The U.S. Supreme Court states that "persons who know enough to blind themselves to direct proof of critical facts in effect have actual knowledge of those facts."[573]

Doctors who continue to administer vaccines in the face of evidence that the vaccines are causing injury but fail to take any steps to confirm or allay their suspicions so that they remain ignorant are complicit in the harm caused by the vaccines. It cannot be long after being a pediatrician that a doctor becomes aware of the damage he is causing by vaccinating the children in his practice. Doctors are not stupid people. Eventually, a pediatrician will go from being a blind doctor to a willfully blind doctor. They are without excuse.

Dr. James C. Meehan, Jr., M.D., posted a statement on Facebook where he calls out such willfully ignorant doctors. He calls on them to stop the child abuse of vaccination. Below is the pertinent part of that post.

> Instead of fighting for truth and safety, you're fighting like rats for your piece of cheese.
>
> I have ZERO RESPECT for vaccine profiteers that are so financially biased, confirmation biased, indoctrinated, and willfully ignorant of the evidence that clearly shows vaccines cause injury, disease and REGRESSIVE AUTISM, that they aggressively lobby lawmakers to make vaccines mandatory, and deny parents the essential knowledge about the risks of toxic ingredients injected into their babies.
>
> Bought by big pharma, the caretakers of children's health have become the perpetrators of harm rather than the protectors. They profit as our precious, perfect children are harmed and killed by vaccines filled with cheap preservatives, neurotoxic

adjuvants, and human cellular material derived from aborted fetal cell lines.

They are complicit accomplices in the murder-by-vaccine crimes that have made American infants THE MOST VACCINATED and THE MOST LIKELY TO DIE in the first year of life.

America's infant mortality rate, the highest rate in ALL developed nations, is a national tragedy. The epidemic of autism, autoimmune diseases, asthma, allergies, ADHD, and pediatric cancers is far worse.

The evidence is everywhere.

Unbelievably, the epidemic of autism is rising exponentially. Today, ONE in 48 children in America suffer autism. At the present rate of increase, by 2032 ONE in TWO children AND 80% OF BOYS could be autistic.

We can't afford to sacrifice our children and the future of our nation to the ignorance and greed of pediatricians and their big pharmaceutical vaccine manufacturer masters demanding parents submit our children to an intolerably dangerous, untested, and unnecessary vaccine schedule of 72+ injections…and rising. There are over 200 vaccines in the pipeline.

Every pediatrician, family practitioner, or vaccine profiteer that isn't rising up against the corruption of the science of vaccines perpetrated by the CDC is betraying their oath to "first, do no harm." They are on the wrong side of history.

Too many have given up objectivity and reason and have simply become sales representatives for the vaccine manufacturers that have so easily bought and conditioned them to believe their lies.

The blood of every vaccine injured or killed child is on the hands of every pediatrician that parroted lies like “vaccines do not cause autism” and “the science is settled.”

The science isn’t settled, it’s corrupt.

The vaccine industry will soon face the backlash as doctors, scientists, and parents across America become aware of your crimes, rise up to oppose your lies, and hold you accountable for the vaccine injury holocaust you’ve caused.

The fraudulent deceit is coming to and end. We won’t allow it to continue.

***

That’s how I see the travesty of the corruption of vaccines that is harming the children of America today. It’s obvious and I’m angry about my how so many of medical colleagues refuse to open the door, expose the abuse, and stop it.

In closing, I beseech my colleagues to open your eyes, minds, and the evidence that for too long you’ve negligently denied.

Confront the reality that you’ve been duped,

> controlled, and indoctrinated.
>
> Free yourselves from the indoctrination. Stand with me.
>
> Demand scientific transparency, integrity, and reform of the vaccine industry.
>
> Join me in this fight to protect children and get yourselves on the right side of history.
>
> Together we must STOP the abuse.[574] (emphasis in original)

Brett Wilcox states: "Rather than jail doctors for refusing to vaccinate their patients as has been done in the past, [J.B.] Handley advocates for the jailing of doctors who—for whatever reason—repeatedly jab sick children." In a blog article titled *Vaccines Don't Cause Autism, Pediatricians Do*, Handley wrote:

> Our community has been giving pediatricians a hall pass for far too long. If a doctor sticks six vaccines into a child while the child is taking antibiotics for an ear infection and Tylenol for a cold, he's not a doctor, he's a criminal, and should be hauled into jail on the spot for assault and battery. If the child also happens to have eczema, long-term diarrhea, and has missed a milestone or two, perhaps the charge should be attempted murder. As you know, pediatricians do just this and more every day. How do we stop this recklessness? If my son's pediatrician had been more careful, better informed of warning signs, less close-minded, and less AAP-party line in his approach to pediatrics, I genuinely believe my son never would have regressed into autism.[575]

But the pharmaceutical companies and their lackey doctors are not backing off. They know that they are engaging in criminal mischief. They also know that they have the upper hand because they have the force of government on their side. So, they are trying to turn the tables and bring the power of government down on those who would expose their malfeasance. Vaccinologists characterize parents of vaccine-injured children raising concerns about vaccine safety as part of a "hate group." Dr. Peter Hotez, M.D., Ph.D., is a vaccine developer, a former president of the Sabin Vaccine Institute, and director of the Texas Children's Center for Vaccine Development. Dr. Hotez labels organizations trying to bring vaccine dangers to light "hate groups" with a "twisted ideology."

> Anti-vaccine organizations camouflage themselves as a political group, but I call them for what they really are: a hate group. ... They are a hate group that hates their family and hates their children.[576]

Dr. Hotez holds that opinion despite having a daughter with autism. His entire career requires him to be an ardent advocate of childhood vaccines. Nothing, it seems, will change his mind. His conscience is seared as with a hot iron. Dr. Hotez is choosing his words carefully. He knows full well that once a group is deemed a 'hate group" by the government, a whole host of laws come into play that can be used to bring legal actions against any such person or organization to shut them down and silence them. Indeed, Dr. Hotez has called on G20 governments to take steps to "snuff out" anti-vaccine movements.[577]

> Given these high stakes, I believe the leaders in the US Government must become more vocal and proactive, while addressing and elevating discussions about vaccine hesitancy and antivaccine movements in international forums. Because there are particular consequences of

reduced vaccine coverage in some of the largest nations comprising the group of 20 (G20), future G20 summits might be an appropriate venue for coordinated action, in addition to the upcoming World Health Assembly in May. An American antivaccine movement is building and we need to take steps now to snuff it out.[578]

24 The Dangerous Quackery of the CDC

Writing for Science Magazine, Meredith Wadman summarized a massive research study[579] in Israel that proves natural immunity is superior to immunity from vaccines.

> The new analysis relies on the database of Maccabi Healthcare Services, which enrolls about 2.5 million Israelis. The study, led by Tal Patalon and Sivan Gazit at KSM, the system's research and innovation arm, found in two analyses that people who were vaccinated in January and February were, in June, July, and the first half of August, six to 13 times more likely to get infected than unvaccinated people who were previously infected with the coronavirus. In one analysis, comparing more than 32,000 people in the health system, the risk of developing symptomatic COVID-19 was 27 times higher among the vaccinated, and the risk of hospitalization eight times higher.[580]

Indeed, studies have shown that "'[i]ndividuals who have recovered from COVID-19 have a substantially lower risk of reinfection with SARS-Cov-2."[581] The NIH confirms this. In a study funded by NIH's National Institute of Allergy and Infectious Diseases (NIAID) and National Cancer Institute (NCI), Daniela Weiskopf analyzed immune cells and antibodies from almost 200 people exposed to SARS-CoV-2 and recovered. She said "our studies showed that natural infection induced a strong response, and this study now shows that the responses last."[582]

The natural immunity from what doctors call COVID-19 is robust and long-lasting. Researchers opine that the natural immunity from COVID-19 should last a lifetime.

> For SARS-CoV, a coronavirus very like SARS-CoV-2 that was originally identified in 2003 and causes severe acute respiratory syndrome (SARS), the continued presence of high concentrations of neutralizing antibodies in blood serum for more than 17 years was reported in 2020. Wang and colleagues' results suggest that long-term immunity might also be expected for SARS-CoV-2.[583]

Epidemiologist Dr. Paul Elias Alexander is a former assistant professor at McMaster University in evidence-based medicine and research methods. He's also a former COVID Pandemic evidence-synthesis consultant advisor to WHO-PAHO Washington, DC (2020) and former senior advisor to COVID Pandemic policy in Health and Human Services (HHS) Washington, DC. He recently published an article for the Brownstone Institute with a list of 141 research studies regarding natural COVID immunity.[584]

Those 141 studies support the claim that natural immunity to COVID is robust and long-lasting, even to the extent of lifetime immunity. For example, one study found that "the cumulative incidence of SARS-CoV-2 infection remained almost zero among previously infected unvaccinated subjects."[585]

Incidentally, the CDC distinguishes between SARS-CoV-2 and COVID-19. The CDC states that SARS-CoV-2 is the virus that causes the disease COVID-19. COVID-19 means "coronavirus disease 2019" whereas SARS-CoV-2 means "severe acute respiratory syndrome coronavirus 2." But that distinction between the two acronyms is not commonly made by the public or the medical community.[586] Most equate SARS-CoV-2 and COVID-19 and use them interchangeably to describe the alleged infectious pathogen that is purported to be transmitted from one person to another.[587] Thus, this author will use those terms interchangeably to refer to the alleged pathogen.

A recent Emory University study debunked the common myth that natural immunity to COVID-19 (i.e., SARS-CoV-2) wanes quickly, leaving the person subject to reinfection.

> Last fall, there were reports that antibodies wane quickly after infection with the virus that causes COVID-19, and mainstream media interpreted that to mean that immunity was not long-lived," said senior author Ali Ellebedy, PhD, an associate professor of pathology & immunology, of medicine and of molecular microbiology. "But that's a misinterpretation of the data. It's normal for antibody levels to go down after acute infection, but they don't go down to zero; they plateau. Here, we found antibody-producing cells in people 11 months after first symptoms. These cells will live and produce antibodies for the rest of people's lives. That's strong evidence for long-lasting immunity."[588]

A study conducted at the Washington School of Medicine in St. Louis found that even "mild cases of COVID-19 leave those infected with lasting antibody protection and that repeated bouts of illness are likely to be uncommon."[589] Another study concluded that substantial immune memory is generated after natural infection with COVID-19.[590]

Dr. Paul Alexander, Ph.D., accused CDC Director Rochelle Walensky, of lying when she stated in an October 2020 published LANCET statement that "there is no evidence for lasting protective immunity to SARS-CoV-2 following natural infection" and that "the consequence of waning immunity would present a risk to vulnerable populations for the indefinite future."[591] Dr. Alexander explains that "[i]mmunology and virology 101 have taught us over a century that natural immunity confers protection against a respiratory virus's outer coat proteins, and not just one, e.g. the SARS-CoV-2 spike glycoprotein. There is even strong evidence for the persistence of antibodies."[592] Dr. Alexander cited 160 research papers in support of his argument.

For example, in a study involving Cleveland Clinic Health System employees, not one of the 1,359 participants who had been previously infected with SARS-CoV-2 (COVID-19) who remained unvaccinated had a SARS-CoV-2 infection over the duration of the five-month study. The study concluded that "[i]ndividuals who have had SARS-CoV-2 infection are unlikely to benefit from COVID-19 vaccination."[593]

Another study compared COVID-19-vaccinated persons against those who were unvaccinated but had been infected and recovered from COVID-19. "This study demonstrated that natural immunity confers longer lasting and stronger protection against infection, symptomatic disease and hospitalization."[594] The study found a 13-fold increased risk for a breakthrough infection of COVID-19 for those in the vaccinated group compared to the unvaccinated group with natural immunity. During the follow-up period, there was a 27-fold increase in symptomatic COVID-19 in the vaccinated group compared to the unvaccinated group. The study was based on positive PCR tests and flu-like symptoms to determine a COVID-19 case. The PCR test is almost meaningless, and flu-like symptoms really means that the persons have the flu. The study, in reality, simply reveals that the COVID-19 vaccines make people ill.

The CDC and the Pharmaceutical companies have a problem because there are increasing numbers of vaccinated persons suffering what the CDC calls breakthrough COVID-19 infections. This is actually antibody-dependent enhancement (ADE), where the person becomes ill because the antibodies enhance disease rather than protect against it. So, on or about August 2021 the CDC announced a booster shot program. The CDC stated that "with the Delta variant, public health experts are starting to see reduced protection against mild and moderate disease. For that reason, the U.S. Department of Health and Human Services (HHS) is planning for a booster shot so vaccinated people maintain protection over the coming months."[595] In reality, it is the COVID-19 vaccine that is causing hospitalizations and deaths from ADE. The booster shots will continue the deadly cycle.

It would seem, therefore, common sense that there would be no need for a person to be vaccinated if he has been infected with COVID-19 and already has a robust natural immunity to the alleged virus. It is especially nonsensical for such persons to be vaccinated in light of the fact that the COVID-19 vaccines have been shown to be ineffective (and indeed drive further illness). But that is not the guidance being given by Dr. Fauci and the CDC. The CDC provides the following advice on its website:

> If I have already had COVID-19 and recovered, do I still need to get vaccinated with a COVID-19 vaccine?
>
> Yes, you should be vaccinated regardless of

whether you already had COVID-19.[596]

The CDC relied on a single research study[597] in giving that advice. That research study is full of holes. The CDC represents the study as meaning "that people get better protection by being fully vaccinated compared with having had COVID-19."[598] But the study is a retrospective study that relies on the accuracy of the records in databases. There was no validation of the data. One significant problem with the survey goes to the heart of its conclusions regarding the infection rate. The study states that "reinfection was not confirmed through whole genome sequencing, which would be necessary to definitively prove that the reinfection was caused from a distinct virus relative to the first infection."[599] Without that confirmation, the study scientists are left to merely guess that "reinfection is the most likely explanation."[600] Guessing is not science. And it seems that they guessed wrong because the study from Israel impeaches their results.

It is pointless to vaccinate someone who has already been infected with COVID-19 (a.k.a. SARS-CoV-2) and has developed a natural immune response. It is also dangerous. Dr. Hooman Noorchashm, an accomplished surgeon and staunch supporter of the new COVID vaccines, states that vaccinating persons with COVID-19 is dangerous if that person has already contracted COVID-19 and has the antibodies for the virus.[601] He has written to the FDA and advised that there should be screening to prevent those who have already contracted COVID-19 from being vaccinated. He stated that such persons are in danger of injury or death from the vaccine. Megan Redshaw, reporting for The Defender, reveals:

> According to Noorchashm, it is scientifically established that once a person is naturally infected by a virus, antigens from that virus persist in the body for a long time after viral replication has

> stopped and clinical signs of infection have resolved. When a vaccine reactivates an immune response in a recently infected person, the tissues harboring the persisting viral antigen are targeted, inflamed and damaged by the immune response.[602]

> Dr. Noorchashm explains:

> "In the case of SARS-CoV-2, we know that the virus naturally infects the heart, the inner lining of blood vessels, the lungs and the brain," explained Noorchasm. "So, these are likely to be some of the critical organs that will contain persistent viral antigens in the recently infected — and, following reactivation of the immune system by a vaccine, these tissues can be expected to be targeted and damaged."[603]

Dr. Noorchashm states: **"It is my professional opinion as an immunologist and physician that this indiscriminate vaccination is a clear and present danger to a subset of the already infected."**[604] That opinion is coming from a doctor who is an advocate in favor of the COVID-19 vaccines.

The CDC recommends vaccinations of persons who already have natural immunity to COVID-19. But both Moderna[605] and Pfizer-BioNTech[606] performed serological tests on all trial participants to specifically screen out those with COVID-19 natural immunity. Those persons necessarily had been infected previously with COVID-19 and had thus developed natural immunity. They were excluded from particpating in the COVID-19 vaccine trials. If the argument is that the COVID-19 vaccine enhances natural immunity, that group would be the ideal group with which to test that hypothesis. The CDC knew that group was not tested and yet still recommends the vaccination of that same group. But if persons with natural immunity are susceptible to a cytokine storm caused by an immediate ADE reaction, as Dr. Hooman Noorchashm has opined, such a group would reveal the danger posed to the naturally immune population. Arguably, Moderna and Pfizer-BioNTech ensured that would not happen by disqualifying all persons with serological tests that showed that the persons already had natural immunity.

Congressman Thomas Massie (R-Ky.), an award-winning scientist, said that the CDC is providing misinformation to the public by recommending that those who have already recovered from COVID-19 should still be vaccinated. Massie told the CDC that their report alleging the efficacy of vaccinating those who already had COVID-19 immunity was flat wrong. How did the CDC respond to Massie's objection? Megan Redshaw reports:

> Massie contacted officials at the CDC about the misinformation. They acknowledged it was false, but instead of correcting it, tried to rephrase their mistake. Massie and other scientists said the new wording still wrongly implies vaccines work in people who previously had COVID.
>
> "And instead of fixing it, they proposed repeating it and just phrasing their mistake differently. **So, at that point, right now I consider it a lie. I think the CDC is lying about the efficacy of the vaccine** based on the Pfizer trials, for those who have already had the coronavirus,"[607] Massie said. (emphasis added)

The CDC is knowingly and intentionally lying to the American people and advising those who already have a natural immunity to COVID-19 to nonetheless be vaccinated. It is ineffective and dangerous for a person who has natural immunity to the illness called COVID-19 to be vaccinated against it. The CDC acknowledges that their advice is wrong, but they are continuing with it.

Why is the CDC recommending COVID-19 vaccinations that have now been proven to be ineffective? Whatever immunity they offer is temporary. Because of their short-lived effectiveness, the CDC is starting a booster shot program. With that in mind, the CDC advises those who have a natural immunity that is robust and long-lasting to receive a COVID-19 vaccine. It makes no sense to advise the injection of a vaccine that has been proven to offer only short-duration benefit (if any) to a person who already has lifelong immunity. There is something else at play here other than the health of the citizens. It is like handing an umbrella to a skydiver with a parachute strapped to his back and telling him the umbrella will slow his descent. The COVID-19 vaccines (like the umbrella) do more harm than good for someone with natural immunity. The primary agenda of the CDC seems to be the vaccination of American citizens and not their good health.

The Israeli COVID-19 study was published on August 26, 2021.[608] The study was worldwide news among epidemiologists. But, on September 9, 2021, when he was asked about the study, Dr. Anthony Fauci feigned ignorance of its implications. Dr. Fauci is the Director of the National Institute of Allergy and Infectious Diseases (NIAID). Dr. Fauci is alleged to be "the nation's top infectious disease expert"[609] and "one of the world's leading clinicians and researchers on the pathogenesis and treatment of immune-mediated diseases."[610] Dr. Fauci is also a member of the White House Coronavirus Task Force. But he did not have an answer to the study that made worldwide news in the scientific community proving that natural immunity to COVID-19 was superior to vaccinated immunity. Let us read the exchange between Dr. Sanjay Gupta, the CNN Chief Medical Correspondent and Dr. Fauci:

> GUPTA: And just real quickly, there was a study that came out of Israel about natural immunity, and

basically, the headline was that natural immunity provides a lot of protection, even better than the vaccines alone. What do people make of that? So as we talk about vaccine mandates, I get calls all the time, people say, I've already had COVID, I'm protected. And now the study says maybe even more protected than the vaccine alone. Should they also get the vaccine? How do you make the case to them?

FAUCI: You know, that's a really good point, Sanjay. **I don't have a really firm answer for you on that.** That's something that we're going to have to discuss regarding the durability of the response. The one thing that paper from Israel didn't tell you is whether or not as high as the protection is with natural infection, what's the durability compared to the durability of a vaccine? So it is conceivable that you got infected, you're protected, but you may not be protected for an indefinite period of time. So, I think that is something that we need to sit down and discuss seriously, because you very appropriately pointed out, it is an issue, and there could be an argument for saying what you said.[611]

Dr. Fauci, "the nation's top infectious disease expert,"[612] does not know what to say about a study that confirms the well-known fact that natural immunity is superior to vaccinated immunity. All of the questions he raised about the study are answered in numerous other studies and research proving robust and long-lasting protection from natural immunity. Juxtaposing that research against the data showing the short-lived COVID-19 vaccine immunity that requires booster shots and the answers to his questions are ineluctable. He is an epidemiological expert. He must already have known the answers to his own questions. His questions were a smokescreen. Dr. Fauci is feigning ignorance of the Israeli study's implications because the study impeaches the CDC protocol calling for the vaccination of those with natural immunity.

Compare Dr. Fauci's response to the Israeli study to that of Former FDA Commissioner Scott Gottlieb, a Pfizer board member. Although Gottlieb's opinion is decidedly against the pecuniary interests of Pfizer, Gottlieb had little trouble acknowledging that the Israeli study showed that natural immunity confers durable protection from COVID-19.

> "The balance of the evidence demonstrates that natural immunity confers a durable protection," Gottlieb said during an Aug. 30 interview, referring to a landmark new preprint Israeli study that found that prior COVID-19 infection confers more protection against the virus than any of the vaccines. "It's fair to conclude that."[613]

In September 2021, a New York attorney, Elizabeth Brehm from the law firm Siri & Glimstead, sent a Freedom of Information request to the CDC asking for "[d]ocuments reflecting any documented case of an individual who: (1) never received a COVID-19 vaccine; (2) was infected with COVID-19 once, recovered, and then later became infected again; and (3) transmitted SARS-CoV-2 to another person when reinfected."[614]

The CDC responded to that request by revealing that "[a] search of our records failed to reveal any documents pertaining to your request. The CDC Emergency Operations Center (EOC) conveyed that this information is not collected."[615]

The CDC makes two revealing admissions. They acknowledge that they do not have any data indicating that natural immunity is inadequate protection. And, more revealing, they divulged that they don't collect that information. Thus, the CDC confessed that they don't care to know the effectiveness of natural immunity. The CDC simply does not care whether innate immunity to COVID-19 protects the person or others with whom the person comes in contact.

Yet, acting out of willful ignorance, the CDC recommends that a person who has already been infected by what is described as COVID-19, who has recovered and has natural immunity, still needs to be vaccinated with the COVID-19 vaccine. But the CDC does not know if that advice is correct, nor it seems does it care. Aaron Siri, the named partner in the law firm that made the FOIA request of the CDC, explained the significance of the CDC's admissions:

> You would assume that if the CDC was going to crush the civil and individual rights of those with natural immunity by having them expelled from school, fired from their jobs, separated from the military, and worse, the CDC would have proof of at least one instance of an unvaccinated, naturally immune individual transmitting the COVID-19 virus to another individual. If you thought this, you would be wrong.
>
> My firm, on behalf of ICAN, asked the CDC for precisely this proof (see below). ICAN wanted to see proof of any instance in which someone who previously had COVID-19 became reinfected with and transmitted the virus to someone else. The CDC's incredible response is that it does not have a single document reflecting that this has ever occurred. Not one.
>
> In contrast, there are endless documents reflecting cases of vaccinated individuals becoming infected with and transmitting the virus to others. Such as

this study.[616] And this study.[617] And this study.[618] And this study.[619] It goes on and on…

But it gets worse. The CDC's excuse for not having a shred of evidence of the naturally immune transmitting the virus is that "this information is not collected." What?! No proof! But yet the CDC is actively crushing the rights of millions of naturally immune individuals in this country if they do not get the vaccine on the assumption they can transmit the virus. But despite clear proof the vaccinated spread the virus, the CDC lifts restrictions on the vaccinated?! That is dystopian.

The facts about natural immunity are simple. Every single peer reviewed study has found that the naturally immune have far greater than 99% protection from having COVID-19, and this immunity does not wane. In contrast, the COVID-19 vaccine provides, at best, 95% protection and this immunity wanes rapidly. I am no mathematician, but a constant 99% seems preferable to a 95% that quickly drops. And, while the vaccinated readily transmit the virus, not so for the naturally immune.

The lesson yet again is not that health authorities should never make mistakes. They will. It happens. The lesson is that civil and individual rights should never be contingent upon a medical procedure. Everyone, the naturally immune or otherwise, who wants to get vaccinated and boosted should be free to do so. But nobody should be coerced by the government to partake in any medical procedure.

The CDC defines immunity as "[p]rotection from an

infectious disease. If you are immune to a disease, you can be exposed to it without becoming infected."[620] But it seems that the CDC does not recognize the efficacy of natural immunity. The CDC recognizes immunity through vaccination to the exclusion of natural immunity. It defines "immunization" as "[a] process by which a person becomes protected against a disease **through vaccination**. This term is often used interchangeably with vaccination or inoculation."[621] The CDC makes no mention of immunization from a disease by recovering from an infection. The CDC has a vaccination agenda that flies in the face of voluminous scientific evidence proving the efficacy of natural immunity.

On December 19, 2022, the Cleveland Clinic, which Newsweek ranked as the second best hospital in the world,[622] published a study of COVID-19 vaccine efficacy.[623] The study involved 51,011 people who worked at the Cleveland Clinic. The researchers found:

> The risk of COVID-19 also varied by the number of COVID-19 vaccine doses previously received. The higher the number of vaccines previously received, the higher the risk of contracting COVID.[624]

The finding by the researchers that "the greater the number of vaccine doses previously received, the higher the risk of COVID-19" was confirmed by two other research papers cited in the Cleveland Clinic study.[625] The added risk was significant. The study found that a vaccinated person getting one shot of COVID-19 vaccine was 1.7 times more likely to be infected with COVID-19 than an unvaccinated person.[626] But the incidence of getting COVID-19 increases with each shot. If a person gets two shots of COVID-19 vaccine, his likelihood of getting COVID-19 is 2.63-fold greater than an unvaccinated person. A person getting three shots raises the likelihood of getting COVID-19 to 3.15 times greater than an unvaccinated person. And if a person is injected more than three times with a COVID-19 vaccine, he is 3.38 times more likely to be infected with COVID-19 than someone who remains unvaccinated.

Thus, there is a direct correlation between the number of COVID-19 shots and the rate of COVID-19 infection. More COVID-19 shots increase the incidence of COVID-19 infection. It seems that the COVID-19 vaccines are driving the COVID-19 infection. But what is actually happening is that the COVID-19 vaccines are making people sick through the mechanism of antibody-dependent enhancement. The victims test positive for COVID-19, and thus they are labeled as COVID-19 "breakthrough" infections.

The increased risk of COVID-19 from the COVID-19 vaccines was known by both Pfizer and the FDA as early as September 17, 2021.[627] Pfizer revealed in its FDA briefing document that a person who received two Pfizer vaccinations against COVID-19 was likelier to get COVID-19 than a person who did not receive any COVID-19 vaccination. Steve Kirsch analyzed the Pfizer data and extrapolated that Pfizers' own data showed that a person who was doubly vaccinated with a Pfizer COVID-19 vaccine was 2.13 times more likely to be infected with COVID-19 than an unvaccinated person.[628]

While knowing that persons were more likely to get COVID-19 if they received a COVID-19 vaccine, the CDC continued to falsely claim "that receiving any vaccine is better than being unvaccinated."[629] The CDC continued to recommend that persons be vaccinated with mRNA COVID-19 vaccines while knowing that those vaccines were ineffective and actually increased the risk of contracting COVID-19. Now, the Cleveland Clinic has come out with a study proving what the FDA, CDC, and Pfizer had known for over a year prior.

It was only on April 19, 2023, that the CDC stopped

recommending the monovalent (original) mRNA COVID-19 for use in the United States. But the CDC continues to recommend the newer bivalent mRNA COVID-19 boosters regardless of whether the person has received the primary monovalent series. The CDC is making that recommendation knowing that the Cleveland Clinic study included persons who received the bivalent booster. That Cleveland Clinic study proves that "the greater the number of vaccine doses previously received, the higher the risk of COVID-19." Yet, the CDC continues to recommend the COVID-19 vaccines.

The CDC is recommending vaccines that it knows will make people sick. It is not that the vaccines are ineffective in protecting a person from COVID-19. Rather, the vaccines are causing the illnesses. A person may test positive for COVID-19, and thus the illness is listed as COVID-19, but what is happening is that the vaccines are causing antibody-dependent enhancement (ADE), which in turn causes the person to have flu-like symptoms. The person may also come down with other debilitating illnesses and even permanent disabilities. The CDC knows this. And that is the plan. The CDC is not run by stupid people. It is run by evil people. The plan is to injure and kill as many people as possible through the COVID-19 vaccine program.

George Orwell explained: "All tyrannies rule through fraud and force, but once the fraud is exposed, they must rely exclusively on force." The fraud behind the unsafe and ineffective COVID-19 vaccines is increasingly being exposed. Since so many people are not being tricked by the fraud, the government has resorted to its only remaining option, force. And that explains President Biden's edicts requiring ordinary citizens, federal workers, military personnel, and medical workers to get vaccinated.

25 COVID-19 Vaccines are Ineffective

On August 26, 2022, the CDC claimed that "[h]ospitalization rates among unvaccinated adults were 3.4 times as high as those among vaccinated adults."[630] But the report's published statistics reveal that 44.1% of persons hospitalized during the period spanning June 20, 2021–May 31, 2022 were fully vaccinated:

> Among hospitalized nonpregnant patients in this same period, 39.1% had received a primary vaccination series and 1 booster or additional dose; 5.0% had received a primary series and ≥2 boosters or additional doses.[631]

According to the CDC published statistics, 44.1% (39.1% + 5.0%) of those hospitalized between June 20, 2021 and May 31, 2022, for COVID-19 had been fully vaccinated and received at least one COVID-19 booster shot. Please understand that those statistics are manipulated to inflate the numbers for COVID-19 unvaccinated patients while deflating the numbers for COVID-19 vaccinated patients.[632]

In a report of Los Angeles County, California, COVID-19 deaths and hospitalizations, it was revealed that the CDC classified COVID-19 hospitalizations and deaths of fully vaccinated persons only if those persons are hospitalized or die 14 days or more after the final dose of a COVID-19 vaccine.[633]

The CDC also decided that someone who dies or is hospitalized after receiving a COVID-19 vaccine will nonetheless be listed as an unvaccinated death or hospitalization if that person died less than 14 days after receiving the first dose of a two-dose series (Moderna and Pfizer) or the first dose of a one dose administration (Johnson & Johnson) or if they cannot determine when the person was vaccinated when referencing the California Immunization Registry.

All other cases falling outside those parameters will be considered partially vaccinated. Partially vaccinated persons would be those who died or were hospitalized ≥14 days after receiving the first dose and <14 days after the second dose in a 2-dose series.

How are partially vaccinated persons treated statistically by the CDC? The CDC states:

> For the purpose of this surveillance, a vaccine breakthrough infection is defined as the detection of SARS-CoV-2 RNA or antigen in a respiratory specimen collected from a person ≥14 days after they have completed all recommended doses of a U.S. Food and Drug Administration (FDA)-authorized COVID-19 vaccine.[634]

Dr. Joseph Mercola explains:

> The CDC is also playing with statistics in other ways to create the false and inaccurate impression that unvaccinated people make up the bulk of infections, hospitalizations and deaths. For example, we now find out the agency is counting

anyone who died within the first 14 days post-injection as unvaccinated.

Not only does this inaccurately inflate the unvaccinated death toll, but it also hides the real dangers of the COVID shots, as the vast majority of deaths from these shots occur within the first two weeks. Now their deaths are counted as unvaccinated deaths rather than being counted as deaths due to vaccine injury or COVID-19 breakthrough infections![635]

***

In other words, if you've received one dose of Pfizer or Moderna and develop symptomatic COVID-19, get admitted to the hospital and/or die from COVID, you're counted as an unvaccinated case. If you've received two doses and get ill within 14 days, you're still counted as an unvaccinated case.

The problem with this is that over 80% of hospitalizations and deaths appear to be occurring among those who have received the jabs, but this reality is hidden by the way cases are defined and counted. A really clever and common strategy of the CDC during the pandemic has been to change the definitions and goalposts so it supports their nefarious narrative.[636]

A breakthrough case is a person who is deemed to be infected with COVID-19 only after being fully vaccinated 14 days or more after receiving all recommended COVID-19 vaccine doses. That means that a partially vaccinated person is NOT listed among the breakthrough cases. That, in turn, means that a partially vaccinated person diagnosed with COVID-19 is NOT listed among the breakthrough COVID-19 cases. Thus, the CDC treats partially vaccinated persons as being unvaccinated COVID-19 cases statistically.

Another confounding factor explained by Dr. Mercola is that to "count as a confirmed vaccinated individual, you must send your vaccination card to your primary care physician's office and have them add it to your electronic medical record. If you got the shot at a pharmacy, you'll need to verify that they forwarded your proof of vaccination to your doctor. Primary care offices are then responsible for sharing their patients' immunization data with the state's immunization information system. Patient-recorded proof of vaccination is only accepted for influenza and pneumococcal vaccines, not COVID-19 injections. What this all means is that, say you got the shot several weeks ago at a drive-through vaccination clinic and get admitted to the hospital with COVID symptoms. Unless your COVID shot status has actually been added into the medical system, you will not be counted as 'vaccinated.'"[637] This all has the effect of artificially inflating the unvaccinated COVID-19 infection tally while showing a misleadingly reduced breakthrough infection rate for those vaccinated.

Likely, the deaths and hospitalizations suffered by those vaccinated for COVID-19 are not because the vaccines have failed to protect those who were vaccinated but rather because the vaccines are causing the deaths and hospitalizations through what is called antibody-dependent enhancement (ADE).[638] Indeed, that is the conclusion of renowned virologist and Nobel Prize Laureate Prof. Luc Montagnier.[639]

The CDC is trying to keep a lid on antibody-dependent enhancement (ADE). ADE can happen many months after vaccination, but ADE can sometimes manifest early. For example, 35 nuns received COVID-19 vaccines, and within two days, 28 nuns fell ill and tested positive for COVID-19, with two nuns dying during those two days.[640] A third nun also died days later. That is clear evidence of ADE within days of being vaccinated. Such evidence of early-onset ADE is information the CDC does not want to be known. And so, from now on, those cases will be listed as unvaccinated COVID-19 cases.

The CDC is trying to bury their statistical sleight of hand down a memory hole. The above language from the CDC that a COVID-19 breakthrough infection is limited to a COVID-19 diagnosis from a person ≥14 days after they have completed all recommended COVID-19 vaccines that had been posted on the CDC website on or before September 3, 2021, at the URL cited in the endnote has been deleted from the CDC website. But Washoe County (Nevada) Health District quotes that deleted CDC language on its COVID-19 Facts page.[641]

The CDC is playing a game of trying to obfuscate the ADE cases (which the CDC calls breakthrough COVID-19 cases) suffered by vaccinated persons while continuing to inflate the alleged COVID-19 cases suffered by the unvaccinated population. The false narrative of a killer SARS-CoV-2 virus causing COVID-19 disease has been generated by two principle methods. 1) false-positive PCR tests which can be manipulated into reporting an artificially high number of false-positives by altering the cycle threshold (CT value), and 2) inflating the case count by a broad definition of what is a COVID-19 case, such as listing a positive PCR test as a COVID-19 case, even if the person never experienced any symptoms. But it seems that inflation strategy began to backfire.

It was becoming an embarrassment to the FDA, CDC, and the vaccine makers because their COVID-19 inflation efforts began to present a very high number of breakthrough infections (which are really ADE cases) for vaccinated persons. To address this, the CDC announced new rules for reporting breakthrough cases of vaccinated persons that they do not apply to unvaccinated persons. First, the CDC instructed local health officials, when reporting breakthrough COVID-19 infections for vaccinated persons, to "submit only specimens with Ct value ≤28 to CDC for sequencing."[642] But the CDC left standing its recommended cycle threshold of 40 cycles for testing unvaccinated patients.[643] Even Anthony Fauci admitted that a cycle threshold more than 35 in a PCR test would return a meaningless false postive test result.[644]

To further lower the reported numbers of breathrough cases, the CDC announced that "[a]s of May 1, 2021, CDC transitioned from monitoring all reported vaccine breakthrough cases to focus on identifying and investigating only hospitalized or fatal cases due to any cause."[645] Neither of these two new strategies were applied to the unvaccinated reporting. There are now different rules for reporting vaccinated COVID-19 cases and unvaccinated COVID-19 cases. The effect is to lower the reported number of vaccinated COVID-19 breakthrough cases while continuing the stratagem of inflating the reported unvaccinated COVID-19 cases. Dr. Joseph Mercola summarizes the consequences of the CDC's data manipulation.

> It's not just the CDC's definition of a breakthrough case that skews the data. Even more egregious and illogical is the fact that the CDC even has two different sets of testing guidelines — one for vaccinated patients and another for the unvaccinated.
>
> Since the beginning of the pandemic, the CDC has recommended a PCR test cycle threshold (CT) of 40. This flies in the face of scientific consensus, which has long been that a CT over 35 will produce 97% false positives, essentially rendering the test useless.

> In mid-May 2021, the CDC finally lowered its recommended CT count, but only for patients who have received one or more COVID shots. So, if you have received a COVID injection, the CDC's guidelines call for your PCR test to be run at a CT of 28 or less. If you are unvaccinated, your PCR test is to be run at a CT of 40, which grossly overestimates the true prevalence of infection.
>
> The end result is that unvaccinated individuals who get tested are FAR more prone to get false positives, while those who have received the jab are more likely to get an accurate diagnosis of infection.[646]

Reporting for *Off Guardian*, Kit Knightly explains how the CDC manipulates data to prop up vaccine efficacy while keeping the COVID-19 scare going. In a series of examples, she describes how under similar circumstances one could be reported as a COVID-19 case when unvaccinated but not reported as a COVID-19 case when vaccinated under the CDC reporting standards.

> Person A has **not been vaccinated**. They test positive for COVID using a PCR test at 40 cycles and, despite having no symptoms, they are officially a "COVID case". [But the person would NOT be a COVID case if he were **vaccinated**.]
>
> Person B has been **vaccinated**. They test positive at 28 cycles, and spend six weeks bedridden with a high fever. Because they never went into a hospital and didn't die they are NOT a COVID case. [But the person would be reported as a COVID case if he were **not vaccinated**.]

> Person C, who was also **vaccinated**, did die. After weeks in hospital with a high fever and respiratory problems. Only their positive PCR test was 29 cycles, so they're not officially a COVID case either. [But the person would be reported as a COVID case if he were **not vaccinated**.][647]

Even those efforts by the CDC to manipulate the data cannot mask the ineffectiveness of the COVID-19 vaccines. With those numbers, how can anyone say that the COVID-19 vaccines effectively stop COVID-19 infection? The major takeaway from these statistics is that massive numbers of vaccinated people are being hospitalized for illnesses attributed to COVID-19. In reality, they are suffering diseases stemming from antibody-dependent enhancement (ADE) caused by the COVID-19 vaccines.

One might argue that the reason that so many vaccinated people are being hospitalized for COVID-19 compared to the unvaccinated is that the population of vaccinated people is greater. But when we look at death rates from COVID-19 and adjust for population, we find that, in fact, those who are vaccinated are dying at a greater rate from COVID-19 than those who are unvaccinated. A former reporter for the New York Times, Alex Berenson, analyzed the official data from the UK government comparing the death rate of those who had been vaccinated with a COVID-19 vaccine with those who remained unvaccinated.[648] He made a startling discovery. Those who had been vaccinated are dying at more than twice the rate of those who remained unvaccinated.[649]

Below is a chart that illustrates the difference in the death rates. The chart reflects a comparison of deaths per 100,000 vaccinated persons against the deaths per 100,000 of unvaccinated persons. The graph shows that vaccinated persons are dying at more than twice the rate of unvaccinated persons. Berenson observed that "overall deaths in Britain are running well above normal."[650] That means that the higher number of deaths among vaccinated persons are an aberration that can only be explained by the variable: vaccination. That, in turn, means that there must be a causal link between vaccination and a higher death rate. Berenson drew the only logical conclusion from that data: **"I don't know how to explain this other than vaccine-caused mortality."**[651]

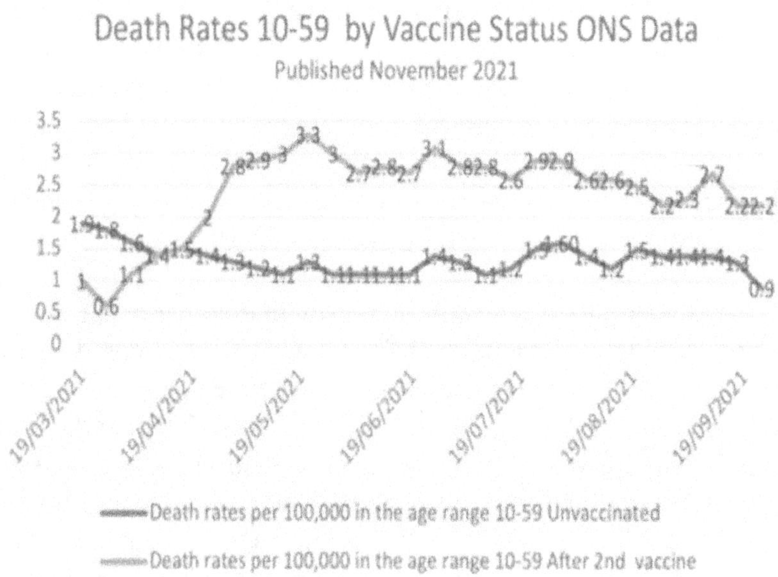

This author looked at the data in the Excel spreadsheet[652] prepared by the UK Government and did a little calculating of my own. My calculations confirm the findings of Alex Benson. Interestingly, the data further shows that across the board the unvaccinated die at a lower rate than the population as a whole. It seems that the unvaccinated are healthier than the general population.

This author found the exact opposite when I looked at the death rate of the vaccinated population. Those who are vaccinated with the COVID-19 vaccine die at a greater rate than the population as a whole. This suggests that the vaccinated population is less healthy than the general population. This data confirms the research done regarding childhood vaccination. Children who receive childhood vaccinations are significantly less healthy than their unvaccinated counterparts.[653]

I took the averages of the deaths per week during the reporting period from January 8, 2021, to September 24, 2021 reported by the UK Government. I found that the average per week mortality rate was 14.6 per 100,000 persons for unvaccinated persons. Multiplying that figure by 52 weeks we arrive at a yearly mortality rate of **0.76%**. That is lower than the average mortality rate of 0.94% for England as a whole.

But when this author looked at the average per week mortality rate for those who received two COVID 19 vaccination shots I found that 26.58 persons out of 100,000 persons who received two doses died per week on average. That is an average yearly mortality rate of **1.4%**. That mortality rate far exceeds the average mortality rate for England of 0.94%.

This author found that on average per week 18.09 persons per 100,00 persons who received one dose of the vaccine died within 21 days of the first dose of the COVID vaccine. That matches the average yearly mortality rate of 0.94% for England.

But what was most remarkable was the mortality rate measured for those who died 21 or more days after the first dose of the COVID-19 vaccine. This author found that on average 30.04 per 100,000 persons died per week who received one dose of the COVID-19 vaccine when their deaths happened 21 days or more after the first dose of the COVID-19 vaccine. That translates to an average yearly mortality rate of **1.6%** for those who make it 21 days or more after the first shot of the COVID-19 vaccine. That is far above the average mortality rate in England of 0.94%.

In conclusion, the official data from the UK Government shows that those vaccinated with two doses of the COVID-19 vaccine have a mortality rate of **1.4%**, which is almost twice the mortality rate (**0.76%**) of those who are unvaccinated. The average death rate for the entire English population, which includes vaccinated and unvaccinated, is 0.94%. Thus, the unvaccinated die at a lower rate than the general population. In contrast, the vaccinated persons die at a greater rate than the general population.

When one realizes that the persons who die after the first shot are not around to get a second shot, one can reasonably conclude that the data for the post-second shot mortality rate understates the deadliness of the COVID-19 vaccines. That is a problem because the standard for reporting vaccine deaths is to report only those deaths 14 days or more after receiving the second shot as deaths of vaccinated persons. A person who only receives one COVID-19 shot or who dies within 14 days of the second shot is considered to be unvaccinated. Those persons fall in the unvaccinated column even though the persons received one or even two vaccination shots. The UK data in this report is unusual in that it separately reports those who died after the first shot.

Dr. Günter Kampf, a Professor at the University Medicine Greifswald, Institute for Hygiene and Environmental Medicine, wrote an article published in *The Lancet* explaining that official government data shows that COVID-19 is being spread mainly through those who have received a COVID-19 vaccination. Dr. Kampf explains:

> In Germany, the rate of symptomatic COVID-19 cases among the fully vaccinated ("breakthrough infections") is reported weekly since July 2021 and was 16.9% at that time among patients of 60 years and older. This proportion is increasing week by week and was 58.9% on 27. October 2021 [...]

providing clear evidence of the increasing relevance of the fully vaccinated as a possible source of transmission.[654]

Below is a chart showing the "[v]accination rates and proportions of fully vaccinated people among symptomatic COVID-19 cases (≥60 years) in Germany between 21 July and 27 October 2021 based on the weekly reports from the Robert Koch-Institute."[655]

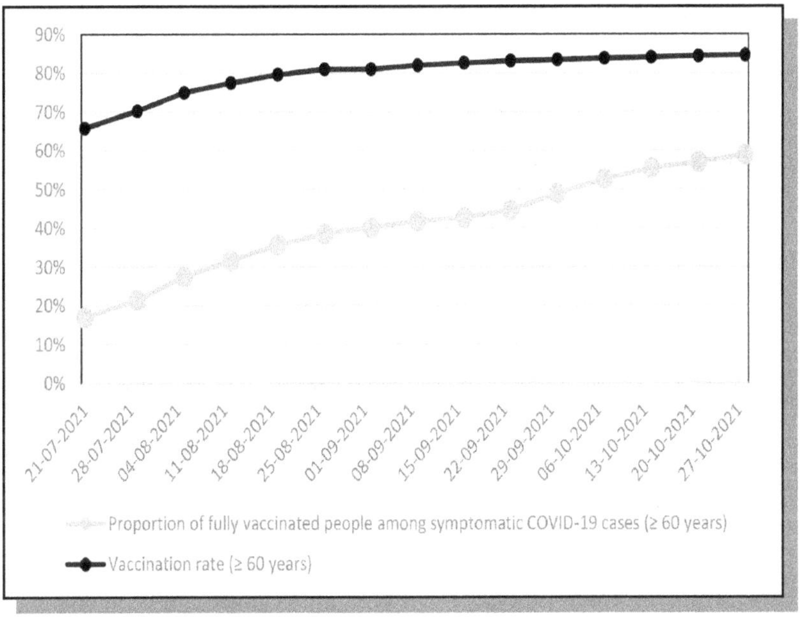

The report upon which the above statistics are based is from the Robert Koch Institute.[656] "The Robert Koch Institute (RKI) is the [German] government's central scientific institution in the field of biomedicine."[657] RKI is tasked with the identification, surveillance, and prevention of diseases to provide the German government with a scientific basis for health-related political decision-making.

Dr. Kampf explains that the RKI study reveals that in Germany, as of October 2021, 58.9% of the symptomatic COVID-19 cases among those ≥ 60 years old are from vaccinated persons. That suggests that the vaccines are driving the infection.

The chart below illustrates that the German data set from the Koch Institute revealed that there were 4,206 cases of the Omicron variant of COVID-19 in Germany between 21 July and 27 October 2021. Of those 4,206 reported cases, 4,020 infected people were fully vaccinated (2,883) or both fully vaccinated and boosted (1,137) (2,883 + 1,137 = 4,020). Only 186 of the reported Omicron COVID-19 cases were unvaccinated. Thus, more than 95% of Germany's reported Omicron COVID-19 variant infections were people who were fully vaccinated or both fully vaccinated and boosted.

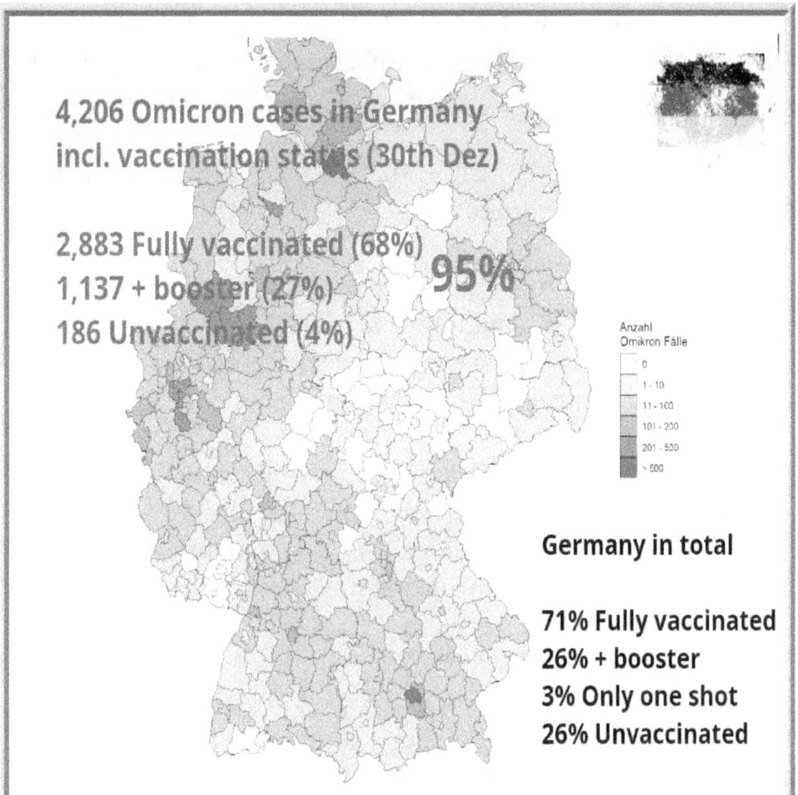

Abbildung 9: Verteilung nach Landkreisen der seit KW 46/2021 mittels variantenspezifischer PCR oder Gesamtgenomsequenzierung detektierter Omikronfälle (B.1.1.529). Es handelt sich um 10.443 Fälle seit dem 21.11.2021 (Datenstand 28.12.2021).

The Delta and Omicron variants of COVID-19 seem to be cover stories to explain away ADE being suffered by COVID-19 vaccine recipients. There is no other reasonable explanation for the fact that RKI has reported that more than 95% of all the Omicron variant cases in Germany are from those who have received two or more doses of the COVID-19 vaccine.[658] Notably, there is no reporting category for those who received only one (1) dose of the COVID-19 vaccine.[659] It is, therefore, likely that single-dose recipients have been included in the "unvaccinated" group. Thus it appears that the vaccines are driving the Omicron variant of COVID-19. Omicron bears all of the hallmarks of ADE, but there is a complete media blackout of ADE. And so, the vaccinated persons diagnosed with COVID-19 are not being described as ADE cases but instead are being mischaracterized as breakthrough Omicron variant cases.

On December 21, 2021, Ethan Huff, writing for NEWSTARGET reported:

> "It appears to be grossly negligent to ignore the vaccinated population as a possible and relevant source of transmission when deciding about public health control measures," Kampf says.
>
> To continue calling the current situation a "pandemic of the unvaccinated" is simply false, Kampf warns. In reality, this is a pandemic of the vaccinated, as the plandemic would already be over had everyone chosen to remain unvaccinated.[660]

Dr. Kampf does not address antibody-dependent enhancement (ADE), which is the actual cause of the illnesses among those vaccinated. What is truly happening is that the vaccinated are suffering the symptoms of antibody-dependent enhancement (ADE). The patients reporting to the hospital with severe illnesses caused by the vaccines are testing positive for COVID-19, thus being labeled as COVID-19 breakthrough cases. In reality, they are suffering from the ADE side effects of the vaccine itself.

The vaccine makers are scamming the public when they claim their vaccines work. Moderna, for example, reported to the FDA that their studies showed a 94.1% efficacy for their Moderna COVID-19 mRNA vaccine. But that figure is the relative risk reduction and not the total (absolute) risk reduction. The total risk reduction for the Moderna vaccine is only 1.25%. That means that one can expect that there will be a reduction of 1.25% in

COVID-19 infections in the population after being vaccinated. Thus you would have to vaccinate 10,000 persons to protect the 125 people at risk from COVID-19. That means that the federal government is needlessly paying to vaccinate 9,875 out of every 10,000 persons. Such a massive vaccine program to protect so few people only benefits the vaccine makers. And when one realizes that the vaccine is driving ADE, which the medical community is reporting as COVID-19, it explains perfectly why the data shows that more vaccinated persons are being infected and hospitalized with COVID-19 than unvaccinated persons.

When a vaccinated person is diagnosed with COVID-19 it is called a breakthrough case. Even with the efforts of the CDC to under-report COVID-19 breakthrough cases involving vaccinated persons, while at the same time inflating the unvaccinated COVID-19 infection numbers, the data shows a growing trend of vaccinated persons being infected, hospitalized, and dying from COVID-19. While the data shows that the vaccines are ineffective, the federal and state governments are still pushing COVID-19 vaccines as safe and effective. For example, the State of Maryland Department of Health vaccine information website states:

> Vaccines are an effective and critical tool to bring the pandemic under control by helping to prevent infection, serious illness, hospitalization and death due to COVID-19. **Although there are cases of people who become sick after they are fully vaccinated, cases where fully vaccinated people are hospitalized or die from COVID-19 are rare and vaccines remain the best way to prevent COVID-19 and its complications.**[661]

The problem with that statement is that it is not true. Writing for the Gateway Pundit, Joe Hoft revealed that the state government statistics from the Maryland Department of Health (MDH) contradict the above statement.[662] The MDH data showed that "[b]etween Sept 22, 2021, and Oct 10, 2021, Maryland had an additional 21,864 Covid-19 cases [of] which 7,233 or 33.1% of the cases were classified as breakthrough cases. ... During this same period, Maryland lost 259 citizens to Covid-19. Of those 259 souls, 77 or 29.7% were fully vaccinated."[663] The MDH has the temerity to claim that it is rare for fully vaccinated people to be hospitalized or die from COVID-19, when its own statistics show that a significant plurality of the population dying from COVID-19 are those who have been vaccinated.

None other than the former CDC Director, Robert Redfield, refuted the false claim made by the State of Maryland Department of Health that it is rare for a fully vaccinated person to die from COVID-19. On or about October 25, 2021, Redfield responded to a question from Martha MacCallum on FOX News about Colin Powell's recent death that his family states was caused by the COVID-19 vaccine:

> I hear a lot of times people feel it's a rare event that fully vaccinated people may die. I happen to be the senior advisor to Governor Hogan in the state of Maryland. In the last 6-8 weeks, more than 40 percent of people who died in Maryland were fully vaccinated."[664]

Jim Hoft explained that "Andy Owen, a spokesperson for the Maryland Department of Health had a different claim that from Sept. 1 to Oct. 15, only about 30% of Marylanders who died of confirmed COVID-19 were fully vaccinated."[665]

Whether it is 30% or 40%, is really of no import. The fact that any vaccinated persons, let alone such a significant plurality of vaccinated people, are being diagnosed as having COVID-19 and dying from it is stark proof that the COVID-19 vaccines are ineffective. Assuming those deaths are actually from ADE caused by the COVID-19 vaccines proves that the vaccines are also unsafe. But what is really disturbing is that in the face of such evidence that a significant number of persons vaccinated with COVID-19 vaccines are dying, state health authorities claim that "cases where fully vaccinated people are hospitalized or die from COVID-19 are rare and vaccines remain the best way to prevent COVID-19 and its complications."[666] That is an unconscionable lie.

That kind of deception by state health officials is being played out all over the country. Hoft explains:

> In Pennsylvania, the acting Sec. of Health Alison Beam stated at a news conference at Lancaster General Hospital, "With nearly seven million Pennsylvanians fully vaccinated, the data makes it clear: the vaccines are safe and effective at preventing severe illness from Covid-19."
>
> However, recent analysis of cases and deaths between September 15 and Oct 4 show that in 132k cases, 26.1% of them were classified as breakthrough and 305 (26.5%) deaths out of a total of 1,153 were in fully vaccinated people. But Sec. of Health Alison Beam makes no mention of that.[667]

Hoft cites a UK Government Health report showing "that between week 37 and week 40 of 2021, there was a total of 2,805 COVID-19 deaths and 2,136 or 76.1% were fully vaccinated. These deaths happened within 28 days of a positive Covid-19 test."[668] Yet, in the face of that data, the British Government health officials still promote the COVID-19 vaccines as effective in preventing COVID-19, and they claim that the COVID-19 vaccines provide a high level of protection against death from COVID-19.[669] The UK Government dares to recommend the COVID-19 vaccines despite official UK Government statistics that reveal that those who had been vaccinated are dying at more than twice the rate of those who remained unvaccinated.[670]

On or about July 27, 2021, Dr. Anthony Fauci, Director of the National Institute of Allergy and Infectious Diseases (NIAID), and member of the White House coronavirus task force, said

> When you look at the virus in the nasal pharynx of a vaccinated person who gets a breakthrough infection with [the] delta [variant of COVID-19], it is exactly the same as the level of virus in a unvaccinated person who is infected. That's the problem.[671]

On or about August 7, 2021, CDC Director Rochelle Walensky stated the following during a CNN interview:

> Our vaccines are working exceptionally well. They continue to work well for Delta with regard to severe illness and death, they prevent it. **But what they can't do anymore is prevent transmission.**[672] (emphasis added)

That was a retraction of Walensky's earlier mistaken claim in March 2021 that vaccinated people almost never carry COVID-19.

The Washington Post reported on an internal document from the CDC:

> It cites a combination of recently obtained, still-unpublished data from outbreak investigations and outside studies showing that vaccinated individuals infected with delta may be able to transmit the virus as easily as those who are unvaccinated.[673]

On or about April 9, 2021, the Prime Minister of England, Boris Johnson, advised persons that they may not meet indoors with vaccinated persons. He admitted that the vaccines do not prevent transmission of COVID-19. He responded to a question that he read out loud during a briefing:

> "Can I now meet my friends and family members indoors if they are vaccinated?" There I am afraid the answer is no, because we're not yet at that stage, we're still very much in the world where you can meet friends and family outdoors, under the rule of six, or two households. And even if your friends and family members may be vaccinated, the vaccines are not giving 100% protection and that's why we need to be cautious. We don't think that they [COVID-19 vaccines] entirely reduce or remove the risk of transmission.[674]

That was not a slip of the tongue or a mistake. Johnson's opinion was based on the data coming from the British health authorities. On or about October 23, 2021, The Prime Minister emphatically repeated that the COVID-19 vaccine "doesn't protect you against catching the disease, and it doesn't protect you from passing it on."[675] Johnson, curiously, went on to promote the COVID-19 vaccine booster, even though the first course of the vaccine has been proven ineffective in preventing infection and the spread of the disease. He trumpeted the new mantra justifying the vaccine booster; it is supposed to lessen the symptoms of COVID-19.

The VAERS system contains hard data on the harm being caused by the COVID-19 vaccines. It is run by the CDC, which is part of the executive branch of government. President Biden is the chief of the executive branch. VAERS is his system. When he issued his order, he and his federal health officials knew that the COVID-19 vaccines were injuring and killing people. A rational

President would have put a halt to the death and injury. But instead, President Biden accelerated the injections by mandating them for executive branch workers.

President Biden's claim that "[t]he vaccines are safe, highly effective,"[676] is provably false. The CDC and the vaccine manufacturers are on record admitting that the COVID-19 vaccines do not prevent the spread of COVID-19. Indeed, before the EUA authorization by the FDA of the Pfizer-BioNtech vaccine, the Daily Mail reported that on or before December 4, 2020, "Pfizer CEO [Albert Bourla] admits he is 'not certain' their COVID-19 shot will prevent vaccinated people from spreading the virus."[677]

As cited above, Moderna Chief Medical Officer Tal Zaks is on record saying that the Moderna vaccine can prevent someone from getting sick from COVID-19 but that there is no evidence that it can prevent someone receiving the vaccine from carrying the virus and infecting others.[678]

The predictions of Moderna and Pfizer have proven correct. A very high percentage of new COVID-19 cases are from vaccinated persons. Britain's Chief Scientific Adviser Patrick Vallance claimed in July 2021 that he mistakenly said that 60% of people being admitted to hospital with COVID-19 are fully vaccinated. He later clarified that he meant to say that 60% of those admitted for COVID-19 to the hospital are unvaccinated.[679] Please don't miss the significance of that admission. It means that the England health authorities recognize that 40% of COVID-19 hospitalizations are from fully vaccinated persons.

There are many anecdotal examples of fully vaccinated persons being subsequently infected with COVID-19. For example, it was reported by COVID Legal USA on March 12, 2021, that there was a COVID-19 infection outbreak at the Cottonwoods Care Centre retirement facility in Kelowna, British

Columbia, even though 82% of the residents were fully vaccinated. Eight out of the twelve COVID-19 confirmed cases were fully vaccinated persons.[680] That means that 66% of confirmed COVID-19 cases were from those who were fully vaccinated.

In a complaint filed in a federal lawsuit, the plaintiffs made the following common-sense observation:

> [T]he logic for the COVD-19 vaccines breaks down when one considers the Defendants' theory of asymptomatic spread. For over a year now, these Defendants and state-level public health authorities have told the American public that SARS-CoV-2 can be spread by people who have none of the symptoms of COVID-19. If that is the case, then a vaccine that merely reduces symptoms yields no benefits - the virus spreads anyway. If that is not the case, and asymptomatic spread is not real, then asymptomatic individuals do not need to be vaccinated with a vaccine that neither prevents infection with SARS-CoV-2 nor prevents its transmission.

What is the point of any employer vaccine mandate when the COVID-19 vaccines have now been proven to be ineffective? There is no reason to get the vaccine if prevention of infections and spread is the objective. Furthermore, there is no justification to require those who are not vaccinated to wear masks, get tested, social distance, and not travel since they are no more likely to spread the alleged SARS-CoV-2 virus than those who are fully vaccinated.

Because it became clear early on that the COVID-19 vaccines did not prevent the spread of SARS-CoV-2, the CDC found it necessary to issue a press release on March 8, 2021, saying that fully vaccinated Americans must "continue to take these COVID-19 precautions when in public."[681] That included wearing masks, staying six feet apart from other people, and avoiding large crowds.

Indeed, the COVID-19 infection rate for vaccinated persons has gotten so out of hand that on July 27, 2021, the CDC had to change its guidance because of the alleged spreading of COVID-19 by vaccinated persons. NBC News reported:

> The Centers for Disease Control and Prevention issued new guidance on Tuesday recommending indoor mask use in areas with high transmission rates after new data suggested fully **vaccinated individuals are not just contracting Covid-19 but could potentially infect others.**
>
> CDC Director Rochelle Walensky said recent studies had shown that those **vaccinated individuals who do become infected with Covid have just as much viral load as the unvaccinated, making it possible for them to spread the virus to others.** Based on that finding, Walensky said the CDC is also recommending that all school children wear masks in the fall.[682] (emphasis added)

Emily Kopp, writing for Roll Call, reported that a confidential congressional briefing revealed that "[t]here are 35,000 symptomatic breakthrough cases each week." Kopp concluded that vaccinated persons can be "superspreaders" of SARS-CoV-2.

> The newly released report showing that vaccinated people can still be superspreaders drove the recent decision by the CDC to once again recommend

masks for vaccinated people indoors where case counts are high or substantial.[683]

On August 6, 2021, the CDC published a report that 346 out of out of 469 COVID-19 cases (74%) in a breakout in Barnsdale County, Massachusetts, were of people who were fully vaccinated.[684] The COVID-19 vaccines are proving to be ineffective in preventing infection.

Dr. Nina Pierpont (MD, Ph.D.), has a BA in biology from Yale University, MA and Ph.D. in population biology/evolutionary biology/ecology from Princeton University, and MD from Johns Hopkins University School of Medicine. Dr. Pierpont has been a Clinical Assistant Professor of Pediatrics at Columbia University's College of Physicians & Surgeons. She is currently in private practice in upstate New York, specializing in behavioral medicine. Dr. Pierpont reviewed the available data, principally from three scientific studies, and concluded that COVID-19 vaccine mandates have no justification because "current vaccines do not prevent transmission of SARS-CoV-2."[685]

Pfizer CEO Albert Bourla, in his attempt to sell the public on their COVID-19 vaccine booster during a news interview, let the cat out of the bag by stating: "We know that two doses of the vaccine offers very limited protection if any."[686] When Pfizer realized the implications of that admission, it immediately filed a copyright claim on that interview and took steps to purge it from the internet. I was able to track down the video of the interview at the Instagram link found in the endnote.[687]

99% of the University of California football team and staff were fully vaccinated.[688] There are approximately 143 players and staff on that team.[689] But on November 13, 2021, it was announced that the team had to cancel its upcoming football game with USC because 47 players and staff members on the University of California football team had tested positive for COVID-19. Many of them were symptomatic for COVID-19, which is why the entire team was tested. That is a 33% COVID-19 infection rate for a single group of fully vaccinated persons. The COVID-19 vaccines are not just ineffective; it seems that the vaccines are driving the infection. It is more likely that the players and coaches are suffering from antibody-dependent enhancement caused by the vaccine.

Indeed, COVID-19 vaccinations are detrimental to the USA's counter-drug mission. For example, on December 25, 2021, Carol Rosenberg and Aishvarya Kavi reported for *The New York Times* that the USS Milwaukee was supposed to deploy to intercept drug traffickers in the Caribbean, but the ship could not do so because of a Covid-19 outbreak onboard the ship.[690] The 105-man crew of the vessel was 100% vaccinated against COVID-19. That is a clear example that the COVID-19 vaccines are ineffective in preventing COVID-19. What was really going on aboard the ship likely was that the sailors were suffering from antibody-dependent enhancement (ADE) caused by the vaccines themselves. The vaccines were making the sailors sick. Oddly, the USS Milwaukee incident comes on the heels of active-duty troops in the Army and Navy being fired because they refused to get vaccinated under President Biden's vaccination mandate for the armed services. Perfectly healthy soldiers and sailors were relieved of duty for exercising their rights to refuse to take experimental vaccines that have now been demonstrated to be both unsafe and ineffective. All the while, the readiness of the armed services is being detrimentally impacted by the growing occurrence of ADE among the soldiers and sailors caused by the mandated vaccines.

On November 10, 2021, U.S. District Court Judge T. Kent Wetherell, II, issued an opinion wherein he denied a request from a plaintiff for a preliminary injunction. He ruled against the doctor requesting a religious exemption. Nonetheless, in the course of rendering his opinion, the judge ruled:

> [T]the evidence I have shows the vaccine is "leaky" and "nonsterilizing" in that **it does not prevent transmission of the virus, nor does it protect vaccinated persons from contracting the virus**. ... [T]he evidence before the court from plaintiff's medical experts suggest **that vaccinated persons actually transmit the virus at a higher rate than unvaccinated**. ... [T]he vaccines are unnecessary for persons who have previously had COVID because **natural immunity provides equivalent or greater protection against severe infection than the vaccines.** ... [T]he irrefutable evidence in this case shows that vaccines simply do not accomplish the purpose of the policy that it's aimed at achieving; that is, "keeping everyone safer," because, again, **they do not protect people from contracting the virus**, nor do they prevent people from getting the virus.[691] (emphasis added)

So prevalent were the breakthrough cases of COVID-19 that the CDC announced that beginning on May 1, 2021, it would no longer monitor or report any breakthrough cases that did not result in hospitialization or death.[692] The CDC and its pharmaceutical overlords could not allow people to use official government statistics to prove that the COVID-19 vaccines are ineffective.

U.S. Senator for Massachusetts, Edward Markey, saw through the CDC's subterfuge. In an official letter of inquiry he demanded to know why the CDC would no longer continue to monitor the breakthrough cases.[693] Senator Markey noted the obvious fact that breakhrough cases are a good measure of COVID-19 vaccine effectiveness. He said that 43.4% of the new COVID-19 infections in Massachusetts were among those who were vaccinated. Notably, Senator Markey asked the CDC: "Is the effectiveness of COVID-19 vaccines decreasing in light of these breakthrough cases?" The answer is clear. Indeed, the evident affirmative answer to that question is why the CDC decided to stop reporting breakthrough COVID-19 cases. The CDC's decision not to report COVID-19 breakthrough cases among the vaccinated population was indicative of a conspiracy between it and the pharmaceutical companies to cover up of the ineffectiveness of the COVID-19 vaccines.

The Expose investigative news service explained that in March 2022, the UK Health Security Agency (UKHSA) announced that starting on April 1st 2022, they would no longer publish the vaccination status of Covid-19 cases, hospitalizations and deaths in England.[694] The UKHSA did that because the reported data showed that the unvaccinated population was suffering fewer hospitalizations and deaths from COVID-19 than those who had recieved the COVID-19 vaccine. Of course, that was not the reason given by the UKHSA. Instead, the UKHSA claimed this was because the UK Government had ended free universal Covid-19 testing, which affected their "ability to robustly monitor Covid-19 cases by vaccination status."[695] But that was a lie.

The Expose revealed the lie of the UKHSA by looking at the statistics from another UK Government agency. The Office for National Statistics (ONS), had published data on deaths by vaccination status.[696] That was the very data that the UKHSA said would no longer be available. *The Expose* reporters examined the ONS data starting from the beginning of April 2022 through the end of May 2022. *The Expose* found the shocking truth that between April 1, 2022, and May 31, 2022, 4,647 of the 4,935 total deaths from COVID-19 during that period were among the vaccinated population. That means that 94% of the COVID-19 deaths in the UK during April and May 2022 were among those vaccinated against COVID-19.

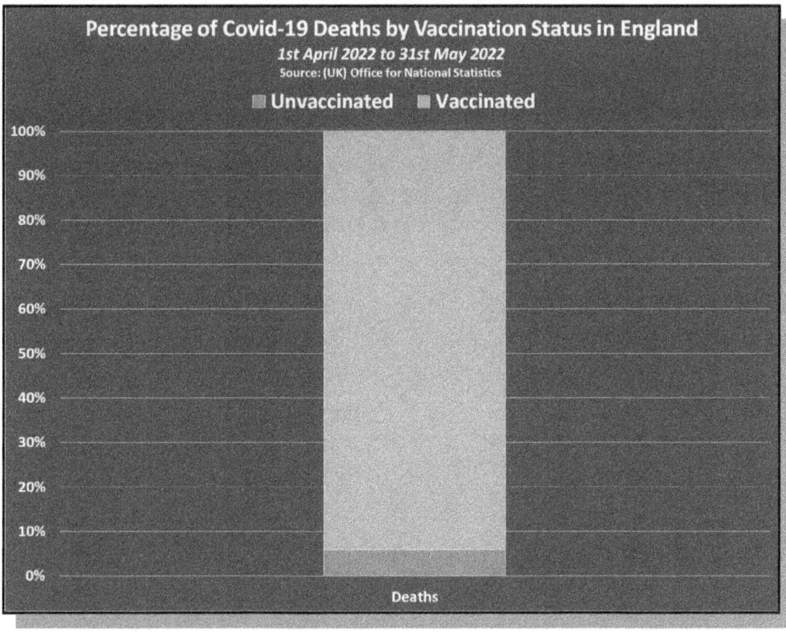

The statistics revealed another shocking detail. It seems that the more shots, the more deadly the vaccines are. Those who received three COVID-19 shots accounted for 4,215 of the 4,647 total deaths among the vaccinated population. That means that those that received three COVID-19 shots accounted for 90% of the vaccinated COVID-19 deaths during April and May 2022. See the graphic below from *The Expose*.

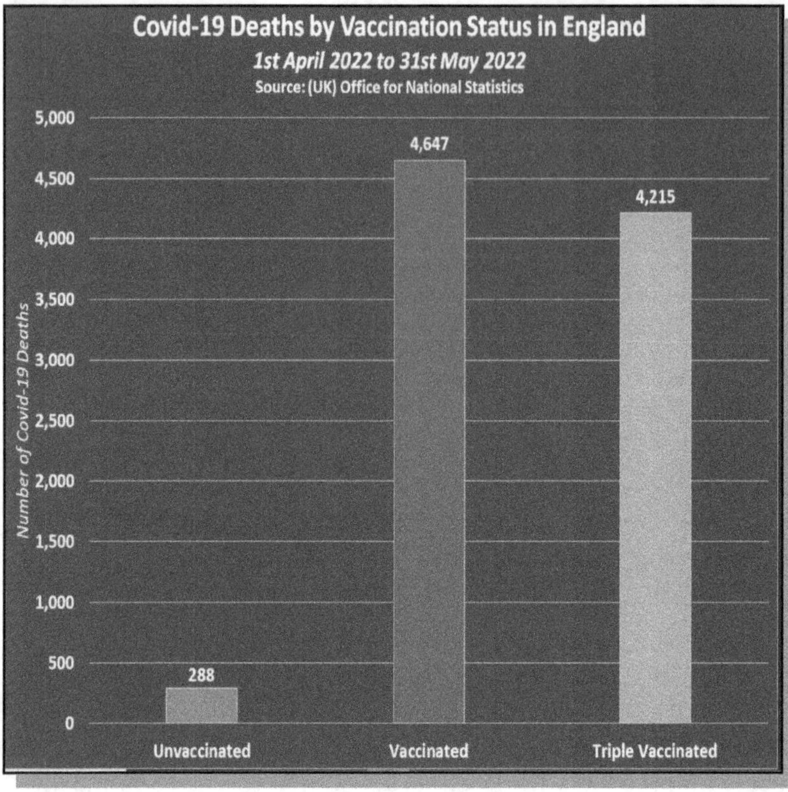

As stated by *The Expose* investigators, "[t]hese aren't the kind of figures you would expect to see if the Covid-19 injections really are up to 95% effective at preventing death, are they?" Indeed, that is likely why the UKHSA decided to stop giving separate statistics revealing the deaths and hospitalizations of vaccinated and unvaccinated persons in the UK.

On March 26, 2023, *The Expose* issued an updated report showing that in the 21 months between April 1, 2021, and December 31, 2022, 86% of the COVID-19 deaths in the UK were among those vaccinated against COVID-19.[697] Those statistics go beyond simply proving that the COVID-19 vaccines are ineffective. Those statistics suggest causation; they suggest antibody-dependent enhancement; the vaccines are dangerous.

The State of Vermont has had a very similar experience to that of England. The Vermont Daily Chronicle reported that 76% of COVID-19 deaths in the State of Vermont during September 2021 were of persons who had received COVID-19 vaccinations.[698] Yet, the State of Vermont Department of Public Health claims that "[v]accines are the best tool we have to protect ourselves against COVID-19, especially from severe illness, hospitalization and death."[699]

In Antwerp, Belgium, 100% of the hospitalized "COVID cases" are fully vaccinated persons. The Hall Turner Radio Show reported that "CEOs and medical directors of Antwerp hospitals met this week and the mood was worrying. They're having another COVID outbreak, but this time, ALL the patients . . . are fully vaccinated."[700] Kristiaan Deckers, Medical Director of the Antwerp GZA, remarked that "the question is whether the vaccines will still work."[701] It was further reported:

> Other officials, who asked to not be named for fear of retribution were far more candid. Said one CEO "Either the vaccines just don't work or, worse, it is the vaccines themselves causing COVID in these people. But if we are publicly quoted as stating the obvious, we will be driven out of our jobs and out of our profession. There is an almost cult-like zeitgeist that no one is allowed to say anything against the vaccines, even if they don't work or are hurting people.[702]

Data from the government health authorities in Scotland showed that the fully COVID-19 vaccinated accounted for 89% of COVID-19 deaths, whilst also accounting for 77% of COVID-19 hospitalizations, and 65% of alleged COVID-19 cases from October 9 through November 5, 2021.[703] According to the data from Public Health Scotland, for December 18, 2021, to January 14, 2022, the COVID-19 case rate was 2.5 times greater for those who received two COVID-19 vaccinations than those who were unvaccinated.[704] Over that same period, there was a 5% greater hospitalization rate for those who had received two COVID-19 vaccines than those who were unvaccinated.[705] From December 11, 2021, to January 7, 2022, there was a 55% greater mortality rate from COVID-19 for those who received two doses of the COVID-19 vaccine compared to those who were unvaccinated.[706]

That was hard data from the health authorities in Scotland. Apparently, someone was not pleased with those revelations. And so, Public Health Scotland deleted the report from the internet. The report from Public Health Scotland, from December 18, 2021, to January 14, 2022, was formerly found at the link in the endnote at the end of this sentence.[707] The report is now gone. But this author found the report using the internet archive Wayback machine. The archive link for the report is at the end of this sentence.[708]

Public Health Scotland has taken further action to conceal the death and destruction caused by the COVID-19 vaccines. On February 16, 2022, Public Health Scotland announced that "[f]rom 16 February 2022, Public Health Scotland (PHS) will no longer report COVID-19 cases, hospitalisations, and deaths by vaccination status on a weekly basis. PHS will continue to provide updates from the latest scientific analyses and reports on the effectiveness of COVID-19 vaccines. … While PHS has stated that the data in the report should not be used as a measure of vaccine effectiveness, PHS is aware of inappropriate use and misinterpretation of the data when taken in isolation without fully understanding the limitations described below."[709]

The Scottish health authorities are taking their toys and going home. They don't think that the public is playing nice with their raw data comparing deaths and hospitalizations of the unvaccinated with the vaccinated population. And so, rather than continue to provide it, they are simply shutting down the flow of information revealing the death and destruction caused by the COVID-19 vaccines.

The government health authorities claim that the data is being inappropriately misinterpreted.[710] I don't think it is inappropriately misinterpreting the data when one concludes that the COVID-19 vaccines are ineffective and dangerous after reading that there is a 55% greater mortality rate from COVID-19 for those who received two doses of the COVID-19 vaccine compared to those who were unvaccinated.

That disturbing statistic may be something that the government of Scotland does not want known, but it is not an inappropriate interpretation to say that it reveals that the COVID-19 vaccines are unsafe and ineffectual.

Below is a graph prepared by Steve Kirsch[711] from the actual Scotland Pubic Health authorities data.[712] This is the information that Public Health Scotland is trying to conceal from the public. Please understand that this data represents COVID-19 per 100,000. The data clearly shows that the vaccinated population did much worse.

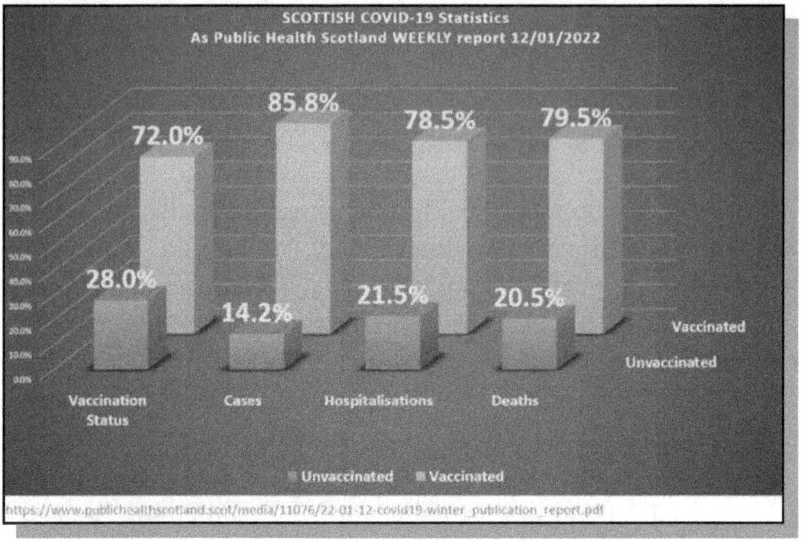

The Public Health Scotland (PHS) COVID-19 Winter Statistical Report dated 12 January 2022 reveals that those who received 2 COVID-19 shots died at a 59% greater rate than those who were unvaccinated. More striking is what a chart in the report reveals when COVID-19 deaths of all persons who received 1, 2, and 3 doses of the COVID-19 vaccine are compared to the unvaccinated persons.[713] When the vaccinated population of those who received 1, 2, and 3 shots is added together, we find that their death rate from COVID-19 was 3.56 times that of the unvaccinated population. Public Health Scotland will no longer provide this information because it reveals that the vaccines are unsafe and ineffective.

We are seeing antibody dependent enhancement (ADE) caused by the vaccine being reported throughout the world, not as

ADE, but rather as COVID-19. ADE being reported as COVID-19 was not unexpected. As noted above, Pfizer explained that ADE will usually be presented as having "severe or unusual manifestations of COVID-19."[714] Thus, what is being announced as "breakthrough" cases of COVID-19 are actually cases of ADE caused by the COVID-19 vaccines. For example, *The Expose* news site reported on the government statistics from Canada[715] showing that the vaccinated population of Canada account for 89% of all COVID-19 cases, 86% of all COVID-19 hospitalizations, and 90% of all COVID-19 deaths.

COVID-19 *Cases* in Canada: Between June 6, 2022 and July 3, 2022 in Canada, "the unvaccinated population accounted for just 11% of Covid-19 cases ... whilst **the vaccinated population accounted for 89%**, 74% of which were among the triple and quadruple jabbed."[716]

COVID-19 *Hospitalizations* in Canada: Between June 6, 2022 and July 3, 2022 in Canada, "the unvaccinated population accounted for just 14% of Covid-19 hospitalisations ... whilst **the vaccinated population accounted for 86%**, 75% of which were among the triple and quadruple jabbed."[717]

COVID-19 *Deaths* in Canada: Between June 6, 2022 and July 3, 2022 in Canada, "the unvaccinated population accounted for just 10% of Covid-19 deaths ... whilst **the vaccinated population accounted for 90%**, 87% of which were among the triple and quadruple jabbed."[718] See the graphic below from *The Expose.*

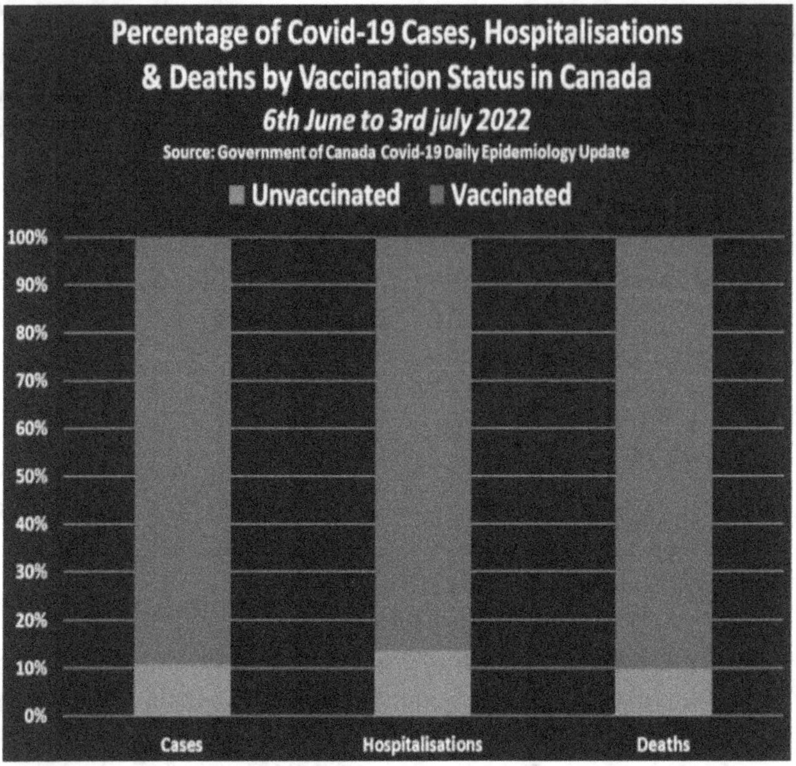

That manifest danger from the COVID-19 vaccines is in the face of evidence that the COVID-19 vaccines are ineffective. There is study,[719] after study,[720] after study,[721] after study[722] proving that vaccinated individuals can still test positive for COVID-19 and manifest illnesses associated with COVID-19. The United Kingdom Health Security Agency COVID-19 Vaccine Surveillance Report published on October 21, 2021, reveals that "[i]n individuals aged greater than 30, the rate of a positive COVID-19 test is higher in vaccinated individuals compared to unvaccinated."[723] But that statement from the British Government understates the ineffectiveness of the COVID-19 vaccinations. Indeed, when looking at the population from 18 years old and up, we find that the infection rate among the vaccinated population is significantly higher than the infection rate for the unvaccinated population. The British Government report reveals that over a monitoring period spanning week 38 to week 41 of 2021, the COVID-19 case rate for the vaccinated group over 18 years old was significantly more than the case rate for the unvaccinated group. There were 5,871 cases of COVID-19 for every 100,000 vaccinated persons more than 18 years old. In contrast, there were only 3,584 COVID-19 for every 100,000 unvaccinated persons more than 18 years old.[724] The workforce would fall largely in the over 18-year-old age bracket. Those statistics mean that a vaccinated person in the workforce is more likely to be infected with COVID-19 than an unvaccinated person.

The method used by the vaccine makers for reporting the efficacy of the COVID-19 vaccines (relative risk reduction) is to subtract the percentage of infected vaccinated persons from the percentage of infected unvaccinated persons and divide that number by the percentage of infected unvaccinated persons (U-V/U). Using that formula, and applying it to the UK government data, this author calculated that the actual effectiveness of the COVID-19 vaccines in the real world is minus-64%.[725] That means that a vaccinated person is 64% more likely to catch COVID-19 than an unvaccinated person.[726]

That calculation of minus-64% COVID-19 vaccine efficacy was from the official reported data of the UK Health Security Agency.[727] That minus-64% means that the immune system of the person who is vaccinated is so debilitated by the vaccine that, on a percentage basis, he is 64% more likely to be infected with COVID-19 than an unvaccinated person. That is data from week 42 of 2021. The UK Health Security Agency data shows that when comparing the number of persons with COVID-19 per 100,000 vaccinated persons to the number of persons with COVID-19 per 100,000 unvaccinated persons, the vaccinated group has significantly higher rate of COVID-19 cases than the unvaccinated group. That indicates that over time the vaccines have a negative efficacy. The COVID-19 vaccines make a person more susceptible to COVID-19. Recall that the efficacy of the COVID-19 vaccines have been calculated to drop at an average rate of 5% per week.[728] As time passes, the likelihood of COVID-19 infection (or more likely, antibody-dependent enhancement (ADE)) increases for the vaccinated persons.

The null hypothesis in a recent study was that areas with low vaccination rates drive the ongoing surge of new COVID-19. The study disproved that null hypothesis. That study by S. V. Subramanian from the Harvard Center for Population and Development Studies published on the NIH website concluded that "increases in COVID-19 are unrelated to levels of vaccination across 68 countries and 2,947 counties in the United States."[729] The study determined that the COVID-19 vaccines are not effective. While the study disproved the null hypothesis, one finds that the data goes beyond showing ineffectiveness of the COVID-19 vaccines. The data showed a positive correlation between vaccine rate and infection rate. The data indicate that COVID-19 vaccines are driving the infection. For example, the study presented data showing that U.S. counties with higher COVID-19 vaccine rates had higher rates of COVID-19 cases. The study states:

> Of the top 5 counties that have the highest percentage of population fully vaccinated (99.9–84.3%), the US Centers for Disease Control and Prevention (CDC) identifies 4 of them as "High" Transmission counties. Chattahoochee (Georgia), McKinley (New Mexico), and Arecibo (Puerto Rico) counties have above 90% of their population fully vaccinated with all three being classified as "High" transmission. Conversely, of the 57 counties that have been classified as "low" transmission counties by the CDC, 26.3% (15) have percentage of population fully vaccinated below 20%.[730]

When looking at the country-level data, the reader finds the same correlation. In disproving the null hypothesis, the study determined there was no relationship between the percentage of the population fully vaccinated and new COVID-19 cases. The study concluded that the COVID-19 vaccines are ineffective. But the data goes beyond showing the vaccines are ineffective. The study shows that vaccines cause a higher rate of COIVD-19 infection. The study showed that the higher the COVID-19 vaccine rate in a country, the higher is its COVID-19 infection rate. The study reveals that "[i]n fact, the trend line suggests a marginally positive association such that countries with higher percentage of population fully vaccinated have higher COVID-19 cases per 1 million people." Thus, the vaccines seem to drive the COVID-19 infection. The study states:

> At the country-level, there appears to be no discernable relationship between percentage of population fully vaccinated and new COVID-19 cases in the last 7 days. In fact, the trend line suggests a marginally positive association such that countries with higher percentage of population fully vaccinated have higher COVID-19 cases per 1 million people. Notably, Israel with over 60% of their population fully vaccinated had the highest COVID-19 cases per 1 million people in the last 7 days. The lack of a meaningful association between percentage population fully vaccinated and new COVID-19 cases is further exemplified, for instance, by comparison of Iceland and Portugal. Both countries have over 75% of their population fully vaccinated and have more COVID-19 cases per 1 million people than countries such as Vietnam and South Africa that have around 10% of their population fully vaccinated.[731]

What accounts for the phenomenon of vaccines that offer no protection? Some think that the answer has been found in a massive study involving approximately 620,000 U.S. Veterans who received COVID-19 vaccines. The researchers determined that "[t]he proportionate reduction in infection associated with vaccination declined for all vaccine types, with the largest declines for Janssen followed by Pfizer-BioNTech and Moderna."[732]

The decline in protection for the Johnson & Johnson (Janssen) COVID-19 vaccine was significant. The protection from COVID-19 dropped from 88% protection against COVID-19 in March 2021 down to 3% protection, just five months later in August 2021. The protection from infection for Pfizer-BioNTech dropped from 91% in March to 50% in August. The Moderna vaccine protection dropped from 92% in March to 64% in August. The vaccines' problem is that they only provide a few months of protection before that protection drops precipitously. What is the point of getting a vaccination that offers only a few short months of protection?

But the waning vaccine efficacy is not why the risk of COVID-19 infection is the same for the vaccinated as it is for unvaccinated. The data indicates that the risk of COVID-19 is actually worse for the vaccinated who are more than 30 years old. It is not that the vaccines are ineffective that is the reason for the COVID-19 infections among the vaccinated; the vaccines drive an illness called antibody dependent enhancement (ADE). ADE is being reported as COVID-19 because the patients are testing positive for COIVD-19.

In October 2021, the U.S. FDA issued an EUA for a COVID-19 vaccine for children five years and older, and the U.S. CDC recommended that EUA COVID-19 vaccine for those children. On March 8, 2022, Florida State Surgeon General Joseph Ladpapo, M.D., Ph.D., contradicted the U.S. CDC and officially recommended against giving the COVID-19 vaccine to healthy children 5 to 17 years old.[733] He made that recommendation based on the limited risk that COVID-19 posed to the young compared to the "higher than anticipated severe adverse events occurred among those receiving the COVID-19 vaccine" in clinical trials.[734] He revealed the troubling fact that the COVID-19 vaccines have no long-term immunity benefit. They don't work as advertised. Dr. Ladpapo explained that a "study conducted out of New York determined that COVID-19 vaccine efficacy declined 84%, from 68% to 12%, over a span of two months for children aged 5 to 11."[735] He further stated that the "same study determined that COVID-19 vaccine efficacy declined 40%, from 85% to 51%, over a span of two months for adolescents ages 12 to 17."[736] Despite that evidence, in June 2022, the FDA authorized a COVID-19 vaccine for children older than six months, and the U.S. CDC recommended that vaccine for those children.[737]

After pushing millions to get vaccinated, the CDC has now implicitly acknowledged that vaccines do not have any beneficial effect on preventing the infection or spread of COVID-19. On September 23, 2022, the CDC guidance was updated to note that **"vaccination status is no longer used to inform source control, screening testing, or post-exposure recommendations."**[738]

The "breakthrough infections" from the alleged COVID-19 virus did not surprise government officials or pharmaceutical companies. It is well known within the field of immunology that no vaccines provide lasting immunity. Thus, the hope of attaining herd immunity through vaccination is propaganda based on mythology.

Catherine J Frompovich interviewed Stanford Research Immunologist Dr. Tetyana Obukhanych, Ph.D. Frompovich asked Dr. Obukhanych the following: "Vaccinated children are coming down with the same infectious diseases for which they have been fully vaccinated. Why do you think vaccine 'immunity'— if we can call it that—is so short lived and not adequate?" Dr. Obukhanych gave the following revealing answer:

> We would expect that vaccinated individuals would not be involved (or very minimally involved) in any outbreak of an infectious disease for which they have been vaccinated. Yet, when outbreaks are analyzed, it becomes apparent that most often this is not the case. Vaccinated individuals are indeed very frequently involved and constitute a high proportion of disease cases.
>
> I think this is happening because vaccination does not engage the genuine mechanism of immunity. Vaccination typically engages the immune response—that is, everything that immunologists would theoretically "want" to see being engaged in the immune system. But apparently this is not enough to confer robust protection that matches natural immunity. Our knowledge of the immune system is far from being complete.[739]

Marcella Piper-Terry is a vaccine researcher, the mother of a daughter recovering from autism, and the founder of VaxTruth.org, who came to the same conclusion arrived at by Dr. Obukhanych.

> There is no such thing as vaccine-induced herd immunity. It doesn't exist. It never has. The vast majority of adults have ZERO immunity from vaccines and we have not been having huge outbreaks of disease. Let's please just stop talking about how we're going to lose herd immunity if we stop vaccinating. We can't lose what we've never had.[740]

Vaccine-induced herd immunity is the mythology behind vaccine mandates. The tyranny of mandates is based on something that is not real. Brett Wilcox explains that vaccine-induced herd immunity is like a superstitious religious belief.

> Whereas the vaccines-are-safe-and-effective dogma assures parents and patients that vaccines safely prevent disease, the doctrine of herd immunity persuades parents and patients that they have a social obligation to vaccinate, that those who fail to vaccinate are "free loaders"—people who freely reap the benefits of vaccines while failing to assume their share of vaccine risks. The two doctrines have now combined in an irrational yet powerful third doctrine: vaccines protect vaccine recipients but only if everyone else vaccinates. Thus, the unvaccinated have morphed from free loaders into diseased and filthy child abusers, child killers, and murderers. It is this third doctrine that vaccine believers and sociopaths wield to justify discrimination, mandatory vaccination, and just plain nasty behavior.
>
> By comparison, ancient believers once threatened to kill non-believers to help them see the value of converting to the religion of their more righteous oppressors. Modern vaccine believers believe their salvation lies in the conversion and baptism by vaccination of all of humanity. Thus, believers view the unvaccinated not only as vectors of disease but also as the indispensible key to their own salvation from the ever-threatening hell of infectious disease.[741]

26 CDC Changes the Definition of Vaccine

The CDC and the vaccine makers understood from the beginning that the COVID-19 mRNA vaccines were ineffective in protecting persons from COVID-19. As the ineffectiveness of the COVID-19 injections in providing immunity was becoming increasingly clear, the CDC realized that the injections did not meet the definition of a vaccine. Indeed, in a Motion for a Preliminary Injunction against HHS filed on July 19, 2021, the plaintiffs alleged:

> [T]he "Pfizer-BioNTech COVID-19 Vaccine" and the "Moderna COVID-19 Vaccine" do not meet the CDC's own definitions. They do not stimulate the body to produce immunity from a disease. They are a synthetic fragment of nucleic acid embedded in a fat carrier that is introduced into human cells, not for the purpose of inducing immunity from infection with the SARS-CoV-2 virus, and not to block further transmission of the virus, but in order to lessen the symptoms of COVID-19. No published, peer-reviewed studies prove that the "Pfizer-BioNTech COVID-19 Vaccine" and the "Moderna COVID-19 Vaccine"

confer immunity or stop transmission.[742]

The lawyers for HHS realized that the plaintiffs were correct. They advised their clients at the HHS component agency, the CDC, that they needed to fix that problem. So many of the laws protecting pharmaceutical companies from liability required that their injections be vaccines. They needed to change the very definition of a vaccine to include an injection that is ineffective in producing immunity to the disease.

The CDC defines immunity as "[p]rotection from an infectious disease. If you are immune to a disease, you can be exposed to it without becoming infected."[743] So far, so good. Up until September 2021, the CDC's definition of "vaccine" was "[a] product that stimulates a person's immune system to produce immunity to a specific disease, protecting the person from that disease."[744] So it was understood by all before September 2021 that a vaccine "stimulates a person's immune system to produce immunity." And immunity means "[p]rotection from an infectious disease. If you are immune to a disease, you can be exposed to it without becoming infected."

CDC Definitions Prior to September 2021

Definition of Terms

Related Information and Materials

Let's start by defining several basic terms:

Immunity: Protection from an infectious disease. If you are immune to a disease, you can be exposed to it without becoming infected.

Vaccine: A product that stimulates a person's immune system to produce immunity to a specific disease, protecting the person from that disease. Vaccines are usually administered through needle injections, but can also be administered by mouth or sprayed into the nose.

Vaccination: The act of introducing a vaccine into the body to produce immunity to a specific disease.

Immunization: A process by which a person becomes protected against a disease through vaccination. This term is often used interchangeably with vaccination or inoculation.

Notice that the CDC defines immunization as only obtained "through vaccination." That implies no natural immune protection from a disease once a person recovers. The CDC implicitly pushes the fallacy that the only efficacious immunization is through vaccination. The CDC misleadingly portrays vaccination, inoculation, and immunization as synonyms.

But in September 2021, the CDC made a notable change. The CDC changed the definition of vaccine to mean instead "[a] preparation that is used to stimulate the body's immune response against diseases."[745] Now, the definition of a vaccine includes a vaccine that merely "stimulates the body's immune response" without actually producing any protection from disease. Now, a vaccine can be ineffective in providing any protection in preventing infection; it only needs to stimulate the body's immune response regardless of whether that stimulation is effective in protecting against disease.

CDC Definitions After September 2021

Definition of Terms

Immunity: Protection from an infectious disease. If you are immune to a disease, you can be exposed to it without becoming infected.

Vaccine: A preparation that is used to stimulate the body's immune response against diseases. Vaccines are usually administered through needle injections, but some can be administered by mouth or sprayed into the nose.

Vaccination: The act of introducing a vaccine into the body to produce protection from a specific disease.

Immunization: A process by which a person becomes protected against a disease through vaccination. This term is often used interchangeably with vaccination or inoculation.

Related Pages

See the Vaccine and Immunization Glossary of Terms

Notice that the CDC maintains that immunization is only through vaccination. The CDC even recommends that those who have recovered from COVID-19 still receive a COVID-19 vaccine. "Getting a COVID-19 vaccine after having COVID-19 provides added protection against the virus that causes COVID-19."[746] Such advice impeaches the germ theory upon which vaccines are based. The whole purpose of a vaccine is to replicate natural immunity by injecting an antigen to stimulate the immune system to protect against future infection. Why get a vaccine when a person has already recovered from the illness and fulfilled the immunity requirement? Vaccinating a person who has recovered from the illness that is the target of the vaccine makes no scientific sense. But it does make perfect Machiavellian genocidal sense.

The Cleveland Clinic did a study that concluded that "[i]ndividuals who have had SARS-CoV-2 infection are unlikely to benefit from COVID-19 vaccination."[747] That study does not stand alone. Other studies confirm the results. The CDC recommendation for someone who has recovered from COVID-19 to be vaccinated against COVID-19 is dangerous quackery.

Studies have shown that children with natural immunity from COVID-19 and then received a COVID-19 vaccine had their immunity from COVID-19 go negative after five months.[748] That means the children who already had natural immunity were more susceptible to the COVID-19 infection after getting the vaccine. Thus, the vaccine harms the patient who already has natural immunity. That harm is caused by vaccine-induced antibody-dependent enhancement.[749]

In an email response to a news inquiry, a spokesman for the CDC stated: "while there have been slight changes in wording over time to the definition of 'vaccine' on the CDC's website, those haven't impacted the overall definition. ... The previous definition…could be interpreted to mean that vaccines were 100% effective, which has never been the case for any vaccine, so the current definition is more transparent."[750]

The real reason for the changed definition is that since the mRNA vaccines have been such a spectacular failure, a change in the definition was necessary to account for that failure. For the CDC to claim that changing the meaning of vaccine from "stimulates a person's immune system to produce immunity" to "stimulate the body's immune response against diseases" is only a slight change that does not impact the definition is dissimulation of the first order.

If the new definition was not a change, then why do it? There is a world of difference between producing immunity and simply responding to a disease. Under the new definition, the body's response could be, and as we have seen with the mRNA vaccines, has been, ineffective in fighting off the disease. Before the definition change, a vaccine was required to offer immunity from the disease; now, all that is needed is for the vaccine to prompt the body's immune system to respond to the disease. Indeed, the body could respond to the disease with a cytokine storm (a.k.a., antibody-dependent enhancement), which may kill the patient, as we have seen with mRNA COVID-19 vaccines. Now, the ineffectiveness of vaccines is built into the definition.

The CDC's redefinition of vaccine is part of the Orwellian newspeak, where our language is being altered to meet the ideological needs of the Zionist ruling class. The power of the these international communists is pervasive. For example, within a little more than a month of introducing the mRNA COVID-19 vaccines, Merriam-Webster Dictionary changed the definition of vaccine to accommodate the ineffective and dangerous new vaccines. That was approximately eight months before the CDC vaccine definition changed.

Before January 18, 2021, the Merriam-Webster Dictionary definition of vaccine was given as:

> [A] preparation of killed microorganisms, living attenuated organisms, or living fully virulent organisms that is administered to **produce or artificially increase immunity to a particular disease.**[751]

But sometime between January 18, 2021, and January 26, 2021, Merriam-Webster changed the definition to remove the requirement that a vaccine must **"produce or artificially increase immunity to a particular disease."** The new definition only requires the vaccine to **"stimulate the body's immune response against a specific infectious agent or disease."** Thus an injection can be ineffective in producing immunity as long as it stimulates the body's immune response. That stimulation of the body's immune response could be quite detrimental, as when the stimulation causes illness due to antibody-dependent enhancement. The new vaccine definition, in pertinent part, states:

> [A] preparation that is administered (as by injection) to **stimulate the body's immune**

> **response** against a specific infectious agent or disease: such as ... an antigenic preparation of a typically inactivated or attenuated (see ATTENUATED sense 2) pathogenic agent (such as a bacterium or virus) or one of its components or products (such as a protein or toxin) ... a preparation of genetic material (such as a strand of **synthesized messenger RNA**) that is used by the cells of the body to produce an antigenic substance (such as a fragment of virus spike protein).[752]

Now, an injection can be a vaccine if it merely stimulates the body's immune response and does not "produce or artificially increase immunity to a particular disease." The Merriam-Webster change was an acknowledgment that the COVID-19 mRNA vaccines are ineffective in producing or increasing immunity to COVID-19. This definition change is evidence that they knew from the beginning that the mRNA COVID-19 vaccines would not stop infection or spread of COVID-19; it would only "stimulate the body's immune response."

Indeed, the Merriam-Webster Dictionary even adds the new mRNA technology to its definition. Merriam-Webster defines a biological weapon (i.e., bioweapon) as "a harmful biological agent (as a pathogenic microorganism or a neurotoxin) used as a weapon to cause death or disease usually on a large scale."[753] An injection that stimulates the body's immune system to attack itself is a bioweapon. That is what the COVID-19 vaccine does. The new definition of vaccine means that if an injection causes harm by stimulating the body's immune system to attack itself through antibody-dependent enhancement, it is still a vaccine. Thus, any bioweapon (e,g,, COVID-19 injection) can masquerade as a vaccine. Since the new definition of a vaccine includes within it the characteristics of a bioweapon, the manufacturers and all who administer the bioweapon are protected from liability by the Public Readiness and Emergency Preparedness Act (PREP Act), which authorizes the Countermeasures Injury Compensation Program (CICP) that grants pharmaceutical companies and medical professionals liability protection for vaccines made and administered under an emergency use authorization(EUA).

27 Antibody Dependent Enhancement

A significant concern of the COVID-19 vaccine makers was the known risk of antibody-dependent enhancement (ADE). ADE will make the recipient of the vaccine ill. The illness can be devastating. Indeed, Peter Loftus wrote in the July 12, 2020, Wall Street Journal about the concerns over ADE during the early stages of the COVID-19 vaccines:

> In 2017, researchers found that some children who got a new vaccine against the tropical disease dengue later came down with a severe case of the illness, forcing production to temporarily stop. Now, researchers developing coronavirus vaccines aim to avoid a similar fate that could set back fast-moving efforts to curb the pandemic.
>
> The researchers say they have designed Covid-19 vaccines in ways that aim to make sure they fight off infections, rather than worsen them.
>
> The large, final-stage trials starting to get under way will look for signs of rare side effects like the ones that arose for vaccines for dengue and other

> respiratory conditions, including other coronaviruses. The rare complication, known as disease enhancement because it worsens the disease the vaccine is supposed to protect against, is a concern for vaccine research generally.[754]

Antibody enhancement can cause severe illness unassociated with the disease that is the target of the vaccine. A person suffering ADE can consequently suffer a cytokine storm with debilitating and potentially deadly inflamation. It was generally known in the scientific community that vaccines against a coronovirus like COVID-19 pose the very real threat of antibody-dependent enhancement. Peter Loftus explains:

> Vaccines are designed to produce immune-system agents, including antibodies, that lock onto a virus and thereby neutralize it. In cases of disease enhancement, however, immune agents act in ways that facilitate replication of the virus.
>
> The complication can dangerously increase the severity of the disease in people exposed to the pathogen after they get the shots.
>
> Aside from affecting Sanofi SA's dengue vaccine Dengvaxia, signs of disease enhancement stymied development of an experimental vaccine against respiratory syncytial virus, or RSV, after studies in children in the mid-1960s detected the side effect.
>
> The safety issue has hovered over efforts to bring to market a vaccine for the new coronavirus because signs of disease enhancement arose in research into vaccines for other coronaviruses.
>
> Researchers studying experimental vaccines

> against the coronavirus that caused an outbreak of severe acute respiratory syndrome, or SARS, in 2002 found that vaccinated mice developed enhanced disease when exposed to the virus. No SARS vaccines have been approved for humans.[755]

Indeed, the very concern about antibody-dependent enhancement has been realized. The death and illness we see worldwide that is being attributed to "breakthrough" cases of COVID-19 are actually the predictable manifestations of ADE caused by the vaccines that were supposed to prevent COVID-19. The initial testing from the COVID-19 vaccine makers revealed that ADE was a problem. For example, On July 15, 2020, Daniel Payne reported that "[a] highly anticipated clinical trial for a potential COVID-19 vaccine managed in part by the American drug company Moderna has resulted in some adverse effects in more than half of the trial's participants, with one test group reporting 'severe' symptoms."[756]

When one reads the actual July 14, 2020, New England Journal of Medicine post of the Moderna study report, one finds that the adverse side effects of pain, myalgia, headache, chills, fatigue, localized symptoms, and systemic symptoms were felt by 80% or more of test subjects for the higher doses after the second vaccination.[757] Furthermore, approximately 85% of the systemic adverse events were moderate to severe for the high dose vaccine after the second dose.[758] And those are only the short term symptoms. We now know that the long term effects of the COVID-19 vaccines have been devastating. As of February 24, 2023, the VAERS system reported 63,862 permanently disabled and 34,576 deaths attributed to the COVID-19 vaccines. That is just the tip of the iceberg because the CDC's contracted study showed that only 1% of vaccine adverse events are reported in VAERS.[759]

A vaccinated person is statistically more likely to be

infected with COVID-19 than an unvaccinated person. What is the cause of this statistical phenomenon that a vaccinated person is more likely to catch COVID-19? The UK Health Security Agency data shows that the COVID-19 vaccine efficacy drops at a steady 5% average rate per week.[760] One would think that fact would only indicate that the vaccine is losing efficacy, ultimately dropping to zero. But that is not the case. The hard data from the UK government indicates that, in fact, the 5% loss of efficacy actually continues past zero. What that means is that the vaccine increases the likelihood of COVID-19.

The UK Health Security Agency COVID-19 data indicates that the COVID-19 vaccines have not merely lost their efficiency; they damage and suppress the immune system. Over time, a vaccinated person is less able to fight off infection and ends up hospitalized. They test positive for COVID-19 and are labeled a breakthrough COVID case. In fact, they are likely a case of antibody-dependent enhancement (ADE), wherein they are ill not because the vaccine did not work but because the vaccine worked to make them sick.

Likely, the deaths and hospitalizations suffered by those vaccinated for COVID-19 are not because the vaccines have failed to protect those who were vaccinated, but rather because the vaccines are causing the deaths and hospitalizations.

On May 17, 2023, researchers published a report announcing that they uncovered the mechanism causing the deterioration of the immune system by the COVID-19 mRNA vaccines. "[R]ecent investigations have found abnormally high levels of IgG4 in people who were administered two or more injections of the mRNA vaccines."[761]

What is IgG4? When someone is vaccinated, there is an immune response. Not all immune responses are beneficial. There can be several immunoglobulin classes in an antibody immune response, including IgA, IgE, IgM, and IgG. The human immunoglobulins G (IgG), in particular, are divided into four subcategories (IgGl, IgG2, IgG3, and IgG4). The increase in IgG4 can pose a problem. The scientists uncovered evidence that "IgG4 can lead to serious illness in several autoimmune disorders as well as cancer." The researchers explain:

> [E]merging evidence suggests that the reported increase in IgG4 levels detected after repeated vaccination with the mRNA vaccines may not be a protective mechanism; rather, it constitutes an immune tolerance mechanism to the spike protein that could promote unopposed SARS-CoV2 infection and replication by suppressing natural antiviral responses. Increased IgG4 synthesis due to repeated mRNA vaccination with high antigen concentrations may also cause autoimmune diseases, and promote cancer growth and autoimmune myocarditis in susceptible individuals.[762]

The research scientists opine that the elevated IgG4 levels in response to COVID-19 mRNA vaccines cause chronic infections.

> In this paper, we provide the scientific rationale suggesting that repeated vaccination with mRNA vaccines could generate an immune tolerance mechanism, thereby favoring unopposed SARS-CoV-2 replication. The long-term consequence of this tolerance could be the establishment of a permissive state of the host leading to chronic infection and other unintended consequences induced by mRNA vaccination in susceptible individuals.[763]

The COVID-19 mRNA vaccines lose efficacy over time and also deteriorate the immune system. The repeated boosting to compensate for the reduced efficacy exacerbates the problem by accelerating an elevation of IgG4 production that suppresses patients' immunity, opening them up to infections and even cancer.

> [The] mRNA and inactivated vaccines temporally impair interferon signaling, possibly causing immune suppression and leaving the individual in a vulnerable situation against any other pathogen. In addition, this immune suppression could allow the re-activation of latent viral, bacterial, or fungal infections and might also allow the uncontrolled growth of cancer cells.[764]

The researchers did not limit their findings only to COVID-19 vaccines. Repeated vaccinations with traditional vaccines had also been found to create dangerous autoimmune responses.

> Repeated vaccination could also lead to auto-immunity: in 2009, the results of an important study went largely unnoticed. Researchers discovered that in mice that are otherwise not susceptible to spontaneous autoimmune disorders, repeated administration of the antigen promotes systemic autoimmunity.[765]

Taiwan health authorities report that the number of people dying in Taiwan after their COVID-19 vaccination exceeds the number of deaths from the virus itself. The health authorities reported that as of October 11, 2021, deaths after COVID-19 vaccination reached 865. In comparison, the deaths from the virus are 845.[766] The COVID-19 vaccines used in Taiwan include Moderna, Pfizer-BioNTech, AstraZeneca, and a Taiwanese vaccine, Medigen.

Ralph Baric, is the William R. Kenan Jr. Distinguished Professor in the Department of Epidemiology, and Professor in the Department of Microbiology and Immunology at the University of North Carolina at Chapel Hill. Dr. Baric stated that with the COVID-19 vaccines "[t]here is the potential for ADE, but the bigger problem is probably Th2 immunopathology."[767] Indeed, that very thing was seen by Dr Ryan Cole, who runs the largest independent testing lab in Idaho. Dr Cole has performed more than 100,000 pathology lab examinations from COVID patients. *The Expose* reported that "[h]e identified what he is seeing as a form of AIDS (reverse HIV he called it – where you lose CD8 killer T cells rather than CD4 Helper T cells)."[768] What does that mean? The researchers for *The Expose* explained that "[t]his suggests that the vaccines are giving people vaccine mediated immune deficiency, which therefore suggests the vaccines are giving people a form of AIDS (Acquired Immune Deficiency Syndrome)."[769]

Most of the serious adverse event outcomes from the COVID-19 known to the FDA and the vaccine manufacturers are not listed in the COVID-19 fact sheets from Pfizer-BioNTech or Moderna.[770] For example, deaths and antibody-dependent enhancement (ADE) were possible "adverse event outcomes" being monitored by the FDA during the COIVD-19 vaccine trials. They knew what to look for because they knew what they were seeing. None of the vaccine makers listed death or ADE in their fact sheets for recipients and caregivers as a risk from its COVID-19 vaccines.[771]

None of the side effects from the COVID-19 vaccines have been a surprise to the vaccine makers or the FDA. Before the FDA issued the EUA for the COVID-19 vaccines, the Vaccines and Related Biological Products Advisory Committee held a meeting on October 22, 2020. Steve Anderson, Director of Biostatistics and Epidemiology for the FDA, gave a slide presentation at that meeting.[772] Anderson inadvertently showed a slide that he had no intention of discussing. The slide appeared for a split second at the 2:33:40 mark in the video before he suspiciously clicked past it and continued his presentation without mentioning any of the facts on the slide. The slide presented the possible adverse events from the COVID-19 vaccines. They knew what to look for because they knew what they were seeing. They were not going to waste their time looking for things that they did not expect to find. They are the very adverse events that are being witnessed in the VAERS reporting. A screenshot of the slide as it flashed on the screen is below:

Below is a screenshot of Anderson's slide. The slide lists ADE, which Dr. Anderson labeled "vaccine enhanced disease," as one of the possible adverse event outcomes being monitored by the FDA during the COVID-19 vaccine trials. The FDA was keyed in and knew from the animal trails for SARS-CoV that ADE was something for which to be on the lookout. And that is why ADE was listed among the possible adverse event outcomes to monitor during the COVID-19 vaccine trials. There is no doubt they found ADE during the trials because we are seeing ADE from the COVID-19 vaccines being administered throughout the country.

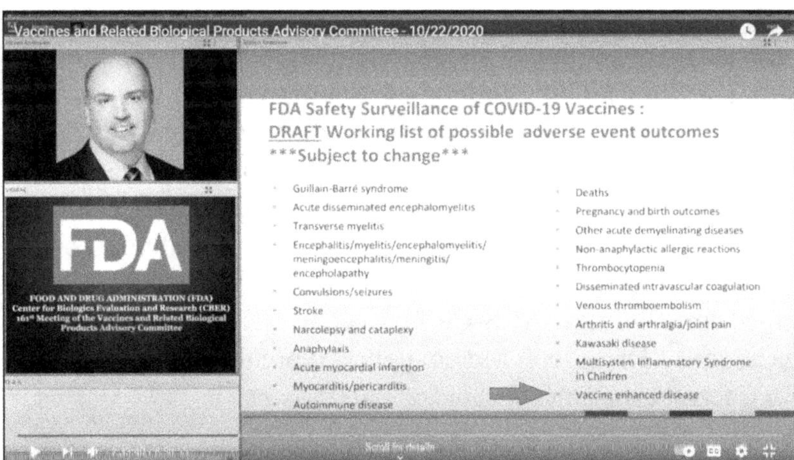

Figure 11: PowerPoint flashed on screen for a split second as Steve Anderson, Director of Biostatistics and Epidemiology for the FDA, gave a slide presentation at the October 22, 2020 Vaccines and Related Biological Products Advisory Committee meeting.

That means that the often announced "breakthrough" cases of COVID-19 are likely not COVID-19 cases but are rather cases of vaccine-associated enhanced disease (VAED), otherwise known as antibody-dependent enhancement (ADE), caused by the COVID-19 vaccines themselves. Indeed, the data coming in from all over the world suggests that the "breakthrough" cases of alleged COVID-19 among the vaccinated population are actually cases of ADE caused by the COVID-19 vaccines.[773]

The Children's Hospital of Philadelphia (CHOP) offers a concise explanation of ADE:

> Many vaccines work by inducing neutralizing antibodies. However, not all antibody responses are created equal. Sometimes antibodies do not prevent cell entry and, on rare occasions, they may actually increase the ability of a virus to enter cells and cause a worsening of disease through a mechanism called antibody-dependent enhancement (ADE).[774]

One would think that all antibodies are good, and thus, you would want to enhance the antibodies. But that is not the case because there are two kinds of antibodies. There are neutralizing antibodies and binding antibodies. Neutralizing antibodies, as the name suggests, neutralize the virus. Binding antibodies do not neutralize the virus; they bind to it and enhance the virus's ability to infect cells. This increases disease. The COVID-19 vaccines cause the production of higher levels of binding antibodies. That causes the disease to spread. This effect was seen when the ADE killed coronavirus (SARS-CoV) vaccine test animals received the vaccines.[775] Dr. Joseph Mercola gives more details of the SARS-CoV ferret experiments:

> In my May 2020 interview above with Robert Kennedy Jr., he summarized the history of

coronavirus vaccine development, which began in 2002, following three consecutive SARS outbreaks. By 2012, Chinese, American and European scientists were working on SARS vaccine development, and had about 30 promising candidates.

Of those, the four best vaccine candidates were then given to ferrets, which are the closest analogue to human lung infections. In the video below, which is a select outtake from my full interview, Kennedy explains what happened next. While the ferrets displayed robust antibody response, which is the metric used for vaccine licensing, once they were challenged with the wild virus, they all became severely ill and died.

The same thing happened when they tried to develop an RSV vaccine in the 1960s. RSV is an upper respiratory illness that is very similar to that caused by coronaviruses. At that time, they had decided to skip animal trials and go directly to human trials.

"They tested it on I think about 35 children, and the same thing happened," Kennedy said. "The children developed a champion antibody response — robust, durable. It looked perfect [but when] the children were exposed to the wild virus, they all became sick. Two of them died. They abandoned the vaccine. It was a big embarrassment to FDA and NIH."[776]

It is not that the vaccines are ineffective that is the reason for the COVID-19 infections among the vaccinated; the vaccines drive an illness called antibody dependent enhancement (ADE).

ADE is being reported as COVID-19 because the patients are testing positive for COIVD-19. Renowned virologist and Nobel Prize Laureate Prof. Luc Montagnier explained that the so-called breakthrough COVID-19 infections being suffered by the fully vaccinated persons are infections caused by the COVID-19 vaccines.[777] Dr. Montagnier said that the high rate of COVID-19 infections among the fully vaccinated population is due to antibody-dependent enhancement (ADE).

Dr. Robert Malone, M.D., M.S., the inventor of the mRNA technology used by Pfizer-BioNTech and Moderna in their COVID-19 vaccines, states that the COVID-19 vaccines are causing ADE. Dr. Malone indicates that the scientific evidence is becoming increasingly clear that the COVID-19 vaccines are causing the virus to replicate at higher levels than would be the case in the absence of the vaccination.[778] He said that this phenomenon of ADE was predictable because ADE has happened in every coronavirus study ever conducted. He said the data indicates that as the immune response from the COVID-19 vaccines wanes after six months, the ADE is kicking in, and we see the result with increased hospitalizations. The hospitalizations are not from breakthrough infections in those vaccinated but rather from ADE brought on by the vaccine itself. The ADE causes the virus to replicate more efficiently than it would otherwise. Dr. Malone further states that those in the vaccinated population are generating the delta variant of COVID-19 due to the COVID-19 vaccine.

One research study explained:

> There are also immunopathological complications associated with the SARS-CoV and MERS-CoV vaccines that require addressing and further optimization. One adverse effect is the induction of antibody-dependent enhancement (ADE) effect, which is usually caused by vaccine-induced

> suboptimal antibodies that facilitates viral entry into host cells.[779]

Since the investigational vaccines for SARS-CoV caused ADE, it is thus not a surprise to find that the SARS-CoV-2 (COVID-19) vaccines also cause ADE.

Researcher Ken Garber explains:

> There are mounting theoretical concerns that vaccines generating antibodies against SARS-CoV-2 may bind to the virus without neutralizing it. Should this happen, the non-neutralizing antibodies could enhance viral entry into cells and viral replication and end up worsening infection instead of offering protection, through the poorly understood phenomenon of ADE. ADE "is a genuine concern," says virologist Kevin Gilligan, a senior consultant with Biologics Consulting, who advises thorough safety studies. "Because if the gun is jumped, and a vaccine is widely distributed that is disease enhancing, that would be worse than actually not doing any vaccination at all."[780]

A study was conducted by Timothy Cardozo of the Department of Biochemistry and Molecular Pharmacology, NYU Langone Health, New York, and Ronald Veazey of the Division of Comparative Pathology, Department of Pathology and Laboratory Medicine, Tulane University School of Medicine, Tulane National Primate Research Center. The scientists determined in their research that the COVID-19 vaccines caused an increase in the risk of more severe diseases caused through ADE. They concluded that recipients of COVID-19 vaccines should be warned about all the dangers of ADE before being vaccinated. The scientists determined that the COVID-19 vaccines worsen COVID-19 disease via antibody-dependent enhancement (ADE). They were concerned that the dangers are kept secret in clinical trial protocols and consent forms.[781] The researcher stated:

> Results of the study: COVID-19 vaccines designed to elicit neutralising antibodies may sensitise vaccine recipients to more severe disease than if they were not vaccinated. Vaccines for SARS, MERS and RSV have never been approved, and the data generated in the development and testing of these vaccines suggest a serious mechanistic concern: that vaccines designed empirically using the traditional approach (consisting of the unmodified or minimally modified coronavirus viral spike to elicit neutralising antibodies), be they composed of protein, viral vector, DNA or RNA and irrespective of delivery method, may worsen COVID-19 disease via antibody-dependent enhancement (ADE). This risk is sufficiently obscured in clinical trial protocols and consent forms for ongoing COVID-19 vaccine trials that adequate patient comprehension of this risk is unlikely to occur, obviating truly informed consent by subjects in these trials.
>
> Conclusions drawn from the study and clinical implications: The specific and significant COVID-19 risk of ADE should have been and should be prominently and independently disclosed to research subjects currently in vaccine trials, as well as those being recruited for the trials and future patients after vaccine approval, in order to meet the medical ethics standard of patient comprehension for informed consent.[782]

Many other researchers have determined that the

COVD-19 vaccines pose a clear danger of ADE. In another study, the researchers concluded:

> Antibody-based drugs and vaccines against severe acute respiratory syndrome coronavirus 2 (SARS-CoV-2) are being expedited through preclinical and clinical development. Data from the study of SARS-CoV and other respiratory viruses suggest that anti-SARS-CoV-2 antibodies could exacerbate COVID-19 through antibody-dependent enhancement (ADE).[783]

Another researcher pleaded for caution in the administration of the COVID-19 vaccine:

> [B]ecause ADE of disease cannot be reliably predicted after either vaccination or treatment with antibodies-regardless of what virus is the causative agent-it will be essential to depend on careful analysis of safety in humans as immune interventions for COVID-19 move forward.[784]

Sadly, the researcher's warning was not heeded. A massive study involving vaccine data from hundreds of countries proves that the COVID-19 vaccines have caused a significant increase in total cases and deaths associated with COVID-19.[785] The study proves that the COVID-19 vaccines are not only ineffective, but they are driving illness and death. The study showed that the COVID-19 vaccines have caused a whopping 38% more COVID-19 cases and an even more astonishing 31% increase in deaths from COVID-19 in the United States.[786] But that is only the tip of the iceberg because many patients suffering ADE may not test positive for COVID-19. They still suffer the consequences of the ailments caused by the vaccine-induced ADE.

As we have learned, there are two kinds of antibodies.

"There are neutralizing antibodies and binding antibodies (aka, non-neutralizing antibodies). We want neutralizing antibodies but not the binding antibodies. Binding antibodies do not 'neutralize' the virus when they bind, and rather, their presence indicates a potential problem."[787] The current vaccines have been touted as successful, but their "success" is based on antibody production. It is not based on challenging the test participants with the virus to see if there is successful protection from the virus or whether there would be an antibody-dependent enhancement that would make the test participant ill.[788] Why was that not done? Presumably, it is because the researchers knew from the SARS-CoV animal studies that the test subjects would suffer ADE. A vaccine producing ADE could never be approved.

The ADE is manifesting among the vaccinated. For example, it was reported on August 26, 2021, that the hospitals in Israel were filling up with vaccinated patients. Dr. Steven Li reported for the Vision Times:

> On Aug. 5, Dr. Kobi Haviv, medical director of Herzog Hospital in Jerusalem, said in a Channel 13 TV News interview, "95% of the severe patients are vaccinated." Furthermore, "85-90% of the hospitalizations are in fully vaccinated people" and the hospital is "opening more and more COVID wards."[789]

ADE was predictable. Pfizer-BioNTech was aware of the risk of ADE. They knew all about it from the SARS-CoV animal trials. Pfizer-BioNTech, in their December 10, 2020 briefing document sent to the FDA in their request for an EUA, claimed that the available data did not show any vacccine-enhanced disease during the short follow up period of their study. But in the next sentence, the company warned that the risk of ADE remains unknown and needs to be evaluated in ongoing trials.

> However, risk of vaccine-enhanced disease over time, potentially associated with waning immunity, remains unknown and needs to be evaluated further in ongoing clinical trials and in observational studies that could be conducted following authorization and/or licensure.[790]

Notice that Pfizer-BioNTech states that there was a risk of ADE "potentially associated with waning immunity."[791] That is precisely what the animal studies showed. And that is why Pfizer-BioNTech said that. Pfizer-BioNTech knew that there was a risk of ADE "with waning immunity." The statement that the risk was unknown is misleading. They knew there was a general risk and that the risk was real; they just did not know it with precision. That is what Dr. Malone explained. He said that this phenomenon of ADE was predictable because ADE has happened in every coronavirus study ever conducted.[792] Pfizer-BioNTech and Moderna certainly knew that. Dr. Malone also revealed that the studies showed that the ADE could be expected to show up as the immune response from the COVID-19 vaccines wanes. He put the time frame at six months for the immune response waning. Moderna and Pfizer-BioNTech knew that also. Indeed, they said that the risk of ADE was "potentially associated with waning immunity."[793] The ADE from the COVID-19 vaccines we are witnessing is not a surprise to the CDC, the FDA, Moderna, or Pfizer-BioNTech. It was predictable. Both Pfizer and Moderna state that the risk of ADE "needs to be evaluated further in ongoing clinical trials and in observational studies that could be conducted following authorization and/or licensure."[794] But no such trials are being conducted. All we hear from both companies and the CDC is that the hospitalizations and deaths of the vaccinated population are from breakthrough infections. They now deny that ADE is a reality.

Identical language about the risk of ADE can be found in the Moderna briefing document. In a later April 30, 2021 post-

EUA authorization report filed with the FDA, Pfizer acknowledged that vaccine-associated enhanced disease (VAED) and vaccine-associated enhanced respiratory disease (VAERD) were listed as "Important Potential Risk[s]" of the COIVD-19 vaccines.[795] Pfizer noted that the VAED may go unreported as such because the patient suffering VAED will usually be presented as having "severe or unusual manifestations of COVID-19."[796] Thus the announced "breakthrough" cases of COVID-19 are likely not COVID-19 cases but are rather cases of VAED, otherwise known by the acronym ADE, caused by the COVID-19 vaccines themselves.

ADE is a known risk for the mRNA coronavirus vaccines. That is why both Pfizer and Modern mentioned it. ADE perfectly explains the VAERS reporting of 595,620 adverse events, including 13,068 deaths, 17,228 permanent disabilities, and 54,142 hospitalizations as of August 13, 2021.[797] The VAERS system reports correlation; it does not mean that causation has been proven. Recall that the HHS-funded study reported that the VAERS database is only catching 1% of all of the vaccine-related adverse events.[798] The means that each of the above numbers can be multiplied by 100 to get the true scope of the damage being done by the COVID-19 vaccines. For example, the 13,068 VAERS deaths represents 1,306,800 actual deaths. The VAERS system reports correlation; it does not mean that causation has been proven. Recall that Megan Redshaw determined that 41% of those getting a COVID-19 vaccine died after becoming ill within 48 hours of injection.[799] We will consider that as establishing a reasonable belief that the COVID-19 vaccines were the cause of the deaths. Thus, we come up with a conservative figure of 535,788 persons we have probable cause to believe died from the COVID-19 vaccines as of August 13, 2021.

Another problem with VAERS is that it is under the auspices and control of the CDC and is consequently subject to their manipulation. For example, the Informed Consent Action

Network (ICAN) discovered that the CDC deleted an adverse event from VAERS. If they got caught deleting one adverse event, there are likely others deleted for which the CDC has not been caught. The deleted report "described an extremely disturbing incident wherein a two-year-old boy 'began bleeding out of the mouth, eyes, nose and ears within six hours' of his first dose of Pfizer's COVID-19 vaccine on November 18, 2021, and died later that night."[800]

The VAERS report (VAERS ID: 1887456) describes a two-year-old child who received a Pfizer/BioNTech COVID-19 vaccine on November 18, 2021. The report states that the child died that same day, November 18, 2021. The VAERS report of the incident was filed two days later, on November 20, 2021, and describes the adverse event:

> Patient began bleeding out the mouth. eyes, nose and ears within six hours of shot Died that night.[801]

ICAN filed a Freedom of Information Act (FOIA) request with the CDC asking for documents explaining why the VAERS report was deleted. By the way, FOIA requests can only be made for documents and not to answer questions. Unsurprisingly, the CDC stated that they had no records that would explain the deletion.

We all know why the VAERS report was deleted. The adverse event is chilling proof of the barbarity and lethality of the COVID-19 vaccines. The CDC's deletion of that report is proof that the CDC is part of the coverup of the deadliness of the COVID-19 vaccines. Likely, that is one of many reports that the CDC has deleted.

Please understand that some pharmaceutical companies are notorious for committing criminal fraud. One of them happens to be the manufacturer of a COVID-19 vaccine. On September 2,

2009, the U.S. Department of Justice announced that Pfizer "agreed to plead guilty to a felony violation of the Food, Drug and Cosmetic Act for misbranding Bextra with the intent to defraud or mislead."[802] As part of that settlement, Pfizer "agreed to pay $2.3 billion, the largest health care fraud settlement in the history of the Department of Justice."[803] Pfizer is a repeat offender.[804] Between 1991 and 2017, Pfizer entered into 34 civil and criminal settlements with the federal and state governments totaling $4.7 billion.[805] Past behavior is the best predictor of future conduct. The VAERS data indicates that Pfizer-BioNTech is responsible for 69% of the COVID-19 vaccine deaths reported in VAERS.[806] Extrapolating from the VAERS data, as explained above, I have probable cause to believe that out of the 535,788 persons who have died from the COVID-19 vaccines as of August 13, 2021, Pfizer and its German partner, BioNTech, are responsible for killing 369,694 of those people.[807] Those figures are as of August 13, 2021; the carnage continued.

The American Liberty Report revealed that "more than 18 million people were injured so badly by their first COVID shot from Pfizer or Moderna that they had to go to the hospital. That's according to the CDC's own internal data, which a court just ordered the federal agency to release to a watchdog group."[808] The CDC started a vaccine monitoring program using a software application called V-safe at the beginning of the COVID-19 vaccine rollout in December of 2020. Ten million people downloaded the V-safe app on their cell phones. Those people then reported adverse events from the COVID-19 vaccines through the V-safe app. The CDC received the data and tracked it for the first 18 months until July 2022. Strangely, the CDC never published the data.

You would think that the data showed that the COVID-19 vaccines were safe, since CDC's main webpage about the mRNA COVID-19 vaccines says, to this day, "COVID-19 vaccines are safe, effective and free."[809] Indeed, that is what the CDC has been saying all along. But that was not true, and the CDC knew it. A court ordered the CDC to release its V-safe data. It showed that there were 800,000 receivng medical care out of 10 million people.[810] That translates to an 8% medical care rate. Approximately 73% of those seeking medical care needed to visit urgent care, the emergency room, or be hospitalized. Extrapolating to the population of 230 million people who received the vaccine in the U.S., we find that 18 million of them received medical care for injuries caused by the COVID-19 vaccines.

The graphic below is from the Informed Consent Action Group (ICAN).[811] It reveals that an additional 2.5 million people were unable to engage in normal activities or missed work or school. That is a total of 3.3 million out of the 10 million people reporting serious adverse events in V-Safe. That is a 33% serious adverse event rate. When extrapolating to the U.S. population who were vaccinated (230 million), we find that 76 million people suffered serious adverse events from the COVID-19 vaccines that required them to miss work or school, be unable to carry on normal activities or seek medical care.

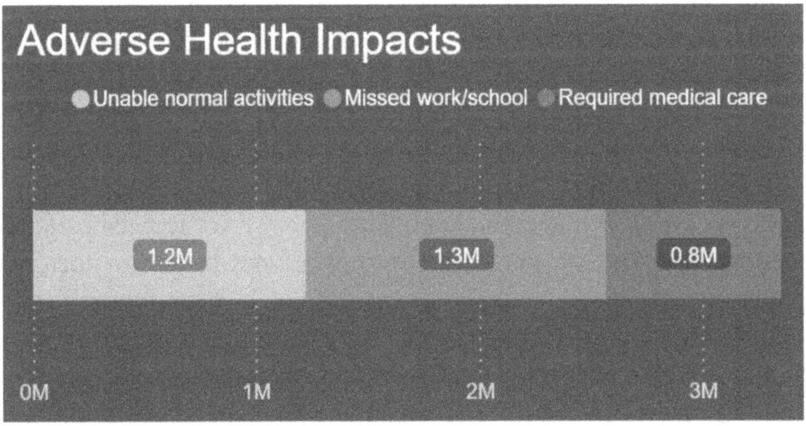

This most recent revelation from the CDC V-safe database is quite incriminating for Inova hospitals. Inova mandates that its employees be vaccinated with the COVID-19 vaccine.[812] Inova claims that the COVID-19 vaccines are safe and effective. Indeed, the claim made on its website is that "Inova has seen minimal side effects in the 100,000+ doses we have administered so far."[813] But we know that cannot be true. We now have the raw data from the CDC V-safe system showing that 8% of those who have received the COVID-19 vaccine have needed medical care for maladies caused by the vaccine.[814] Inova runs five hospitals and approximately 13 urgent care facilities in Northern Virginia. Inova is uniquely positioned to receive a significant number of those vaccine-injured patients. Inova must know about the dangerousness of the COVID-19 vaccines because they would see COVID-19 visits to their hospitals. Yet, Inova claims that it has seen "minimal side effects." The CDC V-safe data impeaches that claim. The V-safe data and the assertions by Inova cannot both be true. Inova is lying.

Why would Inova claim that the COVID-19 vaccines are safe and effective when the evidence shows they are not safe and effective? The answer begins with a survey report published on June 16, 2021, from the Association of American Physicians and Surgeons (AAPS). That survey revealed 58% of the approximately 700 physicians surveyed reported that they were not “fully vaccinated” against COVID-19.[815] The survey revealed that about 53% of the physicians were “aware of patients suffering significant adverse reaction[s]” from a COVID-19 vaccination.

The pharmaceutical companies saw the vaccine hesitancy among doctors as a problem. They could not have a majority of doctors refusing the COVID-19 vaccine because the concern of the physicians would spill over into their recommendations to their patients. The pharmaceutical companies took immediate action and got their lackeys at HHS and CMS to issue a rule mandating all staff at health care facilities that participate in Medicare and Medicaid programs to be vaccinated.[816] That rule applied to 76,000 healthcare providers and facilities and more than 17 million healthcare workers.[817]

The rule issued by the government cracked down on doctors, nurses, and staff, requiring them to be vaccinated against COVID-19. That rule is a virtual guarantee that almost all doctors will be vaccinated because, according to the American Hospital Association, 94% of hospitals have 50% of their inpatient days paid by Medicare and Medicaid and more than three quarters of hospitals have 67% Medicare and Medicaid inpatient days."[818] The hospitals in the U.S. cannot afford to buck against the Centers for Medicare & Medicaid Services (CMS) and lose that income. And so they cracked down on doctors, nurses, and staff, requiring them all to be vaccinated against COVID-19.

Non-compliance with the new vaccination rule comes with heavy sanctions. CMS has issued guidance that if the medical facility does not vaccinate all eligible staff or prove they have an exemption, then they can be cited for noncompliance. Punishment includes cutting off all Medicare and Medicaid funding. "If facility does not return to compliance, it is at risk for additional enforcement actions, including losing Medicare or Medicaid payment."

Inova Hospital's opinion that the COVID-19 is safe and effective is based on its pecuniary interests. More than 50% of the income of their hospital system comes from CMS. The Inova opinion about the COVID-19 vaccines is not based on science. Inova is being paid very well by CMS to opine that the COVID-19 vaccines are safe and effective. Those who run the Inova Hospital system are liars. They lie because their jobs depend on it. If any member of the hospital management team came out against the vaccines, he would immediately be fired. All hospital staff know that.

With that kind of financial carrot and stick, hospital systems like Inova have vigorously enforced the vaccine mandate from HHS and CMS. Upon the issuance of the federal rule, Inova began a program of firing any medical staff who refused to be vaccinated. Inova routinely denied most requests for religious exemptions. Inova and the nation are suffering a nurse shortage. It is indeed bewildering that Inova would terminate qualified nurses, thus exacerbating the already short-staffed Inova hospitals. Inova does not care; it cannot lose CMS money.

The Constitution only places limits on government action. The Federal Government CMS program pressures hospitals like Inova to require staff to be vaccinated on the threat that CMS payments will be withheld. That makes the hospital vaccine requirement "state action." Hospitals are acting as agents of the government, carrying out government edicts. Thus, the constitutional protections and standards for state action apply to the hospital vaccine requirement.[819] That means that a hospital's actions requiring vaccines are limited by the religious protections of First Amendment to the U.S. Constitution. In addition, the U.S. Equal Employment Opportunity Commission (EEOC) states that "Title VII of the Civil Rights Act of 1964 requires employers to make a reasonable accommodation for an employee's sincerely held religious beliefs as long as doing so does not pose an undue hardship on the employer."[820]

Inova's scheme of denying religious exemptions may be illegal. Indeed, Jason Miyares, the Attorney General of Virginia, has opined that Inova's actions of "terminating critical health care professionals" in the way they did could be illegal.[821] General Miyares stated that Inova has repeatedly denied requests for religious exemptions based on an "incorrect judgment of the sincerely held religious beliefs of individuals," and has displayed an "outright failure to accommodate reasonable requests as required by law"[822] General Miyares indicated that Inova is presently under investigation by his office for violations of the Virginia Human Rights Act, Va. Code §§ 2.2-3900, *et seq*.; 2.2-510, *et seq*.

28 COVID-19 Vaccines Are Dangerous

Vaccines are largely ineffective and unsafe. Indeed, it is an established medical fact that the COVID-19 vaccines not only do not prevent illness, they cause illness. Please be mindful that the COVID-19 vaccines were authorized because they purportedly prevented infection and the spread of the disease.

Dr. Peter McCullough, M.D., is an American cardiologist. He is one of the most highly respected and published cardiologists in the U.S. Dr. McCullough, M.D., was vice chief of internal medicine at Baylor University Medical Center and a professor at Texas A&M University. He is editor-in-chief of the journal Reviews in Cardiovascular Medicine and Cardiorenal Medicine. Dr McCullough is an internationally recognized kidney and cardiovascular authority. He has more than 1000 publications. In fact, Dr. McCullough is reputed to be the most cited medical doctor on COVID-19 treatments at the National Library of Medicine, with more than 600 citations. Dr. McCullough has testified before Congress. Dr. McCullough is a medical expert on vaccines. Indeed, he has chaired more than two dozen vaccine safety monitoring boards for the FDA, and National Institute for Health.[823] Dr. McCullough's expert medical opinion is that the COVID-19 vaccines are unsafe and ineffective.[824]

Dr. McCullough was once one of the most published and cited authors in the medical community. Since he has come out explaining the dangers of the COVID-19 vaccines, Baylor and Texas A&M have cut ties with him. He has had his research revealing the dangers of the COVID-19 vaccines suddenly unpublished and deleted.[825]

Dr. Peter McCullough, M.D., gave an informative presentation at the 2022 United Healthcare Summit.[826] During his presentation, Dr. Mcullough cited the sweeping research by the World Council For Health (WCH) that revealed the dangers of the COVID-19 vaccines. This author decided to check his claims about the WCH research findings. I discovered that he was correct. My research took me beyond the WCH findings. It includes some surprising facts and evidence, which will be shocking to some, about the COVID-19 vaccines.

The World Council For Health (WCH) extensively studied the world databases on the COVID-19 vaccine injuries. The WCH studied the WHO VigiAccess, CDC VAERS, EudraVigilance, and UK Yellow Card Scheme to determine whether the COVID-19 vaccines are safe.[827] On June 11, 2022, the WCH announced its results. The WCH found that the databases revealed more than 40,000 deaths linked to the COVID-19 vaccines and called for an immediate recall of those vaccines.[828]

Those reported deaths are just the tip of the proverbial iceberg. Dr. Katrina Lindley explains the deficiency in the reports:

> [S]uch systems of passive surveillance result in significantly fewer ADR [adverse drug reaction] reports than active surveillance reporting. As a result, the actual number of adverse events that occurred in temporal relation to Covid-19 injections is likely to be much higher than revealed by the available official data.[829]

The under-reporting in the databases is quite significant. Indeed, it is exponential. For example, because the VAERS database relies on passive reporting, it suffers from a systemic flaw known to HHS. That flaw is that the VAERS database under-reports the vaccine adverse events by a factor of 100. A Harvard study of the VAERS database that HHS commissioned revealed that "fewer than 1% of vaccine adverse events are reported."[830] That statistical finding in the Harvard study has been confirmed to be accurate in a subsequent scientific study.[831]

The underreporting in VAERS has been verified in other studies. The Journal of the American Medical Association (JAMA) reported that the Vaccine Adverse Events Reporting System (VAERS) reports that occurrence of anaphylaxis from the COVID-19 Vaccines is "4.7 cases/million Pfizer-BioNTech vaccine doses administered and 2.5 cases/million Moderna vaccine doses administered, based on information through January 18, 2021."[832] In a March 30, 2021 posting, the CDC reported similar statistics alleging that "[a]naphylaxis after COVID-19 vaccination is **rare** and occurred in approximately 2 to 5 people per million vaccinated in the United States based on events reported to VAERS."[833] (bold emphasis in original)

The problem with the reports from JAMA and the CDC is that they are contradicted by another, more recent, March 8, 2021 report from JAMA. That study of Mass General Brigham (MGB) employees receiving COVID-19 vaccines, was published by the JAMA reveals that "severe reactions consistent with anaphylaxis occurred at a rate of 2.47 per 10,000 vaccinations."[834]

Elizabeth A. Brehm, wrote a letter on behalf of the Informed Consent Action Network (ICAN) to Dr. Rochelle P. Walensky, the Director of the Centers for Disease Control and Prevention.[835] Brehm pointed out that the MGB study reveals that the VAERS is under-reporting the accounts of anaphylaxis from the COVID-19 vaccines by a factor of between 50 and 120 times.

ICAN complained that "[t]he underreporting of anaphylaxis by the CDC and VAERS is particularly troubling because it is mandatory for medical providers to report anaphylaxis after any COVID-19 vaccine to VAERS."[836] The most salient point in the letter from ICAN is the revelation from the MGB study that "the rate of reporting [of COVID-19 vaccine anaphylaxis adverse reactions] still appears to be only around 0.8 to 2 percent of all cases of anaphylaxis." The ICAN letter goes on to point out the obvious:

> This raises serious concerns regarding (1) under-reporting of other serious adverse events following COVID-19 vaccination, and (2) adverse events following other vaccines for which there has not been the same push to report adverse events. The anaphylaxis study highlights the urgency of the ongoing, well-known problem with adverse event reporting post-vaccination.[837]

The MGB and WCH studies confirm the previous study done by Harvard that indicated that "fewer than 1% of vaccine adverse events" are reported in the VAERS system. Thus, you can multiply any statistic from the VAERS system by 100, and you will have a better idea of the actual number for that category of adverse events. Thus, deaths reported under VAERS would likely be subject to the same under-reporting as would anaphylaxis. As with anaphylaxis, we can expect that only 1% of all deaths from COVID-19 vaccines are being reported in the VAERS system.

The CDC-run Vaccine Adverse Events Reporting Service (VAERS) is a passive reporting system. It relies, for the most part, on reporting of practitioners of adverse events from vaccines. Keep in mind that the VAERS data discloses correlation and it does not prove causation. But that does not mean that the COVID-19 vaccine did not cause the adverse event; it simply means that the causation has not yet been proven with scientific certainty. But the VAERS data establishes probable cause to believe that the COVID-19 vaccines are responsible for a significant plurality of the reported adverse events.

The adverse events listed in VAERS have not been clinically proven to have been caused by the listed vaccine. But we can reasonably infer that those who died within 48 hours of the onset of illness after the vaccination died from the vaccine. Megan Redshaw determined that of those VAERS reported as having died after receiving the COVID-19 vaccine, 19% died within 24 hours of vaccination, 27% died within 48 hours of vaccination, and 41% died after becoming ill within 48 hours of vaccination.[838] We will consider that 41% figure of temporal proximity as establishing a reasonable belief that the COVID-19 vaccines were the cause of those deaths.

It is fair to infer that a very high percentage of those who showed symptoms within 48 hours of receiving the vaccine and later died did so from the vaccine. VAERS reported that of July 15, 2022, there were 29,635 deaths attributed to COVID-19. 41% of 29,635 is 12,150. Thus, one can reasonably conclude there is probable cause to believe that 12,150 persons died from the COVID-19 vaccine. Understanding that the VAERS system only reports 1% of the actual deaths, we find that the deaths from the COVID-19 vaccines are 1,215,000 people as of July 15, 2022.

The World Council For Health (WCH) noted that the Polio Vaccine was recalled in less than one year after ten reported deaths, yet the Covid-19 vaccine, with 29,635 associated deaths, has not been recalled after two years.[839] The WCH concluded that "[t]here is sufficient evidence of adverse events relating to Covid-19 vaccines to indicate that a product recall is immediately necessary."[840] The WCH came to that conclusion based on the associated deaths reported as of July 15, 2022, in VAERS being approximately 29,635. But the argument for an immediate recall becomes more compelling when one considers that there is probable cause to believe that the number of deaths caused by the

COVID-19 vaccines is actually closer to 1.2 million (12,635 x .41 = 12,150) x 100 = 1,215,000.[841]

Similar numbers were arrived at by other researchers. VAERS is a database that reports adverse events associated with vaccines. The appearance of an adverse event in the database does not prove that the vaccine caused the adverse event. Because the VAERS database reports correlation and does not prove causation, we are left to extrapolate causation from the numbers reported in the VAERS database. Researchers led by Dr. Scott McLachlan, Ph.D., determined that the vaccine caused 86% of deaths reported in VAERS.[842] Dr. Jessica Rose, Ph.D., and her team of researchers studied the U.S. VAERS database and determined that VAERS underreported adverse events, including deaths, from the COVID-19 vaccines by a factor of 41. That means the actual adverse events, including deaths, associated with the COVID-19 vaccines are 41 times greater than reported in the VAERS system.[843]

Dr. Rose is a Canadian researcher with a Bachelor Degree in Applied Mathematics and a Master's degree in Immunology from Memorial University of Newfoundland. She also holds a Ph.D. in Computational Biology from Bar Ilan University and two Post Doctoral degrees: one in Molecular Biology from the Hebrew University of Jerusalem and one in Biochemistry from the Technion Institute of Technology.

Assuming the VAERS system underreports adverse events by 41-fold, and the COVID-19 vaccine caused 86% of the deaths reported in VAERS, we can determine the actual number of deaths caused by the COVID-19 vaccines.[844] As of September 23, 2022, the VAERS database reported that 31,214 persons died after being vaccinated with a COVID-19 vaccine. Although the U.S. Government keeps the VAERS database, it also includes deaths from COVID-19 vaccinations in other countries. Approximately 50% of the deaths reported in VAERS are from other countries. That means approximately 15,000 persons died in the U.S. alone from COVID-19 vaccines.

We will start with the 15,000 U.S. figure. Multiplying that figure by 41 we arrive at 615,000. But only 86% of that number can be said to have died from the vaccine. Multiplying 615,000 by .86, we arrive at a final figure of 528,900 as the number of persons who died from the COVID-19 vaccines in the U.S. as of September 23, 2022. If we apply that formula to the total of U.S. and overseas reported deaths in VAERS, we arrive at a figure of 1.1 million deaths caused by the COVID-19 vaccines as of September 23, 2022. That is very close to the estimated 1.2 million deaths caused by the COVID-19 vaccines as of July 15, 2022, which was arrived at above using a different calculation method and assumptions.

As of July 28, 2022, there have been more adverse event reports in VAERS for the COVID-19 vaccines than all other 70+ vaccines combined during the entire 32 year history of the VAERS database. Of the total 2.2 million adverse event reports in VAERS over the last 32 years, 1.3 million of those reports were for adverse events from the COVID-19 vaccines in the past 19 months.[845]

Megan Redshaw also revealed that the VAERS data shows "[t]here were 77 reports of Guillain-Barré Syndrome with 55% of cases attributed to Pfizer, 40% to Moderna and 10% to J&J."[846] Recall that the VAERS database only reflects 1% of actual injuries. Thus, as of April 8, 2021, we can reasonably infer that there have been 7,700 cases of Guillain-Barré Syndrome correlated to COVID-19 vaccines. Guillain-Barré is an autoimmune disorder that causes a person's immune system to damage the body's nerves. This autoimmune response causes severe muscle weakness and sometimes paralysis. The paralysis can be transitory, but it can also be permanent.

Only Janssen (J&J) mentions Guillain-Barré Syndrome in its fact sheet as a risk from its COVID-19 vaccine.[847] Guillain-

Barré Syndrome is not mentioned as an adverse event outcome in either of the COIVD-19 vaccine fact sheets provided to recipients and caregivers from Moderna or Pfizer-BioNTech.[848] But Guillain-Barré Syndrome was listed by the FDA among the possible "adverse event outcomes" being monitored during the COIVD-19 vaccine trials. A slide from a presentation by Steve Anderson, Director of Biostatistics and Epidemiology for the FDA, at the October 22, 2020 Vaccines and Related Biological Products Advisory Committee meeting lists Guillain-Barré Syndrome as one of the possible adverse event outcomes being monitored by the FDA during the COVID-19 vaccine trials.[849] The slide can be seen in the chapter in this book on antibody-dependent enhancement. They knew what to look for because they knew what they were seeing. The slide was shown for only a split second before it disappeared from view, and Dr. Anderson made no mention of it. No doubt they discovered Guillain-Barré Syndrome in all the vaccines, but only Janssen would admit to it.

Why focus only on VAERS data of deaths and Guillain-Barré Syndrome? That is because death and Guillain-Barré Syndrome were the two events that caused the swine flu vaccine to be abruptly pulled from the market. Recall that the swine flu vaccine was administered to 40 million people over a 10 week period in 1976. That vaccine program was stopped within 10 weeks because 25 people died and 500 people developed Guillain-Barré Syndrome.[850]

Guess what else Dr. Anderson listed on his slide among the possible adverse event outcomes from the COVID-19 vaccine trials? — "Deaths."[851] As I said earlier, they knew what to look for because they knew what they were seeing. They were not going to waste their time looking for things that they did not expect to find. And they could not avoid seeing people drop dead. The FDA and the vaccine makers knew that the COVID-19 vaccines would kill people. That revelation in the flashed slide seemed to be inadvertent because the slide with that information disappeared within a split second with no comment on it from Dr. Anderson. Almost certainly, the adverse event outcome of ‘deaths” were found during the COVID-19 vaccine studies because we see COVID-19 vaccine deaths happening throughout the country. But death is not listed as an adverse event in the COVID-19 vaccine fact sheets provided to the recipients and caregivers from the vaccine makers.

The swine flu vaccine program is generally recognized as a “debacle” of epic proportions because of the debilitating injuries and deaths caused by it. But we have the same thing happening with the COVID-19 vaccines but on an exponentially greater level, and yet the COVID-19 vaccines are still being promoted as safe.

The deaths from the COVID-19 vaccines in the U.S. are exponentially greater than the deaths from the swine flu vaccine (25). The same goes for the cases of Guillain-Barré Syndrome from the COIVD-19 vaccine (7,700) versus the swine flu vaccine (500). Those figures are from the early date of April 8, 2021, which was only four months into the COVID-19 vaccine program. No doubt, the cases have continued to mount. Comparing the death rate for the COVID-19 vaccine to the swine flu vaccine, we find that the COVID-19 vaccine is 1,000 times more deadly than the disastrous swine flu vaccine.

So, why was the swine flu vaccine withdrawn from the market, and the exponentially more dangerous COVID-19 vaccine is being promoted as safe and effective? The difference is that the swine flu vaccine was introduced in 1976. That was before Congress passed the National Vaccine Injury Act (NVIA) of 1986. That law granted pharmaceutical companies immunity for injuries caused by their vaccines. The Public Readiness and Emergency Preparedness Act (PREP Act), which authorizes the Countermeasures Injury Compensation Program (CICP) to provide benefits to injured parties, gives pharmaceutical companies even more liability protection than the NVIA. The COVID-19 vaccines presently fall under the PREP Act (CICP).

There is simply no incentive for pharmaceutical companies or government regulators to ensure that vaccines are safe so long as they fall under the protection of the CICP or NVIA. The claims that vaccines are safe and effective are part of a deceptive theater; those behind the curtain know the truth, while the mesmerizing magic show beguiles the audience.

The CDC and the mainstream media persistently promote the COVID-19 vaccines like circus barkers drawing in the suckers to their destruction. President Biden characterizes the COVID-19 vaccines as "safe, free, and effective vaccines."[852] When, on September 9, 2021, President Biden announced his vaccine requirement for federal workers he said: "The vaccines are safe, highly effective."[853]

The President's Executive Order 14043 of September 9, 2021, mandating COVID-19 vaccinations for federal workers, must be considered in light of the carnage that was already known to have been caused by the COVID-19 vaccines by the time he issued the order. As of August 13, 2021, there were reported in the HHS Vaccine Adverse Event Reporting System (VAERS) 13,068 deaths correlated to the COVID-19 vaccines.[854] The Pfizer-BioNTech COVID-19 vaccine accounted for 9,024 of those deaths.[855] A research team from the American Frontline Doctors (AFLD) found that the VAERS database indicates that the total reported vaccine deaths in the first quarter of 2021 represents a 12,000% to 25,000% increase in vaccine deaths, year-on-year.[856] The AFLD determined that there were more deaths (approx. 4,000) from the COVID-19 vaccines reported in VAERS in the first four months of 2021 than deaths reported in VAERS for all other vaccines combined (1,529) over the ten year period from 2009 to 2019.[857] The AFLD research team determined that COVID-19 Vaccines have caused 99% of all reported vaccine deaths in 2021.[858] All other vaccines combined account for the remaining 1% of vaccine deaths. The carnage caused by the COVID-19 vaccines was known when President Biden issued his vaccine mandate for federal workers.

Dr. McCullough explains that the COVID-19 experimental vaccine is "the largest application of a biological product with the greatest amount of morbidity and mortality in the history of our country."[859]

Dr. McCullough details the malfeasance of the government regulatory agencies. "With this program, there is no critical event committee, there is no data-safety monitoring board, and there's no human ethics committee. Those structures are mandatory for all large clinical investigations, and so the word that's really used for what's going on is malfeasance, that's wrongdoing of people in authority."[860]

In an interview, Dr. McCullough gave listeners some perspective on just how dangerous the COVID-19 vaccines are. He explains that "[a] typical new drug at about five deaths, unexplained deaths, we get a black-box warning, your listeners would see it on TV, saying it may cause death," McCullough said. "And then at about 50 deaths it's pulled off the market."[861]

Dr. McCullough juxtaposes that with what he has been able to gather from confidential sources that "[w]e think we have 50,000 dead Americans. Fifty thousand deaths. So we actually have more deaths due to the vaccine per day than certainly the viral illness by far. It's basically propagandized bioterrorism by injection."[862] That statement regarding 50,000 deaths was made on June 11, 2021, which was less than six months after the COVID-19 vaccine rollout.

There is a government database that, unlike VAERS, is not public. That database is found in the Centers for Medicare and Medicaid Services (CMS). A whistleblower, who is a computer programmer with subject matter expertise in the healthcare data analytics field, has filed a sworn affidavit in a lawsuit that the CMS data collated with VAERS data shows 45,000 deaths from COVID-19 vaccines.[863] The affiant stated under oath on July 13, 2021, the following:

> It is my professional estimate that VAERS (the Vaccine Adverse Event Reporting System) database, while extremely useful, is under-reported by a conservative factor of at least 5. On July 9, 2021, there were 9,048 deaths reported in VAERS. I verified these numbers by collating all of the data from VAERS myself, not relying on a third party to report them. In tandem, I queried data from CMS medical claims with regard to vaccines and patient deaths, and have assessed that the deaths occurring within 3 days of vaccination are higher than those reported in VAERS by a factor of at least 5. This would indicate the true number of vaccine-related deaths was at least 45,000. Put in perspective, the swine flu vaccine was taken off the market which only resulted in 53 deaths.[864]

Dr. McCullough's estimate of 50,000 deaths and the CMS expert's estimates of 45,000 deaths from the COVID-19 vaccines may yet still be exponentially under reporting because the sources are relying on government data. Such data suffers from under reporting. The VAERS data study commissioned by HHS concluded that the under reporting in VAERS was by a factor of 100. The VAERS system was only capturing 1% of the adverse events.

The HHS-funded Harvard study revealed that the VAERS data represents only 1% of the total adverse events.[865] As of July 28, 2022, there have been more adverse event reports in VAERS for the COVID-19 vaccines than all other 70+ other vaccines combined during the entire 32 year history of the VAERS database. Of the total 2.2 million adverse event reports in VAERS over the last 32 years, 1.3 million of those reports were for adverse events from the COVID-19 vaccines in the past 19 months.[866]

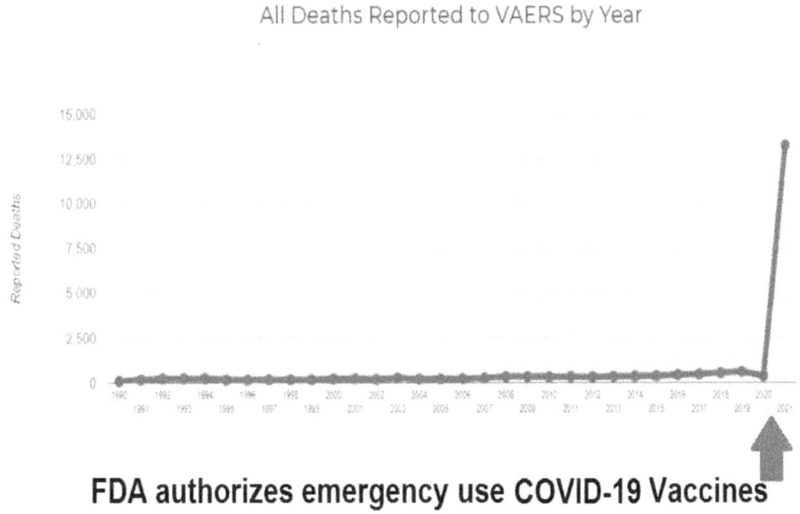

The Expose reported that "[t]he UK Medicine Regulator has confirmed that over a period of nineteen months the Covid-19 Vaccines have caused at least 5.5x as many deaths as all other available vaccines combined in the past 21 years."[867] But when measuring the lethality of the COVID-19 vaccines side-by-side against all other vaccines over the same 19-month period, it was found that the COVID-19 vaccine caused 7,402% (74x) more deaths than all other vaccines combined during that 19-month period.[868] As we saw with the German government statistics, the deaths from vaccines is vastly under-reported. But such under-reporting should be across the board for all vaccines. And so, the statistics about the relative number of deaths should be somewhat accurate. Based on those relative statistics, the COVID-19 vaccines are 74 times more deadly than all other vaccines combined. The below graphic is from *The Expose.*

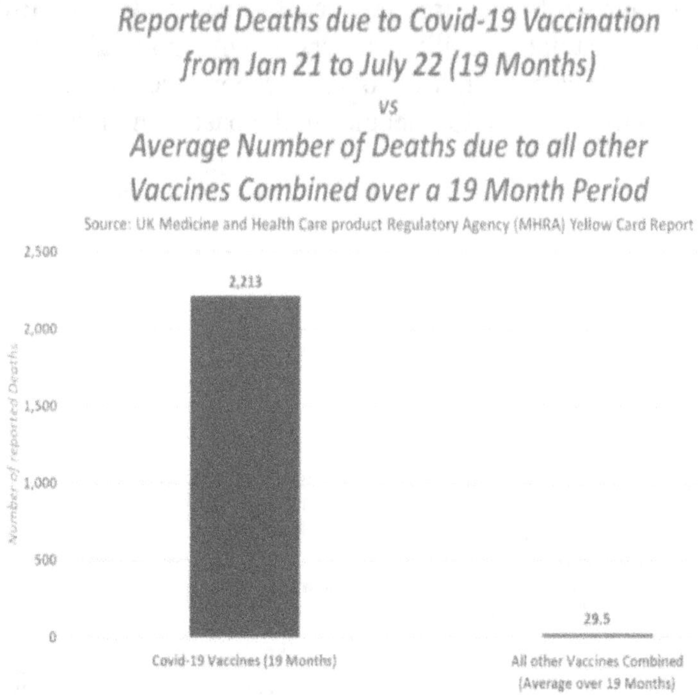

On July 19, 2021, America's Frontline Doctors (AFLDS) filed a motion seeking immediate injunctive relief in the Alabama Federal District Court to stop the Emergency Use Authorization (EUA) of the experimental COVID-19 injections. The plaintiffs averred the following facts in their certified complaint about the relative dangers of the COVID-19 vaccines:

> According to data extracted from the Defendants' Vaccine Adverse Events Reporting System ("VAERS"), 99% of all deaths attributed to vaccines in the first quarter of 2021 are attributed to the COVID-19 Vaccines, and only 1% are attributed to all other vaccines. The number of vaccine deaths reported in the same period constitutes a 12,000% to 25,000% increase in vaccine deaths, year-on-year.[869]

Why are the COVID-19 vaccines so harmful? Dr. Robert Malone has the answer. Dr. Malone is a medical doctor and a world-famous infectious disease expert. Dr. Malone has close to 100 peer-reviewed publications and published abstracts and has over 11,477 citations of his peer reviewed publications. **Most notably, Dr. Malone is the inventor of the mRNA technology used by Pfizer-BioNTech and Moderna in their COVID-19 vaccines.**[870] Vaccines using mRNA technology are not like conventional vaccines, which use weakened forms of the virus. An mRNA vaccine uses only part of the virus's genetic code. An mRNA vaccine carries code into the body, where it enters cells. The mRNA instructs those cells to create spike proteins that are associated with SARS-CoV-2 (the alleged virus that causes COVID-19). These spike proteins are recognized by the immune system, which then attacks them. **Dr. Malone has stated that the spike proteins generated by the cells through the mRNA code are cytotoxic.**[871] That means that the spike proteins are toxic to living cells. Thus, the COVID-19 mRNA vaccines made by Pfizer-BioNTech and Moderna allowed under the EUA cause the body to create spike proteins that kill the cells in the body. That cytotoxicity is the cause of the many adverse events being reported in VAERS. Malone explained that he is a regulatory professional and has connections with persons in senior positions in the FDA. On or about June 13, 2021, Malone stated that he alerted those senior officials in the FDA to the cytotoxicity of the spike protein being generated by the mRNA vaccines "months-and-months ago."[872]

With damning data establishing within the first month that the COVID-19 vaccines are unsafe, the mainstream media quickly sprung into action to do the bidding of the CDC and report that "initial safety data shows everything is going well."[873] For example, Karen Weintraub reported on January 28, 2021, for *USA Today* the following false information:

> Everyone who experienced an allergic response has

> been treated successfully, and no other serious problems have turned up among the first 22 million people vaccinated, according to the Centers for Disease Control and Prevention.[874]

I don't know about you, but I would say that 104 permanent disabilities, 273 life-threatening events, 11 birth defects, 722 hospitalizations, 2,056 visits to the emergency room, and 329 deaths within the first month of the COVID-19 rollout would fall into the category of "serious problems." Indeed, the deaths associated with the COVID-19 vaccines, as reported in VAERS, had exploded to 33,011, and hospitalizations had soared to 186,726 by December 16, 2022.[875] To put those figures into perspective, a typical new drug receives a black box warning after five unexplained deaths. If the deaths raise to 50 the drug is pulled off the market. Yet within one month there were 329 deaths attributed to the COVID-19 vaccines, yet *USA Today* runs a story claiming that the COVID-19 vaccines are "not causing large numbers of unusual or dangerous results."[876] So, how does *USA Today* address those deaths? They dismiss them as not being caused by the vaccine. Weintraub writes:

> Vaccinated people have suffered major health crises and even death within a few days of receiving a shot, but the rate of those events is no higher than would be expected in the general population and cannot be connected to the vaccine, the review found.[877]

That is a complete lie. There is simply no way to reconcile that statement with the fact that there have been more adverse event reports in VAERS for the COVID-19 vaccines than all other 70+ other vaccines combined during the entire 32 year history of the VAERS database.

Interestingly, the CDC and *USA Today* credit the reports of minor responses and allergic reactions as being caused by the vaccines when the person is treated and recovers. But when the person dies or is seriously injured "it cannot be connected to the vaccine." *USA Today* puts the VAERS data in its report; it is there for all to see. But *USA Today* spins the data to the CDC's and mainstream media's preconceived conclusion that the COVID-19 vaccine is safe and effective. Keep in mind this article (more like cheerleading) was early on and floated to minimize the early data of injuries and death and encourage people to be vaccinated.

The same VAERS reporting system that faithfully reports minor injuries is suddenly deemed by *USA Today* not sufficient to conclude that serious injury or death is caused by the vaccine. What a scam. It's a game of heads I win, tails you lose. With that kind of approach, it is easy for *USA Today* to misrepresent that "[a]lthough it's never possible to prove something is completely safe, data from these tracking systems suggests the vaccines are not causing large numbers of unusual or dangerous results."[878]

Keep in mind that conclusion is in the face of an acknowldegment in the *USA Today* report that "[t]he problems in slightly more than 1,000 of those [9,000 VAERSS] reports were considered serious."[879] *USA Today*'s claim that the COVID-19 vaccines are "not causing large numbers of unusual or dangerous results" was refuted, even at that early stage, by the VAERS data. But *USA Today* tried to put a favorable spin on the incriminating data.

Dr. Denis Rancourt, Ph.D., is a former tenured full professor of physics at the University of Ottawa, who has published more than one hundred articles in leading science journals. Dr. Rancourt took the all-cause mortality increases by country and correlated them to the vaccine rollouts in each country. He was able to extrapolate a death rate for the COVID-19 vaccines. In his February 9, 2023 report he concluded that approximately 13 million people have died worldwide from the

COVID-19 vaccines.[880] That figure includes 330,000 deaths in the United States alone. He used robust criteria to establish causation based on the Loannidis criteria of experiment, temporality, and consistency.

While the CDC plays down the hazards of the COVID-19 vaccines, others have taken notice of the VAERS raw data that proves the vaccines are dangerous. For example, on February 15, 2023, the Florida Department of Health issued a health alert to doctors and the public regarding the dangers of the COVID-19 vaccines. Florida health officials are concerned about the significant increase in adverse events reported in VAERS during the COVID-19 vaccine campaign. Some may try to argue that the increase in adverse events was because there was a 400% increase in vaccinations due to the COVID-19 vaccination campaign. The problem is that the Florida Department of Health recorded a troubling 1,700% spike in vaccine adverse events during the 2021 COVID-19 vaccine campaign. In addition, the life-threatening adverse events exploded to an increase of 4,400% during the COVID-19 vaccine program. That means the COVID-19 vaccines are four (4) times more harmful and eleven (11) times more life-threatening than any other vaccine. Below is a chart posted by the Florida Department of Health showing the disturbing spike in reported adverse events.[881]

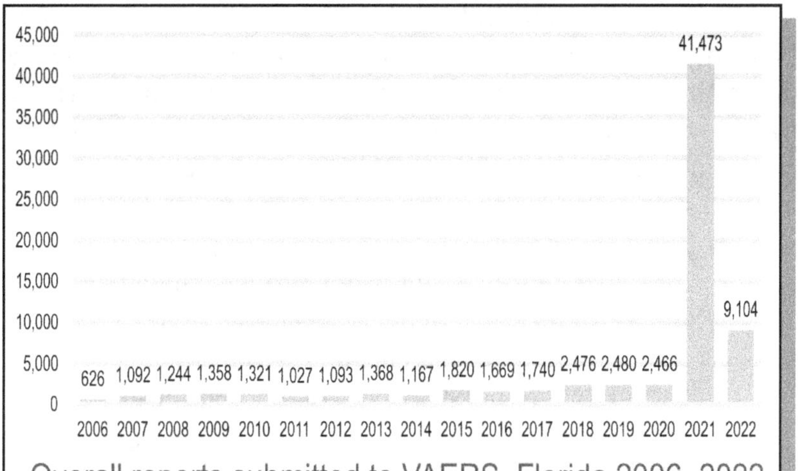

Overall reports submitted to VAERS, Florida 2006–2022

This spike in adverse events prompted Florida Surgeon General, Joseph Ladapo, M.D., to write a letter to Robert M. Calif, MD, Commissioner, U.S. Food and Drug Administration (FDA), and Rochelle P. Walensky, Director, Centers for Disease Control and Prevention (CDC). General Ladapo stated:

> [A]academic researchers throughout our country and around the globe have seen troubling safety signals of adverse events surrounding this vaccine. Their concerns are corroborated by the substantial increase in VAERS reports from Florida, including life-threatening conditions. We have never seen this type of response following previous mass vaccination efforts pushed by the federal government. Even the HINI vaccine did not trigger this sort of response. In Florida alone, we saw a 1,700% increase in reports after the release of the COVID-I9 vaccine, compared to an increase of 400% in vaccine administration for the same period. The reporting of life threatening conditions increased 4,400%.[882]

What was unusual (and refreshing) was that General Ladapo implied that the CDC and the FDA were restricting and diminishing the rights and liberties of U.S. citizens by restricting transparency in the medical community and failing to communicate the risks of the COVID-19 vaccines. He called on them to stop it.

> As a father, physician, and Surgeon General for the State of Florida, I request that your agencies promote transparency in health care professionals to accurately communicate the risks these vaccines pose. I request that you work to protect the rights and liberties that we are endowed with, not restrict, and diminish them.[883]

The Florida Department of Health's health alert did not simply note the correlation between the increase in adverse events and the rollout of the COVID-19 vaccines. The Florida health officials were positing that the COVID-19 vaccines are unsafe. In support of that position, they cited specific research studies that have found that the COVID-19 vaccines cause serious health problems.

> According to a study,[884] mRNA COVID-19 vaccines were associated with an excess risk of serious adverse events, including coagulation disorders, acute cardiac injuries, Bell's palsy, and encephalitis. This risk was 1 in 550 individuals, which is much higher than other vaccines.
>
> A second study,[885] found increased acute cardiac arrests and other acute cardiac events following mRNA COVID-19 vaccination.
>
> Additionally,[researchers in an article in The Journal of the American Medical Association[886]]

> assessed the risk of thromboembolic and thrombocytopenic events related to COVID-19 vaccines and found preliminary evidence of increased risk of both coronary disease and cardiovascular disease.

CDC spokesman Nick Spinelli tried to do damage control and responded to General Ladapo's letter that the Florida Department of Public Health's conclusions were misleading because the data was missing context.[887] He then threw up the smokescreen argument that the VAERS system shows correlation and not necessarily causation. While that statement is true, he is hiding the ball. He conceals that correlation often gives reasonable belief for causation, particularly when there is a temporal relationship between the vaccine and the injury. To say that it cannot be proven that someone dies from a vaccination when they have a heart attack after getting a vaccine is, on its face, accurate. But when there is a pattern of such deaths, and there is no other reasonable cause, it is fair to say that one should be careful about deciding to receive the vaccine. VAERS is not irrelevant, but the CDC argues that VAERS data is only coincidental because there is no sure proof of causation.

The CDC is playing a misleading game. Most of the VAERS reports are submitted by medical professionals who have looked at the circumstantial evidence and determined that there is probable cause (i.e., reason to believe) that the vaccine in question caused the sickness or death they are reporting. It is like a witness who tells police that he heard a gunshot and saw John Doe running from a room carrying a smoking gun. The witness enters the room to see Tom Thumb dead on the floor with a bullet hole in his head. The police would clearly have probable cause to arrest John Doe for the murder of Tom Thumb. But would those facts be enough to prove John Doe's guilt beyond a reasonable doubt? What if John Doe's defense is that Tom Thumb put the gun to his head to commit suicide, and he tried to grab the gun to prevent the suicide, and Tom Thumb suddenly pulled the trigger? John Doe claims he ran from the scene with the gun to report the suicide to the police. If that is true, then John Doe is not guilty of murder. Of course, there is the matter of what other evidence there is in the case and whether the jury believes John Doe's defense.

There is a difference between probable cause to arrest and proof of guilt at trial beyond a reasonable doubt. And that is what the CDC is obfuscating. The CDC is conflating what is necessary to stop the vaccine program, which is equivalent to what is needed to arrest John Doe, with what is required to prove the vaccines cause death and injury, which is equivalent to what is necessary to prove John Doe murdered Tom Thumb.

Just as there is probable cause to arrest John Doe for the murder of Tom Thumb, so also there is probable cause to stop the COVID-19 vaccinations because there is probable cause from the VAERS data showing that the vaccines are unsafe. Just as further investigation will be necessary to prove that John Doe is guilty of murder, so also, further investigation will be necessary to establish with scientific certainty that the vaccines are causing the death and destruction as reported in the VAERS system.

Another important point the CDC is not revealing is that the reported deaths and injuries are just the tip of the proverbial iceberg. Dr. Katrina Lindley explains that the VAERS data under-reports fatalities and injuries because VAERS is a passive reporting system. The reality is that "systems of passive surveillance result in significantly fewer ADR [adverse drug reaction] reports than active surveillance reporting."[888] Consequently, "the actual number of adverse events that occurred in temporal relation to Covid-19 injections is likely to be much higher than revealed by the available official data."[889] But the CDC will not mention that truth.

The CDC is just plain lying about the dangers of the

COVID-19 vaccines. Another CDC spokesman said in an email sent to the media, "COVID-19 vaccines have undergone—and continue to undergo—the most intense vaccine safety monitoring in U.S. history."[890] That is a lie. But the CDC spokeman goes further. He states that "[c]linical research has demonstrated the safety and effectiveness of the recommended COVID-19 primary series vaccines, as well as the recommended updated vaccines."[891] That is another lie. It seems that the CDC is staffed with pathological liars.

Indeed, the deception about the COVID-19 vaccines is so clear and egregious that on December 12, 2022, the Governor of Florida called for a grand jury investigation to bring criminal charges against the officials and companies involved in the death and destruction caused by the vaccines. Arek Sarkissian, reporting for Politico, revealed:

> [Florida] Gov. Ron DeSantis on Tuesday asked the Florida Supreme Court to empanel a grand jury to investigate "wrongdoing" linked to the Covid-19 vaccines, including spreading false and misleading claims about the efficacy of the doses.
>
> Most of the medical community, including the Centers for Disease Control and Prevention, the FDA and Johns Hopkins, have emphasized that the Covid vaccine is safe and effective in preventing the virus and protecting against serious symptoms.
>
> But DeSantis said during a live-streamed round table discussion with Florida Surgeon General Joseph Ladapo that it's against Florida law to mislead the public, especially when it comes to drug safety. He sought to undermine the efficacy of the Covid vaccine and claimed that vaccine manufacturers such as Moderna have made a

fortune on Covid-19 mandates.

> "I think people want the truth that I think people want accountability," DeSantis said. "You need to have a thorough investigation into what's happened with the shots."
>
> In a petition to the state Supreme Court asking for the grand jury, the DeSantis administration said that the "pharmaceutical industry has a notorious history of misleading the public for financial gain" and the grand jury will probe "the development, promotion, and distribution of vaccines purported to prevent COVID-19 infection, symptoms, and transmission."[892]

The Florida Governor stated in his petition that government officials and pharmaceutical companies misled the public about the safety and efficacy of the COVID-19 vaccines. The deception caused people to decide to get the vaccines which caused them injuries. The injuries were foreseeable because government officials and manufacturers knew that the vaccines were dangerous. For example, while the pharmaceutical companies claimed there was no causal link between their vaccines and myocarditis, they knew at the time from their studies and other published studies that, in fact, their vaccines caused myocarditis. The gravamen of the charges in the *Petition For Order To Empanel a Statewide Grand Jury* are as follows:

> Florida law prohibits fraudulent practices, including the dissemination of false or misleading advertisements of a drug and the use of any representation or suggestion in any advertisement relating to a drug that an application of a drug is effective when it is not. § 499.0051(11), Fla. Stat. The pharmaceutical industry has a notorious

> history of misleading the public for financial gain. 42 Questions have been raised regarding the veracity of the representations made by the pharmaceutical manufacturers of COVID-19 vaccines, particularly with respect to transmission, prevention, efficacy, and safety. An investigation is warranted to determine whether the pharmaceutical industry has engaged 1n fraudulent practices. The people of Florida deserve to know the truth.[893]

Sucharit Bhakdi, M.D., is a retired doctor. He is a microbiologist and an expert in immunology. He was a post-doctoral researcher at the Max Planck Institute of Immunobiology and Epigenetics and at The Protein Laboratory in Copenhagen. He was appointed associate professor at the Institute of Medical Microbiology at Giessen University. He was named chair of Medical Microbiology at the University of Mainz. Dr. Bhakdi has published over three hundred articles on immunology, bacteriology, virology, and parasitology, for which he has received numerous awards and the Order of Merit of Rhineland-Palatinate.[894]

Alex Newman, the Senior Editor of The New American magazine, interviewed Dr. Bhakdi.[895] During the interview, the world-renowned microbiologist warned that the COVID-19 virus hysteria is based on lies. The COVID “vaccines” are set to cause a global catastrophe and decimation of the human population. He explains that the PCR test has been abused to artificially inflate the danger of COVID-19 and produce fear in an unscientific way.

Dr. Bhakdi expects massive, deadly clotting and immune system responses that will destroy the human body. During a previous Fox News interview, Dr. Bhakdi warned of impending doom from the vaccines. He calls for criminal prosecutions of the people responsible for the vaccine injuries and death and an immediate halt to the global vaccine experiment.

29 Increased All-Cause Mortality

Vaccine manufacturers often try to obscure their vaccines' dangerousness by arguing that correlation does not necessarily mean causation. That bare statement is true. The correlation is not causation argument offers some logical cover when there is an allegation that a vaccine caused an adverse event or a death. The correlation is not necessarily causation argument can be made in any individual case of death without scientific confirmation that the vaccine caused the death. The vaccine makers often argue a myriad of co-factors for the deaths.

But we must key in on the word "necessarily." While correlation does not "necessarily" prove causation, correlation can nonetheless be convincing evidence of causation where no other variables can explain the adverse event or death. There is a statistic that saps the persuasiveness of the correlation is not necessarily causation argument. The all-cause mortality statistic for an entire population makes it difficult to conceal the deaths caused by a population-wide vaccine program. The occurrence of events (deaths) spread over a large population after the occurrence of an independent variable (vaccination) administered to that same population raises a stronger inference of causation than a single occurrence of an event (death) after a single prior independent variable (vaccination).

The Bradford-Hill criteria are used to determine if there is a causal relationship between a presumed cause and an observed effect. Five Bradford-Hill criteria pertinent to showing if vaccines cause adverse events indicate a causal relationship between COVID-19 vaccinations and excess deaths.[896] 1) Consistency in the reported association between vaccinations and deaths by different authorities at different locations. 2) The association between vaccinations and deaths is strong, involving large populations. 3) There is a specific association between vaccinations and deaths rather than some other factor. 4) There is a temporal relationship between vaccinations and deaths, such that the deaths follow after the vaccinations. 5) It is biologically plausible that vaccinations are causing the deaths.[897]

All-cause mortality covers the gambit of people who die from all causes. A significant increase in all-cause mortality indicates that something acted on the population to bring about that increase. Thus, if a vaccine is dangerous and causes widespread death, the increased deaths will appear in the all-cause mortality rate. Suppose the only change in population behavior is vaccination. In that case, a subsequent increase in deaths would be convincing evidence that the vaccine caused those deaths. The correlation between the population-wide vaccine program and the increased deaths from all causes is compelling evidence that the vaccine is the independent variable causing the deaths since there is no other variable that would explain the excess deaths.

A February 2023 study that compared the average monthly all-cause mortality rate for the years 2016-2019 to the monthly all-cause mortality for the first nine months of 2022 found that the countries that vaccinated their population for COVID-19 during 2021 saw a 0.105% increase in the monthly all-cause mortality rate for every one percent increase in people being vaccinated in that country.[898] That is a direct correlation between COVID-19 vaccines and increased deaths across many countries. More COVID-19 vaccines result in more deaths.

The study looked at the all-cause mortality for the first nine months of 2022 and compared it to the vaccination uptake in 31 European countries by the end of 2021. The 31 countries studied were the EU member states, plus Norway, Iceland, Liechtenstein, and Switzerland. The researchers determined the correlation between vaccination uptake and the mortality rate was significant. It "implies that the mortality increases the higher the vaccination uptake. Specifically, it shows that a one percentage point increase in 2021 vaccination uptake is associated with an increase in 2022 monthly mortality by 0.105 percent."[899]

The vaccine uptake for the COVID-19 vaccines for the countries ranged from Bulgaria, with 27.7% of the country vaccinated, to Portugal, with 83.1% of the population vaccinated. All countries, except Bulgaria, vaccinated more than 50% of their people.

The 0.105% increase in mortality for every one percent increase in vaccinations represents a 10.5% increase in all-cause mortality among the vaccinated population. To understand the significance of the 10.5% increase in all-cause mortality in Western Europe's vaccinated population, we must consider that the background mortality rate from all causes in most Western countries is approximately 1% per year.[900] Eurostat reported that "the number of deaths per 1,000 persons was estimated at 10.4 in the EU in 2019."

For simplicity's sake, we will use 1% as the base mortality rate for Western Europe. That means that year in and year out, approximately 1% of the population in Western Europe die each year. Thus, the statistics from the February 2023 study showing an increase in the all-cause mortality rate of 0.105% for every percentage increase in vaccine uptake indicates that the COVID-19 vaccines are correlated with a rise of 10.5% in all-cause mortality in Western Europe. Assuming a base rate of about 1%, that means there is a death rate of 1.105% for the vaccinated population.

Looking at the U.S, we find the same increase in the mortality rate correlated to the rollout of the COVID-19 vaccines. But U.S. death statistics for 2020, in particular, must be looked at with suspicion. That is because the CDC has been caught fudging the mortality data. For example, The Guardian reported that the CDC was caught over-counting COVID-19 deaths.[901] Once the CDC was confronted with the over-count, it claimed to have corrected it and attributed it to a "coding logic error." Oddly, no "coding logic error" had ever happened before the COVID-19 "pandemic." Usually, a coding error would result in the missed recording of statistics. It is rather suspicious that the "coding logic error" resulted in an artificial increase in COVID-19 deaths.

Also, the CDC has massaged the COVID-19 death data to under-report the vaccinated deaths from COVID-19 by listing vaccinated deaths as unvaccinated deaths. Add to that the efforts made by the CDC to prevent effective treatments like hyrdroxychloroquine and ivermectin for flu-like illnesses while locking down and masking people and administering dangerous and ineffective treatments such as remdesivir, midazolam, and ventilation. It is no wonder that the death rate increased in 2020. With those cautions in mind we will look at what seems to be an increase in mortality in the U.S. after the introduction of the COVID-19 vaccines.

Because of the anomalous government actions during the 2020 "pandemic" and the untrustworthiness of the mortality rates reported by the CDC that year, we will use the average mortality rates in the U.S. from 2015 to 2019. We will compare the average mortality rate from 2015-2019 to the death rates after the introduction of the COVID-19 vaccines to obtain the delta. The average annual mortality rate for 2015-2019 was 0.86%.[902] That means an average of 0.86% of the U.S. population died annually between 2015 and 2019.

The Organisation for Economic Co-operation and Development (OECD) is an intergovernmental organization with 38 member countries. It keeps data on mortality for those countries, which includes the U.S. The data shows a significant increase in all-cause mortality in the U.S. after the rollout of the COVID1-19 vaccines.[903]

That website only provides U.S. all-cause death numbers for 2020, 2021, and 2022. To give the raw death numbers meaning, we must be able to compare them to the deaths for prior years. As noted earlier, the average death rate reported by the CDC for the years 2015 to 2019 was 0.86%.[904] But that number is unhelpful in comparing it to the raw death numbers reported by the OECD. In order to compare the average mortality rate for 2015-2019 to the mortality rate for 2020, 2021, and 2022, we must convert the raw numbers provided by the OECD to a percentage.

The OECD website lists the all-cause deaths and reveals that the 2020 all-cause mortality rate in the U.S. was 1.04%. That figure was arrived at by dividing the all-cause deaths reported by the OECD (3,441,118)[905] by the mid-year U.S. population reported by the U.S. Census Bureau on June 30, 2020 (331,509,617).[906] The OECD website lists the all-cause deaths reveals that the 2021 all-cause mortality rate in the U.S. was 1.04%. That figure was arrived at by dividing the all-cause deaths reported by the OECD (3,457,525)[907] by the mid-year U.S. population reported by the U.S. Census Bureau on June 30, 2021 (332,028,282).[908] The OECD website lists the all cause deaths and reveals that the 2022 all-cause mortality rate in the U.S. was 0.981%. That figure was arrived at by dividing the all-cause deaths reported by the OECD (3,270,300)[909] by the mid-year U.S. population reported by the U.S. Census Bureau on June 30, 2022 (333,282,419).[910]

Thus we find an increase in the mortality rate in the U.S. in 2020 of 0.18% (1.04%–0.86% = 0.18%). Recall that 2020 saw some strange and anomalous actions and reporting of deaths by the CDC, so the numbers cannot be relied upon. What is really interesting is that after the rollout of the COVID-19 vaccines in 2021, we see the same increase in mortality of 0.18% (1.04%–0.86% = 0.18%). You would expect the mortality rate to decrease if you assume the vaccines are effective due to the massive vaccine program. Instead, we find continued carnage at the same rate as 2020. Then, in 2022, we find that there was a continuation of the excess deaths but at a slightly slower clip of 0.12% (0.98%–0.86% = 0.12%).

The 2021 0.18% increase over the 0.86% death rate represents an astounding 20% increase in the mortality rate in the U.S. during 2021. The 2022 0.12% increase over the 0.86% death rate represents a 14% increase in the mortality rate in the U.S during 2022. **What that means in real numbers is that there have been approximately 997,589 excess U.S. deaths correlated to the rollout of the COVID-19 vaccines during 2021 and 2022.**[911] Again, correlation does not necessarily mean causation. But the statistics from the UK where the vaccinated death rate can be compared to the unvaccinated death rate, strengthens the causation argument.

When we focus on the statistics from the UK, the inference of causation becomes clearer. That is because the UK Office for National Statistics (ONS) breaks down its death statistics by vaccination status. Thus, we can compare the all-cause death rate of the vaccinated population against the all-cause death rate for the unvaccinated population and find out from where the excess deaths are coming.

The investigative journalists at *The Expose* examined the official death data from the UK Office for National Statistics (ONS). On March 21, 2023, *The Expose* reported that between

January 1, 2021, and May 31, 2022, the all-cause mortality rate among those who had received a COVID-19 vaccine was 1.36%. But the all-cause mortality rate for those who had not received any COVID-19 vaccine was 0.58%. The mortality rate among the COVID-19 vaccinated population is more than double that of the unvaccinated population. *The Expose* reported:

> 44.48 million people had received at least one dose of a Covid-19 vaccine in England, and 606,537 of those people had sadly died. This, therefore, equates to 1 in every 73 [which is a 1.36% mortality rate for] Covid-19 vaccinated people having sadly died by the 1st of June 2022.
>
> 18.9 million people had not received a single dose of a Covid-19 vaccine in England, and 109,891 of those people had sadly died. This, therefore, equates to 1 in every 172 [which is a 0.58% mortality rate for] unvaccinated people having sadly died by the 1st of June 2022.[912]

The above data presents total all-cause mortality of 1.130% for both vaccinated and unvaccinated combined between January 1, 2021, and May 31, 2022. There were 716,428 total deaths (606,537 vaccinated + 109,891 unvaccinated = 716,428 total deaths). The total vaccinated and unvaccinated population was 63.38 million (44.8 million vaccinated + 18.9 million unvaccinated = 63..38 million total population). That results in a total mortality rate of 1.130% (716,428 ÷ 63.38 million = 1.130%).

The UK's base mortality rate for 2019 and prior was less than 1%. But for simplicity's sake, we will use 1% for the base mortality rate for the UK. Assuming a base mortality rate of 1%, that means there has been about a 13% increase in total mortality in the UK between January 1, 2021, and May 31, 2022, after the rollout of the COVID-19 vaccines. That increased mortality is attributable entirely to the vaccinated population because the unvaccinated population had a mortality rate of approximately 0.58%, which is far below the approximate 1% total expected mortality rate for Wester European countries. *The Expose* explains:

> The official figures unfortunately confirm that mortality rates per 100,000 are the lowest among the unvaccinated population in every single age group in England. And the data reveals the gap between the unvaccinated and vaccinated populations in terms of mortality rates is widening by the month.[913]

When you break out just the vaccinated group, we find a mortality rate of 1.36%. Comparing that to the expected base mortality rate of approximately 1%, we see a whopping 36% increase in mortality among the vaccinated population. *The Expose* comes to the ineluctable conclusion:

> There is no other conclusion that can be found for the fact mortality rates per 100,000 are the lowest among the unvaccinated other than that the Covid-19 injections are killing people.[914]

To put that in perspective, a study of 1,118 unique armed conflicts spanning 193 countries between 1990 and 2017 found that the increase in civilian mortality during a war is 81.5 per 100,000 population.[915] That is an increased mortality rate of 0.0815% during a war. That increased war mortality is due to a break-down in infrastructure that increases communicable and non-communicable diseases, respiratory infections, maternal, neonatal, and nutritional diseases, respiratory infections and tuberculosis, enteric infections, and maternal and neonatal disorders, increased cardiovascular diseases, diabetes and kidney diseases, neoplasms, and digestive diseases, etc.

During a war, the civilian mortality rate increases by 0.0815%. Assuming the background mortality rate in the European Union of approximately 1%, we arrive at a total civilian mortality rate during a war in Europe of approximately 1.0815%. The COVID-19 vaccines are inferred to cause a greater mortality increase of 10.5% among the vaccinated population of Western Europe. That suggests that the COVID-19 vaccines had a devastating effect on the population of Europe. The inference from the all-cause mortality statistics is that the COVID-19 vaccines caused the mortality rate to increase in the vaccinated population to 1.105% which is more than what would be expected in the civilian population during a war.

According to the European Centre for Disease Prevention and Control, as of March 2023, approximately 330 million persons in the EU have received at least two doses of a COVID-19 vaccine.[916] Ordinarily, about 3.3 million of those people would die from all different causes each year. But extrapolating a death rate of 0.105% increase in the monthly all-cause mortality rate for every one percent of the persons vaccinated, we can expect that an additional 10.5%, or 346,500 persons will have died from the COVID-19 vaccine in 2022.

While correlation does not "necessarily" mean causation when the correlation across so many different countries only shows a rise in mortality, the inference of causation is robust. It certainly raises to the level of at least probable cause. Dr. John Campbell, Ph.D., opined that the correlation from the February 2023 study was so strong that he declared it a "slam dunk."[917]

Mathematician Igor Chudov conducted a separate study and analyzed the correlation between COVID-19 booster shots and the rise in all-cause mortality across approximately 29 countries (including the USA). He used the average weekly mortality rates of 2017-2019 to establish the baseline and compared it to the weekly mortality increase during weeks 10 to 35 in 2022. On August 30, 2022, Chudov announced his findings.[918] He was shocked by what he found. He discovered an almost linear correlation between the rate of COVID-19 booster shots and a rise in national mortality rates. The P value for the correlation was 0.0002. A P value that is below 0.05 is considered statistically significant. A P value that is 0.0002 is considered to be an ironclad correlation that could not be by random coincidence.

Chudov was careful to say that he was merely reporting the correlation. Chudov stated that the proper interpretation "is that there is an EXTREMELY PROMINENT RELATIONSHIP between boosters and deaths in 2022." (emphasis in original). The correlation showed: "More boosters – more deaths!" Chudov concluded:

> Despite my stating clearly that I uncovered a *correlation*, not a *causation*, I personally believe that boosters ARE a cause of increased mortality. There are many reasons to believe this to be highly likely.[919] (italics and emphasis in original)

Igor Chudov conducted another analysis of UK data. This time it was limited to UK mortality data. He analyzed the unique data from the UK, which tracked the COVID-19 vaccinated population. The UK Government has data where it collects and reports weekly excess mortality by vaccination status.[920] To arrive at the excess mortality, the UK government used the average mortality rate between 2015 to 2019 as their base mortality rate.

The UK Government tracks the vaccination rates among quintiles that rank a population according to economic disparities. Igor Chudov downloaded and analyzed the May to September 2022 UK Government data. He found a direct correlation between an increase in the vaccination rate and an increase in the excess death rate.

The lowest rank of the five quintiles was the most economically deprived and was found to have the lowest vaccine rate of 79.40%. That lowest quintile was shown to have an excess death rate of 7.85%. There was a steady increase in the death rate as the vaccination rate increased with the economic status of the quintile. The highest excess death rate of 12.55% was found at the highest quintile, with a COVID-19 vaccine rate of 93%. When you look at the chart below, you can see a steady increase in the death rate as there is an increase in the vaccination rate.

Deprivation Level	Vaccination Rate %	Excess Mortality %
Most Deprived	**79.4%**	**7.85%**
More Deprived	**84.5%**	**9.22%**
Median	**88.7%**	**11.36%**
More Wealthy	**91.1%**	**12.37%**
Most Wealthy	**93.0%**	**12.55%**

As you can see from the above chart, there is a direct correlation between the COVID-19 vaccination rate and the mortality rate. More COVID-19 vaccines mean more deaths. Chudov analyzed those statistics and found that the R^2 was 0.9471. That means that the increase in the COVID-19 vaccination rate explains 95% of the increase in the death rate across the quintiles.

Chudov further calculated the P value for the statistics to be 0.0052. That means there is only a 0.5% chance that the increase in the death rate correlated to the increase in the vaccine rate was due to chance. Chudov plotted the data on a chart, illustrating the obvious correlation between increased COVID-19 vaccination and deaths. Chudov concluded that "this makes a very strong case that excess mortality in the UK in May-Sep 2022 is caused by Covid vaccines."[921]

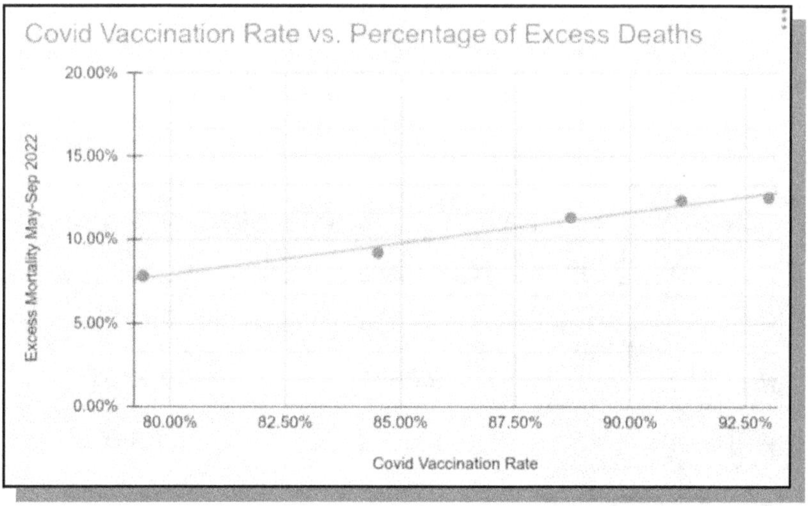

Chudov also uncovered evidence from another statistician showing a significant drop in the UK birthrate in 2022 compared to 2021. The statistician did some digging and found a correlation between the increase in the COVID-19 vaccination rate and a decline in the birth rate.[922] That correlation was based on the UK deprivation statistics. The study showed that the proportion of women giving birth in the two wealthier quintiles of the UK population, which had the higher COVID-19 vaccination rate, dropped in 2022. But the proportion of women giving birth in the two more deprived quintiles of the population, which had a lower vaccination rate, increased in 2022. That was notable because it is the reverse of the historical precedent between 2017 and 2020, where the two higher quintiles had a steadily growing proportion of mothers giving birth, and the two most deprived quintiles had a steadily reduced proportion of mothers giving. That suddenly flipped in 2022, directly correlating to the COVID-19 vaccination program and a reduced overall birth rate. Chudov suggested that the COVID-19 vaccines are acting as a depopulation scheme. Chudov commented:

> We have an interesting situation: Covid vaccines appear to cause a decline in birth rate, and at the same time, an increase in the death rate. A decline in births and a simultaneous increase in deaths is called depopulation. So, is Covid vaccine a depopulation vaccine?[923]

Up to this point, we have been comparing total all-cause mortality differences. But the devastating effect of the vaccines can be seen more clearly when looking at just the sliver of increase in excess deaths from all causes. For example, according to official government data from the Australian Organisation for Economic Co-Operation and Development (OECD), the increase in excess deaths became exponential upon the rollout of the COVID-19 vaccines in 2021. *The Expose* reports that "the Australian Government confirms the first 38 weeks of 2021 saw a shocking 1,452% increase in excess deaths following the rollout of the COVID-19 injections compared to the same period in 2020."[924] *The Expose* limited its analysis to the first 38 weeks of 2020, 2021, and 2022 because it only had official government statistics for excess death data available for the first 38 weeks of 2022.

When comparing the excess deaths during the first 38 weeks of 2022, when the vaccine rollout was in full swing, compared to the first 38 weeks of 2020, during the height of the alleged COVID-19 pandemic, *The Expose* discovered a whopping 5,162% increase in excess deaths in 2022 compared with 2020.

> By 2022, the nation was hit by a devastating blow, with a shocking 5,162% increase in excess deaths in the first 38 weeks of the year following the repeat rollout of the COVID-19 injections compared to the first 38 weeks of 2020, at the alleged height of the pandemic.[925]

If the vaccines were effective, you would expect just the opposite. You would expect that there would be more excess deaths during the height of the COVID-19 pandemic, with the number dropping into negative territory after the protective effect of the vaccines saving lives during 2021 and 2022. But in (the first 38 weeks of) 2021, after the COVID-19 vaccine rollout, there was a whopping 1,452% increase in excess deaths over (the first 38 weeks of) 2020 pandemic levels. And there was an explosion of 5,162% increased excess deaths in (the first 38 weeks of) 2022 over the excess death rate during (the first 38 weeks of) 2020, which was the height of the alleged COVID-19 pandemic. That can mean only one thing. The COVID-19 vaccines are killing people.

Denis Rancourt, Ph.D., is an accomplished interdisciplinary scientist and physicist and a former tenured Full Professor of Physics and lead scientist, originally at the University of Ottawa. Dr. Rancourt studied all-cause mortality for the years beginning in 2020. He concluded, "[t]here was no pandemic causing excess mortality."[926] He explained that the 2020 excess mortality was the result of a "multi-pronged state and iatrogenic attack against populations, and against societal support structures, which caused all the excess mortality, in every jurisdiction."[927] He attributed the rise in all-cause mortality starting in 2021 to the COVID-19 vaccines. He stated, "we quantified many instances in which a rapid rollout of a dose in the imposed vaccine schedule was synchronous with an otherwise unexpected peak in all-cause mortality." Dr. Rancourt determined that the vaccines killed 3.7 million people in India alone. He further determined:

> In Western countries, we quantified the average all-ages rate of death to be 1 death for every 2000 injections, to increase exponentially with age (doubling every additional 5 years of age), and to be as large as 1 death for every 100 injections for those 80 years and older. We estimated that the vaccines had killed 13 million worldwide.[928]

Dr. Rancourt conducted a later study that was published on September 17, 2023.[929] The Data from that extensive research study involved 17 countries, which comprised 9.10% of the worldwide population and 10.3% of the worldwide COVID-19 injections. The study showed a significant rise in all-cause mortality that synchronized with the rollout of the COVID-19 vaccines. The researchers concluded that "[i]t is unlikely that the rise in all-cause mortality (ACM) coinciding with the rollout and sustained administration of COVID-19 vaccines in all 17 countries could be due to any cause other than the vaccines."[930] The study deduced that the 13.25 billion COVID-19 vaccine injections worldwide caused a statistically inferred increase of 17 million worldwide deaths from all causes as of September 2, 2023. The researchers stated: "This would correspond to a mass iatrogenic [caused by medical treatment] event that killed (0.213 ± 0.006) % of the world population (1 death per 470 living persons, in less than 3 years)."[931]

We have more than statistical inference of causation. There is medical proof that the COVID-19 vaccines are killing people. Renowned cardiologist Dr. Peter McCullough, Yale epidemiologist Dr. Harvey Risch, and former Senior Pandemic Advisor to the Secretary of Health and Human Services, Paul E. Alexander, Ph.D. along with other doctors and researchers, conducted a study to determine the causal link between the reported COIVID-19 vaccine deaths in VAERS and the COVID-19 vaccine. They reviewed 325 autopsy cases and one necropsy case of persons who died after receiving a COVID-19 vaccine. The doctors determined that "[a] total of 240 deaths (73.9%) were independently adjudicated as directly due to or significantly contributed to by COVID-19 vaccination."[932] The average time in which the persons died after vaccination was 14.3 days. The study proves causation; it attests that COVID-19 vaccines are killing people. A pre-print of the study was posted on The Lancet website on July 5, 2023, pending peer review.[933] But after a high volume of downloads, after only 24 hours, The Lancet removed the pre-print from its website. The coverup continues.

30 Prion Disease

Dr. Peter McCullough called the COVID-19 vaccines bioterrorism.[934] That was not hyperbole. Other highly respected doctors share that opinion. Dr. Barthelow Classen likens the COVID-19 vaccines to bioweapons. Dr. Barthelow Classen, M.D., has published a report revealing that the Pfizer-BioNTech COVID-19 vaccine uses an RNA sequence known to cause prion diseases such as Alzheimer's and amyotrophic lateral sclerosis (ALS).[935] Dr. Classen states that "[t]he current analysis indicates Pfizer's RNA based COVID-19 vaccine contains many of these RNA sequences that have been shown to have high affinity for TDP-43 or FUS and have the potential to induce chronic degenerative neurological diseases."[936] Dr. Classen reveals that the manifestation of the disease may take many years after the vaccination to develop in the vaccine recipient.

Other researchers have confirmed the findings of Dr. Classen. Jeff Childers reports a study revealing that COVID-19 vaccines have been shown to cause mad-cow disease.[937] That study "cited three previous studies from 2020 and 2021 finding a link between the mRNA jabs and prion diseases like Mad Cow."[938] The researchers identify the prion disease as a virulent kind of mad-cow disease, which Childers calls "Turbo Mad Cow."

Dr. Classen opines that the mRNA COVID-19 vaccines have the earmarks of bioweapons that are purposely designed to harm.

> Many have raised the warning that the current epidemic of COVID-19 is actually the result of a bioweapons attack released in part by individuals in the United States government. Such a theory is not far fetched given that the 2001 anthrax attack in the US originated at Fort Detrick, a US army bioweapon facility. Because the FBI's anthrax investigation was closed against the advice of the lead FBI agent in the case, there are likely conspirators still working in the US government. In such a scenario the primary focus of stopping a bioweapons attack must be to apprehend the conspirators or the attacks will never cease. Approving a vaccine, utilizing novel RNA technology without extensive testing is extremely dangerous. The vaccine could be a bioweapon and even more dangerous than the original infection.[939]

Dr. Stephanie Seneff, Ph.D., who is a senior research scientist at MIT Computer Science and Artificial Intelligence Laboratory, opines that "[g]iving young people COVID vaccines will likely cause an 'alarming increase in several major neurodegenerative diseases.'"[940] Dr. Seneff elaborated:

> [B]oth the mRNA vaccines and the DNA vector vaccines may be a pathway to crippling disease sometime in the future. Through the prion-like action of the spike protein, we will likely see an alarming increase in several major neurodegenerative diseases, including Parkinson's

> disease, CKD, ALS and Alzheimer's, and these diseases will show up with increasing prevalence among younger and younger populations, in years to come.[941]

Dr. Seneff affirms the opinion of Dr. Classen that it takes years before the prion disease causes degeneration of the brain sufficient for a diagnosis of permanent brain damage.

> Unfortunately, we won't know whether the vaccines caused this increase because there will usually be a long time separation between the vaccination event and the disease diagnosis.[942]

Dr. Seneff explains how the delay in the manifestation of brain damage works to the advantage of pharmaceutical companies. She said it is "very convenient for the vaccine manufacturers, who stand to make huge profits off of our misfortunes — both from the sale of the vaccines themselves and from the large medical cost of treating all these debilitating diseases."[943]

31 Myocarditis

Peter McCullough, M.D., and Dr. Jessica Rose, Ph.D., researched the sudden appearance of myocarditis in young people. Dr. McCullough is a highly-published world-renowned cardiologist, and Dr. Rose is a Canadian researcher with a Bachelor's Degree in Applied Mathematics and a Master's degree in Immunology from Memorial University of Newfoundland. She also holds a Ph.D. in Computational Biology from Bar Ilan University and two Post Doctoral degrees: one in Molecular Biology from the Hebrew University of Jerusalem and one in Biochemistry from the Technion Institute of Technology. Drs. McCullough and Rose determined that the COVID-19 vaccines caused myocarditis. While their study focused on young people, their conclusions also apply to the population as a whole. The October 1, 2021, McCullough & Rose report revealed the following startling facts.

> Within 8 weeks of the public offering of COVID-19 products to the 12-15-year-old age group, **we found 19 times the expected number of myocarditis cases in the vaccination volunteers over background myocarditis rates for this age group.**[944]

The VAERS system only reports about 1% of the actual adverse events.[945] VAERS is a reporting system that shows correlation. Further analysis is required to prove causation. Drs. McCullough and Rose did that further analysis and opined that the VAERS data indicates a cause and effect between the vaccinations and teenage myocarditis. Their report indicates: "It is noteworthy that 'Vaccine-induced myocarditis' was in fact used as the descriptor by medical professionals as the reason for the myocarditis in the VAERS database."[946] Their report labeled the myocarditis caused by the vaccines "COVID-19-Injection-Related Myocarditis (CIRM);" the report concluded:

> Thus, due to both the problems of under-reporting and the known lag in report processing, this analysis reveals a strong signal from the VAERS data that the risk of suffering CIRM [COVID-19-Injection-Related Myocarditis] – especially males is unacceptably high. Again, children are not a high-risk group for COVID-19 respiratory illness, and yet they are the high-risk group for CIRM.[947]

The McCullough & Rose report caused quite a stir in the medical community. After the preliminary draft of their report was peer-reviewed and approved for publication, it was posted by the publisher on its NIH website. Shortly thereafter, the publisher, Elsevier, without giving a reason, suddenly withdrew the publication. Dr. McCullough is reportedly pursuing legal action against Elsevier for its unlawful actions.

In its guidance dated October 4, 2022, the U.S. CDC recommended COVID-19 vaccines for all persons over six months old.[948] That is a bizarre recommendation when viewed in light of a January 25, 2022, study published in the Journal of the American Medical Association (JAMA).[949] That study was conducted by the FDA and CDC using the VAERS data. The study confirmed the findings of Drs. Rose and McCullough. The joint CDC/FDA study showed that the incidence of autoimmune heart disease (myocarditis) among those vaccinated against COVID-19 was 13,200% higher than among the unvaccinated.[950]

On October 7, 2022, Dr. Ladpapo, M.D., Ph.D., in his capacity as Florida Surgeon General, contradicted the U.S. CDC and announced that the risks of COVID-19 vaccines outweigh the benefits for 18 to 39-year-old males. He came to that conclusion based on a scientific study of the mortality risk of the COVID-19 vaccines. That study "found there is an 84% increase in the relative incidence of cardiac-related death among males 18-39 years old within 28 days following mRNA vaccination."[951]

Dr. Toby Rogers points out that "Pfizer's clinical trial in kids was intentionally undersized to hide harms. This is a well-known trick of the pharmaceutical industry. The FDA even called them out on it earlier this summer and asked Pfizer to expand the trial, and Pfizer just ignored them because they can."[952] Dr. Rogers explains the trick: "To put it simply, if the rate of particular adverse outcome in kids as a result of this shot is 1 in 5,000 and the trial only enrolls 1,518 in the treatment group then one is unlikely to spot this particular harm in the clinical trial. Voilà "Safe & Effective (TM)".[953]

Another trick vaccine makers use is to have a brief period to monitor test participants for adverse events. Pfizer only followed cohort 1 for two months and cohort 2 for 17 days for adverse events. But many adverse events take much longer to show up. Dr. Rogers observed: "As the old saying goes, 'you can have it quick or you can have it done right, but you cannot have both.' Pfizer chose quick."[954]

Such short observation periods acts to conceal the harm done to the heart. Dr. Rogers explains that "the harms of myocarditis from these shots will likely unfold over the course of years." The Pfizer study seemed designed to conceal the danger of myocarditis. For example, "they estimate 'excess' (read: caused by the shot) myocarditis using data from the private 'Optum health claim database' instead of the public VAERS system."[955] That is odd indeed. Why use a private database and eschew using the government-administered VAERS database? There was something in the VAERS system that Pfizer and the FDA did not want known.

Drs. Peter McCullough and Jessical Rose found out why the FDA and Pfizer steered clear of the VAERS database. Drs. McCullough and Rose revealed how the VAERS database showed a substantial cause and effect relationship between the COVID-19 vaccines and myocarditis.[956]

That information reported by McCullough and Rose was in the VAERS database and was known to the FDA when it authorized the use of the unsafe and ineffective COVID-19 vaccines for children 5 through 11 years of age. That seems to be why the FDA and Pfizer steered clear of the VAERS data and instead used the private data from Optum Health.

Another fact that the McCullough & Rose report revealed was that the incidence of myocarditis among teenagers is much worse than even the raw statistics obtained from the Vaccine Adverse Events Reporting Service (VAERS) indicate. The report states:

> Because of the spontaneous reporting of events to VAERS, we can assume that the cases reported thus far are not rare, but rather, just the tip of the iceberg. Again, under-reporting is a known and serious disadvantage of the VAERS system.[957]

Myocarditis can cause irreversible heart damage. Once the heart muscle is damaged, it cannot be repaired by the body. It is a devastating condition. Dr. Rogers explains that "over the course of several years many of those children will die. Dr. Anthony Hinton ('Consultant Surgeon with 30 years experience in the NHS') points out that myocarditis has a 20% fatality rate after 2 years and a 50% fatality rate after 5 years."[958] One person observed: "You can't have 'mild myocarditis' — in the same way you can't be 'a little bit pregnant.'"[959] Dr. Aaron Kheriaty, M.D., stated that "there is no such thing as "mild" myocarditis. Inflammation of the heart is always medically serious. Anyone attempting to minimize it is not giving medical information but selling something."[960] The Associated Press (AP) tried to debunk the seriousness of vaccine induced myocaditis and contacted Dr. Kheriaty. He told the AP that "'mild myocarditis' is like saying 'mild heart attack [myocardits is] always medically serious, even on the mild end of the spectrum."[961]

On November 16, 2021, this author received the fact check inquiry from the Associated Press (AP). I wrote an article about vaccine-induced myocarditis. The article was titled: *The FDA and Pfizer Concealed Evidence That COVID-19 Vaccines Will Cause Myocarditis in Children.*[962] In that article, I explained how severe myocarditis could be. The AP claimed that my contention that myocarditis is a dangerous heart condition was "not correct." The AP claimed that it had "gotten confirmation from Dr. Eric Adler and Dr. Leslie Cooper, professors of medicine and practicing cardiologists, that most myocarditis cases are indeed mild or asymptomatic."

The AP experts' opinion raises an issue. How can a doctor know to look for myocarditis if it is asymptomatic? It would seem that the only time that asymptomatic myocarditis would be detected is after the person suddenly and unexpectedly dies or is hospitalized. Otherwise, if the patient is asymptomatic, there is no complaint for the doctor to examine the patient for myocarditis. It seems that asymptomatic myocarditis is a very serious and perilous condition indeed. That is why we have an epidemic of young people with asymptomatic myocarditis who are dying suddenly.

I replied in an email to the inquiry by asking: "Have you spoken with Dr. Anthony Hinton? He is a surgeon with 30 years' of experience. He opines that "myocarditis has a 20% fatality rate after 2 years and a 50% fatality rate after 5 years?" I also emailed the AP the following additional information.

> Myocarditis is caused by vaccine induced blood clotting. The mechanism for the COVID-19 vaccine causing myocarditis and other organ damage is blood clotting caused by the spike protein generated by the cells coded with the mRNA from the COVID-19 vaccine. Dr. Charles Hoffe, M.D., explains in straightforward terms how the mRNA COVID vaccines cause the body to create the spike proteins that in turn cause widespread microscopic blood clotting.
>
> Dr. Hoffe reveals that when someone is given an mRNA vaccine, "it is literally collected by your lymphatic system and fed into your circulation. So these little packages of messenger RNA — and by the way, in a single dose of a Moderna vaccine, there are 40 trillion mRNA molecules that are injected into your arm … they go into your blood stream in these little packages that are designed to be absorbed into your cells."[963]
>
> Dr. Hoffe reveals that the absorption of the mRNA is most notable in the capillary networks, which are the tiniest blood vessels in the body. Because they are so small, the blood slows down while flowing through the capillaries. The little packages of mRNA from the vaccine are absorbed into the cells around the blood vessels (the vascular

endothelium). There, the mRNA packages are absorbed, and the body goes to work reading the mRNA code. The blood vessel cells (the endothelium) begin manufacturing trillions and trillions of COVID spike proteins. There are 40 trillion mRNA packets per vaccine dose; each of those gene packets can produce many, many spike proteins.

The theory behind the mRNA COVID-19 vaccines is that your body will recognize the spike protein created by your cells as a foreign protein and make antibodies against it. Theoretically, you are then protected against COVID-19. But Dr. Hoffe explains the problem with how the mRNA acts in the body. The spike proteins are jutting from the cell walls in the very tiny capillaries in the body and block the blood flow.

> In a virus — in a coronavirus — that spike protein becomes part of the viral capsule — like the cell wall around the virus called the viral capsule. But it's not in a virus — it's in your cells. So therefore it becomes part of the cell wall of your vascular endothelium — which means that these cells that line your blood vessels, which are supposed to be smooth so that your blood flows smoothly, now have these little spiky bits sticking out. So it is absolutely inevitable that blood clots will form — because your blood platelets circulate around in your blood vessels —

> and the purpose of blood platelets is to detect a damaged vessel and block that vessel to stop bleeding. So when the platelet comes through the capillary, it suddenly hits all these COVID spikes that are jutting into the inside of the vessel — it is absolutely inevitable that a blood clot will form to block that vessel. That's how platelets work.

Dr. Hoffe is presently treating patients suffering from COVID-19 vaccine injuries. He reveals the health dangers of mRNA vaccines.

> So the most alarming thing about this is that there are some parts of your body — like your heart and your brain, and your spinal cord and your lungs, which cannot regenerate — when those tissues are damaged by blocked vessels, they are permanently damaged. So I now have 6 people in my medical practice who have reduced effect tolerance, which means they get out of breath much more easily than they used to....literally what's happened to them is they have plugged up thousands of tiny capillaries in their lungs — and the terrifying thing about this is....that once you block off a significant number of blood vessels in your lungs, your heart is now pumping against a much greater resistance to

trying and get the blood through your lungs — a condition called pulmonary artery hypertension. A condition of high blood pressure in your lungs because the blood can't get through because so many of the vessels are blocked. People with pulmonary artery hypertension usually die of right sided heart failure within three years.

So the huge concern about this mechanism of injury is that these shots are causing permanent damage — and the worst is yet to come. Some tissues in your body like intestine and liver and kidneys that can regenerate to quite a good degree — but brain and spinal cord and heart muscle and lungs do not. When they are damaged, it's permanent — like all these young people who are now getting myocarditis from these shots — they have permanently damaged hearts — it doesn't matter how mild it is, they will not be able to do what they used to be able to do….but with each successive shot, the damage will add and add and add. It's going to be cumulative because you are getting progressively more damaged capillaries.

I also pointed the AP to the following information from the

Myocarditis Foundation:

> A rare form of heart disease, myocarditis develops when the heart muscle becomes inflamed and enlarged, thus weakening the heart. Naturally, the risk of sudden death for people with myocarditis is a reason for concern.[964]

I further supplied the AP with a link to a published article and emiled the AP the following quote from the article:

> Immediate complications of myocarditis include ventricular dysrhythmias, left ventricular aneurysm, CHF, and dilated cardiomyopathy. The mortality rate is up to 20% at 1 year and 50% at 5 years. Despite optimal medical management, overall mortality has not changed in the last 30 years.[965]

The AP contacted Michael Kang, the author of the article I had sent them; and Kang claimed that I had misrepresented the figures in the article. I did not misrepresent anything. I simply quoted the passage from Michael Kang's article. The AP had orignally emailed this author and asked me for further evidence supporting my article about myocarditis; and I gave it to them. Quoting Kang's own words does not constitute misrepresentation. Kang stated that his article was written "as a general review of viral myocarditis and does not pertain to vaccine induced myocarditis."[966] The AP reported:

> With regards to the myocarditis death rate, Kang said his article was referencing the most severe forms of myocarditis. Those numbers pertain to smaller, older studies, in which patients had extreme forms of the disease, "not what we are seeing with the covid19 vaccine," Kang said in an

email.[967]

How can Kang say that somehow the conclusion in his article, which is based on "overall mortality" statistics that he said in the article have "not changed in the last 30 years" do not apply to myocarditis induced by the COVID-19 vaccines? What study has he done to distinguish virus-induced myocarditis (the subject of his article) from COVID-19 vaccine-induced myocarditis? And when you read his article in context, his statistics were clearly about the "overall mortality" for myocarditis and not the most severe forms of myocarditis, as Kang now claims. Indeed, he describes his statistics as "overall mortality" rates for myocarditis.

In the context of the quote about mortality, Kang begins discussing acute myocarditis, which he describes as the "first two weeks," which he distinguishes from chronic myocarditis, which he describes as "lasting more than 2 weeks." Acute in the context of the article means "immediate," it does not mean severe. His article addresses three phases of myocarditis "acute, subacute, or chronic." Subacute is between acute and chronic, and is a temporal measure.

Interestingly, Kang's article undermines one of the premises of the AP fact-check, that myocarditis does not result in permanent heart damage. Kang states in his article:

> Myocarditis begins with the direct invasion of an infectious agent and its subsequent replication within or around the myocardium causing myonecrosis. **This leads to the destruction of the cardiac tissue** from the infiltration and replication of the infectious agent.[968] (endnotes omitted)

Once heart tissue is destroyed, it cannot regenerate. The AP fact check conflated the issue by framing it as whether someone can recover from myocarditis. Certainly someone can recover from myocarditis. Myocarditis is inflammation of the heart. That inflammation often causes damage to the heart tissue. The issue is not whether one can recover from myocarditis but whether when the heart is damaged by myocarditis, can the body repair that damage. The answer to that question is no. Other organs in the body can repair themselves; the heart and brain cannot repair themselves. Once the heart tissue is damaged, that damage is permanent.

The AP fact check cites Dr. Eric Adler, who states, "[t]hough dead heart tissue is indeed felt to be non-recoverable there are lots of examples of damaged hearts that recover to normal function over time or with medical therapy."[969] A heart that is damaged is quite simply not the same as it was before the damage. Just because some people can make it by and exist with a damaged heart does not mean it is a minor life inconvenience. Especially when those who do not recover sometimes die. And indeed, many do not get treatment because the onset of the damage kills them before they can receive medical care; they just die suddenly. The AP article downplays the dangers of myocarditis, seemingly to offset the concern of getting myocarditis from the COVID-19 vaccine. The argument of the AP seems to be that myocarditis is not all that bad, so don't worry if the COVID-19 vaccine causes it. That approach is reckless.

When Kang discussed severe forms of myocarditis, he said that "[p]atients with severe disease have a poor prognosis without a transplant."[970] That is dire indeed! Contrast that with what Kang said about mild myocarditis: "Patients with mild myocarditis usually have a good outcome."[971] And what does he think is a good outcome? He states, "[t]he long-term prognosis was usually good, with a 3 to 5-year survival ranging from 56 to 83%, respectively." He meant that the survival rate was 83% after 3 years dropping to 56% after 5 years.

Thus, according to Kang, mild myocarditis outcome is

"usually good" because 83% survive for 3 years and 56% survive after 5 years. That is only just a little bit better than the "overall mortality" of "50% at 5 years."

It seems that Kang's fancy dancing cannot get him out from underneath the statistics for "overall mortality" for myocarditis that is "20% at 1 year and 50% at 5 years." He pointed out that "[d]espite optimal medical management, overall mortality has not changed in the last 30 years." But suddenly, when he is called on the carpet, Kang maintains that those rock-solid numbers with a 30-year pedigree have no applicability to COVID-19 vaccine-induced myocarditis.

This dangerous effect of the COVID-19 vaccines is well known to the vaccine makers and the FDA. The AP fact-check article did not mention the information I provided from Dr. Hoffe, Dr. Hinton, or the Myocarditis Foundation. Instead, the AP focused on Michael Kang. It was as though once the AP found someone who would cave in and agree with their premise, no further fact-checking was necessary. The AP gave the impression that my article was based solely on the statistics in Kang's article. But that is not the case and is not what I said. I cited Kang, along with Dr. Hoffe and Dr. Hinton. But the AP steered clear of those other doctors.

In a December 6, 2021 interview with Bret Weinstein, world-renowned cardiologist Dr. Peter Mcullough revealed that the usual rate of myocarditis in a given year in the United States is 640 cases. In 2021, VAERS reported 11,000 cases of myocarditis associated with the COVID-19 vaccines. That represents a 17-fold increase in myocarditis due to the COVID-19 vaccines. He further revealed that approximately 13% of myocarditis cases involve permanent damage to the heart. He also stated that the CDC and FDA were reprehensibly reckless when they falsely claimed that myocarditis caused by the COVID-19 vaccine was rare and mild.

I was on national TV in June when the FDA and CDC reviewed myocarditis. And they said two things that I think were completely incorrect from a public health perspective. I'm trained in public health. At this point time my career I have over 650 publications in the National Library of Medicine and Pubmed. I'm an editor of a major cardiology journal, former editor of another journal, I'm the principal editor of my own textbook. I am in academic medicine right now and anybody you're talking to on COVID-19, I imagine I'm probably at the top of the academic pile, right now, of scholarship.

I can tell you those two statements by our public health officials who are junior to me in their scholarship and accomplishments, both of those statements I think are reprehensible and reckless. They said that myocarditis is mild. And they said it was rare. Well it wasn't mild then because 90% of the kids are in the hospital. By regulatory standards, anything that causes hospitalization, as you know, is a serious adverse event. It's never classified as mild, never!

And then they said it was rare because they took 200 cases and they divided by the universe and people who got the vaccine. Well, we can't do that in safety because we didn't assess everybody from myocarditis, so we don't know if it's rare. And when we see a signal like this in safety pharmacovigilance we use the term, tip of the iceberg. So I was on national TV saying, listen it's not mild because the kids are being hospitalized, and two, it's not rare, it's the tip of the iceberg. And boy was I right. Being at now 11,000 cases in

> VAERS. And you're right, it's underreported.
>
> And interestingly, it's who reports it. There's a paper that's published in the American College of Pediatrics that asked the question in 2016 who reports to VAERS. And you know who reports to VAERS? The answer was about about 14% of the time it's actually the patient or the patient's family that reports to VAERS. 86% of the time it's another entity that actually really was concerned that the product, in this case, the vaccine, caused the problems. That means doctors, nurses, people [who] administered the vaccine, and pharmaceutical companies who receive this and they're concerned about their products. So I have to tell you this VAERS data is real. And I've heard people say that "oh anybody can report things to VAERS." I filled out the various sheets, But I'll tell you every single page says "warning," This falsification is punishable by imprisonment or federal fines. I tell you right now the VAERS system 11,000 cases. That's serious, and the number almost certainly is going to be much larger.[972]

Vaccine-induced myocarditis is widespread, affecting athletes' ability to continue competing in their sport. For example, Free West Media reported on April 2, 2022, that 15 tennis players dropped out of the Miami Open due to unexplained illnesses.[973] Fans and the news media were baffled and unable to explain the weird turn of events. Two favorites to win the tournament, Paula Badosa and Jannik Sinner, dropped out after becoming “unwell.” Badosa was soon to be ranked third in the world.

Jannik Sinner could only compete for 22 minutes before he bent over on the court and could not continue. His opponent,

Francisco Cerundolo described it as very strange. Free West Media offered no analysis about what caused the sudden wave of resignations from the tournament from physical infirmities.

None of the withdrawals or retirements have been attributed by the media to vaccine injury. Indeed the mainstream media is not discussing the reasons for the withdrawals and retirements from the tournament.[974] Some of the stated injuries suggest that some of the withdrawals and retirements were not from the vaccine. Some of the reasons given were "foot injury," "thigh injury," and "low back injury." Oddly there were three withdrawals or retirements for "abdominal injuries," which could mean anything from a muscle pull to intestinal discomfort. But some reasons for the withdrawals and retirements from the tournament raise suspicion that they were caused by vaccine injury. For example, M. Vondrousova withdrew due to a "viral illness," C. Tauson retired due to "heat illness," V. Azarenka retired due to "personal reasons."

One of the common side effects of the COVID-19 mRNA vaccines is blood clotting, which often causes muscle and joint pain, which could be masked by being reported as an "injury" to a muscle or joint.

J.D. Rucker, writing for The Liberty Daily, was not so reticent to comment on the cause of the Miami Open carnage. J.D. Rucker opined:

> Nobody is pointing to the obvious. All of the players must be "fully vaccinated" [against COVID-19] in order to compete. Just as we've noted for several months, most major sports have been hit with "inexplicable" medical conditions popping up in young and otherwise healthy athletes, including our report that three cyclists fell in March alone.[975]

Folks, this is the [COVID-19] jab. There is no other viable possibility, especially when we consider how even the CDC and other agencies have acknowledge the Covid "vaccines" cause increases in heart problems for young people, including myocarditis, pericarditis, and heart attacks.

There has never been as much gaslighting and propaganda geared towards covering up the truth than with these [COVID-19] injections. Leaders across the country and around the world have so much wrapped into the vaccines, one has to wonder who's pulling the strings. Some of it is personal; any politician who comes out with the truth about the jabs will be pushed out of office faster than Will Smith's exit from Hollywood's elite club. The same is true for journalists. Corporate media is just as invested and possibly even more complicit in spreading the lies.

But it may be worse than that. Like so many things we've witnessed over the last three years, there appears to be a coordinated effort to suppress the truth. Pandemic Panic Theater is still in action despite the odd February push by Democrats to lift most face mask and vaccine mandates. There are already talks of 5th and 6th jabs even as the 4th jab gets rolled out in the United States.

Is this all part of The Great Reset agenda? Is it all about control? Depopulation? The answer to all three questions is very likely, "Yes."

These [COVID-19] injections are dangerous. Athletes across the globe are falling. Average

> people are experiencing horrible adverse reactions. Tens, perhaps hundreds of thousands of people are dying from them. It could even be millions; the data is so obscured. All the while, politicians and corporate media are pretending it all away is if there's nothing to see here.[976]

Retsef Levi, Ph.D., is the J. Spencer Standish (1945) Professor at the MIT Sloan School of Management. He is a specialist in operations research, which concerns safety and quality in the manufacture of biological drugs and health policy. After analyzing the death and destruction caused by the COVID-19 vaccines, most notably the significant spike in myocarditis among the young, Dr. Levi issued a formal statement calling for the cessation of all such vaccines:

> I'm filming this video to share my strong conviction that at this point in time all covid mRNA vaccination programs should stop immediately. They should stop because they completely failed to fulfill any of their advertised promise regarding efficacy. And more importantly, they should stop because of the mounting and undisputable evidence that they caused unprecedented level of harm, including the death of young people and children.[977]

32 Graphene

Yumiko Urasaki and Yuko Nomura, Nikkei staff writers, reported on August 26, 2021, that the Japanese Ministry of Health, Labor, and Welfare had pulled 1.6 million vials of the Moderna vaccine from circulation in Japan because the vaccine was found to contain a substance that reacts to magnets.[978] The article states that "Prime Minister Yoshihide Suga told reporters on Thursday afternoon that he had instructed the ministry to look into the case with safety as the top priority."[979]

Some suggest the vials could have been contaminated with some kind of metal. But Tyler Durden, reporting for Zero Hedge, states that "[s]ome believe the reported magnetism can be explained by graphene oxide, a magnetic nanoparticle studied[980] for its use as a drug delivery platform[981] and other biomedical applications."[982] Indeed, graphene oxide has been studied as an ingredient for use in hydrogels.[983] Hydrogels are used to protect the otherwise fragile mRNA in the COVID-19 vaccines. One of the characteristics of graphene oxide is that it develops a rare form of magnetism when it is stacked and twisted.[984]

Angus Liu reported on February 17, 2021. for Fierce Biotech, that "Scientists at China's National Center for

Nanoscience and Technology (NCNST) have designed a hydrogel to deliver an mRNA vaccine with an immune-stimulating adjuvant."[985] China's National Center for Nanoscience reported that their new hydrogel contains graphene oxide.[986] Liu reported:

> [T]he NCNST team designed a hydrogel with graphene oxide and low-weight polyethyleneimine. The graphene oxide can efficiently load drug substances thanks to its large surface area, and the polyethyleneimine binds the mRNA content for translation.[987]

The article by Liu was written on the day that the NCNST published their findings about the efficacy of their graphene oxide infused hydrogel, February 17, 2021. But certainly, the use of graphene oxide was likely already incorporated into the COVID-19 vaccines. Please be mindful that communist countries are parasitic. They steal technology developed by the west. The alleged development by the NCNST of hydrogel using graphene oxide was, in all likelihood, reverse engineering of that technology developed by Moderna, Pfizer-BioNTech, and others.

Why is this a problem? Graphene Oxide is cytotoxic. That means it is a poison that kills cells. If the hydrogels used in the COVID-19 vaccines contain graphene oxide, that would make the vaccines dangerous to those being injected. Do the COVID-19 vaccines contain graphene oxide? There is at least probable cause to believe that they do.

Robert Young, M.Sc., D.Sc., Ph.D., used phase-contrast microscopy, transmission and scanning electron microscopy, and energy-dispersive x-ray spectroscopy to analyze the following COVID-19 vaccines: Pfizer-BioNTech mRNA Vaccine, the Moderna-Lonza mRNA-1273 Vaccine, the Serum Institute Oxford Astrazeneca Vaccine, and the Janssen COVID -19 Vaccine. Dr. Young concluded:

> The Pfizer, Moderna, Astrazeneca and Janssen drugs are NOT "vaccines" but complexed Graphene Oxide nano particulate aggregates of varying nano elements attached to genetically modified nucleic acids of mRNA from animal or vero cells and aborted human fetal cells.[988]

Dr. Young found the presence of graphene oxide using advanced microscopy. Some would consider that presumptive proof but not confirmatory. Some suggest that mass spectrometry analysis is necessary to confirm of Dr. Young's findings. It is fair to say that Dr. Young's advanced microscopy evidence, along with the other circumstantial evidence, establishes at least probable cause that the COVID-19 vaccines contain graphene oxide.

The companies making the COVID-19 vaccines tested by Dr. Young did not list graphene oxide as an ingredient in any publicly available documents. Dr. Young concluded that graphene oxide in the COVID-19 "vaccines" renders them poisonous to the body's cells. The toxicity of graphene oxide is a generally known fact among scientists, which may explain why the companies did not reveal it as an ingredient in their COVID-19 "vaccines." Dr. Young explains:

> [T]he ingredients in these so-called vaccines are highly magneticotoxic, cytotoxic and genotoxic to plant, insect, bird, animal and human cell membranes and their genetics.

Dr. Andreas Noack is one of the foremost experts on graphene in the world. He has studied data from Professor Pablo Campra from the University of Almeira. Dr. Campra used micro-raman spectroscopy to analyze the contents of the Pfizer-BioNTech COVID-19 vaccine. Dr. Noack reviewed Dr. Campra's findings and found that the Pfizer-BioNTech COVID-19 vaccine contains graphene hydroxide. Dr. Noack is an expert in the field and he opined that the graphene was in the form of graphene hydroxide rather than graphene oxide. Dr. Noack confirmed the findings of Dr. Young, other than his distinction that the vaccines contained graphene hyrdroxide.

On November 23, 2021, Dr. Noack posted a video presentation during which he explained that the graphene hydroxide in the vaccine is a nanoparticle that is 50 nm long and 0.1 nm thick.[989] Dr. Noack explains that the nanoparticles of graphene hydroxide act as kind-of razor blades slicing and dicing as they move through the body. Graphene hydroxide is not biodegradable. It remains circulating in the blood indefinitely. Dr. Noack explains that the heart and brain are organs that are particularly susceptible to damage from graphene hydroxide. Dr. Noack opines that is why there has been a rash of young athletes dropping dead from heart attacks. The blood of the young athletes is efficiently coursing throughout the body causing unseen damage until they unexpectedly drop dead. Dr. Noack explains that doctors performing autopsies on victims of the vaccine are not going to find the graphene hydroxide because they are looking for something biological as the cause of death. Graphene hydroxide is not biological so it will not be visible in their tests.

On November 27, 2021, Dr. Noack's wife announced that shortly after Dr. Noack posted his video and it went viral, he was attacked and killed.[990] The timing of the attack suggests that it was in retribution for his revelations about graphene hydroxide in the Pfizer-BioNTech COVID-19 vaccine. They determined to silence Dr. Noack. They could not allow Dr. Noack, an authoritative and unimpeachable expert in graphene, to reveal the dangerousness of the COVID-19 vaccines.

33 COVID-19 Vaccine Blood Clotting Danger

Dr. Charles Hoffe, M.D., explains in straightforward terms how the mRNA COVID vaccines cause the body to create the spike proteins that in turn cause widespread microscopic blood clotting. Dr. Hoffe reveals that when someone is given an mRNA vaccine, "it is literally collected by your lymphatic system and fed into your circulation. So these little packages of messenger RNA — and by the way, in a single dose of a Moderna vaccine, there are 40 trillion mRNA molecules that are injected into your arm ... they go into your blood stream in these little packages that are designed to be absorbed into your cells."[991]

Dr. Hoffe reveals that the absorption of the mRNA is most notable in the capillary networks, which are the tiniest blood vessels in the body. Because they are so small, the blood slows down while flowing through the capillaries. The little packages of mRNA from the vaccine are absorbed into the cells around the blood vessels (the vascular endothelium). There, the mRNA packages are absorbed, and the body goes to work reading the mRNA code. The blood vessel cells (the endothelium) begin manufacturing trillions and trillions of COVID spike proteins. There are 40 trillion mRNA packets per vaccine dose; each of those gene packets can produce many, many spike proteins.

The theory behind the mRNA COVID-19 vaccines is that your body will recognize the spike protein created by your cells as a foreign protein and make antibodies against it. Theoretically, you are then protected against COVID-19. But Dr. Hoffe explains the problem with how the mRNA acts in the body. The spike proteins are jutting from the cell walls in the very tiny capillaries in the body and block the blood flow.

> In a virus — in a coronavirus — that spike protein becomes part of the viral capsule — like the cell wall around the virus called the viral capsule. But it's not in a virus — it's in your cells. So therefore it becomes part of the cell wall of your vascular endothelium — which means that these cells that line your blood vessels, which are supposed to be smooth so that your blood flows smoothly, now have these little spiky bits sticking out. So it is absolutely inevitable that blood clots will form — because your blood platelets circulate around in your blood vessels — and the purpose of blood platelets is to detect a damaged vessel and block that vessel to stop bleeding. So when the platelet comes through the capillary, it suddenly hits all these COVID spikes that are jutting into the inside of the vessel — it is absolutely inevitable that a blood clot will form to block that vessel. That's how platelets work.[992]

Dr. Hoffe is presently treating patients suffering from COVID-19 vaccine injuries. He reveals the health dangers of mRNA vaccines.

> So the most alarming thing about this is that there are some parts of your body — like your heart and

your brain, and your spinal cord and your lungs, which cannot regenerate — when those tissues are damaged by blocked vessels, they are permanently damaged. So I now have 6 people in my medical practice who have reduced effect tolerance, which means they get out of breath much more easily than they used to....literally what's happened to them is they have plugged up thousands of tiny capillaries in their lungs — and the terrifying thing about this is....that once you block off a significant number of blood vessels in your lungs, your heart is now pumping against a much greater resistance to trying and get the blood through your lungs — a condition called pulmonary artery hypertension. A condition of high blood pressure in your lungs because the blood can't get through because so many of the vessels are blocked. People with pulmonary artery hypertension usually die of right sided heart failure within three years.

So the huge concern about this mechanism of injury is that these shots are causing permanent damage — and the worst is yet to come. Some tissues in your body like intestine and liver and kidneys that can regenerate to quite a good degree — but brain and spinal cord and heart muscle and lungs do not. When they are damaged, it's permanent — like all these young people who are now getting myocarditis from these shots — they have permanently damaged hearts — it doesn't matter how mild it is, they will not be able to do what they used to be able to do....but with each successive shot, the damage will add and add and add. It's going to be cumulative because you are getting progressively more damaged capillaries.[993]

34 Scuttling the Control Group to Hide Injuries

The only way to scientifically measure the onset of ADE and blood clotting is to conduct a placebo trial and monitor the vaccinated group with a placebo group. Both Moderna and Pfizer-BioNTech know that. They also knew that such a study would be devastating to the continued viability of their vaccines. So what did they do? After the EUAs for the Moderna and Pfizer vaccines were granted, both Moderna and Pfizer vaccinated the placebo group in their trials.[994] There are no longer control groups against which to compare the onset of ADE or blood clotting in a follow-up investigation. The vaccine companies knew that they needed to monitor their trial groups over the long term. They said so in their briefing documents. They said the risk of ADE "needs to be evaluated further in ongoing clinical trials and in observational studies that could be conducted following authorization and/or licensure." They already had the groups in place with whom they could study ADE. They knew that was the way to determine if there was ADE. The pharmaceutical companies purposely scuttled the placebo group to conceal that their vaccines cause ADE.

Steven Goodman, Professor of Epidemiology and Population Health and Medicine at Stanford University explains that "losing the those control groups makes it more difficult to answer some important questions about COVID-19 vaccines."[995] He said we now have no way of knowing how long the protections last or the efficacy against variants. There is no way to measure differences in any of the parameters by age, race, or infirmity. And there is no way to measure ADE or blood clotting quantitatively. The usefulness of the study has been destroyed. And that is the reason that the companies vaccinated the control group. Writing for *Natual News*, Lance Johnson explains that without the placebo group, "[t]here is no data to guarantee the safety and effectiveness of these shots and there is no longer any route to obtain that data from a clinical standpoint."[996] Johnson, writing his article on August 10, 2021, after the government granted the EUA for the Pfizer-BioNTech COVID-19 vaccine but before the approval of Pfizer's COMIRNATY (COVID-19 Vaccine, mRNA), opined that there is no way to scientifically or legally approve a vaccine that does not have a control group for long-term monitoring. But that is just what the FDA did. Pfizer had an EUA for their predecessor COVID-19 vaccine known as the Pfizer-BioNTech COVID-19 vaccine. The EUA "Pfizer-BioNTech COVID-19 vaccine" is legally distinct but with substantially the same ingredients as the approved "COMIRNATY (COVID-19 Vaccine, mRNA)." An emergency use authorization (EUA) is not the same as approval. On what basis did the FDA approve COMIRNATY (COVID-19 Vaccine, mRNA) when there was no control group?

Figure 1 below is from page 15 of the FDA briefing document for the Pfizer COVID-19 vaccine.[997] It shows the planned follow-up period for further monitoring of the test subjects to continue for two (2) years. But Pfizer has now made it impossible for any follow-up comparison of ADE or myocarditis between the vaccinated and placebo groups by purposely vaccinating the placebo groups.

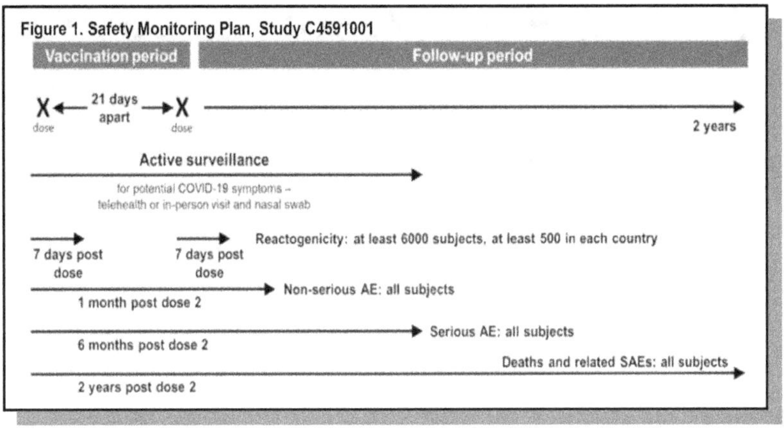

Figure 1. Safety Monitoring Plan, Study C4591001

The briefings for both the Moderna and Pfizer-BioNTech COVID-19 vaccines included the following proviso from the FDA:

> FDA does not consider availability of a COVID-19 vaccine under EUA, in and of itself, as grounds for immediately stopping blinded follow-up in an ongoing clinical trial or grounds for offering vaccine to all placebo recipients.[998]

Yet, both Moderna and Pfizer-BioNtech disregarded that guidance from the FDA and instead purposely sabotaged their studies by vaccinating the control groups and thus making it impossible to do long-term efficacy and safety studies on their vaccines. The charts below from the Canadian Covid Care Alliance[999] illustrate what happened.

WHAT WAS SUPPOSED TO HAPPEN

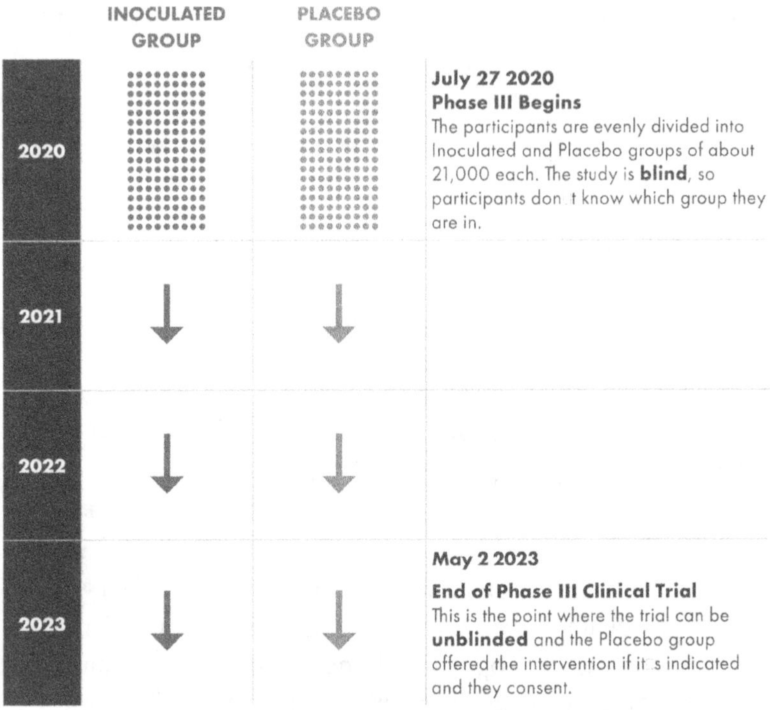

WHAT ACTUALLY HAPPENED

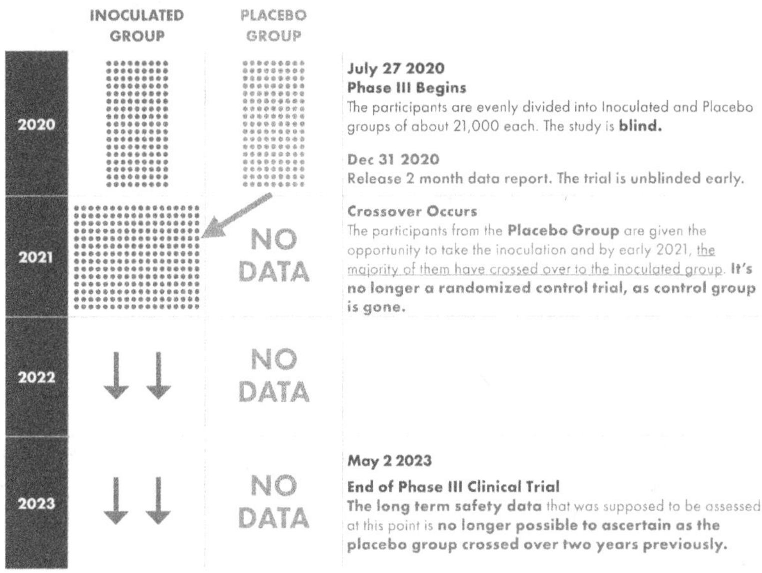

35 Bait and Switch #1

On or before August 23, 2021, the FDA announced that they do not know if the Pfizer-BioNTech or the Comirnaty COVID-19 vaccines worked to stop transmission. The FDA said it could only hope that the vaccines would do so.

> Most vaccines that protect from viral illnesses also reduce transmission of the virus that causes the disease by those who are vaccinated. While it is hoped this will be the case, **the scientific community does not yet know if the Pfizer-BioNTech COVID-19 Vaccine or Comirnaty will reduce such transmission.**[1000]

The FDA lied. Before the FDA said, on or before August 23, 2021, they did not know if the Pfizer-BioNTech COVID-19 vaccines would reduce transmission, the CDC, on March 8, 2021, was already on record saying that fully vaccinated persons should be "mindful of the potential risk of transmitting the virus to others."[1001] Indeed, the CDC was convinced that the COVID-19 vaccines did NOT work because it advised fully vaccinated residents of non-healthcare congregate settings to "quarantine for 14 days and be tested for SARS-CoV-2 following an exposure to someone with suspected or confirmed COVID-19."[1002] The only reason to quarantine a fully vaccinated person exposed to COVID-19 would be if the vaccine does not prevent infection and does not prevent the transmission of COVID-19.

That means that while the FDA was claiming it was not sure if the Pfizer-BioNTech COVID-19 vaccine would reduce transmission, the CDC was already on record saying it was so sure it did not prevent transmission it was recommending quarantining for 14 days fully vaccinated persons who had been exposed to someone even suspected of having COVID-19. The left hand did not know what the right hand was doing. Which is worse, the deception by the FDA or the dystopian quarantining recommendation by the CDC?

The COVID-19 vaccine was supposed to prevent someone from getting COVID-19.[1003] The whole purpose of the COVID-19 vaccine is to prevent COVID-19 infection. Indeed, that was the primary focus of the study that resulted in the Emergency Use Authorization (EUA) by the FDA for the Moderna and the Pfizer-BioNtech COVID-19 vaccines. But early in the COVID-19 vaccine program, on March 8, 2021, the CDC implicitly admitted that the COVID-19 vaccines are ineffective in preventing the infection and spread of COVID-19.[1004] On March 8, 2021, the CDC listed the following official recommendations for **fully vaccinated people**:

> For now, **fully vaccinated people** should continue to:
>
> - Take precautions in public like **wearing a well-fitted mask and physical distancing**
> - **Wear masks**, practice **physical distancing**, and adhere to other prevention measures when visiting with unvaccinated people who are at increased risk for severe COVID-19 disease or who have an

unvaccinated household member who is at increased risk for severe COVID-19 disease

- **Wear masks, maintain physical distance**, and practice other prevention measures when visiting with unvaccinated people from multiple households
- **Avoid medium- and large-sized in-person gatherings**
- **Get tested if experiencing COVID-19 symptoms**
- Follow guidance issued by individual employers
- Follow CDC and health department travel requirements and recommendations[1005]

There is no way that if a person obtains immunity from COVID-19, as the vaccines were purported to do, the CDC would recommend that a person who is fully vaccinated continue to:

- **Wear a mask;**

- **Practice physical distancing;**

- **Avoid medium and large-sized in-person gatherings;**

- **Get tested if experiencing COVID-19 symptoms;**

- **Follow other prevention measures to stop the spread of COVID-19.**

The CDC claimed on March 8, 2021, that "a growing body of evidence suggests that fully vaccinated people are less likely to have asymptomatic infection and potentially less likely to transmit SARS-CoV-2 to others." Notice that the CDC used the terms "less likely" to be infected and "potentially less likely" to transmit

SARS-CoV-2. What do those unscientific weasel terms mean? The CDC was beginning a campaign of equivocation. The vaccines were proving ineffective. And the CDC was implicitly admitting it. The CDC said: "How long vaccine protection lasts and how much vaccines protect against emerging SARS-CoV-2 variants are still under investigation."

The CDC said they used the terms "less likely" to be infected and "potentially less likely" to transmit SARS-CoV-2 because they did not know at that time if the vaccines worked. But even that is a lie because they did know. The evidence was clear by that point that the vaccines offered no protection, and that is why the CDC continued to recommend that a vaccinated person still take precautions to prevent getting and spreading SARS-CoV-2. The CDC stated on March 8, 2021:

> Until more is known and vaccination coverage increases, some prevention measures will continue to be necessary for all people, regardless of vaccination status.[1006]

That was a damning admission in light of the EUA authorization for the vaccines being based on the promise that the vaccines would **"prevent"** COVID-19. Indeed, on December 11, 2020, the FDA explicitly stated that it issued the EUA for the first COVID-19 vaccine from Pfizer-BioNTech "for the **prevention** of coronavirus disease 2019 (COVID-19) caused by severe acute respiratory syndrome coronavirus 2 (SARS-CoV-2)."[1007]

The COVID-19 vaccines were promoted to the public as a preventive measure. But while the unofficial public pronouncements were that the COVID-19 vaccines were effective in preventing COVID-19, the CDC and FDA began the strange process of official equivocation about the effectiveness of the vaccines in preventing COVID-19. They very soon began to admit what they knew from the beginning. The vaccines were ineffective in preventing COVID-19.

The CDC described the "less likely" to be infected and "potentially less likely" to transmit SARS-CoV-2, "residual risk." Don't be fooled. Residual risk is a real risk. The CDC was admitting that the COVID-19 vaccines do not work. The CDC makes the astounding statement:

> The benefits of reducing social isolation and relaxing some measures such as quarantine requirements may outweigh **the residual risk of fully vaccinated people becoming ill with COVID-19 or transmitting SARS-CoV-2 to others.**[1008]

That March 8, 2021, statement is proof that the CDC knew and admitted within the first three months of the COVID-19 vaccine programs that "fully vaccinated" people were at risk of "becoming ill with COVID-19 or transmitting SARS-CoV-2 to others." They knew that the vaccines did not work. Yet, the CDC kept up its vaccination campaign.

The CDC claimed that the residual risk is low for infection of a fully vaccinated person. But the claim that the residual risk is low makes no sense in light of the CDC's advice that a person should be monitored following any exposure to someone with "suspected or confirmed COVID-19."

> Fully vaccinated people who do not quarantine should still monitor for symptoms of COVID-19 for 14 days following an exposure. If they experience symptoms, they should isolate themselves from others, be clinically evaluated for COVID-19, including SARS-CoV-2 testing, if indicated, and inform their health care provider of their vaccination status at the time of presentation

to care.[1009]

That advice would makes no sense unless the CDC had already established that vaccinated persons have, in-fact, been infected with SARS-CoV-2 after being vaccinated. Thus, to the satisfaction of the CDC, the vaccine had been proven to be ineffective in preventing COVID-19. Furthermore, the advice makes no sense unless the vaccine had been proven ineffective in preventing the spread of SARS-CoV-2. Indeed, the vaccine is so ineffective that the CDC recommended quarantining for 14 days a fully vaccinated person working in a jail or group home who had been exposed to someone suspected of having COVID-19.

> Fully vaccinated residents of non-healthcare congregate settings (e.g., correctional and detention facilities, group homes) should continue to quarantine for 14 days and be tested for SARS-CoV-2 following an exposure to someone with suspected or confirmed COVID-19. This is because residential congregate settings may face high turnover of residents, a higher risk of transmission, and challenges in maintaining recommended physical distancing.[1010]

That advice to quarantine a fully vaccinated person who has been exposed to someone suspected of being infected with SARS-CoV-2 confirms that the CDC knew that the COVID-19 vaccines were ineffective against contracting and spreading SARS-CoV-2.

You only quarantine a person with a real risk of transmitting the disease. The fact that the CDC advised that a fully vaccinated person be quarantined upon being exposed to a person even suspected of having COVID-19 means that the CDC believed that a fully vaccinated person can be infected with SARS-CoV-2 and then spread that disease to others. That advice by the CDC testifies that the CDC believed at the early date of March 8, 2021, that the COVID-19 vaccines were ineffective in preventing the infection and spread of SARS-CoV-2.

The CDC knew that the COVID-19 vaccines had been proven to be ineffective. The CDC admitted that fact. The CDC explained that a "fully vaccinated" person can still become ill with COVID-19 and transmit SARS-CoV-2. The CDC stated that the only reason to relax some liberty restrictions for COVID-19 vaccine recipients is NOT that the vaccine is effective in preventing the infection and spread of SARS CoV-2 but to "improve COVID-19 vaccine acceptance and uptake" by the general public.

> Additionally, taking steps towards relaxing certain measures for vaccinated persons may help improve COVID-19 vaccine acceptance and uptake.[1011]

The CDC admitted that the loosening of restrictions for fully vaccinated persons does not mean that those who have been vaccinated cannot still be infected with SARS-CoV-2 or spread the disease to someone else. The CDC only relaxed restrictions on vaccinated persons to encourage more people to get vaccinated. The CDC was clear that fully vaccinated persons can still get infected with SARS-CoV-2 and should remain on guard for the risk of transmitting the virus to others.

> Therefore, there are several activities that fully vaccinated people can resume now, at low risk to themselves, **while being mindful of the potential risk of transmitting the virus to others.**[1012]

The CDC then completely lets the cat out of the bag with the following advice for fully vaccinated persons:

> Fully vaccinated people should not visit or attend

> a gathering if they have tested positive for COVID-19 in the prior 10 days or are experiencing COVID-19 symptoms, regardless of vaccination status of the other people at the gathering.[1013]

> That advice from the CDC assumes two things.

> **1) Fully vaccinated persons can get infected with SARS-CoV-2.**

> **2) Fully vaccinated persons can transmit SARS-CoV-2.**

That CDC advice, given on March 8, 2021, proves that the CDC knew within three months of the vaccine program that the COVID-19 vaccines did not work.

After investigating a COVID-19 outbreak in Barnstable County, Massachusetts, where 74% of the 469 persons infected with COVID-19 were fully vaccinated, the CDC Director, Rochelle P. Walensky, MD, MPH, issued a statement on July 30, 2021.[1014] In that news release Director Walensky admonished fully vaccinated persons to wear masks indoors because the COVID-19 vaccinations offer little or no protection against contracting COVID-19. A little-known fact is that those not listed among the fully vaccinated in the Barnstable outbreak may have been vaccinated, just not fully vaccinated. Many excluded from the fully vaccinated statistic were partially vaccinated, or their vaccination status was unknown.[1015]

Furthermore, the CDC Director acknowledged in the July 30, 2021, Barnstable press release that "vaccinated people infected with Delta can transmit the virus."[1016] Director Walensky revealed in the news release that the Barnstable outbreak was just one of many outbreaks the CDC was investigating nationwide. We have since learned that those other outbreaks nationwide were populated, for the most part, by those who had been fully vaccinated. Thus, the CDC and the medical establishment were fully aware by at least July 2021 that the COVID-19 vaccines do not prevent infection or spread. And, indeed, it was looking very much like the COVID-19 vaccines were causing illnesses. The alleged breakthrough cases were likely antibody-dependent enhancement caused by the vaccines.

Once the flames of COVID-19 fear were fanned, the population was primed to get their COVID-19 vaccines when they were rolled out on December 11, 2020. The ordinary people did not know the vaccines did not work and that they were dangerous. It is not that the government officials slowly learned after the vaccine rollout that the vaccines were ineffective and unsafe. They knew that from the beginning. They lied to the public. They are pretending that they only learned about the danger and ineffectiveness of the vaccines after their rollout. The purpose of the vaccines was to kill and injure. The officials behind the COVID-19 vaccine program are evil minions of the Devil who hate God. God reveals: "all they that hate me love death." Proverbs 8:36.

Dr. Deborah Birx was the U.S. Government Coronavirus Response Coordinator in the Trump Administration from February 27, 2020, until January 20, 2021. Dr. Birx was instrumental in pushing for COVID-19 vaccinations. On July 22, 2022, Neil Cavuto, a journalist for Fox News, "asked Dr. Birx why the unvaccinated should take the vaccine if it does not prevent COVID." Astonishingly, Dr. Birx started by recommending the COVID-19 vaccines but then admitted that she knew from the outset that the vaccines would not protect against infection. She said: "I knew these vaccines were not going to protect against infection, and I think we overplayed the vaccines. ... Let's be clear, 50% of the people that died from the Omicron surge were older vaccinated."[1017]

While Dr. Birx knew the vaccines were ineffective in protecting against infection, she told the public a different story. She claimed that the COVID-19 vaccines were safe and effective while knowing they were not. On December 16, 2020, ABC News reported that Dr. Birx said:

> I understand how this vaccine was made. I understand the safety of the vaccine. And critically, I understand the depth of the efficacy of this vaccine. This is one of the most highly-effective vaccines we have in our infectious disease arsenal. And so that's why I'm very enthusiastic about the vaccine.[1018]

She further stated on that day:

> I want to make it clear there's two very important sides to that equation. There is herd immunity, which would prevent community spread, and then there's absolute clarity on what people need, in an equity way, to prevent severe disease, hospitalizations and fatalities.[1019]

One day earlier, on December 15, 2020, Laurence Smith of WDRB in Kentucky interviewed Dr. Birx. Her focus in the interview was on the steps needed to stop the spread of COVID-19. The key to stopping the spread of COVID-19, according to Dr. Birx, was to get as many people vaccinated as possible so that herd immunity could be achieved. She told Smith:

> While we have so much viral spread, it's really important to get control of this viral spread. ... And we can get to spring together by being vigilant now and being vaccinated when it's our turn. ... To truly achieve herd immunity, it's going to take through the summer and potentially even into the fall.

> That's getting 70-80% of Americans immunized.[1020]

She knew when she made those statements that the vaccines would not stop the spread of the alleged SARS-CoV-2 virus. Stopping the spread of a virus through herd immunity from a vaccine is premised on the theory that the vaccine will protect those in the herd against infection. Immunity is "[p]rotection against infectious disease."[1021] By definition, immunity means a person can resist a particular infection.[1022] If a person is immune from a disease, he is in a state where he "is not susceptible to [that] infection or disease."[1023] If a person is immune to a disease, that disease does not affect that person; he will not become ill from that disease.[1024]

But Dr. Birx's recent 2022 admission that she knew from the outset the vaccines would not protect against infection means that when she made the statements in 2020 about the COVID-19 vaccines providing immunity, she knew the vaccines would not protect against infection. She knew the vaccines were ineffective in stopping the spread of the alleged virus. That means that she intentionally lied on December 15th and 16th, 2020, when as Coronavirus Response Coordinator she claimed that the COVID-19 vaccines would give recipients immunity.

Why would Dr. Birx continue to recommend the COVID-19 vaccines during her July 22, 2022 interview when she knew from the beginning that "these vaccines were not going to protect against infection"? During her July 22, 2022 interview she justified the recommendation by changing the standard for the efficacy of the vaccines from preventing infection to reducing the severity of disease and hospitalizations. That is the pharmaceutical industry's tried and true bait-and-switch scheme. They sell to the public vaccines on the promise of preventing infection and the spread of disease. And when the vaccines are shown not to work, that evidence forces them to admit that the vaccines do not prevent disease. They then switch to a different efficacy standard of lowering the severity of the disease. That is the duplicitous game they are now playing with the COVID-19 vaccines.

Dr. Birx always knew that the COVID-19 vaccines would not work; they do not prevent infection, and she admitted they have been overplayed. Yet, knowing that, Dr. Birx still recommends today that people get vaccinated. "A double minded man is unstable in all his ways." James 1:8. As we have seen, the vaccines are not efficacious, even under the new phony efficacy standard. Indeed, the vaccines are driving the disease. People are getting very sick and suffering ADE from the vaccines.

President Joe Biden has repeatedly stated that the COVID-19 vaccines prevent the spread of SARS-CoV-2. Indeed, that was the alleged purpose of his unconstitutional executive orders requiring federal workers, federal contractors, and the private sector to receive the COVID-19 vaccine. In an October 7, 2021 speech Joe Biden stated:

> We still had more than a quarter of people in the United States who were eligible for vaccinations but didn't get the shot.
>
> And we know there is no other way to beat the pandemic than to get the vast majority of Americans vaccinated. It's as simple as that.
>
> And to — **to spread to our children, to spread throughout society and at our hospitals the risk of other variants** — it's all dangerous and obvious, but we're still not there.
>
> We have to beat this thing. So, while I didn't race to do it right away, that's why I've had to move toward requirements that everyone get vaccinated

or I had the authority to do that. That wasn't my first instinct.

My administration is now requiring federal workers to be vaccinated. We've also required federal contractors to be vaccinated. If you have a contract with the federal government, working for the federal government, you have to be vaccinated.

We're requiring active duty military to be vaccinated. We're making sure healthcare workers are vaccinated, because if you seek care at a healthcare facility, you should have the certainty that the pro- — **the people providing that care are protected from COVID and cannot spread it to you.**

The Labor Department is going to shortly issue an emergency rule — which I asked for several weeks ago, and they're going through the process — to require all employees [employers] with more than 100 people, whether they work for the federal government or not — this is within a — in the purview of the Labor Department — to ensure their workers are fully vaccinated or face testing at least once a week.

In total, this Labor Department vaccination requirement will cover 100 million Americans, about two thirds of all the people who work in America.

And here's the deal: These requirements are already proving that they work.

***

> But don't take it from me. Not from some, you know, liberal think tank this comes from. But here's what Wall Street is saying:
>
> Goldman Sachs, quote: "Vaccinations will have a positive impact on employment." **It means less spread of COVID-19, which will help people return to work.**[1025]

On October 10, 2022, we found out that Pfizer never tested their vaccine for whether it would prevent transmission of the alleged SARS-CoV-2 virus. The CEO of Pfizer, Albert Bourla refused to testify before the European Parliament. Janine Small, President of International Markets at Pfizer testified in his stead. She testified before the European Parliament that Pfizer never tested their vaccine to determine if it would prevent the spread of the virus. At the hearing, Bob Roos, a Dutch European Parliament member, asked Small "was the Pfizer COVID vaccine tested on stopping the transmission of the virus before it entered the market?"[1026] Small answered: "No. We had to really move at the speed of science to really understand what is taking place in the market."[1027] That astounding admission hit the public like a bomb because it undermines the basis for vaccine mandates.

On May 16, 2021, Anthony Fauci appeared on CBS's "Face the Nation." The host, John Dickerson, interviewed him. During the interview, Dr. Fauci announced without equivocation that the COVID-19 vaccines are effective in stopping the spread of SARS-CoV-2. He stated that "even though there are breakthrough infections with vaccinated people ... [it is] not impossible but very, very low likelihood — that they're going to transmit it." He elaborated:

> When you get vaccinated, you not only protect your own health and that of the family but also you contribute to the community health by **preventing**

> **the spread of the virus** throughout the community. ... In other words, **you become a dead end to the virus.** And when there are a lot of dead ends around, the virus is not going to go anywhere. And that's when you get a point that you have a markedly diminished rate of infection in the community.[1028]

We now know Dr. Fauci's statements were not true because Pfizer never did any studies to determine the effectiveness of the vaccines in stopping the spread of SARS-CoV-2. There was simply no evidence from which Dr. Fauci could say otherwise. He was lying.

Indeed, we have proof that when he made those statements, he knew they were not true. We know that Fauci intentionally lied because four months earlier, on January 19, 2021, he said in an article that he knew the COVID-19 vaccines (and indeed all injectable vaccines) typically do not result in immunity that interrupts infection or transmission through mouth and nose. Mouth and nose (i.e., mucosal) transmission is the alleged means by which the COVID-19 virus is spread. Dr. Fauci was the co-author of the January 19, 2021 article in which he said:

> **Administration of parenterally administered vaccines alone typically does not result in potent mucosal immunity that might interrupt infection or transmission.** ... For these reasons, additional data regarding protection from infection should be generated as soon as possible.[1029] (emphasis added)

His statement in the January 19, 2021 article was the opposite of his May 16, 2021 statement. There is no way to reconcile the two statements. Dr. Fauci lied to encourage people to get vaccinated, falsely telling them by doing so they would help others by stopping the spread of SARS-CoV-2. He knew what he was saying was a lie, and did not care who was injured by being injected with the ineffective and unsafe COVID-19 vaccines.

But that admission by Pfizer and Dr. Fauci's deception really miss the elephant in the room. That elephant in the room is the issue of whether the COVID-19 vaccines even prevents infection from the beginning. Pfizer did not test for whether the vaccine would prevent transmission because they knew to begin with that it would not stop infection. Pfizer knew that their COVID-19 vaccine was ineffective in doing what vaccines are supposed to do, provide immunity from infection. Pfizer's vaccine does not work and they know it.

Logically, if the vaccine cannot prevent transmission, that means it cannot prevent infection. In order for someone to spread the virus they must be infected from the begining. Thus, the key issue is stopping the infection. Of course, if the vaccine stops infection, it will necessarily stop the spread. Because if a person is not infected with a disease, he cannot transmit the disease; a person cannot spread something he does not have. All government officials knew from the beginning that the COVID-19 vaccines would not prevent infection and consequently would not prevent the spread of the virus.

Joseph Choi reported for The Hill the following December 3, 2020, statement from Pfizer CEO Albert Bourla:

> Pfizer chairman Albert Bourla told Dateline host Lester Holt that the pharmaceutical company was "not certain" if the vaccine prevented the coronavirus from being transmitted, saying, "This is something that needs to be examined."[1030]

But just six weeks later, on January 13, 2020, the official Pfizer Twitter account strongly implied that, indeed, their vaccine does stop transmission of the SARS-Cov2 virus. "The ability to vaccinate at speed to gain herd immunity and stop transmission is our highest priority."[1031]

To erase all doubt about Pfizer's public position, on June 8, 2021, Albert Bourla stated on Twitter: "Although data shows that severe #COVID19 is rare in children, widespread vaccination is a critical tool to help stop transmission."[1032] Bourla later deleted that Tweet, but it was recovered using the Internet Archive Wayback Machine. Recall that Janine Small, President of International Markets at Pfizer, testified on October 10, 2022, before the European Parliament that Pfizer never tested their vaccine to determine if it would prevent the spread of the virus. Boural knew that and even said on December 3, 2020, that Pfizer was not sure if the vaccine prevented SARS-Cov2 from being transmitted, saying preventing transmission was something that needed to be examined. Yet, both Pfizer and its CEO, knowing that their vaccine was ineffective in preventing virus transmission, nonetheless had no qualms in lying to the public and misrepresenting it as effective. They are liars.

Senator Matthew Canavan, during an Australian Senate Education Employment and Legislation Committee hearing, asked the Australia Country Medical Director for Pfizer, Dr. Krishan Thiru, whether Pfizer tested its COVID-19 vaccine to determine if it could stop or reduce the transmission of the virus before its approval and rollout of the vaccine in 2020.[1033] Dr. Thiru employed obfuscation in refusing to answer the question. Senator Canavan also asked Dr. Thiru on what evidence Pfizer Tweeted on January 13, 2020, that the Pfizer vaccine is intended to fulfill its high priority to gain herd immunity and stop transmission. Dr. Thiru again employed obfuscation in refusing to answer the question. Senator Canavan asked the Pfizer representative whether Pfizer CEO Albert Bourla's statement that widespread vaccination is a critical tool to help stop transmission was true. Dr. Thiru danced around the question but suggested in his answer that the

Pfizer vaccine is NOT a critical tool to help stop the transmission of the SARS-CoV-2 virus.

Please understand that the SARS-CoV-2 virus does not actually exist. It has never been isolated.[1034] Vaccinated people who are testing positive for SARS-CoV-2 do not actually have "breakthrough" COVID-19. They are testing positive for SARS-CoV-2 because the tests are rigged to provide false positive results.[1035] The "breakthrough" patients actually are suffering from an autoimmune disease known as antibody-dependent enhancement (ADE) caused by the COVID-19 vaccines.[1036] ADE is being falsely labeled as COVID-19, when in fact it is an autoimmune disease caused by the vaccine. Indeed, it seems that is the purpose of the vaccine; it is a kill shot.[1037]

Please be mindful that the COVID-19 vaccines were authorized because they purportedly prevented infection and the spread of the disease. Dr. Hilary Marston of the National Institute of Allergy and Infectious Disease at the NIH, gave a presentation during an October 22, 2020 meeting of the Vaccines and Related Biological Products Advisory Committee.[1038] That meeting was before the issuance of the EUAs for the COVID-19 vaccines. During her presentation, she explained that the primary endpoint for all COVID-19 vaccine studies was to prevent COVID-19. Below is one of her slides where it states: **"Primary Endpoint: Prevention of symptomatic COVID-19 disease (PCR confirmed)."**[1039] The PCR tests for SARS-CoV-2, the alleged virus thought to cause COVID-19.

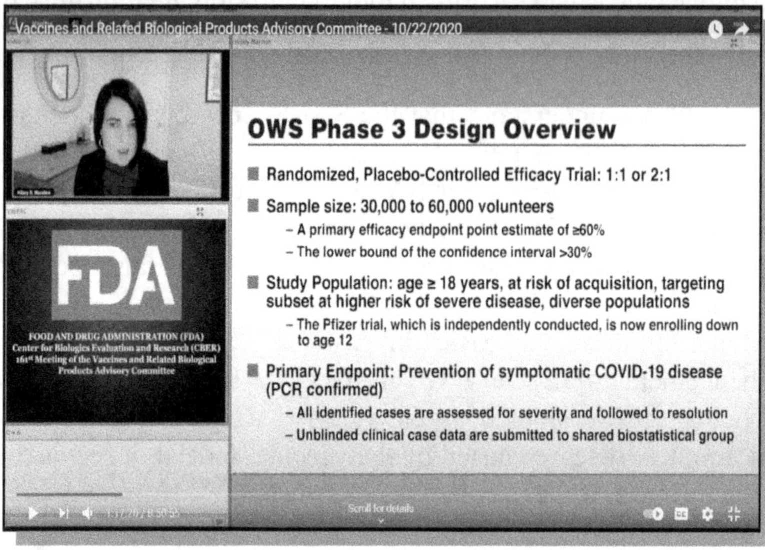

Indeed, the pertinent criteria announced by the FDA for the EUA granted to the Pfizer-BioNTech COVID-19 vaccine said nothing about lessening symptoms. The criteria for the EUA was simply that the vaccine may be effective in "preventing" COVID-19.

> Based on the totality of scientific evidence available to FDA, it is reasonable to believe that Pfizer-BioNTech COVID-19 Vaccine may be effective in **preventing COVID-19**, and that, when used under the conditions described in this authorization, the known and potential benefits of Pfizer-BioNTech COVID-19 Vaccine when used to **prevent COVID-19** outweigh its known and potential risks.[1040]

And when on August 23, 2021, the FDA approved the substantially similar COMIRNATY (COVID-19 Vaccine, mRNA), it said nothing about lessening symptoms. The FDA only mentioned the alleged effectiveness of the approved vaccine to prevent COVID-19. The FDA stated that that "[t]he [approved] vaccine has been known as the Pfizer-BioNTech COVID-19 Vaccine, and will now be marketed as Comirnaty (koe-mir'-na-tee), for the **prevention of COVID-19** disease in individuals 16 years of age and older."[1041]

When it became clear, though, that the vaccines were ineffective in preventing COVID-19, the standard for effectiveness had to be changed to something else. The standard for effectiveness is now no longer prevention of COVID-19 infection or preventing the spread of COVID-19. The standard has shifted to lessening the symptoms of COVID-19. It seems that the vaccine manufacturers and the CDC knew from the beginning that the COVID-19 vaccines would be ineffetive in preventing the spread of the disease. Indeed, as early as October 26, 2020, prior to the EUA issuance, Anthony Fauci, Director of the National Institute of Allergy and Infectious Diseases (NIAID), stated that preventing infection with COVID-19 was only a secondary endpoint. The primary purpose of the vaccine was not to prevent infection or spread but rather only to lessen symptoms.[1042]

Dr. Fauci claimed at the time that preventing COVID-19 was only a secondary endpoint of the vaccines. He made that statement just four (4) days after his subordinate, Dr. Hilary Marston, gave a presentation during an October 22, 2020 meeting of the Vaccines and Related Biological Products Advisory Committee, where she explained that the **primary endpoint** of the COVID-19 vaccine trials was the **prevention** of COVID-19.[1043] When people in government are conspiring to commit fraud, it is sometimes hard to keep everyone on the same sheet of music.

Before the FDA issuance of the EUA for the Moderna vaccine, Moderna Chief Medical Officer Tal Zaks stated on or before November 23, 2020: "our results show that this vaccine can prevent you from being sick, it can prevent you from being severely sick. **They do not show that it prevents you from**

potentially carrying this virus transiently and infecting others."[1044] Yet, the basis on which the EUA was granted to Moderna was that it was allegedly effective in preventing infection. There was no basis for authorizing the EUA on the vaccine's ability to only lessen the symptoms of COVID-19, while not preventing infection. Moderna limited the measure of efficacy for their COVID-19 vaccine, in pertinent part, as follows: "**The primary efficacy endpoint was efficacy of the vaccine to prevent protocol-defined COVID-19 occurring** at least 14 days after the second dose in participants with negative SARS-CoV-2 status at baseline."[1045] The EUA was based on the representation by Moderna that their study proved that the vaccine would prevent infection. But the Moderna's Chief Medical Officer Tal Zaks knew from the beginning that the vaccine was ineffective in preventing infection, and he said so.

The efficacy studies done for the EUA only measured the prevention of COVID-19. There was no publication of any studies that were the basis for EUA that measured lowering symptoms. For example, When you read page 35 of the Pfizer-BioNtech publication titled *Fact Sheet for Healthcare Providers Administering Vaccine*, it reveals that the only criterion reported for establishing the effectiveness of the COVID-19 vaccine is the subsequent infection rate in the study groups.[1046] The study compared the COVID-19 infection rate among the vaccine group and the placebo group to come up with an effectiveness of 95% for the COVID-19 vaccine. The study announced that the "Vaccine Efficacy" was based upon a finding of the "First COVID-19 Occurrence From 7 Days After Dose 2."[1047]

That fact sheet indicates that "FDA issued this EUA, based on Pfizer-BioNTech's request and submitted data. Although limited scientific information is available, based on the totality of the scientific evidence available to date, it is reasonable to believe that the Pfizer-BioNTech COVID-19 Vaccine **may be effective for the prevention of COVID-19** in individuals as specified in the Full EUA Prescribing Information."[1048]

On or about November 23, 2021, the FDA claimed that "[v]accinating children ages 5 years and older can help protect them from getting COVID-19, spreading the virus to others, and getting sick if they do get infected."[1049] The FDA used the qualifying word "help," but the statement was intended to deceive people into believing that the vaccine would protect persons from being infected, getting sick, or spreading the alleged virus. It had become apparent by the time the FDA posted that statement that the vaccines did none of those things. On or about March 30, 2022, the CDC finally admitted in writing that the COVID-19 vaccines do not prevent infection. On its frequently asked questions page, the FDA posted the question: "Why should I get vaccinated if I might get COVID-19 anyway?" To which the FDA responded, in pertinent part: "Like all vaccines, COVID-19 vaccines are not 100% effective at preventing infection. Some people who are up to date with their COVID-19 vaccinations will get COVID-19 breakthrough infection."[1050]

Since it has become clear that the COVID-19 vaccine does not prevent infection, the FDA has switched from saying that the COVID-19 vaccine will prevent infection to instead saying that "COVID-19 vaccination significantly lowers your risk of severe illness, hospitalization, and death if you get infected."[1051] But people were prodded to get vaccinated to prevent infection. When that was seen not to be true, the FDA pivoted from preventing infection to claiming instead that "COVID 19-vaccines are effective at protecting people from getting seriously ill, being hospitalized, and dying."[1052] But preventing serious illness, hospitalization, and death were not the efficacy criteria of the vaccine studies. The vaccine studies and approval under the EUA were based on the vaccine's purported ability to prevent COVID-19.

Ponder the sheer nonsense of measuring any medication's

efficacy by whether it lowers the risk of hospitalization or death. Even Kool-Aid could be touted by that low bar as a wonder drug. Indeed, the CDC has created a measure of efficacy that is almost impossible to verify. If one receives a COVID-19 vaccine and then gets sick from COVID-19 and survives, the doctor will claim that the person survived the bout from COVID-19 because of the vaccine. But that can never be known, and the doctor knows it. Indeed, suffering during any illness is subjective. After the person survives the alleged COVID-19 bout, he will be told by his doctor that it was a good thing he was vaccinated; otherwise, it could have been much worse. The doctor will convince the patient that the vaccine lowered the severity of the symptoms. But the doctor is just making it up. If the person is not hospitalized, the doctor will say the vaccine kept his patient out of the hospital. If the person is hospitalized, the doctor will lower the bar further and say the vaccine saved his life. It is a subjective game that the COVID-19 vaccine always wins. It is a medical scam.

This bait and switch strategy was brought to light publically when on January 30, 2021, Andrew Court reported for The Daily Mail that "Democrat Rep. Stephen Lynch has tested positive to COVID-19 after receiving both shots of the Pfizer vaccine."[1053] In a that news article it was explained that the reason that Rep. Lynch was infected with COVID-19 after being vaccinated is that "Pfizer's vaccine does not necessarily prevent COVID-19 infection, but is said to be 95 percent effective in stopping the serious symptoms that are caused by the coronavirus."[1054]

Pfizer-BioNtech announced that their COVID-19 vaccine was 95% effective in "preventing" COVID-19. They did NOT announce that it was 95% effective in reducing symptoms of COVID-19. The FDA allowed the EUA of the Pfizer COVID-19 vaccine because the COVID-19 vaccine study claimed a 95% effectiveness in "preventing" the recipients from getting COVID-19 after they had been vaccinated.[1055] Indeed, the FDA states the reason for the EUA of the Pfizer-BioNtech COVID-19 vaccine was that it is theorized to be effective in "preventing" the SARS-CoV-2 infection. The FDA explicitly states:

> Pfizer-BioNTech COVID-19 Vaccine is authorized to **prevent** coronavirus disease 2019 (COVID-19) caused by severe acute respiratory syndrome coronavirus 2 (SARS-CoV-2) in individuals 16 years of age and older.[1056]

The argument that the COVID-19 vaccines lessen symptoms is a smokescreen. The report from Britain's Chief Scientific Adviser, Patrick Vallance, proves it. In July 2021, he stated that 40% of all COVID-19 patients being admitted to hospitals with COVID-19 are fully vaccinated.[1057] That fact alone proves that the COVID-19 vaccines do not lessen symptoms. Persons are admitted to the hospital when they have severe symptoms. The fact 40% of those being hospitalized for COVID-19 are fully vaccinated indicates that the patients are suffering severe symptoms and thus the vaccines do not lessen the symptoms. You cannot have droves of vaccinated people jamming into hospitals after coming down with COVID-19 and maintain that the vaccines lessen symptoms.

Indeed, the FDA explicitly stated on or before August 20, 2021, that it did not know if the Pfizer-BioNTech COVID-19 vaccine reduces symptoms. The FDA has stated that the Pfizer-BioNtech COVID-19 vaccine has been authorized under the EUA hoping that it will **"prevent"** COVID-19 and NOT in the hope it will reduce the severity of COVID-19.

> To date, only a small number of severe cases have occurred during the study, which makes it **difficult to evaluate whether the vaccine reduces the severity of COVID-19.** Pfizer-BioNTech COVID-19 vaccine is **authorized to prevent**

> **coronavirus disease** 2019 (COVID-19) caused by severe acute respiratory syndrome coronavirus 2 (SARS-CoV-2) in individuals 16 years of age and older.[1058]

The CDC has expressed hope that the COVID-19 vaccines will prevent infection, but the evidence is that the vaccines do no such thing. The CDC claims that a person who is vaccinated is unlikely to be infected with COVID-19, but then they give the following guidance, which suggests that they know that the likelihood of a vaccinated person getting COVID-19 is significant:

> Fully vaccinated people who have come into close contact with someone with COVID-19 should be tested 3-5 days following the date of their exposure and wear a mask in public indoor settings for 14 days or until they receive a negative test result. They should isolate if they test positive.[1059]

That advice indicates that the CDC has no confidence in the efficacy of the COVID-19 vaccines in preventing the disease.

CDC Director, Dr. Rachelle Walensky has even less faith in the COVID-19 vaccines. She revealed that not only do the vaccines not lessen the symptoms, but NPR reports that "Walensky noted that data from Israel suggests 'increased risk of severe disease amongst those vaccinated early.'"[1060]

Writing for Roll Call, Emily Kopp reported on July 30, 2021, that data presented at a confidential congressional briefing showed that "[u]p to 15 percent of deaths in May were among vaccinated people."[1061]

A government report from Public Health England reveals that persons who have been vaccinated are six (6) times more likely to die from the delta variant of the SARS-COV-2 than those who are unvaccinated.[1062] The report shows that 26 out of 4,087 fully vaccinated persons died from the variant. Whereas 34 out of 35,521 unvaccinated persons died from the variant.[1063] That is a 665% greater death rate among the vaccinated group. So much for lessening symptoms.

If it has now been shown that the vaccine is truly ineffective in "preventing" a vaccine recipient from getting COVID-19, it should be announced as ineffective. The vaccine should be taken off the market. Apparently, that will not happen. Instead, there is now being announced a new criterion for effectiveness that was never studied. And that new criteria is lessening of symptoms. But that is also a deception because the data proves the vaccines don't do that either. This bait and switch strategy for vaccines has been around since the 1800's. Dr. Suzanne Humphries reveals that "[w]hen it was clear that the smallpox vaccine was not able to prevent disease, the medical profession tried to justify vaccination by changing the goal posts from lifelong 'perfect' immunity to "milder disease.'"[1064] Dr. Humphries revealed that bait and switch from immunity to milder symptoms was used to justify getting ineffective pertussis and influenza vaccines in 2013.

The CDC seems incapable of telling the truth. After it went through all the machinations to change the criteria from preventing infection and spread to lessening symptoms, it is now faced with vaccines that nobody wants. Why would anyone get vaccinated against COVID-19 if the vaccine does not prevent the infection or spread of the illness? Faced with that reality, what did the CDC decide to do? It seems the CDC is hoping that most will forget that the COVID-19 vaccines do not prevent infection or spread because the CDC is now going back to claiming that is what the COVID-19 vaccines will do.

The agency is like a snake oil salesman hawking his wares without much thought to the reality of what it says. As we have seen above, the CDC knows the COVID-19 vaccines do not prevent COVID-19. Yet, on or before March 17, 2023, the CDC posted on its website that "COVID-19 vaccination is recommended for everyone ages 6 months and older in the United States for the **prevention** of COVID-19."[1065] You read that correctly. The CDC is now touting the COVID-19 vaccines as preventatives against COVID-19, while knowing they do no such thing. Below is a cropped screenshot from the CDC website.

> Recommendations for COVID-19 vaccine use
>
> **Groups recommended for vaccination**
>
> COVID-19 vaccination is recommended for everyone ages 6 months and older in the United States for the prevention of COVID-19. There is currently no FDA-approved or FDA-authorized COVID-19 vaccine for children younger than age 6 months.

The CDC is suddenly changing its tune and is now saying that the COVID-19 vaccines prevent COVID-19. But the medical community and the general public understand that the COVID-19 vaccines do NOT prevent a person from getting COVID-19. For example, in an October 27, 2022, article in Medical News Today, which incidentally was medically reviewed for accuracy by Meredith Goodwin, M.D., FAAFP, Helen Miller explains what everyone now knows:

> The COVID-19 vaccine does not prevent COVID-19. A person who is fully vaccinated can still contract the SARS-CoV-2 virus, which causes COVID-19, and may go on to develop the disease.[1066]

What is the point of getting a vaccine that does not prevent the disease? Miller explains that the purpose of the vaccine is not to prevent COVID-19 but rather to "strengthen immunity against the virus and help prevent serious illness, hospitalization, and death."[1067] That is what the CDC had previously said. But the CDC is now stating that the COVID-19 vaccines do not just prevent serious illness from COVID-19, but any degree of the disease; the CDC claims now that the COVID-19 vaccines prevent COVID-19, which is false.

It gets worse. On or before December 22, 2022, the CDC posted a statement that "COVID 19-vaccines are effective at preventing severe illness from COVID-19 and **limiting the spread of the virus** that causes it."[1068] One of the vaccines that the CDC recommends is the Pfizer-BioNTech COVID-19 vaccine. Pfizer-BioNTech is on record in testimony before the EU Parliament that it never tested its vaccine for whether it would prevent the spread of the virus. Indeed, it has been proven that none of the COVID-19 vaccines prevent the spread of SARS-CoV-2. But the pathological liars at the CDC say that the ineffective COVID-19 vaccines prevent the spread of SARS-CoV-2. Below is a cropped screenshot from the CDC website.

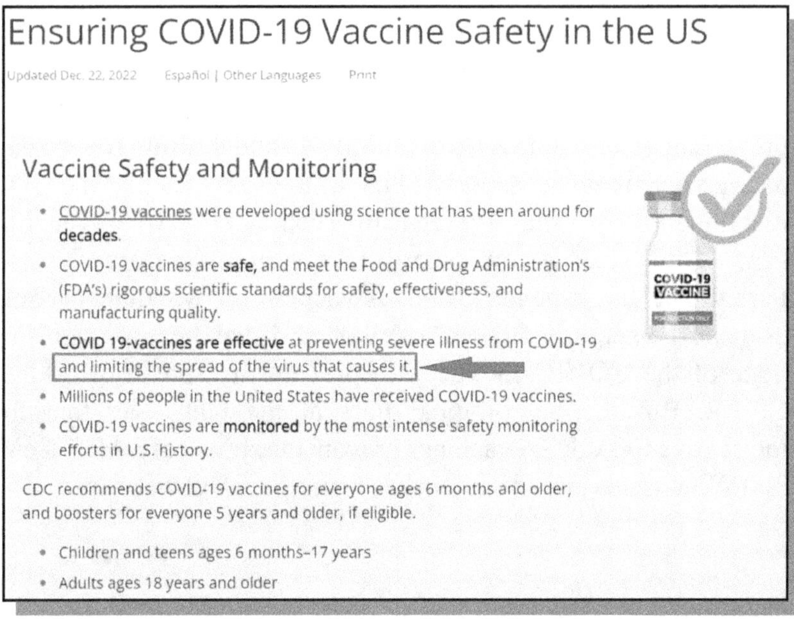

Ensuring COVID-19 Vaccine Safety in the US

Updated Dec. 22, 2022 Español | Other Languages Print

Vaccine Safety and Monitoring

- COVID-19 vaccines were developed using science that has been around for **decades**.
- COVID-19 vaccines are **safe,** and meet the Food and Drug Administration's (FDA's) rigorous scientific standards for safety, effectiveness, and manufacturing quality.
- **COVID 19-vaccines are effective** at preventing severe illness from COVID-19 and limiting the spread of the virus that causes it.
- Millions of people in the United States have received COVID-19 vaccines.
- COVID-19 vaccines are **monitored** by the most intense safety monitoring efforts in U.S. history.

CDC recommends COVID-19 vaccines for everyone ages 6 months and older, and boosters for everyone 5 years and older, if eligible.

- Children and teens ages 6 months–17 years
- Adults ages 18 years and older

Dr. John Campbell, Ph.D., was incredulous at what the CDC said on its website. He could not believe that the CDC said that the COVID-19 vaccines prevent the spread of the SARS-CoV-2 virus that causes COVID-19 because the evidence clearly establishes that the vaccines do no such thing. Dr. Campbell sated:

> [COVID-19] vaccines are safe, according to the Centers for Disease Control. [That statement] was taken from their website not an hour ago. ... "COVID 19 vaccines are effective at preventing some severe illness from COVID-19 and limiting the spread of the virus that causes it."[1069]

Dr. Campbell then sardonically states:

> Now, you might have thought that COVID vaccination has minimal if any effect for any period of time at preventing the spread of COVID-19. You might have thought that; I might have thought that, but, hey, we're both wrong because the CDC states here in black and white, taken from their website not an hour ago that, and I've made a note. Note: "and limiting the spread of the virus that causes it."[1070]

Dr. Campbell then exhales as he tries to stop laughing before he continues to speak in exasperated disbelief.

> This is the CDC. This is the CDC on Tuesday, the 28th of March 2023, saying the COVID vaccine prevents the spread of COVID-19.[1071]

Dr. Campbell then drops his head in his hands in shock and disbelief at what he has just read on the CDC website. He continues then to sarcastically explain the incredible statements by the CDC:

> That's what it says. It prevents the spread of COVID-19! That's what they say on their website, today! And we can't argue with it, it must be right because it's on the CDC website. So, there we go, make a note of that. The vaccine prevents the spread.[1072]

Dr. Campbell then shakes his head as he says in an exasperated, cynical, mocking tone: "Unbelievable! Because I thought it didn't really prevent the spread but there you go. [You] can't be right all the time. So that's what they're saying."[1073]

On or before March 2021, Johns Hopkins said that an effective vaccine "will protect someone who receives it by lowering the chance of getting COVID-19." But that the "more important" benefit of the COVID-19 vaccines was that they are "highly efficacious at preventing serious illness, hospitalization and death."[1074] On July 28, 2022, the Johns Hopkins article was updated to include the following statement: "Johns Hopkins Medicine views the FDA-approved mRNA vaccines from Pfizer and Moderna as highly effective at preventing serious disease, hospitalization, and death from COVID-19."[1075]

The authors of that Johns Hopkins article knew with certainty when they wrote that statement it is not true that the COVID-19 vaccines were "highly effective at preventing serious disease, hospitalization, and death from COVID-19" because it had become quite evident by the time that they wrote that that the vast majority of the people dying from COVID-19 were vaccinated.

Johns Hopkins is an elite medical center at the forefront of the medical establishment and has medical data from governments worldwide at its fingertips. The UK has monthly mortality data regarding deaths from COVID-19 that are regularly published and made available online. That data revealed a steady rate of COVID-19 deaths among the vaccinated population each month. It is more accurate to describe those people as persons who tested positive for SARS-CoV-2 before dying because SARS-CoV-2 does not exist. The UK data shows that during the 21 months between April 1, 2021, and December 31, 2022, 86% of the COVID-19 deaths in the UK were among those vaccinated against COVID-19.[1076] Clearly, it is not true that the COVID-19 vaccines are "highly effective at preventing serious disease, hospitalization, and death from COVID-19." when 86% of those who are dying with COVID-19 have gotten the COVID-19 vaccine.

Johns Hopkins has followed the CDC lead and has now

changed its tune regarding the efficacy of the COVID-19 vaccines in preventing COVID-19 and the spread of the virus that causes it. The change is subtle but real. On or before November 1, 2022, the same article cited above was again updated to place highlights around a statement that "evidence continues to indicate that getting a COVID-19 vaccine is the best protection against getting COVID-19, whether you have already had COVID-19 or not."[1077] Johns Hopkins further now states that "[g]etting vaccinated provides greater protection to others since the vaccine helps reduce the spread of COVID-19." But we know that both statements are not true.

Johns Hopkins has gone from saying that the COVID-19 vaccines merely "lower the chance of getting COVID-19" to saying with certainty that "getting a COVID-19 vaccine is the best protection against getting COVID-19." That flies in the face of the evidence that has now become so apparent. Adding insult to injury, Johns Hopkins now says that the vaccine "helps reduce the spread of COVID-19." The evidence is now in. It is clear that the vaccines do no such thing. Indeed, Pfizer-BioNTech is on record admitting they never even tested their COVID-19 vaccine to determine whether it would reduce the spread of COVID-19.

In the same article in which Johns Hopkins states that the COVID-19 vaccines help reduce the spread of COVID-19, Johns Hopkins implicitly acknowledges that the vaccines do no such thing. In the article, Johns Hopkins explains that it follows the CDC's recommendation for those vaccinated to wear masks and remain physically distant from others in all of their facilities. If the vaccines effectively prevented the spread of SARS-CoV-2, no such steps would be necessary to prevent the transmission of the alleged virus.

36 Planned Obfuscation

The FDA tries to cover its and vaccine makers' deception by distinguishing between SARS-CoV-2 and COVID-19. While the distinction is technically correct, it is a contrivance that is part of their plan to hoodwink the masses. The FDA states that the SARS-CoV-2 virus causes an illness known as COVID-19. And so, the claims by the government officials and the pharmaceutical companies that the COVID-19 vaccines will prevent COVID-19 should not be interpreted to mean that it will prevent infection from the SARS-CoV-2 virus. If you are confused by that distinction, it is because it is part of their plan to baffle you with baloney.

The public and the medical community do not generally make a distinction between the SARS-CoV-2 virus and the COVID-19 disease.[1078] It is not uncommon to read references to the "COVID-19 virus," even by experts.[1079] For example, Johns Hopkins, which Newsweek rated as the #4 rated medical facility in the world,[1080] considers SARS-CoV-2 and COVID-19 as meaning the same thing. On November 1, 2022, Johns Hopkins stated that "[g]etting vaccinated provides greater protection to others since the vaccine helps reduce the spread of COVID-19."[1081] Johns Hopkins considers COVID-19 a virus that can be spread. Indeed, expert virologists consider the many alleged virus variants

"COVID-19 variants."[1082] Even the CDC refers to a SARS-CoV-2 breakthrough infection in a person up to date with his COVID-19 vaccinations as a "COVID-19 breakthrough infection."[1083]

Despite the common interchangeable usage of COVID-19 and SARS-CoV-2 to describe the same pathogen, the FDA distinguishes the alleged virus (SARS-CoV-2) from the illness it is alleged to cause (COVID-19). By doing that, the FDA can claim that the COVID-19 vaccines are not required to prevent the infection or spread of a pathogen (in this case the SARS-CoV-2). The distinction, in the end, does not help the FDA or the pharmaceutical companies because the vaccines do not prevent COVID-19 either. Indeed, the evidence is that the vaccines cause antibody-dependent enhancement that is often manifested in a diagnosis of COVID-19.

If you are confused at this point it is because the pharmaceutical companies have created a scheme that is confusing by design. Moving on, let's consider the following statement on April 23, 2023, from Peter Marks, MD, Ph.D., Director, FDA Center for Biologics Evaluation and Research. It will shock you. The FDA now admits that, from the outset, the FDA did not require the COVID-19 vaccine makers to demonstrate that their vaccines would prevent the infection or transmission of any pathogen. The FDA uses the distinction between COVID-19 and SARS-CoV-2 to throw sand in your eyes so that you do not realize there is no justification for their actions. Dr. Marks states:

> It is important to note that FDA's authorization and licensure standards for vaccines do not require demonstration of the prevention of infection or transmission. A vaccine can meet the licensure standard if the vaccine's benefits of protecting against disease outweigh the vaccine's risks for the licensed use. There is no requirement that the vaccine also prevents infection with the pathogen

> that can cause the disease or transmission of that pathogen to others. Similarly, a vaccine can meet the EUA standard without any evidence that the vaccine prevents infection or transmission. To that end, there is no requirement that the clinical trials supporting a vaccine's licensure or authorization be designed to determine whether the vaccine prevents infection of a pathogen or transmission of that pathogen to others.[1084]

There you have it in black and white. The FDA did not require the COVID-19 vaccine makers to demonstrate that their vaccines worked to prevent the infection or transmission of any pathogen. But the public was never told that. It is only now, after the FDA was pushed to explain the ineffectiveness of the vaccines, that they decided to let the cat out of the bag and admit that the vaccines were never intended to stop the infection or transmission of any pathogen. The government treats the public the same malevolent way a psychopathic adult would take advantage of the naive trust of children: "You silly kids, you should have known the vaccines weren't designed to work."

If the public had understood that the vaccines were not designed to prevent infection or transmission of the alleged virus, they would never have gotten injected with the vaccine. Vaccine mandates were premised on obtaining herd immunity from the alleged virus. There would be no justification for vaccine mandates if the vaccines do not stop the infection and spread of the virus. And so, the fact that the vaccines were not designed to prevent infection or transmission needed to be kept secret. The pharmaceutical companies and the government began a campaign of deception portraying the COVID-19 vaccines as safe and effective in stopping the infection and transmission, all the while knowing full well the vaccines at the outset were not even designed to do either.

Indeed, on or before December 22, 2022, the CDC posted a statement that "COVID 19-vaccines are effective at preventing severe illness from COVID-19 and **limiting the spread of the virus** that causes it."[1085] So, here you have the CDC saying that the vaccines would stop the spread of the virus, but the FDA claims that no demonstration of the prevention of infection or transmission of a pathogen was ever required or proven. Everyone was led to believe that the COVID-19 vaccines would protect the vaccinated from the virus and stop its spread. The CDC lied. Everyone was fooled.

The public has been hoodwinked by subtlety. "Now the serpent was more subtil than any beast of the field which the LORD God had made." Genesis 3:1. The nuanced distinction between COVID-19 and SARS-CoV-2 is not adhered to by government officials or the pharmaceutical companies in their public statements or official documents. It seems that the FDA and pharmaceutical companies used the terms interchangeably to confuse the public, while concealing that they considered them to have two different meanings. It was a trick to fool the public. For example, NIAID Director Anthony Fauci is on record deceptively saying on May 16, 2021, that "[w]hen you get vaccinated ... you contribute to the community health by **preventing the spread of the virus** throughout the community. ... In other words, **you become a dead end to the virus**."[1086] Dr. Fauci falsely portrays the vaccines as effective in stopping the infection and spread of the SARS-CoV-2 virus.

On March 9, 2021, the CDC Director, Dr. Rochelle Walensky, said, "our data from the CDC today suggests that **vaccinated people do not carry the virus**, don't get sick — and it's not just in the clinical trials, but it's also in real world data."[1087] Walensky was talking about protection against the SARS-CoV-2 virus. She elaborated that since those vaccinated against COVID-19 do not carry the virus, it eliminates the risk that they would be contagious to others.[1088] Walensky and Fauci were both lying. On April 1, 2021, Walensky retracted her statement and admitted that "some people who are fully vaccinated could get Covid-19."[1089]

Notice that Walensky did not make any distinction between the SARS-CoV-2 virus and COVID-19 illness. She understood that in both instances, she was discussing the spread of the alleged virus known to the public as both COVID-19 and SARS-CoV-2. Notice that her retraction was made six weeks prior to Dr. Fauci's May 16, 2021, assurance that the vaccinated persons "**become a dead end to the virus**." Government officials were misrepresenting the vaccines as preventing the infection and spread of the SARS-CoV-2 virus while knowing full well that the vaccine makers were not required to (and did not) prove either.

On August 23, 2021, the FDA cited the Pfizer Comirnaty vaccines as a strategy to gain herd immunity to the SARS-CoV-2 virus. "Public health vaccination goals of immunizing 75% of the population (to achieve herd immunity) have not yet been achieved."[1090] The FDA clearly described the Pfizer Comirnaty COVID-19 vaccine under review as providing widespread immunity against infection and spread, known as herd immunity, of the SARS-CoV-2 virus. But that was a deception because FDA Director of the Center for Biologics Evaluation and Research Peter Marks revealed on April 23, 2023, that "the FDA's authorization and licensure standards for vaccines do not require demonstration of the prevention of infection or transmission."[1091]

Pfizer suggested that widespread uptake of its COVID-19 vaccine would provide herd immunity to the SARS-CoV-2 virus. Its October 21, 2021 FDA briefing document stated that its vaccine would reduce infection and transmission rates.

> Maximizing the proportion of the population that is vaccinated is critically important to help reduce rates of infection, decrease transmission, prevent

the emergence of new variants of concern, and hasten the end of the pandemic.[1092]

We now know that Pfizer lied in that October 21, 2021, briefing document claiming that its vaccine would "decrease transmission" because on October 10, 2022, Pfizer went on record, through the admission of Janine Small, President of International Markets at Pfizer, in testimony before the European Parliament that Pfizer never tested its vaccine to see if it would stop the transmission of the virus.[1093] Furthermore, the FDA now says that "there is no requirement that the clinical trials supporting a vaccine's licensure or authorization be designed to determine whether the vaccine prevents infection of a pathogen or transmission of that pathogen to others."[1094]

Moderna used COVID-19 to describe the SARS-CoV-2 virus in its public pronouncements. For example, the Moderna FAQ website stated: "To safely achieve herd immunity against COVID-19, a large amount of a population needs to be vaccinated."[1095] Notice that Moderna discusses immunity to COVID-19, which is the word used to describe the virus known as SARS-CoV-2. The common parlance within the government and the pharmaceutical companies has been to use both "COVID-19" and "SARS-CoV-2" to describe the alleged virus.

As we have seen from the pronouncements from the government and pharmaceutical companies, when the distinction between SARS-CoV-2 and COVID-19 got in the way of their goal of hoodwinking the public, the distinction was ignored, and they announced that the vaccines protect against the infection and transmission of the virus itself. But when the evidence surfaced that the COVID-19 vaccines do not prevent infection or spread of the virus, the FDA claimed that is because the vaccines were only designed to prevent the illness (COVID-19) caused by the virus (SARS-CoV-2) and were not required to prevent the infection and spread of the virus itself. It's a game of heads, I win, tails, you lose.

In any event, the distinction between SARS-CoV-2 and COVID-19 is a distinction without a difference because the vaccines neither stopped the alleged SARS-CoV-2 virus nor the alleged COVID-19 illness. The vaccines do not work.

The evidence is now clear. The COVID-19 vaccines were not designed to stop infection or transmission of any virus or illness. The COVID-19 vaccines are bioweapons designed to injure and kill. The vaccine makers and government officials are playing a game of nuanced obfuscation to conceal their culpability.

37 Bait and Switch #2

On August 23, 2021, the FDA published a notice that it had approved a COVID-19 vaccine manufactured by Pfizer-BioNTech. The notice was given wide publicity throughout the nation. The notice stated:

> On August 23, 2021, FDA approved the biologics license application (BLA) submitted by BioNTech Manufacturing GmbH for COMIRNATY (COVID-19 Vaccine, mRNA) for active immunization to prevent COVID-19 caused by SARS-CoV-2 in individuals 16 years of age and older.[1096]

The letter contains the following pertinent information:

> [T]he EUA will remain in place for the Pfizer-BioNTech COVID-19 vaccine for the previously-authorized indication and uses.[1097]

Please notice that there are two vaccines discussed in the letter with two distinct legal identities. The FDA pointed out in a footnote in the authorization letter that the vaccines are not identical. "The products are legally distinct with certain differences that do not impact safety or effectiveness."[1098] The two distinct vaccines are:

1) COMIRNATY (COVID-19 Vaccine, mRNA) and

2) Pfizer-BioNTech COVID-19 vaccine.

The Pfizer-BioNTech COVID-19 vaccine remains unapproved and under its original emergency use authorization (EUA). At the same time, the FDA has approved COMIRNATY (COVID-19 Vaccine, mRNA).[1099]

Vaccines can be authorized for use in an emergency by the FDA while undergoing experimental trials. Authorization for use in an emergency is not the same as approval. Such investigational vaccines are not approved by the FDA. COVID-19 vaccines are "investigational vaccines" authorized under an emergency use authorization (EUA). An investigational vaccine is, by definition, an experimental vaccine. The FDA explains that "[a]n investigational drug can also be called an experimental drug."[1100] Investigational vaccines being used under an EUA are "still in the testing and evaluation phase and are not licensed for use in the general public."[1101]

The Pfizer-BioNTech Comirnaty COVID-19 vaccine FDA is an FDA approved form of the vaccine, but that approved vaccine is not available in the U.S. Thus, all formulations that are packaged differently and are not labeled Comirnaty are experimental vaccines under the EUA. According to the NIH, "[a]n investigational product refers to a preventative (vaccine), a therapeutic (drug or biologic), device, diagnostic, or palliative used in a clinical trial. An investigational product may be an unlicensed product **or a licensed product when used or assembled (formulated or packaged) differently from the approved form.**"[1102]

The FDA states that "Comirnaty has the same formulation as the EUA vaccine and is administered as a series of two doses, three weeks apart."[1103] The FDA further explains that "[t]he [approved] vaccine has been known as the Pfizer-BioNTech COVID-19 Vaccine, and will now be marketed as Comirnaty (koe-mir'-na-tee), for the prevention of COVID-19 disease in individuals 16 years of age and older."[1104] But keep in mind that, while the two vaccines have the same formula, they are not identical. They have "certain differences," which were not specified; and they are "legally distinct."

Thus, we have two substantially similar vaccines, one being administered under an EUA and another under FDA approval. The problem is that the approved vaccine, COMIRNATY (COVID-19 Vaccine, mRNA), is now manufactured in Germany by Pfizer and BioNTech, a company that works in partnership with Pfizer.[1105] A footnote in the FDA notice states:

> Although COMIRNATY (COVID-19 Vaccine, mRNA) is approved to prevent COVID-19 in individuals 16 years of age and older, there is not sufficient approved vaccine available for distribution to this population in its entirety at the time of reissuance of this EUA.[1106]

That means that it is not yet available in the U.S. Thus, all of the COVID-19 vaccines now being administered in the U.S. under the Pfizer-BioNTech partnership are being administered under the EUA. The effect of that is that the public thinks that it is getting an approved vaccine under the legal standards for an approved vaccine, but in reality, they are receiving an EUA vaccine that comes with all of the legal vulnerabilities of an EUA vaccine.

Why did the FDA not simply approve the Pfizer-BioNTech

COVID-19 vaccine? Why are there two vaccines with the same formula made by the same company given different treatment? It makes no logical sense unless you understand the stratagem of Pfizer and the FDA. The FDA has slickly approved a vaccine that is not available. If the vaccine were to be made available, Pfizer-BioNTech and all other COVID-19 makers would lose their EUA's. The COVID-19 vaccines allowed under EUAs would all be taken off the market. That is because one of the legal requirements for an EUA is "that there is no adequate, approved, and available alternative to the product for diagnosing, preventing, or treating such disease or condition."[1107] That means that if the COMIRNATY (COVID-19 Vaccine, mRNA) is made available, all other EUA vaccines would immediately be removed from the market. That would hit Moderna particularly hard since their COVID-19 vaccine is the only product they sell. Indeed, Moderna's COVID-19 vaccine is the first product they have ever sold.

Albert Bourla, Chairman and Chief Executive Officer of Pfizer, gives a hint to the reason for the strange approval of a vaccine with the same formula as an identical vaccine that remains unapproved: "I am hopeful this approval will help increase confidence in our vaccine."[1108] It is a confidence game, which is popularly known as a con-game. The approval of the COMIRNATY (COVID-19 Vaccine, mRNA) is to increase the "confidence" in the Pfizer-BioNTech COVID-19 vaccine being administered under the EUA. People will be convinced to get the Pfizer-BioNTech COVID-19 vaccine under the mistaken belief that it is approved by the FDA, when in fact it is only authorized under the EUA.

Indeed, the FDA approval of the unavailable COMIRNATY (COVID-19 Vaccine, mRNA) is being used by President Biden to push the COVID-19 vaccine mandate he instituted on September 9, 2021. "[M]any said they were waiting for approval from the Food and Drug Administration — the FDA.

Well, last month, the FDA granted that approval. ... The vaccine has FDA approval."[1109] It is significant that President Biden did not mention that the FDA approved vaccine to which he referred is not available in the United States.

All the news services reported the approval of the Pfizer COVID-19 vaccine without mentioning that the only vaccine available in the U.S. is the EUA Pfizer experimental vaccine. Fox Business News segued into the motive behind the approval. "Full licensure has been widely anticipated to boost confidence in those otherwise hesitant to receive the shot under emergency approval."[1110] That was the pattern for all of the mainstream news outlets. One of the primary subscription services, the Associated Press (AP) news service, is an example of the kind of propaganda about the Pfizer approval being pushed. The AP did not mention anything about the only available COVID-19 vaccines in the U.S. being EUA experimental vaccines. Instead, the AP pushed the narrative that "[t]he U.S. gave full approval to Pfizer's COVID-19 vaccine Monday, potentially boosting public confidence in the shots and instantly opening the way for more universities, companies and local governments to make vaccinations mandatory."[1111] The mainstream media outlets are giving people the false impression that the Pfizer COVID-19 vaccine they will be getting is approved. It is not.

Moderna's COVID-19 vaccine has since also been approved by the FDA (Moderna's SPIKEVAX). Neither Moderna's SPIKEVAX nor Pfizer's Comirnaty are available in the United States.[1112] Pfizer-BioNTech states in its fact sheet for its COVID-19 vaccine for children that "there are no approved COVID-19 vaccines."[1113] That was not a misstatement. Pfizer specifically mentioned the FDA approved COMIRNATY in the fact sheet.

Dr. Paul E. Alexander is an expert in clinical epidemiology; he is a former COVID Pandemic Advisor to the

WHO and the Pan American Health Organization; he was a former senior advisor on the COVID Pandemic in the Department of Health and Human Services during the Trump administration. He opines that the COVID-19 vaccines are ineffective and unsafe and should be stopped. He explains that the spike protein that is being created by the body via the mRNA code in the COVID-19 vaccines is "the business end of the virus that causes the pathology."[1114] The spike protein is what is killing people and making them ill. That confirms the opinion of Dr. Robert Malone, the inventor of the mRNA technology used in several COVID-19 vaccines. Dr. Malone has stated that the spike proteins generated by the cells through the mRNA code are cytotoxic.[1115] Dr. Alexander reveals that the approval of the COMIRNATY (COVID-19 Vaccine, mRNA) is a trick to convince people to be vaccinated with the unapproved and experimental Pfizer-BioNTech COVID-19 vaccine that is being allowed under the EUA. It is a Machiavellian bait and switch. The people will think they are receiving an approved vaccine when, in reality, they will be getting the experimental vaccine.

What does that all mean? The key to understanding what is going on is in the footnote in the FDA approval letter. "The products are **legally distinct** with certain differences that do not impact safety or effectiveness."[1116] Maintaining separate legal identities for the two vaccines with the same formula has the effect that those injured by the EUA Pfizer-BioNTech COVID-19 vaccine will be subjected to the exacting standards and limited compensation of the Public Readiness and Emergency Preparedness Act (PREP Act), which authorizes the Countermeasures Injury Compensation Program (CICP) to provide benefits to injured parties. A notable limitation under the CICP is that an injured party will be subjected to the statute of limitations that forecloses all legal actions not filed within one year of vaccination.[1117] That is compared with the statute of limitations for an approved vaccine under the National Vaccine Injury Compensation Program (VICP) of 3 years from the occurrence of the first symptom of injury from the vaccine.[1118] Experts specializing in vaccine injury cases say that the bar for obtaining compensation is very high under the PREP Act.[1119] Over the last ten years, 94% of injured patients who filed claims under the PREP Act received no compensation.[1120] In reference to the virtually insurmountable hurdles erected under the CICP, Renée Gentry, director of the Vaccine Injury Litigation Clinic at the George Washington University Law School, said COVID-19 vaccine claimants have two rights: **"You have the right to file," she said. "And you have the right to lose."**[1121] Altom Maglio, whose 22 lawyer law firm, Maglio Christopher & Toale, specializes in vaccine injury cases, says that you're out of luck if you've suffered an injury related to any of the COVID-19 vaccines in receiving any compensation for your injury.[1122] That all is not intended to suggest that the VICP is fair. The VICP has its own problems which are beyond the scope of this chapter. Two out of three claims filed under the VICP are denied.[1123]

Visitors to the Health Resources & Services Administration website to find information about filing a VICP claim are met with a notice ribbon announcing: **"For claims associated with the COVID-19 vaccine or other COVID-19 related countermeasures, please file your Request for Benefits with the Countermeasures Injury Compensation Program."**[1124] The ribbon provides a link directly to the CICP website. The premise of that advisory is that all COVD-19 vaccines are experimental vaccines allowed under an EUA. There is no separate advice on the FDA website for the approved COMIRNATY (COVID-19 Vaccine, mRNA) vaccine. That indicates that all vaccines administered in the United States for COVID-19 are experimental vaccines being administered under that EUA and are thus not allowed recovery ordinarily available for an approved vaccine under the VICP program.

It is unclear how the approval of the COMIRNATY (COVID-19 Vaccine, mRNA) was accomplished in nine months, particularly when, as of August 13, 2021, there were reported in the HHS Vaccine Adverse Event Reporting System (VAERS) 13,068 deaths correlated to the COVID-19 vaccines.[1125] Recall that the FDA states that "Comirnaty has the same formulation as the EUA vaccine."[1126] The Pfizer-BioNTech COVID-19 vaccine accounted for 9,024 of those deaths.[1127] A study funded by HHS determined that the VAERS program only reports 1% of the adverse events from vaccines.[1128] Thus, we can extrapolate that the 9,024 deaths reported for the Pfizer-BioNTech COVID-19 vaccine in VAERS represent 902,400 deaths.

Please be mindful that VAERS is a system of correlation. HHS explains that an adverse event may be reported to VAERS for "clinically important adverse events that occur after vaccination of adults and children, even if you are not sure whether the vaccine caused the adverse event."[1129] Thus, a person does not have to be "sure" of causation. But just because causation is not certain does not mean that causation cannot be inferred. One can infer probable causation even when it is not scientifically proven causation. The correlation of the reported adverse events to the vaccines is verified by the judgment of medical professionals. Eighty percent (80%) of the correlations reported in VAERS are based on the judgment of medical professionals that the adverse event was closely related to the vaccine and was probably caused by it. Otherwise, it would not have be reported in VAERS. Indeed, there is a disincentive against reporting a questionable adverse event. On the HHS VAERS website, it warns: "Knowingly filing a false VAERS report is a violation of Federal law (18 U.S. Code § 1001) punishable by fine and imprisonment."[1130] Once the report is sent to VAERS, the CDC reviews and verifies it before it is logged and posted on the VAERS database. The adverse events reported on VAERS have not been scientifically proven to have been caused by the vaccines. And certainty of causation is not the test for reporting. The HHS website advises that the reporter to VAERS does not have to be "sure" of causation, and causation does not have to be "clear." But

HHS otherwise implies that the reporter have a reasonable basis for believing the vaccine caused the injury reported to VAERS. If a medical professional does not reasonably believe that the vaccine caused the reported injury, reporting that injury to VAERS as an adverse event could be punishable under federal law "by fine and imprisonment." The 1% of total vaccine injuries that make it into the VAERS database are mainly based on the judgment of medical professionals that the vaccine probably caused the reported injuries.

The unexpected approval by the FDA of the COMIRNATY (COVID-19 Vaccine, mRNA) changes nothing regarding the continued experimental status of the Pfizer-BioNTech COVID-19 vaccine. The COMIRNATY (COVID-19 Vaccine, mRNA) and the Pfizer-BioNTech COVID-19 vaccine have "certain differences," and they are "legally distinct." The COMIRNATY (COVID-19 Vaccine, mRNA) is not being administered in the U.S. The Pfizer-BioNTech COVID-19 experimental vaccine and the other COVID-19 experimental vaccines are the only vaccines available to any worker in the United States. None of them are approved by the FDA, and all of them are experimental vaccines. The argument against administering an experimental vaccine without informed consent is pertinent because all COVID-19 vaccines in the U.S. remain unapproved and experimental vaccines. They are all being administered under EUAs, and are not FDA approved, including the Pfizer-BioNTech COVID-19 vaccine.

The Food and Drug Administration has also approved the Moderna COVID-19 vaccine branded SPIKEVAX.[1131] The unapproved EUA vaccine from Moderna is being marketed under the name "Moderna COVID-19 vaccine." The CDC explains that "[a]fter receiving FDA approval on January 31, 2022, the Moderna COVID-19 vaccine for people ages 18 years and older began to be marketed under the SPIKEVAX brand name. No change was made to the vaccine's formula with the name change."[1132] According to the CDC, the approved SPIKEVAX is the same vaccine as the unapproved vaccine being administered under the EUA. While Moderna's SPIKEVAX and Pfizer-BioNTech's COMIRNATY are approved, those approved branded vaccines are not available in the United States.[1133] As of January 2023, one can only obtain the EUA versions of those vaccines in the United States. The following explanation for the unavailability of the approved Moderna SPIKEVAX was posted on the Wisconsin Department of Health Services website:

> The Moderna COVID-19 vaccine branded as SPIKEVAX was approved by the FDA on January 31, 2022, as a two-dose series for individuals aged 18 years and older. No change was made to the vaccine's formula for this age group. At this time, there is no concrete timeline for when the brand name vaccine, SPIKEVAX, will be available directly to consumers. Moderna continues to distribute EUA labeled vaccine to fulfill the U.S. Government contractual agreements.[1134]

38 Never-Ending Boosters

The ineffectiveness of the COVID-19 vaccines has caused medical authorities to call for booster shots. The continued ineffectiveness of the boosters will be met with calls for more boosters. What a racket! The Inova Hospital system in Northern Virginia is an example of how hospitals have forfeited their independence and fallen into lockstep with the CDC's vaccine protocols. Inova provided a handout to its medical staff titled "Bivalent COVID-19 Booster Recommendations and Team Member Clinics." It states that Inova uses "the same consistent process we have used in making decisions about our COVID-19 vaccine requirements, including best evidence, safety, and impact to our patients and team members." Although the bivalent booster is not required at this time, based on that "best evidence," Inova is "strongly recommending" the Pfizer bivalent COVID-19 booster.

It seems that Inova is acting as an arm of the federal government. It is in lockstep with the edicts and pronouncements of the CDC. For example, on September 1, 2022, the CDC recommended the bivalent COVID-19 boosters manufactured by Moderna and Pfizer-BioNTech with the following statement:

This recommendation followed a comprehensive

scientific evaluation and robust scientific discussion.[1135]

Inova, suspiciously, used the same language in its promotional email recommending the Pfizer BioNTech COVID-19 bivalent boosters to staff:

> *This recommendation followed a comprehensive scientific evaluation and robust scientific discussion*, both nationally and locally at Inova.

Incidentally, the “comprehensive scientific evaluation” involved eight (8) mice in the case of the Pfizer-BioNTech bivalent booster and ten (10) mice in the case of the Moderna bivalent booster. By the way, all Moderna mice that were boosted with the Ba.5 based bivalent booster, got sick with Covid when they were challenged with the Ba.5 (omicron) variant virus.[1136] How did Moderna get around that problem? They claimed that, while the boosted mice got infected with the Ba.5 virus, they had fewer viral particles in the lungs than the unboosted mice. But the fact remains that they got infected. And the boosted mice showed no reduction in viral particles in their noses, indicating that the booster did little to nothing to prevent infection.

Thus, the study showed that the bivalent COVID-19 vaccine was ineffective. Based on that outcome, the CDC recommended the Moderna COVID-19 bivalent booster. That is what passes as “comprehensive scientific evaluation.” It seems that Inova is like a blind mouse following the lead of the CDC. The problem is that the CDC is also a blind mouse; we have two blind mice. “[I]f the blind lead the blind, both shall fall into the ditch.” Matthew 15:14.

The "best evidence" alleged by Inova for the Pfizer bivalent booster consists of tests done on eight mice. Read the Pfizer report for yourself. Kena A. Swanson, Ph.D, Vice President,

Viral Vaccines Vaccine Research and Development for Pfizer prepared the report, which reveals on pages 25 and 26 "N=8 mice."[1137] Inova claims that they are making a strong recommendation that its staff receive the bivalent booster on the "best evidence." But that evidence consists of no data on its effect on human beings. How can Inova strongly recommend a treatment of any kind based solely on lab results involving eight mice?

It gets worse. The eight-mice study showed that the mice receiving the Pfizer bivalent booster had wildly inconsistent reactions to the shot. One mouse measured 300 titers of antibodies, while another mouse reacted with 22,000 titers of antibodies.[1138] That is a 7,300% difference in antibody reaction to the vaccine.[1139] We have no idea what such a wide disparity would look like if the subjects were human beings and not mice. Would a person at the low end have no protection? Would a person at the high end suffer a cytokine storm? We don't know. But Inova is comfortable "strongly recommending" the bivalent vaccine without knowing what it might do to people. Inova should be embarrassed. This is shameful. It is well beyond incompetence. It is fraud. It is reckless disregard for the well-being of others.

What is truly scary is that Inova's conclusion that the Pfizer bivalent vaccine is safe and effective was based on "the same consistent process we have used in making decisions about our COVID-19 vaccine requirements." That becomes a scary statement in light of what we know about the "best evidence" of the bivalent safety and effectiveness used by Inova to recommend it. Inova's judgement on the mandated COVID-19 vaccine regimen is also well beyond incompetence. The evidence is clear that Inova has committed fraud and recklessly disregarded its staff's well-being.

Inova seems to be pushing the COVID-19 vaccine on those who have no need for it. For example, Inova advises that "it is recommended that you still get the vaccine even if you previously had COVID-19."[1140] Germ theory is that if someone has recovered from a virus, they have immunity from that virus. There is no need to be vaccinated against that which one already has immunity.[1141] That is basic immunology. But if you doubt that truth, the Cleveland Clinic did a study to determine if it is necessary to administer a COVID-19 vaccine to a previously infected person. The scientists concluded that "[i]ndividuals who have had SARS-CoV-2 infection are unlikely to benefit from COVID-19 vaccination."[1142] Incidentally, the study revealed that "[n]ot one of the 1359 previously infected subjects who remained unvaccinated had a SARS-CoV-2 infection over the duration of the study."[1143] There are many other studies that have come to the same conclusion. For example, the National Institute of Health funded a study that concluded that natural COVID-19 infection induced a strong and long-lasting immune response.[1144]

Studies have shown that children who already had immunity from COVID-19 and then received a COVID-19 vaccine had their immunity from COVID-19 go negative after five months.[1145] That means the children who already had natural immunity were more susceptible to the COVID-19 infection after getting the vaccine. The vaccine does more harm than good when someone already has innate immunity. This is a result of antibody-dependent enhancement caused by the vaccine.[1146] The vaccines make people sick. Inova's claim of following the "best evidence" is simply newspeak for ignoring the best evidence.

39 Killing Children to Save Them

The FDA's 242-page manual titled *Communicating Risks and Benefits: An Evidence-Based User's Guide* explains that the "number needed to treat" (NNT) is one of the three most important statistics for describing the risk and benefits of any drug or vaccine.[1147] Toby Rogers, Ph.D., explains that the CDC and the FDA violated their own standards and the fundamental norms of science by not revealing the NNT when reviewing the Emergency Use Authorizations (EUA) and Biologics License Application from Pfizer-BioNTech when reviewing its COVID-19 vaccine for use in children ages 5 to 11.

Dr. Rogers explains that the pharmaceutical industry hates talking about NNT. They hate talking about NNT even more when it comes to COVID-19 vaccines because the NNT is so high that the COVID-19 vaccines could not pass any honest risk-benefit analysis.[1148]

The NNT can be reported for any number of variables, such as deaths, ICU admissions, hospitalizations, etc. Taking death as an example, the death NNT for 5 to 11 year-olds from COVID-19 would tell the researchers and the public how many children need to be vaccinated to prevent a single death from

COVID-19.

The lower the risk from the disease, the higher the NNT. Children ages 5 to 11 are at extremely low risk of hospitalization, ICU admission, or death from COVID-19. Indeed, there were no hospitalizations, ICU admissions, or deaths in either the vaccine group or the control group in the Pfizer-BioNTech trials involving 5 to 11 year-olds. Dr. Rogers explains:

> [The NNT] is calculated by dividing 1 by the Absolute Risk Reduction. But there was no risk reduction in hospitalizations, ICU admissions, nor death for 5 to 11 year olds. So if one remembers grade school math, 1/0 is "undefined" since one cannot divide by zero.
>
> This means one could vaccinate every child age 5 to 11 in the U.S. and not prevent a single hospitalization, ICU admission, or death from coronavirus — according to Pfizer's own clinical trial data as submitted to the FDA.
>
> It appears Pfizer was not even trying to conduct a responsible clinical trial of its mRNA shot in kids ages 5 to 11. Pfizer submitted an EUA application to the FDA showing no health benefit in children ages 5 to 11 and the FDA's Vaccines and Related Biologics Products Advisory Committee approved it anyway, 17 – 0 with 1 abstention.[1149]

Dr. Rogers assumed a very generous 80% efficacy in preventing hospitalizations and deaths of 5 to 11-year-olds. He extrapolated that efficacy rate from the FDA claim that Pfizer-BioNTech has an 80% efficacy rate for COVID-associated hospitalizations for ages 20+ years old. The FDA used that 80% figure to estimate the efficacy rate for the Pfizer-BioNTech

COVID-19 vaccine for 5 to 11-year-olds. Using the FDA's very optimistic benefit of the Pfizer-BioNTech COVID-19 vaccine, Dr. Rogers calculated the death NNT for children 5 to 11 years old.

Dr. Rogers used the optimistically reported efficacy of 80% from the FDA and applied that figure to the reported fatalities for COVID-19 for 5 to 11-year-olds and calculated the death NNT for the Pfizer-BioNTech COVID-19 vaccine was 630,775. That means that the vaccine must be given to 630,775 children to save one child.

But that astronomical death NNT does not tell the whole story. We must compare that death NNT to the death risk from the vaccine. Dr. Rogers used the nearest age group vaccine risk data (12 to 15-year-olds) available and applied that data to the 5 to 11-year-olds. This is known as immuno-bridging of data. The VAERS data under-reports adverse events by a factor of 100. But Dr. Rogers multiplied the reported death numbers by a more conservative 41 times. By doing that, he determined that there were 5,248 deaths in the 12-15-year-old age group from the COVID-19 vaccines. Dr. Rogers compared the death rate to the death NNT and concluded:

> Simply put, the Biden administration plan would kill 5,248 children via Pfizer mRNA shots in order to save 45 children from dying of coronavirus.
>
> **For every one child saved by the shot, another 117 would be killed by the shot.**
>
> The Pfizer mRNA shot fails any honest risk-benefit analysis in children ages 5 to 11.
>
> ***
>
> The Biden Administration, the FDA, and the CDC

claim they "follow the science" and yet they violate their own standards and scientific norms in order to exaggerate the benefits and hide the harms from vaccines.

The FDA refused to calculate an [NNT], not because it forgot, but because agency officials knew the number and corresponding side effects are so high it would destroy the case for mRNA vaccines in children this age.[1150] (emphasis added)

40 Sudden Adult Death Syndrome

The ADE and myocarditis suffered by vaccine recipients is causing them to unexpctedly die in large numbers. The sudden deaths of young people in the prime of health cannot be ignored. Edward Dowd, in his book, "Cause Unknown," *The Epidemic of Sudden Deaths in 2021 and 2022*, reveals that in 2006, a systematic review was done of sudden cardiac death by young athletes over a period of 38 years.[1151] Experts at the Division of Pediatric Cardiology at the University Hospital of Lausanne, Switzerland, looked at the data on deaths between 1966 and 2004. They found that there were 1,101 total cases of sudden cardiac deaths over that period. That amounts to an average rate of 29 sudden cardiac deaths per year.

Fast forward to 2021 and 2022, and we find that the rate of cardiac deaths among young athletes exceeds 29 deaths per "month." Indeed, Dowd reveals that not a single month during 2021 and 2022 had fewer than 29 cardiac deaths among young athletes. For example, in December 2021, there were 90 deaths, and about the same number the next month.[1152]

The prevalence of those deaths is forcing the hand of the media to report on them. But the mass media is trying to conceal the cause of the sudden deaths of thousands of young people by labeling the deaths sudden adult death syndrome (SADS). It is sometimes also called sudden arrhythmic death syndrome (SADS). The medical establishment and the media engage in all sorts of conjecture, including blaming the sudden premature deaths on a genetic condition.[1153] But they do not ever mention the elephant in the room, the COVID-19 vaccines, as a suspected cause for the deaths. Ethan Huff, writing for Natural News, explains:

> In an attempt to explain away the rash of deaths occurring in otherwise healthy-seeming adults who got "vaccinated" for the Wuhan coronavirus (COVID-19), the medical establishment has coined a new term called "Sudden Adult Death Syndrome," or SADS, that it is pretending appeared out of nowhere with no explanation.[1154]
>
> Much like Sudden Infant Death Syndrome (SIDS), which was also made up out of thin air to explain away infant deaths caused by vaccines, SADS is being called a "mystery" condition that could strike anyone at any time for no apparent reason.[1155]

It is quite strange that the apparent culprits, the COVID-19 vaccines, are not even mentioned in the major media. They report the sudden premature deaths and essentially leave the readers to guess why young people are keeling over dead in the prime of their lives. Ethan Huff explains the obvious:

> They will never admit to it, but the sudden rise in SADS directly coincides with the unleashing of Operation Warp Speed, which has turned hundreds of millions of Americans into deadly spike protein factories. These spike proteins are ripping apart their cardiovascular systems and leaving them prone to early death.[1156]

41 How the Vaccine Makers Scammed the Public

The 94.1% efficacy result for the Moderna COVID-19 mRNA vaccine reported by the FDA is misleading because they are not telling you that it is a relative risk reduction and not an absolute (total) risk reduction.[1157] The vaccine manufacturers used misleading statistics to report the effectiveness of their vaccines. The vaccine manufacturers and often persons running studies, including the study of 620,000 veterans discussed earlier in this book, are reporting the relative efficacy of the COVID-19 vaccines.

In the Moderna study, the subsequent COVID-19 infection rate for the vaccinated group was 0.079%. The COVID-19 infection rate for the placebo group was 1.33%. That means that the rate of those who were infected by COVID-19 after receiving the vaccine was reduced by 1.25% as compared to those who were infected by COVID-19 after receiving a placebo (1.33% – 0.079% = 1.25%). Thus, the vaccine has an absolute efficacy of 1.25%. One can expect that there will be a reduction of 1.25% in COVID-19 infections in the population after being vaccinated. Out of a group of 10,000 people who are vaccinated with the Moderna mRNA COVID-19 vaccine, there will be approximately 125 fewer illnesses from COVID-19.

But that is not how Moderna reported the results. Instead of a 1.25% efficacy rate, which is the absolute (total) efficacy rate, the FDA review indicates that Moderna reported a 94.1% efficacy rate, which is a relative efficacy rate.[1158] The relative efficacy rate is misleading because it gives the false impression that out of 10,000 people, 9,410 people would be protected from getting COVID-19. How did Moderna come up with the 94.1% figure? They divided the rate of subsequent COVID-19 infection in the vaccinated group (0.079%) by the rate of subsequent COVID-19 infection in the placebo group (1.33%) and then subtracted that difference (0.059) from one (1) to arrive at (0.941) to arrive at 94.1%. After rounding, the FDA reported the interim effectiveness for the Moderna mRNA COVID-19 vaccine of 94.1%. But that is not the absolute (total) efficacy, which is what people want to know. That 94.1% figure is a relative risk reduction, which is different from a absolute (total) risk reduction.

The false impression given by that figure is that the vaccine will effectively protect 9,410 out of 10,000 people from COVID-19. In reality, 9,867 are at no risk of getting COVID-19 (10,000 – 133 = 9,867). That means that out of every 10,000 people vaccinated with the COVID-19 vaccine, it will only prevent 125 people from becoming ill from COVID-19 (133 - 8 = 125). According to the study, a total of only 133 people out of every 10,000 are at risk to get COVID-19, and the vaccine will protect 125 of those 133 people. When the relative efficacy rate of 94.1% is reported, most people do not understand that it ignores the 9,867 people out of 10,000 who are at no risk of getting COVID-19 and do not need to be vaccinated. Thus, the true efficacy rate is the absolute efficacy rate. The absolute efficacy rate takes into account the entire population of people. The absolute (total) efficacy rate for the vaccine is only 1.25 % (125 people out of 10,000). That is the efficacy rate the public should have been informed about, and not 94.1 %, which gives the false impression that the vaccine will protect 9,410 people out of 10,000.

Dr. Ron Brown of the University of Waterloo explains that Moderna's and Pfizer-BioNTech's reporting of their vaccine's relative efficacy rate (a.k.a. risk reduction) is misleading to the public.[1159] Researchers often use relative risk reduction, but it should not be announced to the public as the vaccine's efficacy because it always gives an elevated sense of the vaccine's efficacy.[1160] The public was thus given an artificially inflated impression of effectiveness of the COVID-19 vaccinesis.[1161] Dr. Brown stated that absolute risk reduction should be given to clinicians and the public. Indeed, in a draft advisory, the FDA stated that relative risk reduction should never be given to the public without also mentioning the absolute risk reduction.[1162] The FDA explained, "that research suggests that consumers do not understand relative frequencies." The FDA explained that "[c]onsumers may also find the efficacy or risk probability described as a relative frequency harder to comprehend and more favorable as compared to the absolute frequency."[1163] The concern of the FDA is that the consumer will view the benefit from a vaccine much greater than it is in reality if they are only informed of the relative efficacy rates. The FDA recommended that the public always be given the absolute efficacy rate.

Dr. Brown states that "selective reporting of vaccine efficacy measures can cause a type of outcome reporting bias that misrepresents health information disseminated to the public."[1164] Dr. Brown presents an example in an article he prepared to show how misleading relative risk reduction can be. Dr. Brown explains how a risk reduction of only 1% can be sold to the public as a risk reduction of 50%:

> [The figure below] shows an example of a vaccine clinical trial for an infectious disease. The vaccine and placebo groups in Figure 1 each have 100 randomly assigned individuals with no history of infection, and an event is defined as the incidence of infection among all individuals during the

course of the trial. The percentage of events in the vaccine group is the experimental event rate (EER) or the risk of infection in the vaccine group (1/100 = 1%), and the percentage of events in the placebo group is the control event rate (CER) or the risk of infection in the placebo group (2/100 = 2%). Absolute risk reduction (ARR) is the disease risk difference between the placebo and vaccine groups, i.e., the CER minus the EER (2% - 1% = 1%). The ARR is also known as the vaccine disease preventable incidence (VDPI). Relative risk reduction (RRR) or vaccine efficacy (VE) is the reduced risk from vaccination, the ARR or VDPI, relative to or divided by the risk in unvaccinated individuals, the CER (1%/2% = 50%)

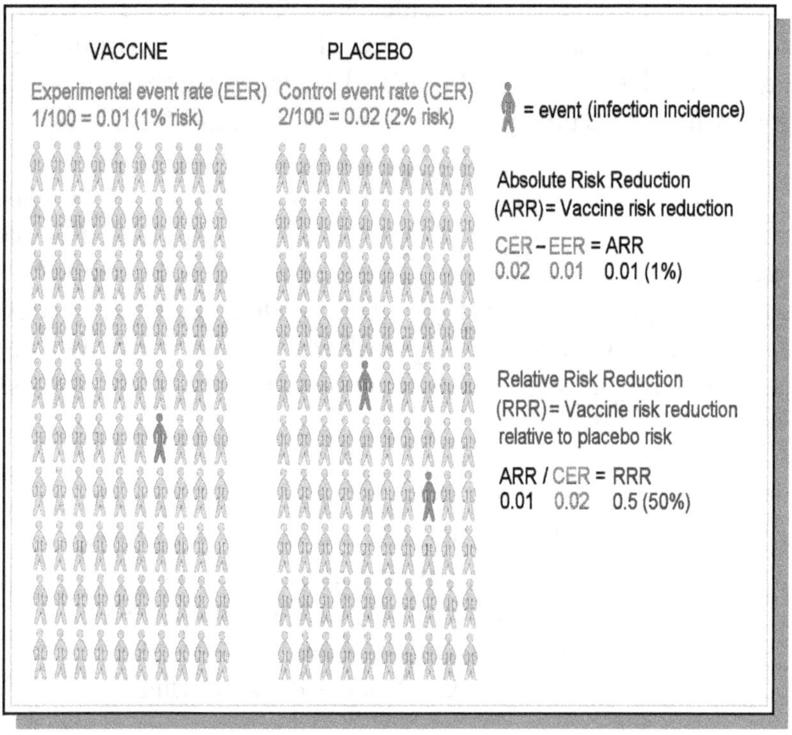

The same issue explained above with the Moderna report, Dr. Brown found in the Pfizer-BioNTech study. He explains how the absolute risk reduction of the Pfizer-BioNTech COVID-19 vaccine of 0.7% tells a very different story from the much-publicized relative risk reductions of 95.1% for that vaccine. While the relative efficacy rate was widely publicized, the absolute efficacy rate was not shared with the public.

The COVID-19 vaccines are unsafe and ineffective. As we have seen, the manufacturers and some insiders in the federal regulatory agencies knew before the EUA was issued that the vaccines would not prevent COVID-19 infections. If that is the case, why did the FDA give them EUA status? The vaccines were given EUA status based on the clinical studies performed by the vaccine manufacturers. An objective review of the data in the studies and the protocols reveals that they were rigged to falsely show that the vaccines were effective.

Dr. David Martin reveals that Moderna concealed the evidence that their vaccine was ineffective by waiting 14 days to perform a confirmatory RT-PCR test on the test subjects.[1165] They reported that the Moderna study shows that within 7 days of both the first and the second vaccinations, the group receiving the Moderna COVID-19 vaccines displayed greater systemic symptoms of COVID-19 than the control group.[1166] But Moderna ignored those systemic COVID-19 symptoms by reporting them not as symptoms of COVID-19 caused by the vaccine but systemic adverse reactions to the vaccine.

Moderna avoided reporting the COVID-19 systemic symptoms caused to the vaccine recipients within 7 days of receiving the first and the second vaccinations as being "confirmed COVID-19 cases" by not testing the vaccine recipients with the RT-PCR test during that time. By not performing the RT-PCR test, Moderna was able to report the COVID-19 symptoms during that 7 day period under a category of "systemic adverse reactions" to the vaccine instead of "systemic symptoms" of COVID-19 caused by the vaccine that were confirmed COVID-19 cases. Moderna did not do any confirmatory RT-PCR tests on the test subjects until 14 days following the second vaccination. Thus, by waiting until 14 days after the second vaccination to conduct the confirmatory RT-PCR tests, Moderna was able to report that their vaccine was 94.1% (interim results were 94.5%) effective in preventing COVID-19.

The FDA reported that Moderna limited the measure of efficacy for their COVID-19 vaccine as follows: "The primary efficacy endpoint was efficacy of the vaccine to prevent protocol-defined COVID-19 occurring at least 14 days after the second dose in participants with negative SARS-CoV-2 status at baseline."[1167]

What is a confirmed COVID-19 case? Moderna defined it thusly in its study submitted to the FDA:

> For the primary efficacy endpoint, the case definition for a confirmed COVID-19 case was defined as:
> • At least TWO of the following systemic symptoms: Fever (=38°C), chills, myalgia, headache, sore throat, new olfactory and taste disorder(s), or
> • At least ONE of the following respiratory signs/ symptoms: cough, shortness of breath or difficulty breathing, OR clinical or radiographical evidence of pneumonia; and
> • NP swab, nasal swab, or saliva sample (or respiratory sample, if hospitalized) positive for SARS-CoV-2 by RT-PCR.[1168]

Notice in the chart below the systemic symptoms for

COVID-19 **(fever, chills, myalgia, and headache)** were significantly greater within 7 days of the second vaccination. But Moderna did not perform any confirmatory RT-PCR test during that period. Consequently, those systemic symptoms of COVID-19 were reported not as systemic symptoms of COVID-19 caused by the vaccine that were confirmed COVID-19 cases but as "systemic adverse reactions" to the vaccine.

Moderna reported that an astounding **81.9%** of the vaccinated group aged 18-64 years old suffered systemic adverse events after the second vaccination. That is more than double the systemic adverse events occurring in the placebo group. Even more telling is that **17.4%** of the vaccinated group aged 18-64 years old suffered grade 3 systemic adverse events after the second vaccination. A grade 3 adverse event is defined as a severe adverse event. That is more than eight (8) times the grade 3 severe systemic adverse events in the placebo group. Furthermore, 10 people in the vaccine group suffered a grade 4 systemic adverse event. A grade 4 adverse event is a life-threatening adverse event. That is more than five (5) times the rate of the placebo group's grade 4 systemic adverse events.

Table 23. Frequency of Solicited Systemic Adverse Reactions Within 7 Days Following Either the First or Second Dose of Vaccine, Participants Age 18-64 years, Solicited Safety Set*a

Adverse Reaction	Vaccine Group Dose 1 n/N (%)	Placebo Group Dose 1 n/N (%)	Vaccine Group Dose 2 n/N (%)	Placebo Group Dose 2 n/N (%)
Any Systemic	6503/11405 (57.0)	5063/11406 (44.4)	8484/10358 (81.9)	3967/10320 (38.4)
Grade 3	363/11405 (3.2)	248/11406 (2.2)	1801/10358 (17.4)	215/10320 (2.1)
Grade 4	5/11405 (<0.1)	4/11406 (<0.1)	10/10358 (<0.1)	2/10320 (<0.1)

The chart below is from the Moderna COVE Study Group and published in the New England Journal of Medicine.[1169] I annotated it to indicate certain percentages and circle the "systemic symptoms" of COVID-19 as defined by Moderna but reported by Moderna as "systemic adverse events."

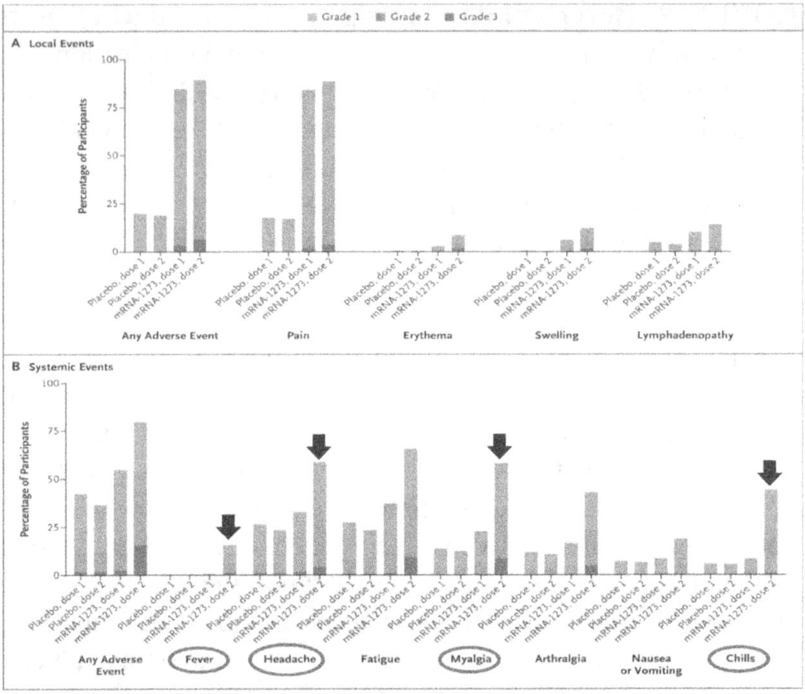

Shown is the percentage of participants who had a solicited local or systemic adverse event **within 7 days** after injection 1 or injection 2 of either the placebo or the mRNA-1273 vaccine. The above chart was provided by the Moderna COVE Study Group and published in the New England Journal of Medicine. It was annotated by Edward Hendrie with arrows to indicate the percentages for participants suffering adverse events from the second COVID-19 vaccine dose for systemic symptoms and red circles indicating the systemic symptoms of COVID-19 as defined by Moderna.

For the primary efficacy endpoint of preventing COVID-19, Moderna defined, in pertinent part, the case definition for a **confirmed COVID-19 case** in their report presented to the FDA to obtain Emergency Use Authorization (EUA) as:

- At least TWO of the following systemic symptoms: **Fever** (=38°C), **chills**, **myalgia**, **headache**, sore throat, new olfactory and taste disorder(s), and
- Positive test for SARS-CoV-2 by RT-PCR.

Notice that within **7 days** a significantly greater percentage of the COVID-19 vaccine recipients displayed COVID-19 **"systemic symptoms"** (circled in red) than the placebo group. But they were not reported as COVID-19 infections because no RT-PCR test was done to confirm them as COVID-19 cases. By not performing the RT-PCR test the symptoms could be reported under a category of **"systemic adverse reactions"** to the vaccine instead of **"systemic symptoms"** of COVID-19 caused by the vaccine that were confirmed COVID-19 cases. Moderna did not do any RT-PCR tests until **14 days** following the second vaccination. Thus, by waiting until **14 days** after the second vaccination to conduct the RT-PCR tests, Moderna was able to report that their vaccine was 94.1% effective in preventing COVID-19.

Peter Doshi, Ph.D., is Associate Professor of Pharmaceutical Health Services Research at the University of Maryland School of Pharmacy. He is also a senior editor at the British Medical Journal (aka, BMJ).

Dr. Doshi wrote an opinion in the BMJ wherein he criticized the Pfizer COVID-19 safety and efficacy trials. He noted several irregularities in the study. Dr. Doshi explains:

> All attention has focused on the dramatic efficacy results: Pfizer reported 170 PCR confirmed covid-19 cases, split 8 to 162 between vaccine and placebo groups. But these numbers were dwarfed by a category of disease called "suspected covid-19"—those with symptomatic covid-19 that were not PCR confirmed. According to FDA's report on Pfizer's vaccine, there were **"3410 total cases of suspected, but unconfirmed covid-19 in the overall study population, 1594 occurred in the vaccine group vs. 1816 in the placebo group."**
>
> With 20 times more suspected than confirmed cases, this category of disease cannot be ignored simply because there was no positive PCR test result. Indeed this makes it all the more urgent to understand. A rough estimate of vaccine efficacy against developing covid-19 symptoms, with or without a positive PCR test result, would be a **relative risk reduction of 19%** (see footnote)—far below the 50% effectiveness threshold for authorization set by regulators.[1170]

You read that correctly; there were 3,410 cases of suspected COVID-19 with no indication in the report whether or not they were tested. The report only indicated that the participants were not confirmed to be COVID-19 via a PCR test. It gets worse. That information was not revealed in the 92-page report filed by Pfizer-BioNTech. Dr. Doshi reveals:

> There is a clear need for data to answer these questions, but Pfizer's 92-page report didn't mention the 3410 "suspected covid-19" cases. Nor did its publication in the New England Journal of Medicine. Nor did any of the reports on Moderna's vaccine. The only source that appears to have reported it is FDA's review of Pfizer's vaccine.[1171]

One can reasonably infer that the reason Pfizer did not reveal the 3,410 cases of suspected COVID-19 is that the revelation of that data would undermine the safety and efficacy of the COVID-19 vaccine under study.

Dr. Doshi was also troubled by the unusually unbalanced and unexplained numbers of people excluded from the efficacy analysis. There were five (5) times more people lost in the vaccine group due to protocol deviations than the control group. 311 were excluded from the vaccine group vs. 60 on placebo. Dr. Doshi was perplexed:

> What were these protocol deviations in Pfizer's study, and why were there five times more participants excluded in the vaccine group? The FDA report doesn't say, and these exclusions are difficult to even spot in Pfizer's report and journal publication.[1172]

Not mentioned by Dr. Doshi was that in the Pfizer trial, as in the Moderna trial, those that had suspected COVID-19 within seven (7) days of vaccination were not publically reported by Pfizer. The FDA auditors found that data. The FDA explained that "[s]uspected COVID-19 cases that occurred within seven (7) days after any vaccination were 409 in the vaccine group vs. 287 in the placebo group."[1173] You read that correctly; there were more suspected COVID-19 cases within seven (7) days in the vaccinated group than in the placebo group. They manifested clinical symptoms of COVID-19. They got ill from the vaccine. Those persons were likely not given confirmatory COVID-19 PCR tests and thus were left in the suspected category, just as was done in the Moderna trial. That way, Pfizer could be sure not to contradict their desired outcome of preventing COVID-19. But the suspected COVID-19 cases within seven (7) days were not reported by Pfizer in their published reports. The government auditors were left to guess that "[i]t is possible that the imbalance in suspected COVID-19 cases occurring in the seven (7) days postvaccination represents vaccine reactogenicity with symptoms that overlap with those of COVID-19."[1174] But that is just a guess by the auditors, as Pfizer, apparently, provided no explanation.

There is a reason that Moderna and Pfizer did not PCR test those who showed symptoms of COVID-19 within seven (7) days of vaccination. They knew the results would likely be positive. Indeed, that is what we see in the real world. For example, 35 nuns received the COVID-19 vaccine, and within two days, 28 nuns fell ill and tested positive for COVID-19, with two of the nuns dying during those two days.[1175] A third nun also died days later. That is clear evidence of ADE within days of being vaccinated. It is the very evidence that both Moderna and Pfizer sought to conceal in their studies.

The Canadian Covid Care Alliance (CCCA) scrutinized the Pfizer data and confirmed Dr. Doshi's findings. The CCCA found that the relative risk reduction reported by Pfizer was inaccurate. The CCCA discovered:

> The Pfizer trials DID NOT test all participants for COVID-19. Instead, they instructed their investigators to test only those with a COVID-19

> symptom and left it up to their discretion to decide what those were.[1176]

That means that asymptomatic infection would have been missed entirely. A high level of subjectivity was introduced to the study. An investigator had the ability to sway the results. The lack of objective, systematic testing made the results unreliable.[1177]

"The basis for the Emergency Use Authorization was the Confirmed COVID cases of 8 vs 162, which meant a Relative Risk Reduction of 95%. But **when dealing with such a small number of cases, any change can impact the results significantly.**" The inoculated group lost **80** persons to follow up. The placebo group lost **86** persons to follow up. There were **1,594** persons in the inoculated group that were suspected of having COVID-19 but were not tested. There were **1,816** persons in the placebo group that were suspected of having COVID-19 but were not tested. Those numbers render the reported 95% efficacy meaningless. The CCCA explains:

> **Lost to follow up** means **they lost touch with those subjects** and can't confirm whether they got sick or not. They don't know.
>
> **Suspected, but unconfirmed** means these people were **symptomatic for COVID-19**, but were never tested. (Discretion for testing was left up to the investigator.)
>
> The fact that the Lost to Follow Up and Suspected but Unconfirmed numbers are higher - and here they are even significantly higher - than the End Point numbers means that **this data is unreliable. The study should not have been accepted in this state.** In normal scientific practice they should have returned to investigate further.[1178]

The improprieties in the study inflated the RRR. When the excluded numbers are factored back into the equation, the true RRR was actually 19% and not the reported 95%. Thus the study actually proved that the vaccines were ineffective. And that is just what we see in the real-world results after the EUA was granted. Below is a chart from the CCCA illustrating how the failure to test the suspected cases of COVID-19 affected the results.

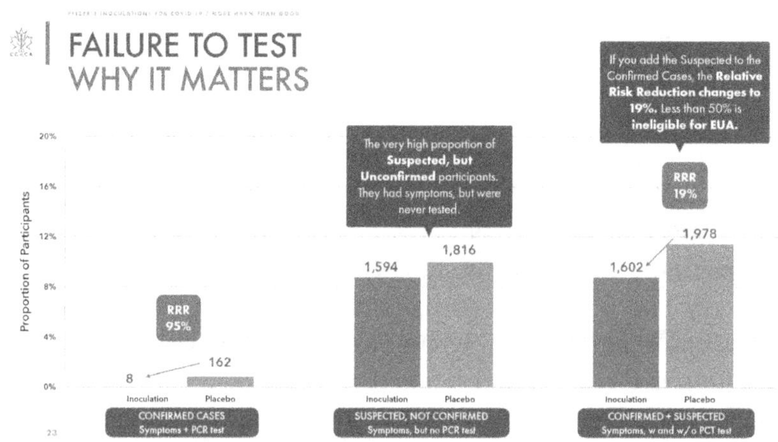

Dr. Doshi was further troubled by the fact that the adjudication committee for the Pfizer adjudication committee consisted of three Pfizer employees. The study could hardly be unbiased when it is being run by Pfizer employees being paid by the company that is banking on a favorable outcome.

Brook Jackson, a whistleblower who helped run one of Pfizer's clinical trials, revealed that the Pfizer trials were rigged. Vaccinated individuals who had COVID-19 were not being tested for COVID-19 to conceal the vaccine's ineffectiveness.[1179] Both Moderna and Pfizer concealed data showing injuries caused by their vaccines. For example, injuries caused by the vaccines were concealed and not reported by the scheme of removing those in the trials who were vaccine injured. For example, 302 vaccinated subjects were dismissed from one of the Pfizer study groups. Another stratagem is for the principal medical investigator (PI) to aggressively reclassify each serious complication as unrelated to the vaccines.[1180] For example, in one Pfizer study group, 21 vaccinated study participants died, but their deaths were reported as being "unrelated to the vaccines."[1181] The pharmaceutical companies set parameters for the trials that avoided long-term follow-up on study participants. Thus, preventing the reporting of incriminating safety data. Adding insult to injury, the pharmaceutical companies refused to pay for medical treatment for the injured trial participants, as they had initially contracted to do.

Pfizer has been caught lying about the severity of the injuries suffered by trial participants during its COVID-19 vaccine trials. And medical doctors are so afraid of attributing vaccine injuries to the vaccines that they will resort to saying the patients are crazy rather than get to the cause of the injury. Maddie de Garay is an example. U.S. Senator Ron Johnson tweeted the plight of Maddi de Garay. "After being part of a Covid vaccine trial for 12-15 year-olds, Maddie has been to the ER 9 times and hospitalized 3 times for a total of 2 months. Doctors even wanted to put her in a mental hospital saying her symptoms were caused by anxiety."[1182] Pfizer is doing all it can to cover up Maddie's injuries and others like her. Young Maddie has lost bowel and bladder control and lost the ability to walk and is now bound to a wheelchair, yet Pfizer listed her adverse reaction to their vaccine as "functional abdominal pain."[1183]

Twelve-year-old Maddie de Garay volunteered for the Pfizer vaccine trial. Her mother, Stephanie de Garay, explained that Maddie volunteered for the Pfizer vaccine trial "to help everyone else, and they're not helping here. Before Maddie got her final dose of the vaccine, she was healthy, got straight As, had lots of friends, and had a life." Megan Redshaw reported on Maddie for The Defender:

Upon receiving the second shot, Maddie immediately felt pain at the injection site and over the next 24-hours developed severe abdominal and chest pain, de Garay said at the press event. Maddie told her mother it felt like her heart was being ripped out through her neck, and she had painful electrical shocks down her neck and spine that forced her to walk hunched over.

Maddie's parents took her to the emergency room as instructed by the vaccine trial nurse administrator. Her labs were taken, she was checked for appendicitis, given an IV with medicine and sent home. The diagnosis in the discharge summary read "adverse effect of vaccine initial encounter." Maddie's condition continued to worsen. Over the next two and a half months her abdominal, muscle and nerve pain became unbearable, her mother said.

She developed gastroparesis, nausea and vomiting, erratic blood pressure, memory loss, brain fog, headaches, dizziness, fainting, seizures, verbal and motor tics, menstrual cycle issues, lost feeling from the waist down, lost bowel and bladder control and had an nasogastric tube placed because she lost her ability to eat.[1184]

Below is Maddie de Garay's vaccine card introduced as an exhibit as part of her Mother's, Stephanie de Garay's, public comment to the FDA as a supporting document to prove that Maddie was in the trial and got the actual vaccine. It is posted on the FDA website.[1185]

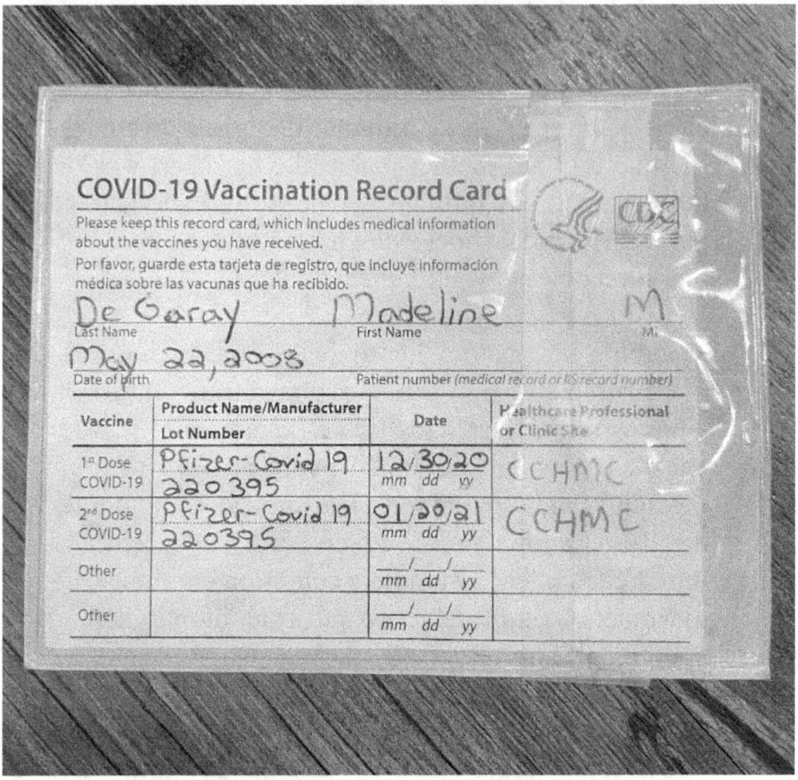

The Canadian Covid Care Alliance studied the raw data from the Pfizer COVID-19 trials. The researchers found that data hidden in the report proves that vaccinated persons are more likely to suffer physical harm and death from the vaccine compared to unvaccinated persons.[1186]

PFIZER TRIALS DID NOT PROVE SAFETY THEY PROVED HARM

ILLNESS

	BNT162b2	Placebo	Risk Change
Efficacy (Meaning number of people diagnosed with COVID-19)	77	850	**-91%**
Related Adverse Event (Meaning an investigator has assessed it as related to the BNT162b2 injection)	5,241	1,311	**+300%**
Any Severe Adverse Event (Interferes significantly with normal function)	262	150	**+75%**
Any Serious Adverse Event	127	116	**+10%**

DEATHS

BNT162b2	Placebo
20	14

These are the results of Pfizer's own randomized control trial.

LEVEL 1 EVIDENCE OF HARM.

Pfizer published its study results on November 30, 2020, but four months earlier, on or before July 22, 2020, the U.S. government had already placed a $1.95 billion order for the Pfizer COVID-19 vaccine.[1187] At that time Pfizer had just begun to enter its late-stage, 30,000-person study. The study had not begun and no data had even been generated. But recall, Pfizer ran the study and was able to rig it to say what they wanted it to say. The skids were greased. There were 1.95 billion reasons for making sure the Pfizer COVID-19 vaccine study showed safety and efficacy. "The love of money is the root of all evil." 1 Timothy 6:10.

Amazingly, the financial deals were being struck when the U.S. government did not know what it was buying. Indeed, the dose level has not even been determined because the late-stage trials have not been conducted. On July 22, 2020, Jared S. Hopkins and Chris Wack, writing for the Wall Street Journal, reported, "Pfizer and BioNTech said they expect to seek emergency use authorization or some form of regulatory approval as early as October."[1188] To do that meant that the favorable results from the testing must have been baked into the study. Hopkins and Wack noted that "[v]accines typically take years to develop and prove they work safely, and many fail during the process."[1189] But in July of 2020, Pfizer confidently expected "approval as early as October." So was the FDA, as the Federal Government had already agreed to pay billions of dollars to buy the untested vaccine. Hopkins and Wack explain that "[t]he U.S. Food and Drug Administration has the authority to quickly authorize drugs and vaccines on an emergency basis."[1190] The deal with Pfizer is not the only drug vaccine deal signed. Hopkins and Wack explain:

> As part of its Operation Warp Speed program, the U.S. has already struck agreements with other vaccine developers to secure doses, including a $1.2 billion deal with AstraZeneca PLC for at least 300 million doses of a vaccine developed by University of Oxford researchers. A $1.6 billion agreement with Novavax Inc. will fund clinical studies of its experimental vaccine and establish large-scale manufacturing of doses."[1191]

How were the vaccine manufacturers cutting the time for development so drastically? Simple, they were ramping up the manufacturing of their vaccines as they were testing them. I kid you not. Hopkins and Wack revealed that in July 2020, "Covid-19 vaccine developers are also combining phases of studies and studying their vaccines at the same time they are ramping up manufacturing capabilities, industry and health officials say."[1192] That means that the pharmaceutical companies already manufactured the same vaccine that they had not yet finished testing for safety and efficacy. Pfizer Chief Business Officer John Young admitted this. Young stated: "This is unprecedented, and that is the only way you can really move at this kind of speed—is to do so many stages over your development and manufacturing process in parallel, rather than doing them sequentially."[1193] Pfizer is not financially stupid. This was not a gamble; this was a sure thing. The fix was in, and Pfizer knew it. With the COVID-19 vaccines, the drug companies were expecting favorable results from their trials. And, as we now know, they got them. Of course, they did. They preordained the favorable results. The pharmaceutical companies are experts in those kinds of shenanigans. And they expected a big pay-off. They were not disappointed. In 2021 alone, Pfizer hauled in $36.8 billion in sales for its COVID-19 vaccine. That made the Pfizer COVID-19 vaccine the most profitable pharmaceutical product over a one year period in the history of pharmaceuticals.[1194]

Johnson & Johnson began planning to manufacture their COVID-19 vaccine within the first few months of the alleged COVID-19 pandemic. Matt Grossman reported on March 30, 2020, for The Wall Street Journal that "Johnson & Johnson said it would try to scale its global manufacturing capabilities to make more than 1 billion doses of a Covid-19 vaccine by the end of next year."[1195] That was well before they even began human testing their vaccine.

In a July 16, 2020, Wall Street Journal article, it was revealed that J&J had invested in "manufacturing sites" and "filling sites" and everything necessary to deliver one billion vaccines. That was after their initial March 2020 plans and still before their vaccine had even undergone human testing. J&J did not even know if their vaccine would cure or harm the patient. Why would J&J spend millions of dollars building manufacturing facilities for an untested vaccine? Because they knew that the vaccine would be approved. The skids were greased, and it didn't care if the vaccine was safe or effective; it knew that the vaccine would be allowed under an EUA, which protected J&J from civil liability for injuries caused by the vaccine. The July 16, 2020, Wall Street Journal article reveals:

> Johnson & Johnson ... said Thursday it plans to begin the first human studies of its experimental coronavirus vaccine next week, as it races to make the shot available starting early next year.

> The New Brunswick, N.J., company's initial study will aim to enroll more than 1,000 healthy adults, starting first in Belgium on July 22 and then the following week in the U.S. Researchers will assess the vaccine's safety and ability to induce an immune response, J&J Chief Scientific Officer Paul Stoffels said Thursday on a conference call with analysts. The company also plans studies in additional countries.
>
> The more definitive testing will take place as soon as September. J&J said it is still having discussions with the U.S. National Institutes of Health for a large phase 3 clinical trial that could begin in late September, which would test whether the vaccine protects people from Covid-19, the disease caused by the new coronavirus.
>
> J&J could get an answer about whether the vaccine safely prevents Covid-19 by the end of the year, Dr. Stoffels said. If successful, the company expects the shot to become available in early 2021, and J&J plans to manufacture up to one billion doses by the end of next year.
>
> "We have the manufacturing sites, we have the filling sites, we have everything that's needed to deliver that one billion vaccines" next year, Dr. Stoffels said.[1196]

It has been now confirmed that the COVID-19 vaccines from Moderna, Pfizer-BioNtech, and Johnson & Johnson (Janssen) do not prevent COVID-19. The vaccines were authorized to be used on an emergency basis to prevent COVID-19, but they have been shown not to do that. So, the pharmaceutical companies just changed the rules for what it means to be effective. Now the standard is no longer whether the vaccine prevents COVID-19 but, instead, whether it lessens the symptoms of COVID-19. When Democrat Rep. Stephen Lynch tested positive to COVID-19 after receiving both shots of the Pfizer vaccine, the Daily Mail explained that "Pfizer's vaccine does not necessarily prevent COVID-19 infection, but is said to be 95 percent effective in stopping the serious symptoms that are caused by the coronavirus."[1197]

Moderna knew from the outset that their vaccine would not prevent COVID-19. A careful reading of Moderna's study indicates that its vaccine likely causes COVID-19. Indeed, there have been many reported cases since the use of both the Moderna and Pfizer-BioNtech vaccines were authorized under the FDA's EUA where the recipient of a COVID-19 vaccination became subsequently ill from COVID-19 and the COVID-19 illness was determined to have been caused by the COVID-19 vaccination.

The insiders seemed to have known from the beginning that the COVID-19 vaccines would not prevent COVID-19 and very likely cause COVID-19. Before either vaccine was authorized, Anthony Fauci explained that reducing symptoms of COVID-19 was the "primary endpoint" of the vaccines. Fauci said that getting rid of the virus through immunity was only a "secondary endpoint." On October 28, 2020, Carol Crist, writing for WebMD, summarized Dr. Fauci's argument as meaning that "with reduced severe symptoms, the coronavirus would pose a lower threat as a pandemic. Then scientists could focus on developing a solution that would reach the full goal of preventing initial infection."[1198]

On October 29, 2020, Dr. Fauci explained: "If the vaccine also allows you to prevent initial infection that would be great," Fauci said. "But what I would settle for, and all my colleagues would settle for, is the primary endpoint, which is to prevent clinically recognizable disease. That's what we hope happens."[1199]

Dr. Fauci said that reducing symptoms of COVID-19 was the "primary endpoint" of the COVID-19 vaccines and not the prevention of COVID-19. But Fauci's statement is contradicted by the FDA. The FDA reported that the primary efficacy endpoint when reviewing the data in deciding whether to grant Moderna's petition to obtain an Emergency Use Authorization (EUA) for their COVID-19 vaccine was its ability to prevent COVID-19. The FDA review states that **"[t]he primary efficacy endpoint was efficacy of the vaccine to prevent protocol-defined COVID-19."**[1200] The protocol-defined COVID-19 included a positive PCR test for SARS-CoV-2, the alleged virus purported to cause COVID-19.

Moderna, J&J, and Pfizer-BioNtech got their COVID-19 vaccines authorized by the FDA under EUAs based on their alleged effectiveness in preventing COVID-19. They then promoted the vaccines to the public on that basis. When the vaccines are increasingly proving ineffective in preventing COVID-19, they just change the standard for success to lessening symptoms. They knew full well that the FDA could not approve an EUA for lessening symptoms and nobody would take a vaccine that would not prevent the targeted disease. So they used the classic bait and switch strategy with a willing accomplice in the FDA.

42 Hydroxychloroquine

The pharmaceutical companies and the FDA had a problem on their hands. To have the COVID-19 vaccines allowed under an emergency use authorization (EUA), Section 564 (21 U.S. Code § 360bbb–3 (c)(3)) required them to prove that "that there is no adequate, approved, and available alternative to the product for diagnosing, preventing, or treating such disease or condition." There were several drugs, most notably hydroxychloroquine (HCQ), that had proven to be safe and effective treatment against viral infections, including COVID-19. HCQ has a 60 year track record of safety and efficacy.[1201]

HCQ FOR COVID-19

280 TRIALS, 4,563 SCIENTISTS, 398,415 PATIENTS

64% IMPROVEMENT IN 31 EARLY TREATMENT TRIALS RR 0.36 [0.28-0.46]

75% IMPROVEMENT IN 13 EARLY TREATMENT MORTALITY RESULTS RR 0.25 [0.16-0.40]

46% IMPROVEMENT IN 8 EARLY TREATMENT RCT RESULTS RR 0.54 [0.35-0.84]

21% IMPROVEMENT IN 190 LATE TREATMENT TRIALS RR 0.79 [0.74-0.84]

23% IMPROVEMENT IN 44 RANDOMIZED CONTROLLED TRIALS RR 0.77 [0.65-0.93]

SUMMARY OF RESULTS REPORTED IN HCQ STUDIES FOR COVID-19. 08/28/21. HCQMETA.COM

HCQ had to be removed as an effective treatment for COVID-19 in order for the COVID-19 vaccines to be given their EUAs. And so, on June 15, 2020, the FDA issued a decision letter revoking the EUA for hyrdroxychloroquine (HCQ), stating that "it is no longer reasonable to believe that oral formulations of HCQ and CQ may be effective in treating COVID-19, nor is it reasonable to believe that the known and potential benefits of these products outweigh their known and potential risks."[1202]

The decision letter had attached to it a memorandum explaining the alleged scientific basis for the decision. The memorandum stated that Biomedical Advanced Research and Development Authority (BARDA) considered several studies in determining that HCQ was not a safe and effective treatment for COVID-19.

There is a notable conflict of interest. Moderna, one of the manufacturers of an mRNA COVID-19 vaccine, published a 2019 letter to shareholders from Stéphane Bancel, Chief Executive Officer, in which she revealed:

> The Phase 1 study of mRNA-1893 is ongoing and is being advanced with funding from the U.S. Department of Health and Human Services (HHS); the Office of the Assistant Secretary for Preparedness and Response; and the Biomedical Advanced Research and Development Authority (BARDA).[1203]

You read that correctly. Moderna received funding from BARDA to develop its mRNA vaccine technology. That technology was used to make their COVID-19 vaccine. That COVID-19 mRNA vaccine could not have been granted an EUA from the FDA unless there was no adequate, approved, and available alternative to the vaccine. HCQ was such an alternative. BARDA, who funded the Moderna mRNA research, steps in and issues a memorandum stating that studies show that HCQ is not a safe and effective alternative treatment for COVID-19. That cleared the path being blocked by HCQ for the FDA to grant the EUA to Moderna.

Let us read the BARDA memorandum. One of the studies BARDA said it evaluated but said it "will not be included in this Memerorndum."[1204] The study was not included in the BARDA memorandum because before publishing the BARDA memorandum that study was publicly exposed as a fraudulent study. That study that purported to prove that HCQ was ineffective and unsafe in treating COVID-19 was shown to be an embarrassing fraud and was retracted by The Lancet.[1205]

The fake study falsely showing hydroxychloroquine was unsafe and ineffective was published in The Lancet and The New England Journal of Medicine. The Lancet and The New England Journal of Medicine are the top two most respected medical journals in the world. The study published by those two journals was exposed as based upon fabricated data and performed by a false-front company.

The Guardian investigated the study, known as the Surgishere Study, and determined that it was a fabricated study performed by a scam organization whose principal employees included a sci-fi writer and adult content model. *The Guardian* reported:

> A search of publicly available material suggests several of Surgisphere's employees have little or no data or scientific background. An employee listed as a science editor appears to be a science fiction author and fantasy artist whose professional profile suggests writing is her fulltime job. Another employee listed as a marketing executive is an adult model and events hostess, who also acts in videos for organisations.[1206]

The discovery that the study was completely made up from fabricated data forced The Lancet and The New England Journal of Medicine (NEJM) to retract their publication of the study. The odd thing is that it only took a modicum of review to discover the fraud. That is something that could easily have been done by the editors of The Lancet and the NEJM.

The article had the effect of halting all studies by the World Health Organization (WHO) into the effectiveness of hydroxychloroquine.[1207] The WHO subsequently reintroduced HCQ into its Solidarity Trial. The Solidarity Trial is a story in and of itself and will be discussed below.

Many governors in the United States prohibited hydroxychloroquine to treat COVID-19 based upon that fraudulent study. Those governors continued their bans on HCQ long after the study was exposed as a fraud.

What is amazing is that the study was announced by the NEJM as being retracted not because the data was shown to be fabricated (which it was), but rather "because all the authors were not granted access to the raw data and the raw data could not be made available to a third-party auditor, we are unable to validate the primary data sources underlying our article." But the article was a complete fraud. It should be announced as such. But, instead, it was announced as being retracted because the data could not be verified. That is how the NEJM rolls.

What did The Lancet say? In much the same way as the NEJM, The Lancet stated that "our reviewers were not able to conduct an independent and private peer review and therefore [the authors] notified us of their withdrawal from the peer-review process."

Both The Lancet and the NEJM rushed a fraudulent study to press without adequate peer review and a shocking lack of due diligence because it supported the narrative that hydroxychloroquine was unsafe and ineffective. Indeed, a typical medical study sometimes takes years to get through the peer-review process for publication. But this article was seemingly not reviewed at all. Why would the world-renowned NEJM and The Lancet publish garbage? That was answered by Dr. Douste-Blazy, who spilled the beans and revealed the control of pharmaceutical companies over The Lancet and NEJM. Philippe Douste-Blazy, MD, is a cardiologist and former French Health Minister who served as Under-Secretary-General of the United Nations. He was a candidate in 2017 for the Director of the World Health Organization. Vera Sharav reported in the Alliance for Human Research Protection the following information from Dr. Douste-Blazy:

> In a videotaped interview on May 24, 2020, Dr. Douste-Blazy provided insight into how a series of negative hydroxychloroquine studies got published in prestigious medical journals.

> He revealed that at a recent Chatham House top secret, closed door meeting attended by experts only, the editors of both The Lancet and the New England Journal of Medicine expressed their exasperation, citing the pressures put on them by pharmaceutical companies.
>
> **He states that each of the editors used the word "criminal" to describe the erosion of science.**[1208] (emphasis added)

He who pays the piper calls the tune. Digging further, we find that the fraudulent study itself was financed by a pharmaceutical company that is trying to market a substitute for hydroxychloroquine as a treatment for COVID-19.[1209] Sharav reveals:

> Dr. Mandeep Mehra, the lead co-author [of the fraudulent article] is a director at Brigham & Women's Hospital, which is credited with funding the study. Dr. Mehra and The Lancet failed to disclose that Brigham Hospital has a partnership with Gilead and is currently conducting TWO trials testing Remdesivir, the prime competitor of hydroxychloroquine for the treatment of COVID-19, the focus of the study.[1210]

Sharav explains that within days of the study being published "Dr. Anthony Fauci, head of the National Institute of Allergy and Infectious Diseases (NIAID) declared on CNN [about HCQ] 'The scientific data is really quite evident now about the lack of efficacy.'"[1211] And right on cue, there was a media blitz against hydroxychloroquine. Sharav reports:

> A media blitz against hydroxychloroquine (HCQ) created panic: clinical trials aimed at testing

hydroxychloroquine for COVID-19 were suspended by International public health institutions including the World Health Organization the UK government regulatory agency and the French government.[1212]

Sharav concluded:

WHY are very powerful corporate-government stakeholders so intent on killing a drug with a 70 year track record? Because the drug works against the pandemic; it is readily available, and costs very little. Therefore, it poses a financial threat to both pharma companies and their partners in government and academia, those who are intent on profiting from the COVID-19 pandemic.

As uncovered by Science Defies Politics: 16 of the panel members selected by NIH to formulate the official COVID-19 Treatment Guidelines – including two of the three co-chairs – were paid by Gilead. They issued guidelines that raised fear, uncertainty, and doubt about the use of HCQ combined with AZ, while raising no fear, doubt, or uncertainty about using Gilead's unproven, unapproved, drug remdesivir; a drug that has shown mediocre performance in clinical trials. Seven of the NIH panelists failed to disclose their financial ties to Gilead. ...

The medical scientific literature is infested with financially motivated, shoddy, studies aimed at promoting products and, when a life-saving, non-patentable product, proves effective, scientists are hired to author study reports that are designed to tarnish scientists' reputations, and to proclaim

> findings that refute legitimate findings. In this case, studies designed to "debunk" the effectiveness of hydroxychloroquine against COVID-19.
>
> Examples of countries and physicians who have witnessed the effectiveness of the HCQ – Az combination as a treatment for COVID-19, are viewed by corporate-government collaborating partners as posing a major threat to their marketing agendas.[1213]

Two other studies cited in the BARDA Hydroxychloroquine (HCQ) memorandum are known as the UK Recovery trial and the WHO Solidarity trial. BARDA alleged that "the RECOVERY Trial results offer persuasive evidence of a lack of benefit of HCQ in the treatment of hospitalized patients with COVID-19."[1214] The WHO Solidarity trial was ongoing and not yet completed, but it was nonetheless cited in the memorandum. Odd that BARDA would cite a study the outcome of which was at that time unknown. Both trials showed HCQ to be unsafe and ineffective in treating COVID-19. But medical and scientific experts who have reviewed the trials have concluded that they were rigged to falsely show that HCQ was unsafe and ineffective. For example, Dr. Merul Nass, M.D. studied both trials and concluded that "[i]n the UK Recovery trial, and in WHO Solidarity trial, HCQ is used in a non-therapeutic, toxic and potentially lethal dose."[1215] She concluded that the patients in those studies were being poisoned with toxic levels of HCQ for the purpose of falsely showing that HCQ was unsafe and ineffective. She states that "WHO and other national health agencies, universities and charities have conducted large clinical trials that were designed so hydroxychloroquine would fail to show benefit in the treatment of Covid-19, perhaps to advantage much more expensive competitors and vaccines in development. ... In so doing, these agencies and charities have de facto conspired to increase the number of deaths in these trials."[1216]

With HCQ out of the way, the FDA could issue an EUA for the experimental COVID-19 vaccines. On December 11, 2020, the Food and Drug Administration (FDA) issued an Emergency Use Authorization (EUA) for emergency use of Pfizer-BioNTech COVID-19 Vaccine for the prevention of COVID-19. In its announcement, it stated one of the required legal bases was fulfilled, that being "There is no adequate, approved, and available alternative to the emergency use of Pfizer-BioNTech COVID-19 Vaccine to prevent COVID-19."[1217]

Let us explore the WHO Solidarity trial and see how it was rigged to falsely show that HCQ was unsafe and ineffective.

Dr. Claus Kohnlein, the author of *Virus Mania*, reveals how the World Health Organization (WHO) has scammed the public into thinking that hydroxychloroquine is unsafe and ineffective as a therapy for COVID-19.[1218] Dr. Kohnlein explains how the WHO published a study, known as the Solidarity Trial,[1219] during which the study scientists gave the study participants toxic dosages of hydroxychloroquine (HCQ) to falsely show it is unsafe and ineffective.

The phony WHO study presents a graph comparing the mortality percentage of those alleged to have COVID-19 who took hydroxychloroquine and those alleged to have COVID-19 in the control group who did not take hydroxychloroquine. You will notice immediately that those that took the hydroxychloroquine died at a higher rate than those that received no medication. This is supposed to be scientific proof for the public and the medical community that hydroxychloroquine is unsafe and ineffective in treating COVID-19.

(b) Hydroxychloroquine vs its control

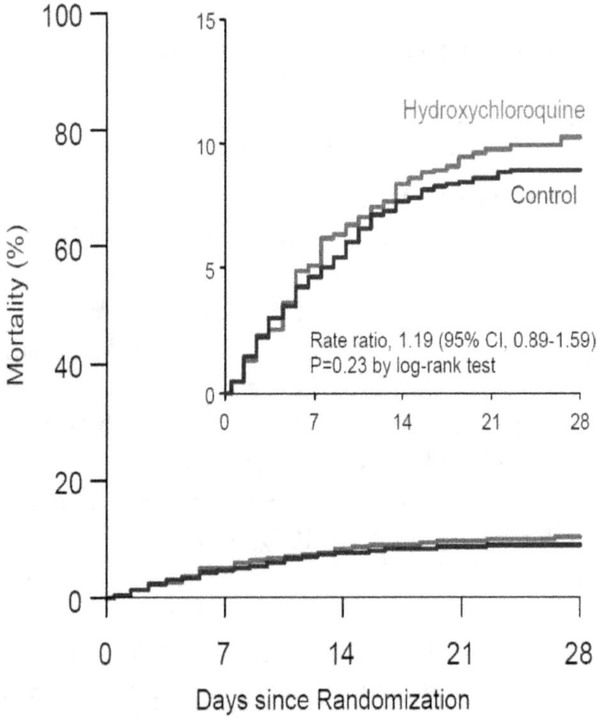

Numbers at risk at the start of each week, and numbers dying

Hydroxyc.	947	48	889	31	854	13	838	6	833	6
Control	906	42	853	27	823	8	814	4	809	3

Kaplan-Meier graphs of in-hospital mortality. The inset shows the same data on an expanded y-axis

Hidden deep in the study is the little-publicized fact that the patients receiving the hydroxychloroquine were given toxic doses. That is correct. The doctors were poisoning the patients. Hydroxychloroquine is very safe when the dose is kept between 200 mg and 400 mg per day. But hydroxychloroquine has a narrow therapeutic index. That means that while hydroxychloroquine is otherwise safe, it does not take very much over the therapeutic dosage to be toxic.

Studies have shown that a toxic daily dosage of hydroxychloroquine is 20 mg per kg weight of the patient. Four grams 4 g of Hydroxychloroquine is considered a potentially lethal dose (4 g = 4,000 mg). The WHO study involved males and females from all over the world. The average weight of all persons in the world, male and female, is 136 pounds (62 kg). That means that the toxic dosage for hydroxychloroquine for the average person in the world is 1.24 g (62 kg x 20 mg = 1,240 mg). A common symptom of hydroxychloroquine poisoning is cardiac arrhythmia leading to death.

What dosage of hydroxychloroquine was administered to the WHO study group? the study reported:

> Hour 0, four tablets; Hour 6, four tablets; Hour 12, begin two tablets twice daily for 10 days. Each tablet contained 200mg Hydroxychloroquine sulphate (155mg base/tablet; a little-used alternative involved 155mg chloroquine base/tablet).[1220]

They administered to each of the study patients a dosage of 2.4 g (2,400 mg) of hydroxychloroquine sulphate (which contained 1,860 mg of hydroxychloroquine base) in the first 24 hours of the study. That dosage of 1.86 g (1,860 mg) HCQ base is more than 9 times the recommended dosage, which is 200 mg, and more than the daily toxic dosage, which is 1.24 g (1,240 mg). The doctors were poisoning the patients in the study.

The doctors followed that initial poisoning with 10 days of 800 mg Hydroxychloroquine sulphate (620 mg HCQ base), which is more than three (3) times the recommended daily dosage. The doctors were conducting the study across 30 countries and involving more than 405 hospitals. Weren't they concerned that somebody might notice that they were using suspiciously high dosages of hydroxychloroquine? Of course they were. They tried to cover themselves with the following statement:

> Despite concerns that the loading dose could be temporarily cardiotoxic, in neither trial was there any excess mortality during the first few days, when blood levels were highest. Neither trial recorded dosage/kg, obesity, or cardiac parameters, and cardiac deaths were too few to be reliably informative.[1221]

They knew full well that they were poisoning the study patients. They identified the first-day "loading" dosage as "temporarily cardiotoxic." They started the study patients off by exceeding the toxic dose of Hydroxychloroquine. They admitted that that dose was "cardiotoxic." They were poisoning their study patients and gave no explanation for why they would do such a thing. But they made sure they kept their study patients on the edge of death over the next ten (10) days by continuing to administer more than three (3) times the recommended daily dosage of hydroxychloroquine.

The study scientists argued that there was no "excess mortality during the first few days" and the few who died of cardiac arrest didn't matter to the study. What they did not say was that the cumulative effect of the hydroxychloroquine over the next 10 days acted to cull the herd in the hydroxychloroquine group just enough to show that hydroxychloroquine was unsafe and ineffective.

The doctors discuss the "few" who died from cardiac arrest. They cleverly avoid discussing those who died because the toxic dosages of hydroxychloroquine compromised the immune systems of the study patients. Hydroxychloroquine is a drug that is sometimes used to modulate the immune system. That is why hydroxychloroquine is used to treat autoimmune diseases like lupus.[1222] The doctors conducting the study knew that hydroxychloroquine is immunosuppressive when it is dispensed in high dosages. Suppressing a patient's immune system would make the patient less able to fight off an infectious disease.

The study doctors did not want to give the recommended dosage of 200 mg per day because they knew it would not kill anyone and it would likely show hydroxychloroquine to be both safe and effective. Instead, they decided to poison their patients the first day with a "cardiotoxic" dosage of hydroxychloroquine and then keep the toxic level up for ten (10) straight days. They knew full well that they would kill some of them but "too few to be reliably informative."[1223]

We do not know the numbers of those who died of cardiac arrest from hydroxychloroquine poisoning because the study did not report that result. All who died were listed as having died of COVID-19. Certainly, the toxic dosages of hydroxychloroquine increased the deaths by suppressing the immune systems of the patients, 65% of whom were over 50 years old and in frail health. The deaths for the Hydroxychloroquine group included those who died from the effects of hydroxychloroquine poisoning, but they were reported as COVID-19 deaths. The scientists claimed that only a few died from cardiac arrest. But they make no mention of the immunosuppressive qualities of the toxic hydroxychloroquine dosages. Are we supposed to believe mad scientists who poison study patients to be honest in reporting what happened in the study?

The worldwide medical establishment had to prove that

hydroxychloroquine was an ineffective treatment so that they could push the emergency use of the dangerous COVID-19 vaccines on the public with the argument that "[t]here is no adequate, approved, and available alternative to the emergency use of [Pfizer-BioNTech and Moderna] COVID 19 Vaccine[s] to prevent COVID-19."[1224]

Keep in mind that he who pays the piper calls the tune. The Bill and Melinda Gates Foundation is the second-largest donor in the world to the WHO, which in turn funded the fraudulent Solidarity Trial. Only the U.S. Government surpasses the Bill and Melinda Gates Foundation in funding the WHO. The Bill and Melinda Gates Foundation has donated billions for the administration of vaccines, including the COVID-19 vaccines, worldwide.[1225]

Bill Gates was the #2 largest donor ($228 million) to the World Health Organization in 2018, only behind the U.S. Government ($281 million). Interestingly, the #4 donor to the WHO is GAVI ($158 million). We will find out more about GAVI below. And, of course, the WHO is one of the vehicles pushing vaccine mandates. The World Health Organization (WHO) is on record saying that "[v]accination mandates can be ethically justified."[1226] The WHO offers guidance on when such mandates would be appropriate.

> Mandatory vaccination should be considered only if it is necessary for, and proportionate to, the achievement of one or more important societal or institutional objectives (typically but not exclusively public health objectives, which may also be in service of social and economic objectives).[1227]

The WHO is not keen on allowing religious exemptions. Indeed, the WHO does not even mention religious exemptions in its vaccine mandate policy brief.[1228] The WHO calls it a "conscientious objection." The WHO says that any "conscientious objection" should be limited by "strict scientific and prudential limits."[1229] The WHO argues:

> There should ... be strict scientific and prudential limits to appeals for accommodation or "conscientious objection," especially when such accommodation might be used by individuals to 'free ride' the public health good of community protection (i.e., taking advantage of the benefit without contributing towards the cost of its production) or if they threaten public health and others' right not to be infected with a virulent infectious disease.[1230]

Under the WHO standard, no "conscientious objection" can be allowed for a vaccine mandate because the very reason to justify the mandate furnishes the basis to deny the request for a religious exemption. The WHO standard does not consider the sincerity of the religious objection. It only considers whether there is a threat to public health. But that determination had already been made when the mandate was announced. That seems to be the idea; nobody gets a so-called "free ride." There can be no religious exemption allowed under a vaccine mandate because the only consideration is the threat to public health, and the decision to grant the religious exemption is guided only by scientific and prudential limits. Limiting the consideration of the exemption request to scientific and prudential matters precludes consideration of the sincerity of the person's religious beliefs.

You must look at the donations coming from the Bill and Melinda Gates Foundation as strategic investments with a big payoff in the future. Bill Gates is probably the single person on the planet who will benefit the most financially by the imposition of the COVID-19 vaccine. Gates and his foundation have close financial ties with Moderna, one of the COVID-19 vaccine manufacturers.[1231] The mainstream media tries to keep a lid on that information. But it is a fact that is published on the Moderna website.[1232] The Bill & Malinda Gates Foundation is listed as one of Moderna's strategic collaborators.[1233] Indeed, Bill gates admitted in a CNBC interview he has turned an initial $10 billion investment in vaccine manufacturing into $200 billion.[1234]

Bill Gates has a clever scheme where he uses his charity to fund vaccine development by pharmaceutical companies in which he has invested. When the vaccines bring in billions of dollars, he, in turn, reaps the financial reward. In his CNBC interview, he admitted to making $200 billion on vaccines.

The Bill and Melinda Gates foundation is the #2 Donor ($1.5 Billion) to Global Alliance for Vaccines and Immunization (GAVI).[1235] That is more than the U.S. Government ($1.4 billion) and a little less than the #1 donor, Great Britain ($2 billion). One of the GAVI programs is the Advance Market Commitments (AMCs). The World Bank explains that the AMC is a way to encourage pharmaceutical companies to make vaccines by guaranteeing that there will be funds to purchase the vaccines.[1236] The top 14 donors funding the GAVI AMC are nations. Under the AMC, tax dollars are used to fund the purchase of vaccines using GAVI as the intermediary. The Pharmaceutical companies are all too happy to participate in the AMC as they directly benefit financially.[1237] Under the AMC, donor countries agree to purchase a number of vaccine doses meeting certain specifications.

That explains how before the issuance of the emergency use authorization (EUA), the U.S. government agreed to buy 100 million doses of the experimental COVID-19 vaccine from Pfizer/BioNTech for nearly $2 billion.[1238] Thus the vaccines were purchased in advance of the authorization guaranteeing a market for the vaccines. All that was needed was for the government and the media to whip up the fear of COVID and offer the free vaccines purchased ahead of time with tax dollars. When the uptake slowed, corporations, state and federal governments started issuing mandates requiring vaccination.

Bill Gates continues to push for mandatory COVID-19 vaccinations. But he decided that when it was his turn to be vaccinated he hired someone to stand in for him.[1239] On January 12, 2020, Bill Gates sent out the following Tweet:

> One of the benefits of being 65 is that I'm eligible for the COVID-19 vaccine. I got my first dose this week, and I feel great. Thank you to all of the scientists, trial participants, regulators, and frontline healthcare workers who got us to this point.[1240]

Bill Gates
@BillGates · Follow

One of the benefits of being 65 is that I'm eligible for the COVID-19 vaccine. I got my first dose this week, and I feel great. Thank you to all of the scientists, trial participants, regulators, and frontline healthcare workers who got us to this point.

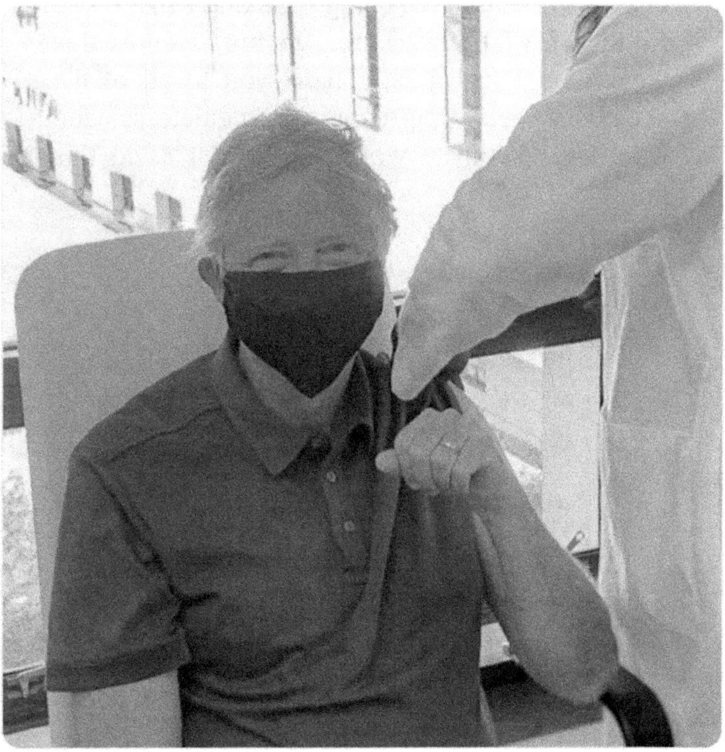

12:01 PM · Jan 22, 2021

In the tweet, Bill Gates appended a photograph purporting it to be him getting the COVID-19 vaccine.[1241] The problem is that the photo is not Bill Gates. Indeed when comparing the picture with known pictures of Bill Gates, it is apparent that the person that Bill Gates is alleging is him is actually an imposter.

It isn't easy to find a modern photograph of Bill Gates where he is not wearing his ubiquitous glasses. But this author found one.[1242] The hair on the imposter is gray. Bill Gates has gray hair, but it is salt and pepper gray. Notice also the right ear is different. The imposter's ear sticks out much more than Gates' ear.

One could argue that the ear sticking out is due to the face mask pulling on the imposter's ear. But notice it is the top of the ear that is protruding. That is not what happens when an ear loop pulls hard from behind the ear. Assuming extreme pressure from the ear loop, the pressure from the pull would be uniform and not cause the top of the ear to stick out while the bottom of the ear remains against the head, as we see happening in the imposter's photograph.

There is another point of comparison, however, that cannot be explained away. That physical feature nails the fact that it is not Bill Gates in the picture allegedly getting the COVID-19 vaccination. One of the most distinctive physical features of Bill Gates is his neck. Bill Gates has a great deal of loose skin around his neck. That loose skin completely obscures his Adam's apple. On the other hand, the imposter has much tighter skin around his neck, which displays a visible Adam's apple.

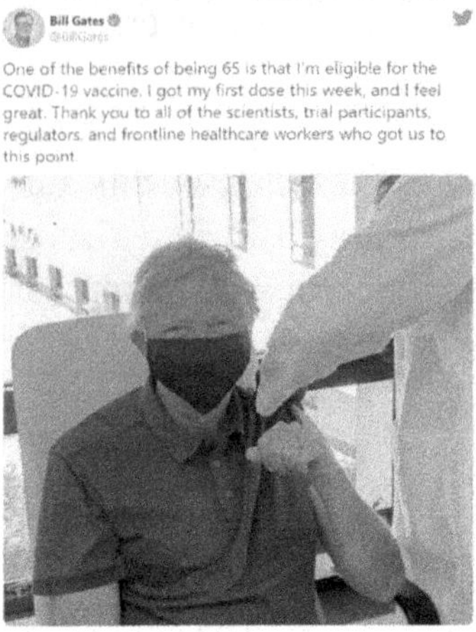

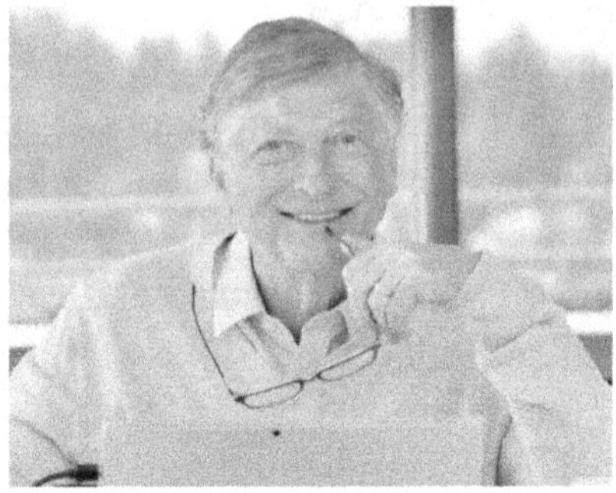

Imposter
January 22, 2021

Bill Gates
December 30, 2019

The hair of the imposter is completely gray. Whereas Bill Gates has salt and pepper gray hair.

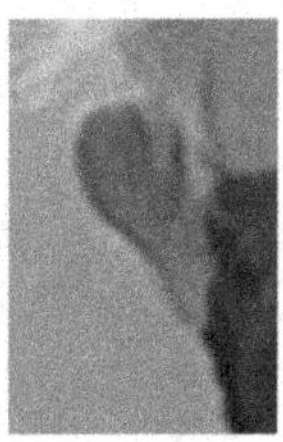

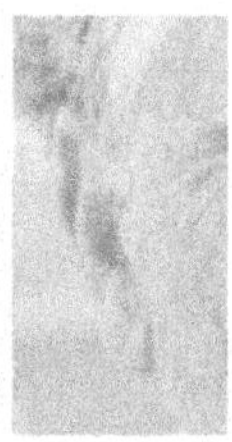

The right ear of the imposter is quite different from the right ear of Bill Gates. One could argue it is due to the mask that is pulling on the ear. Experiment with that theory yourself, and you will find that a mask loop pulling at the base of the ear will not cause the ear to stick out. In any event, that explanation does not explain the striking difference between the distinctive neck of Bill Gates and the imposter.

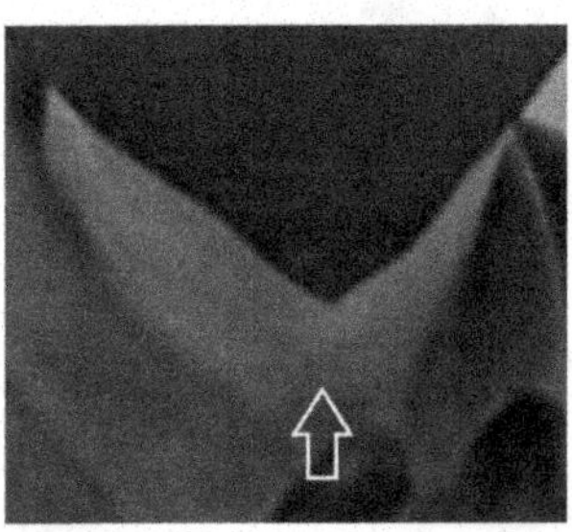

Visible Adam's Apple

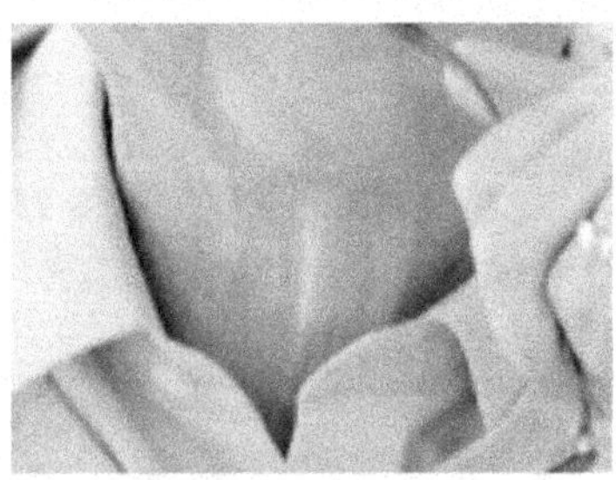

No Visible Adam's Apple

The imposter has tight skin around his neck that shows a distinct Adam's apple. Bill Gate has significant excess skin around his neck where no Adam's apple is visible.

Please keep in mind that Bill Gates, himself, posted the picture of the imposter on his official Twitter account. He portrayed it as being him getting a COVID-19 vaccination.

Why would Bill Gates hire an imposter to stand in for him to get a COVID-19 vaccine? Why would he falsely publicize on Twitter that he got a COVID-19 vaccine? The answer is obvious. He knows that the vaccine is unsafe and ineffective. He will not allow himself to be poisoned with an experimental vaccine. But Bill Gates must portray to the world that he got the vaccine to quiet his critics and falsely represent the COVID-19 vaccine as safe and effective.

What possibly can be clearer evidence that the COVID-19 vaccines being pushed by Bill Gates are unsafe and ineffective than the fact that the very man who pushes most for mandatory COVID-19 vaccines and serves to make the most money from those vaccines would hire an imposter to pretend to be him getting the vaccine? He knows he is peddling deadly poisons and will not allow that poison to be injected into him.

You should always be suspicious when politicians and other notables who benefit financially and politically from vaccine uptake are seen in publicity events getting vaccine injections. In 1995, Dr. Archie Kalokerinos, an Australian Doctor, opined that Gerald Ford received a saline solution injection instead of the H1N1 Swine Flu shot he was seen receiving at a news conference. Dr. Kalokerinos explained:

> I was in America when President Ford was about to vaccinate the entire population of America, every man, woman and child, black, white and brindle against swine flu, because some idiot had told him there was going to be a massive epidemic that was going to kill millions of people. And my views received considerable publicity. In fact I

ended up appearing on Cathy Cosby's television program, and I said it would be mass murder and I specifically described how people who had heart problems could drop dead. There was a man watching the programme in New York who did not like a particular gentleman by the name of Gambino. Gambino was 69 years old and a mafia boss. He thought this is a great idea. So he got someone to persuade Gambino to have his flu shot and Gambino promptly dropped dead. The heading of the newspapers went something like "Mafia flu jab conspiracy". It was fairly obvious that the person who advised Gambino knew what would happen or was hoping that Gambino would drop dead. It caused a hell of a row. But President Ford said "I'll settle all this", and he called a special news conference and in front of the whole of America rolled up his sleeve and had his shot. Now there is no doubt he did not have swine flu vaccine. They would not have given it to him, no way! But then he invited all the news media people that were there to line up and have theirs. Only one man volunteered and he was the White House press secretary, the rest refused to have it. And of course the other part of the story, which is history now, is that people started to sue or drop dead in the buildings where they had received their injections. There have been several huge settlements, I think they are still going on now, haven't finally been settled yet.[1243]

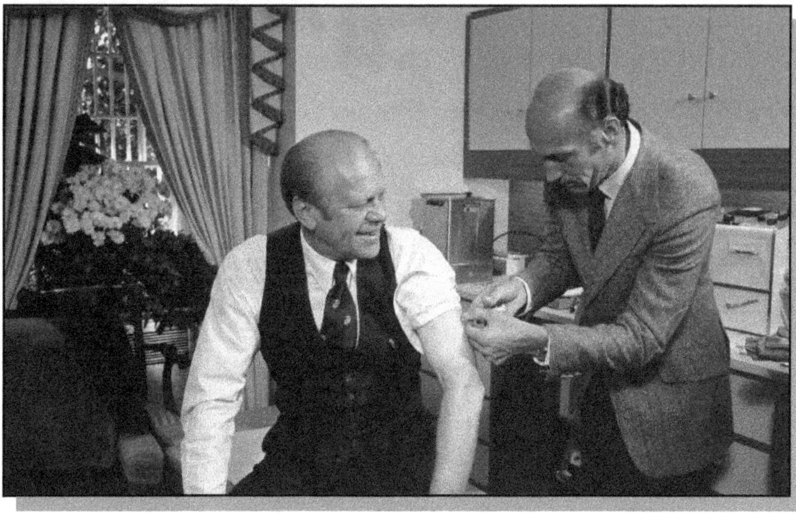

Figure 55: President Ford allegedly receives a saline injection portrayed as a swine flu inoculation from his White House physician, Dr. William Lukash, October 14, 1976 (White House photograph B1874-07A)

It turns out that, indeed, Carlo Gambino reportedly died on October 15, 1976, after receiving his swine flu vaccine injection. Time Magazine reported:

> Unverified Mob talk last week went so far as to suggest that Galente ordered his spies within the Gambino family to persuade the capo di tutti capi to take a swine-flu shot, knowing that a frail individual with a heart ailment and hardening of the arteries might succumb. According to federal sources, Gambino did get his flu shot shortly before his death.[1244]

43 Suppression of Hydroxychloroquine

In a video conference on the Charlie Kirk Show posted on July 30, 2020, Kirk interviewed nine (9) doctors with more than 200 years of combined medical experience.[1245] They all made the point that hydroxychloroquine is a safe and effective cure for the flu-like illness that has been described as COVID-19.

The YouTube video of the July 30, 2020, Charlie Kirk Show with the nine doctors revealing the benefits of hydroxychloroquine, was deleted by YouTube on or before August 10, 2020, with the following notice: "This video has been removed for violating YouTube's Community Guidelines." Google, which owns YouTube, will stop at nothing to keep this important information hidden from the public.

YouTube cannot claim medical expertise that exceeds the 200 years of medical experience represented by the nine doctors in the video. No, this has nothing to do with the merits of the video. This was purely a powerplay in shutting down a disfavored remedy that undermines the vaccine and patent medicine profits of the drug companies from whom Google receives massive advertising revenues. YouTube is simply the piper obeying the dictates of the pharmaceutical companies and the government, who, by paying that piper, get to call the tune. But the video was backed up on BitChute, and it can be viewed at the link in the endnote at the end of this sentence.[1246]

Many of the doctors on the Charlie Kirk Show had attended a previously held a press conference on July 27, 2020, extolling the safety and effectiveness of hydroxychloroquine. After receiving millions of views in the first day, the video was taken down and scrubbed from the internet. Jon Passantino and Oliver Darcy from CNN, of course, described the information from the doctors as "false and dubious claims." Passantino and Oliver stated:

> A video featuring a group of doctors making false and dubious claims related to the coronavirus was removed by Facebook, Twitter, and YouTube after going viral online Monday.[1247]

Passino and Oliver also stated that the claim that "recent studies showing hydroxychloroquine is ineffective for the treatment of the flu-like illness known as Covid-19 are 'fake science' sponsored by 'fake pharma companies'" was a dubious claim made by the assembled doctors. As explained above, it turns out that the study the doctors claimed was fake was, in fact, fake. Although the study the doctors claimed was bogus was withdrawn after proof of its fakery was made public, the CNN article by Passino and Oliver remains posted without any correction. The doctors were correct, but CNN ignored the evidence.

Full Court Press to Censor Doctors

The nine doctors on Charlie Kirk show promoting the effectiveness of hydroxychloroquine posted the research supporting their claims for the safety and effectiveness of hydroxychloroquine on a website at:

www.americasfrontlinedoctors.com. But within days of their announcement of that resource website, their webhost, Squarespace, shut down the website. Christopher Zara reported for Fast Company:

> But after news of the video spread on Tuesday, the website suddenly became unreachable. Squarespace, which hosts the website, now presents visitors with a message saying it has "expired."[1248]

One of the doctors on the Charlie Kirk Show revealed the astounding truth that "doctors can't freely speak by the way. So many doctors have, I mean, thousands have come to me and said I work for such and such institution if I speak out, I've heard many doctors say I would be fired instantly."

This is censorship on a massive scale to keep the public ignorant about a cure for the flu-like illness known as COVID-19. Why? Because there are very powerful pharmaceutical interests that are pushing for patent medicines and vaccinations to treat COVID-19.

Government officials are working hand in hand with the major media companies to suppress knowledge of and access to a drug that is safe and effective in treating COVID-19. Their actions are killing people. Former University President Everett Piper stated in an August 10, 2020, Washington Times article that the effort by governors, in particular, Governors Andrew Cuomo of New York, Gavin Newsom of California, and Gretchen Whitmer of Michigan, the CDC, the mainstream media, and media-tech companies to keep Hydroxychloroquine and information about HCQ from people as a treatment for COVID-19 has resulted in the deaths of more than 120,000 people in the United States.

On July 23, 2020, the Association of American

Physicians & Surgeons (AAPS) provided the U.S. Department of Health & Human Services and the Food and Drug Administration copious amounts of data showing, among other things, that countries using hydroxychloroquine (HCQ) are attaining far lower mortality rates than the United States. "The mortality rate from COVID-19 in countries that allow access to HCQ," said the AAPS, "is only one-tenth the mortality rate of countries where there is interference with this medication, such as the United States."

***

[T]he Henry Ford Health System in Michigan, which recently published a study involving thousands of patients where HCQ proved to be both very safe and highly effective in treating COVID-19. This study reports reducing mortality by 50%. Did you catch that? Fifty percent.

***

[T]he Palmer Foundation report published last week highlighting the Indian slum of Dharavi. This is Asia's biggest and densest slum, housing more than a million people. In the early days of the pandemic, Dharavi suffered a cluster outbreak. Doctors report containing it by using proactive measures, "including the use of hydroxychloroquine for prophylaxis (preventive) treatment." As a result, Dharavi's COVID-19 infection rate dropped drastically from April through June, and in July, new infections were very low, almost reaching zero on July 9."

Yes, you read that correctly. "Almost reaching zero."

***

Harvey, A. Risch, MD, Ph.D., professor of epidemiology at Yale School of Public Health (generally not known as a bastion of conservative political thought), who recently wrote in Newsweek magazine: "I am … flummoxed to find that, in the midst of a crisis, I am fighting for a treatment that the data fully support but which, for reasons having nothing to do with a correct understanding of the science, has been pushed to the sidelines. As a result, tens of thousands of patients with COVID-19 are dying unnecessarily."

Yes, you read that correctly. "Tens of thousands of patients are dying unnecessarily."

***

Dr. Risch then goes on to cite study after study showing the efficacy of HCQ. There is a study involving 400 high-risk patients treated by Dr. Vladimir Zelenko, with zero deaths. There are four studies totaling almost 500 high-risk patients treated in nursing homes and clinics across the U.S., with no deaths. There is a controlled trial of more than 700 high-risk patients in Brazil, with significantly reduced hospitalization and two deaths among 334 patients.

There is another study of 398 matched patients in France, also with significantly reduced hospitalization. And there is the reverse natural experiment in Switzerland where on May 27 the Swiss national government banned outpatient use of hydroxychloroquine. By June 10, COVID-19 deaths had increased four-fold and remained elevated. On June 11, the Swiss government revoked the ban, and on June 23, the death rate reverted to what it had been beforehand.[1249]

44 Ivermectin

The FDA and the vaccine makers have another problem. And that problem is that scientific studies have proven that ivermectin is a safe and effective (and inexpensive) treatment for COVID-19. To continue the EUA for the COVID-19 vaccines, they need to maintain that "that there is no adequate, approved, and available alternative to the product for diagnosing, preventing, or treating such disease or condition." The FDA controls what is approved. All the FDA needs to do is not approve ivermectin, and the EUA for the COVID-19 vaccines continue. And so, ivermectin must go. Thus, the FDA has announced:

> The FDA has not authorized or approved ivermectin for the treatment or prevention of COVID-19 in people or animals. Ivermectin has not been shown to be safe or effective for these indications.[1250]

On what basis does the FDA make that judgement that ivermectin is not safe or effective? The FDA claims:

> Currently available data do not show ivermectin is effective against COVID-19. Clinical trials

assessing ivermectin tablets for the prevention or treatment of COVID-19 in people are ongoing. Taking large doses of ivermectin is dangerous.[1251]

That statement by the FDA is not true. There have been 63 studies of the safety and effectiveness of ivermectin in treating COVID-19.[1252] Meta-analysis of those studies found an average of 69% improvement for early treatment and 86% improvement for prophylaxis.[1253] Those numbers are probably conservative because researchers found a negative bias against ivermectin in a review of the studies. The researchers determined that the statistical probability for the studies to falsely portray a positive outcome for ivermectin is one in one trillion.

- Meta analysis using the most serious outcome reported shows 69% [54-79%] and 86% [75-92%] improvement for early treatment and prophylaxis, with similar results after exclusion based sensitivity analysis and restriction to peer-reviewed studies or Randomized Controlled Trials.
- Statistically significant improvements are seen for mortality, hospitalization, recovery, cases, and viral clearance. 29 studies show statistically significant improvements in isolation.

	Studies	*Prophylaxis*	*Early treatment*	*Late treatment*	*Patients*	*Authors*
All studies	63	**86%** [75-92%]	**69%** [54-79%]	**40%** [24-52%]	26,422	613
Peer-reviewed	44	**86%** [73-92%]	**70%** [52-81%]	**43%** [21-59%]	17,082	479
Randomized Controlled Trials	31	**84%** [25-96%]	**64%** [48-74%]	**30%** [2-50%]	6,561	359

Percentage improvement with ivermectin treatment

- There is evidence of a negative publication bias, and the probability that an ineffective treatment generated results as positive as the 63 studies is estimated to be 1 in 1 trillion.

In the face of that evidence of ivermectin efficacy, the FDA claims that "[c]urrently available data do not show ivermectin is effective against COVID-19."[1254] There is no other way to put it: the FDA is lying.

The FDA misleadingly portrayed ivermectin as a treatment for animals, with the message: "You are not a horse. You are not a cow. Seriously, y'all. Stop it."

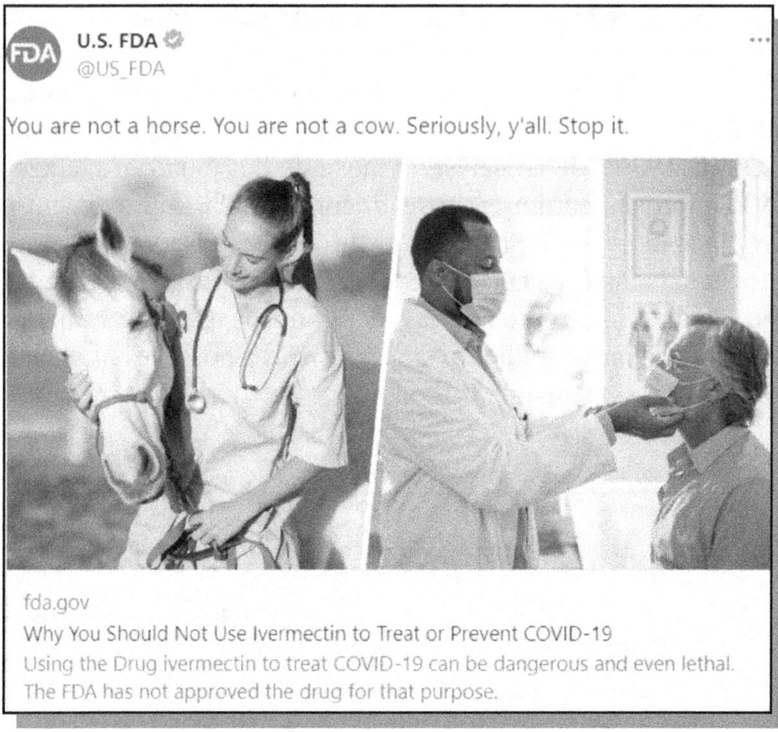

August 21, 2021, FDA Twitter Post

The FDA's campaign against ivermectin was utterly fraudulent. The misleading campaign, complete with a picture of a horse, suggested it was a veterinary medicine and not fit for humans. The FDA ominously warned that "[u]sing the drug ivermectin to treat COVID-19 can be dangerous and even lethal." In reality, ivermectin is an FDA approved drug that has been proven safe and effective for human use. In 2015, the Nobel Prize for Medicine was given for the discovery of ivermectin.

In the case of *Apter v. HHS*, several doctors sued the FDA for its recommendation against taking ivermectin as a remedy for COVID-19. The doctors bringing the lawsuit alleged that the FDA's recommendation that ivermectin not be used to treat COVID-19 interfered with the doctors' ability to exercise professional medical judgment in practicing medicine. The FDA recommendation against ivermectin also harmed the doctors' reputations. One doctor was referred for discipline to two state medical boards for prescribing ivermectin to treat COVID-19. Those disciplinary charges were founded on the FDA recommendation against ivermectin. The doctors further stated that pharmacies followed the FDA recommendation and refused to fill ivermectin prescriptions for their patients. One of the doctors lost her admitting privileges at a hospital after she tweeted about using ivermectin to treat patients with COVID-19. Another doctor lost his position at a medical school and a hospital because he promoted the use of ivermectin.

Andrew L. Schlafly, the Counsel for the Association of American Physicians and Surgeons (AAPS) wrote a powerful and to-the-point amicus curiae brief filed in *Apter v. HHS*, in the U.S. District Court for the Southern District of Texas. In 12 pages, he deconstructed the FDA's campaign against ivermectin and revealed that the FDA emperor has no clothes. The AAPS brief states, in pertinent part:

> Defendant FDA has improperly exploited misunderstandings about the legality and prevalence of off-label uses of medication, in order to mislead courts, state medical boards, and the public into thinking there is anything improper about off-label prescribing. Not only is off-label prescribing fully proper, legal, and commonplace, but it is also absolutely necessary in order to give effective care to patients. It has never been proper for the FDA to interfere with that essential part of

the practice of medicine, and the FDA knows it. Yet it has engaged in a campaign of interference with the proper use by physicians of ivermectin, which has long been approved as fully safe for human use.

***

Defendant FDA lacks both the authority and the expertise to practice medicine, interfere with the practice of medicine, guide the practice of medicine, or advise about the practice of medicine. Federal law is clear about this, and common sense reinforces it. FDA employees are not practicing physicians, and are not treating patients. FDA employees, for the most part, are not even licensed physicians.

***

It follows, from the recognition by the Supreme Court that off-label uses are ethically required, that it is wholly improper for the FDA to interfere with such off-label practices. Ivermectin has long been a medication fully approved as safe for humans. That is where the FDA's authority begins and ends. Beyond that, it is exclusively a matter of state law in authorizing physicians to prescribe approved-as-safe medications for the benefit of their patients. When a physician is fully licensed by a state to practice medicine, then he has the authority without interference by the FDA to prescribe an approved-as-safe medication such as ivermectin to treat Covid-19 or any other illness.

***

> The FDA is without authority to interfere with prescriptions by physicians of this approved as-safe medication for treating Covid-19 or any other condition.[1255]

Despite the soundness of the doctors' arguments, the federal district court ruled against the doctors in *Apter v. HHS*.[1256] The district court decided that the FDA has the authority to recommend against ivermectin. The doctors appealed. And the U.S. Court of Appeals for the Fifth Circuit reversed the district court ruling. The court of appeals ruled that the FDA acted outside its authority by recommending against taking ivermectin.[1257] The legal term for acting outside one's authority is *ultra vires*. The court ruled that the FDA has no authority to endorse, denounce, or advise medication. The FDA may inform, announce, and apprise—but it cannot go beyond that to recommend for or against a medical treatment.

The court of appeals ruled that recommendation and medical advice are the province of the medical profession. The court concluded that the "FDA is not a physician. It has authority to inform, announce, and apprise—but not to endorse, denounce, or advise." What the FDA did by giving medical advice for the public not to take ivermectin was the practice of medicine, and the FDA was not qualified to do that. The FDA acted *ultra vires*. Even tweets posted on Twitter violated the law. The court stated that "[e]ven tweet-sized doses of personalized medical advice are beyond FDA's statutory authority." The FDA acted illegally by advising the public not to take ivermectin to treat COVID-19.

45 Fake News About Ivermectin

The media campaign against Hydroxychloroquine and Ivermectin knows no bounds. The conspirators behind the COVID-19 vaccine gambit must not allow a safe and effective remedy for COVID-19. Writing for National File, Andrew White reported that "*Rolling Stone* recently ran a story about an Oklahoma hospital that was supposedly overwhelmed with ivermectin overdoses. Shortly thereafter, the hospital issued a statement completely rebuking the claims made in the *Rolling Stone* story."[1258] White explained:

> *Rolling Stone* ran a story in which they claimed that a hospital in Oklahoma was so overwhelmed with ivermectin overdoses that they were unable to treat patients for gunshot wounds. "The rise in people using ivermectin, an anti-parasitic drug usually reserved for deworming horses or livestock, as a treatment or preventative for Covid-19 has emergency rooms "so backed up that gunshot victims were having hard times getting" access to health facilities, an emergency room doctor in Oklahoma said.
>
> This week, Dr. Jason McElyea told KFOR[1259] the

overdoses are causing backlogs in rural hospitals, leaving both beds and ambulance services scarce," wrote *Rolling Stone*'s Peter Wade.[1260]

Shortly afterwards, the Northeastern Health System – Sequoyah issued a statement completely rebuking the *Rolling Stone* article. In the statement, it was revealed that the doctor quoted in the *Rolling Stone* story was not even employed with NHS Sequoyah, had not worked at the location in months, and had not treated any patients related to ivermectin. The statement further debunks the *Rolling Stone* piece by stating that no patients have been turned away and that no ivermectin overdoses had occurred.

> Although Dr. Jason McElyea is not an employee of NHS Sequoyah, he is affiliated with a medical staffing group that provides coverage for our emergency room.
>
> With that said, Dr. McElyea has not worked at our Sallisaw location in over 2 months.
>
> NHS Sequoyah has not treated any patients due to complications related to taking ivermectin. This includes not treating any patients for ivermectin overdose.
>
> All patients who have visited our emergency room have received medical attention as appropriate. Our hospital has not had to turn

> away any patients seeking emergency care.
>
> We want to reassure our community that our staff is working hard to provide quality healthcare to all patients. We appreciate the opportunity to clarify this issue and as always, we value our community's support.

> After the hospital issued the rebuking statement, *Rolling Stone* was forced to correct their story, but critics found the move dissatisfying. "*Rolling Stone* casually drops in an update to their article which is the statement from NHS that effectively boils down to "Everything you're going to read below is based off an unsubstantiated report from a guy that doesn't work with us and is lying to everyone reading this.", one user tweeted regarding the sham story.[1261]

Why would *Rolling Stone* not retract the story? Why was the discredited story repeated by the mainstream media outlets? The reason is that it is part of a smear compaign to discredit ivermectin as a safe and effective treatment for COVID-19.

Why would the mainstream media want to smear ivermectin? The FDA and the vaccine makers have a problem. And that problem is that scientific studies have proven that ivermectin is a safe and effective (and inexpensive) treatment for COVID-19. To continue the EUA for the COVID-19 vaccines, they need to maintain that "that there is no adequate, approved, and available alternative to the product for diagnosing, preventing, or treating such disease or condition."[1262] The FDA controls what is approved. All the FDA needs to do is not approve ivermectin, and the EUA for the COVID-19 vaccines continue. And so, ivermectin must go. Thus, the FDA has announced that "The FDA has not authorized or approved ivermectin for the treatment or prevention of COVID-19 in people or animals."[1263] The FDA falsely claims that there is no available data to show that ivermectin is effective against COVID-19.[1264] That is a lie. Sixty-three studies have established the safety and effectiveness of ivermectin in treating COVID-19.[1265]

46 Operation Mockingbird Vaccine

At the same time that the government and media are suppressing ivermectin and hydroxychloroquine, the media is working with the government to promote the COVID-19 vaccines. The media is completely under the control of the government. It is a virtual propaganda arm of the government. It is infiltrated by the CIA. It has been revealed in past Congressional testimony that the CIA has code-named their control of the media *Operation Mockingbird*.

Barbara Honegger, who was Assistant to the Chief Domestic Policy Adviser to the President, was present at a cabinet meeting during the first weeks (February 1981) of the Reagan Administration in the Roosevelt Room in the West Wing of the White House when CIA Director William Casey stated: "We'll know our disinformation program is a success when everything the American public believes is false."[1266] Honegger reported the statement to her close friend Senior White House correspondent Sarah McClendon, who in turn made it public without naming Honegger as the source.

In or about 2013, people posted on the internet their skepticism of the authenticity of the Casey quote. On November 25, 2014, Barbara Honegger came forward to verify its genuineness by revealing that she was the source for the quote. Honegger stated:

> I am the source for this quote, which was indeed said by CIA Director William Casey at an early February 1981 meeting of the newly elected President Reagan with his new cabinet secretaries to report to him on what they had learned about their agencies in the first couple of weeks of the administration. The meeting was in the Roosevelt Room in the West Wing of the White House, not far from the Cabinet Room. I was present at the meeting as Assistant to the chief domestic policy adviser to the President. Casey first told Reagan that he had been astonished to discover that over 80 percent of the 'intelligence' that the analysis side of the CIA produced was based on open public sources like newspapers and magazines. As he did to all the other secretaries of their departments and agencies, Reagan asked what he saw as his goal as director for the CIA, to which he replied with this quote, which I recorded in my notes of the meeting as he said it. Shortly thereafter I told Senior White House correspondent Sarah McClendon, who was a close friend and colleague, who in turn made it public. Barbara Honegger.[1267]

Note the two significant things revealed by CIA Director Casey: 1) The CIA relies on public sources for over 80 percent of its intelligence; and 2) he, as Director of the CIA, stated that his goal was to provide disinformation to the American public, and that his success in that goal would be when everything the public believed was false. Why wouldn't Director Casey make it his goal to fix the woeful intelligence gathering of the CIA that he was astonished to discover? Because he understood that intelligence gathering is not the primary purpose of the CIA, and therefore it was not a priority to fix that deficiency. The CIA's chief purpose is to provide disinformation to the American public as a means of controlling the people. His goal, as director, was to further the CIA's principal purpose.

How is the CIA able to run a disinformation campaign to the degree that it can influence the American public? Dave McGowan, in his book, *Derailing Democracy*, quotes William Colby, former CIA Director, saying: "The Central Intelligence Agency owns everyone of any significance in the major media."[1268] A CIA operative discussed with Philip Graham, editor of the Washington Post, how easy it was for the CIA to buy influence over journalists willing to peddle CIA propaganda and cover stories. "You could get a journalist cheaper than a good call girl, for a couple hundred dollars a month."[1269]

Michael Collins Piper, in his book *Final Judgement*, reveals the CIA subversion of the American media, particularly with regard to covering up the CIA and Israeli Mossad connection to the assassination of President John F. Kennedy.[1270] Piper explained that the subversion of the American media by the CIA is pervasive. Piper cited award winning author David Wise, who, in his book, *The American Police State: The Government Against the People*, exposed the role of the CIA in manipulating the media:

> The CIA's contacts with the publishing world were not confined to attempts to suppress books. Through the U.S. Information Agency as a 'cut-out,' the CIA subsidized major publishers to produce books, some of which were then sold in the United States bearing no government imprint to warn the unsuspecting purchaser. In 1967 publisher Frederick A. Praeger conceded he had published 'fifteen or sixteen' books for the CIA. By the mid-sixties, more than $1 million had been spent by the government on its 'book development'

> program. The Senate intelligence committee estimated that by 1967, the CIA had produced, sponsored, or subsidized 'well over 1,000 books' here and abroad.[1271]

Wise reveals that "the CIA operated two news services of its own in Europe. These 'proprietaries,' or CIA cover companies, serviced American newspapers; one had more than thirty U.S. subscribers."[1272] The thirty U.S. subscribers to whom Wise refers are newspapers and other publishing concerns. Those U.S. media outlets then parrot the CIA propaganda, which, in turn, influences public opinion and behavior.

Indeed, it seems that the Washington Post had developed into a virtual department of the CIA. Alex Constantine reveals:

> Former Washington Post publisher Philip Graham "believing that the function of the press was more often than not to mobilize consent for the policies of the government, was one of the architects of what became a widespread practice: the use and manipulation of journalists by the CIA" This scandal was known by its code name Operation MOCKINGBIRD. Former Washington Post reporter Carl Bernstein cites a former CIA deputy director as saying, "It was widely known that Phil Graham was someone you could get help from."[1273]

Carl Bernstein, in his 1977 article for Rolling Stone, *The CIA and the Media*, recounts a briefing of members of the Senate Intelligence Committee by William B. Bader, former CIA intelligence officer, who was hired by the Senate to head the Senate investigation into CIA influence in the media. Bader told the Senate Committee members: "There is quite an incredible spread of relationships. You don't need to manipulate Time magazine, for example, because there are [Central Intelligence]

Agency people at the management level."[1274] Bader's investigation provided a low-end estimate of 400 journalists who were CIA shills. Those 400+ "working journalists" included all areas of news reporting, from top management to reporters, editors, correspondents, and photographers. The CIA influence also reached into book publishers, trade publications, and newsletters.[1275] Bernstein explained that "Colby, Elder and Rogovin also implored individual members of the [Senate] committee to keep secret what the staff had found. 'There were a lot of representations that if this stuff got out some of the biggest names in journalism would get smeared,' said another source."[1276] Bernstein revealed that a senator who was the object of the Agency's lobbying later said: "From the CIA point of view this was the highest, most sensitive covert program of all.... It was a much larger part of the operational system than has been indicated."[1277]

Why is the CIA so adamant that the lid be kept on their influence over the media? Because the media is parroting propaganda that influences the very thoughts of the population. The media is used not to inform the people, but rather as a tool of control over the masses. The CIA subversion of the media has turned the idea of a free press into a charade. Thomas Jefferson once said that "the man who reads nothing at all is better educated than the man who reads nothing but newspapers." That statement is as true today as it was in Jefferson's day.

The CIA subversion of the media is effective because it is generally not known. The general population of the United States believes that the major media outlets are providing them with unbiased news. In fact, nothing could be further from the truth. The false belief that the news media is independent and free from government influence is why the government propaganda spewed from the major media outlets is so effective. The major media outlets are part and parcel of a mass mind control operation. Michael Rivero explains:

> As terrible as it is to live in a nation where the press in known to be controlled by the government, at least one has the advantage of knowing the bias is present, and to adjust for it. In the United States of America, we are taught from birth that our press is free from such government meddling. This is an insidious lie about the very nature of the news institution in this country. One that allows the government to lie to us while denying the very fact of the lie itself.[1278]

One must understand that the CIA is simply a tool of mass disinformation under the control of the Jewish elite. Government is force; we must look behind the labels (e.g., CIA) to those who control that force. The CIA, as all agencies of government, are the means of control, but the true controllers are hidden behind the scenes, pulling the strings in secret.

Edward Bernays was named one of the 100 most influential Americans of the 20th century by Life magazine. Bernays was the nephew to the wicked founder of psychoanalysis, Sigmund Freud. Bernays was a Jewish expert on propaganda, who was in the service of the powerful elite. Bernays famously wrote in 1928:

> The conscious and intelligent manipulation of the organized habits and opinions of the masses is an important element in democratic society. Those who manipulate this unseen mechanism of society constitute an invisible government which is the true ruling power of our country. We are governed, our minds are molded, our tastes formed, our ideas suggested, largely by men we have never heard of. This is a logical result of the way in which our democratic society is organized. Vast numbers of human beings must cooperate in this manner if

> they are to live together as a smoothly functioning society. Our invisible governors are, in many cases, unaware of the identity of their fellow members in the inner cabinet. They govern us by their qualities of natural leadership, their ability to supply needed ideas and by their key position in the social structure. Whatever attitude one chooses toward this condition, it remains a fact that in almost every act of our daily lives, whether in the sphere of politics or business, in our social conduct or our ethical thinking, we are dominated by the relatively small number of persons a—trifling fraction of our hundred and twenty million—who understand the mental processes and social patterns of the masses. It is they who pull the wires which control the public mind.[1279]

Be mindful that Bernays was a proponent of propaganda as a tool to manipulate the behavior of the masses. He was in the service of the very "invisible governors" whom he praised for their "natural leadership" and "ability to supply the needed ideas." Bernays explained matter-of-factly that "it is they who pull the wires which control the public mind." Bernays felt that these governors were necessary for "the orderly functioning of our group life."[1280]

In order for the "invisible governors" to manipulate the population through propaganda, it is necessary for them to control the mass media. Evidence presented before United States Congress in 1917 proved that J.P. Morgan, who was the American agent for the international Jewish (Rothschild) banking interests, purchased control over the major media companies in the United States.[1281] That control continues today. According to some researchers, Jews own or control 96% of the world's major media outlets to include newspapers, television, movies, and other media.[1282]

On February 17, 1917, Congressman Oscar Callaway presented the following facts before the United States Congress which explained the successful efforts of J.P. Morgan and his cabal to control public opinion in order to involve the United States in World War I.

> Mr. CALLAWAY. Mr. Chairman, under unanimous consent, I insert in the record at this point a statement showing the newspaper combination, which explains their activity in this war matter, just discussed by the gentleman from Pennsylvania,
>
> [Mr. Moore]: In March, 1915, the J.P. Morgan interests, the steel, shipbuilding, and powder interests, and their subsidiary organizations, got together 12 men high up in the newspaper world and employed them to select the most influential newspapers in the United States and sufficient number of them to control generally the policy of the daily press of the United States.
>
> These 12 men worked the problem out by selecting 170 newspapers, and then began, by an elimination process, to retain only those necessary for the purpose of controlling the general policy of the daily press throughout the country. They found it was only necessary to purchase the control of 25 of the greatest newspapers.
>
> The 25 papers were agreed upon; emissaries were sent to purchase the policy, national and international, of these papers; an agreement was reached; the policy of the papers was bought, to be paid for by the month; an editor was furnished for each paper to properly supervise and edit

> information regarding the questions of preparedness, militarism, financial policies, and other things of national and international nature considered vital to the interest of the purchasers.
>
> This contract is in existence at the present time, and it accounts for the news columns of the daily press of the country being filled with all sorts of preparedness argument and misrepresentations as to the present condition of the United States Army and Navy and the possibility and probability of the United States being attacked by foreign foes.
>
> This policy also included the suppression of everything in opposition to the wishes of the interests served. The effectiveness of this scheme has been conclusively demonstrated by the character of stuff carried in the daily press throughout the country since March, 1915. They have resorted to anything necessary to commercialize public sentiment and sandbag the national congress into making extravagant and wasteful appropriations for the Army and Navy under the false pretense that it was necessary. Their stock argument is that it is "patriotism." They are playing on every prejudice and passion of the American people.[1283]

How successful have the Jews and their fellow conspirators been in controlling public knowledge and opinion? Read and weep over the sad truth as John Swinton, the former Chief of Staff for the New York Times, explains the state of the supposed free press in the United States in a speech before the New York Press Club in 1953.

> There is no such thing, at this date of the world's

> history, in America, as independent press. You know it and I know it. There is not one of you who dares to write your honest opinions, and if you did, you know beforehand that it would never appear in print. I am paid weekly for keeping my honest opinion out of the paper I am connected with. Others of you are paid similar salaries for similar things, and any of you who would be so foolish as to write honest opinions would be out on the streets looking for another job. If I allowed my honest opinions to appear in one issue of my paper, before twenty-four hours my occupation would be gone. The business of the journalists is to destroy the truth; to lie outright; to pervert; to vilify; to fawn at the feet of mammon, and to sell his country and his race for his daily bread. You know it and I know it and what folly is this toasting an independent press? We are the tools and vassals of rich men behind the scenes. We are the jumping jacks, they pull the strings and we dance. Our talents, our possibilities and our lives are all the property of other men. We are intellectual prostitutes.[1284]

On March 26, 2022, Dr Joseph Mercola wrote an article for *The Expose*.[1285] In it, he reveals that the U.S. Government has coopted mainstream news organizations. The federal government paid news agencies to push the COVID-19 vaccines through interviews of "experts." That resulted in many news articles and broadcasts that were essentially COVID-19 vaccine advertisements disguised as news.

HHS released documents to *The Blaze* in response to a Freedom of information Act request. Those documents revealed that the government had paid more than $1 billion to hundreds of media organizations to produce TV, print, radio, and social media advertising to convince the public to vaccinate. Dr. Mercola states:

> Virtually every one of the news organizations paid by HHS, including ABC, NBC, CBS, CNN, MSNBC, The Washington Post, Los Angeles Times and the New York Post, covered stories about the vaccines and did not disclose they had accepted taxpayer dollars to support the vaccine effort.[1286]

While the media companies protest that their news organizations are immune from the influence of government advertisers, the reality is quite different. He who pays the piper calls the tune. The media is subservient to its financial overlords.

> It's not hard to imagine that a large news organization promoting vaccinations through their advertising department would not look kindly on editorial staff who choose to report facts that do not align with large sums of money spent by advertisers. You can guess what the editorial staff may be told to write.[1287]

There were many examples of news stories that seemed more like government propaganda than news reports. News articles about the COVID-19 vaccines were sprinkled with quotes from NIAID Director Anthony Fauci, CDC director Dr. Rochelle Walensky, and HHS Secretary Xavier Becerra falsely touting the safety and effectiveness of the vaccines.[1288] Often, news articles and broadcasts were thinly disguised advertising published as "news." Government officials, particularly Anthony Fauci, acted as shills pushing the COVID-19 vaccines on behalf of the pharmaceutical companies.[1289]

Even supposedly conservative news outlets were coopted to push the vaccine. For example, a Newsmax article in November

2021 ran an editorial against the vaccine mandate. But in the article, the author supported the vaccine campaign by falsely claiming that the vaccine has been proven safe and effective. The piece contained the message that "Newsmax has encouraged citizens, especially those at risk, to get immunized."[1290]

Dr. Mercola reveals that "[t]he government collaborated with social media influencers … and engaged 'experts' to be interviewed and promote the mass vaccination campaign in the news." For example, articles in the *Los Angeles Times* featured "experts" advising people how to convince their vaccine-hesitant friends and relatives to change their minds.[1291] A *Washington Post* article promoted "the pro-vaccine messages people want to hear."[1292]

So, we have the government purchasing unsafe and ineffective vaccines, promoting them, and even abusing its authority by mandating them. The public is injured and killed by those vaccines.[1293] At the same time, pharmaceutical companies make immense profits from the carnage while enjoying immunity from liability granted to it by the government. The public pays through its taxes for its own destruction, with the pharmaceutical companies laughing all the way to the bank.

47 Canceling Doctors

State medical boards are at the ready to take action against doctors who go against the grain and try to treat their patients using drugs proven to be safe and effective (but officially disfavored) like ivermectin and hydroxychloroquine and eschewing toxic and ineffective (but officially favored) drugs like remdesivir. For example, the State of Maine medical board has suspended Dr. Meryl Nass's medical license.[1294]

Dr. Nass is a board-certified internist and a biological warfare epidemiologist and expert in anthrax.[1295] She has been a consultant to the government accountability office and the U.S. Director of National Intelligence on the prevention and mitigation of biological warfare and pandemics.[1296] She is also a scientific advisory board member of Robert Kennedy Jr.'s Children's Defense Fund. Dr. Nass has been successfully treating COVID-19 patients with hydroxychloroquine and ivermectin.

None of the patients under Dr. Nass's care have complained about her treatment advice. She has written extensively to expose the massive corruption in the medical community and the Federal Government by their suppression of safe and effective drugs for treating COVID-19. The suppression of safe drugs by the Federal Government and state medical boards is matched by their recommended treatment of patients using dangerous and ineffective drugs and vaccines like Remdesivir and the COVID-19 vaccines. And that is why the state medical board is coming after her.

Because she is a voice of reason in a sea of corruption, she finds herself in the Orwellian position of having her medical license suspended by the same unscrupulous Maine State Board of Medicine trying to suppress safe and effective treatments for COVID-19. The allegation by the state medical board is not that she has engaged in any malpractice. Indeed, no complaint has been brought against her by any of her patients. The board is retaliating against her as an object lesson to all physicians who would dare to buck the pharmaceutical companies' efforts to push their unsafe and ineffective drugs on the unsuspecting public. At the same time, they suppress safe and effective alternatives.

The State Board of Medical Licensure alleges that Dr. Nass's advocacy for the treatment of COVID-19 with ivermectin and hydroxychloroquine constituted "public dissemination of misinformation." They are using the tried and true method of the communist international to brand her as a crazy person for the temerity to go against their efforts to suppress safe and effective treatments. Dr. Nass has been ordered to undergo a psychological examination by a psychologist chosen by the state medical board to ensure she is fit to continue treating patients. This is a direct attack on her First Amendment Right to freely and publically express her medical opinion regarding the effective treatment of a disease.

The persecution of Dr. Nass reveals the corruption of state medical boards by medical professional non-profit organizations like the American Medical Association (AMA), the Board of Internal Medicine, the Board of Pediatrics, and the Federation of State Medical Boards. These organizations act as fronts for powerful pharmaceutical companies. Those private non-profit organizations have no legal authority over a physician, but they have a corrupting influence over state medical licensure boards. Those non-profit medical professional organizations have acted to suborn the state medical boards to suppress safe, effective, and inexpensive drugs and, in turn, promote the use of unsafe, dangerous, and expensive drugs and vaccines that enrich the pharmaceutical companies.

48 Child Abuse by Government Edict

The CDC Advisory Committee on Immunization Practices (ACIP) voted 15-0 to add the dangerous and ineffective COVID-19 vaccine to the childhood immunization schedule. Why would they do that? Steve Kirsch explains why the ACIP made the decision.

> The "emergency" can now end. They needed the emergency to be able to create EUA approval which gave them liability protection as long as the emergency existed. The emergency is no longer needed.
>
> The vaccine makers can now manufacture fully "approved" vaccines and have complete liability protection forever.
>
> The ACIP vote is just a recommendation. The CDC must add it to the schedule, but that's a slam dunk.[1297]

It is all about money and protecting the vaccine makers from liability for the death and destruction their ineffective and poisonous vaccines cause. When a product has a record like that of the COVID-19 vaccines, sowing carnage in its wake, the makers of that poisonous concoction will want liability protection. Of course, that is all part of the COVID-19 gambit.[1298]

Meryl Nass correctly summed up the ACIP decision:

> This is regulatory agencies and their advisory committees gone amuck. Time for the people to stop consenting. Now there is no question whether these are public health professionals carefully considering decisions for 334,000,000 people. They are careerists who love vaccines and are blind to the consequences of their actions. Blind is putting it charitably.[1299]

Steve Kirsch justifiably vents his righteous indignation at the corrupt cretins on the ACIP committee:

> These people do not want to see any data that shows the vaccines are not safe.
>
> I tried to ask the Chair of the ACIP committee, Grace Lee, if she wanted to see the Israeli safety data showing the vaccines aren't safe. She refused to answer my Yes or No question on this important data and called the cops on me (even though I didn't violate any laws). I have it all on video.[1300]

Steve Kirsch correctly points out that "[t]his means COVID shots will be required in certain states."[1301] States can set their own vaccination requirements and are not required to follow the CDC schedule. But Kirsch points out that many states simply adopt the entire CDC childhood schedule as a requirement to attend public school. Kirsch concludes:

> We all knew this was going to happen. I still don't

> know of a single healthy kid who died from COVID. We do know of healthy kids who die from the shot. This is insanity and few members of Congress have the guts to speak out about this.[1302]

Be mindful that the bivalent COVID-19 booster that the children will receive contains not one but two mRNA components. One component is for the original SARS-CoV-2 strain and the other contains mRNA for the BA.4 and BA.5 lineage of the omicron variant of SARS-CoV-2.[1303]

The Pfizer BioNTech bivalent booster containing the original mRNA for the SARS-CoV-2 strain along with the mRNA for the omicron variant was only tested in eight mice.[1304] And that booster was shown to be dangerous in those mouse tests.[1305] They plan on giving that booster to children. Below is the slide from the October 19, 2022 ACIP meeting showing their plans to give that dangerous booster to children.[1306]

Notice that they are going to be giving the Moderna bivalent booster to the 6-11-year-olds. When the mice injected with the Moderna bivalent booster were exposed to the omicron variant Ba.5, the mice got COVID! The Moderna vaccine was proven in the test on mice not to work. Igor Chudov reports "that all 10 of the [Moderna] bivalent-boosted mice got sick and had significant viral counts, not only in the noses but also in the lungs."[1307]

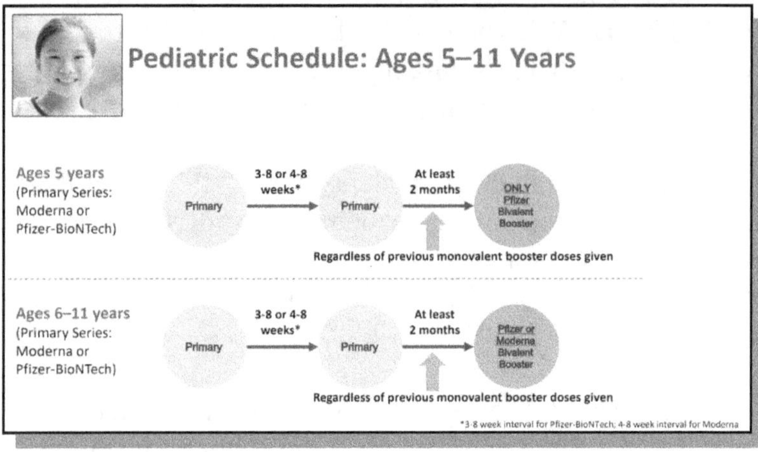
Pediatric Schedule: Ages 5–11 Years
Ages 5 years
(Primary Series:
Moderna or
Pfizer-BioNTech)
Primary
3-8 or 4-8
weeks*
Primary
At least
2 months
ONLY
Pfizer
Bivalent
Booster
Regardless of previous monovalent booster doses given
Ages 6–11 years
(Primary Series:
Moderna or
Pfizer-BioNTech)
Primary
3-8 or 4-8
weeks*
Primary
At least
2 months
Pfizer or
Moderna
Bivalent
Booster
Regardless of previous monovalent booster doses given
*3-8 week interval for Pfizer-BioNTech; 4-8 week interval for Moderna

49 None Dare Call it Genocide

Sir John Harrington famously said: "Treason doth never prosper. What's the reason? Why if it prosper, none dare call it treason." Giuseppe Vafanculo put a twist on that famous quote, reframing it: "None dare call it Genocide." Those behind the COVID-19 vaccine malice have prospered; thus, none dare call it genocide. But that is what it is. And there is proof it was premeditated.

Deadly Vaccine Batches

On October 31, 2021, investigative reporters from *The Expose* published a research investigation revealing that official data from the U.S. Government Vaccine Adverse Event Reporting Service (VAERS) showed 5% of the COVID-19 vaccines lots caused 100% of the COVID-19 deaths.[1308] The Expose report uncovered evidence that the vaccine makers, Moderna and Pfizer, each distributed a small set of immediately dangerous vaccine batches entirely differently from their more benign vaccine batches. The more immediately dangerous vaccine lots were distributed more widely across the United States. In contrast, the more benign vaccine lots that caused few injuries or adverse events were not given the same broad distribution.

The fact that the vaccine companies distributed the more immediately deadly "hot shot" batches differently from the more initially benign batches means that the companies knew that those immediately deadly batches were distinctly different before distribution. That means that it was planned out in advance to distribute widely the death and hospitalizations from the COVID-19 vaccines. This proves intent!

The Expose researchers asked:

> Why is it that the most harmful and deadly Covid-19 vaccines were distributed across the entire USA, whilst the least harmful and deadly were only ever distributed to a few states? Was this done on purpose?[1309]

The answers to their questions are obvious; think about it logically.

- The evidence establishes that the most immediately harmful "hot lots" of COVID-19 vaccines were **distributed more broadly** to more states than the more benign (in the short term) lots of COVID-19 vaccines.

- That necessarily means that the companies **purposely manufactured non-uniform formulations of their vaccines** while representing to the public that all COVID-19 vaccines from a given manufacturer were uniform in their formulation.

- That also means that the vaccine makers **identified** the more immediately dangerous vaccines as such.

- In order to identify the more immediately hazardous vaccines required that the vaccine makers **know** that certain lots were more immediately hazardous formulations of the COVID-19 vaccines.

• They **distributed** those known dangerous vaccine lots **differently**.

• That different distribution scheme means that the vaccine makers distributed the more immediately dangerous lots differently because they had a **purpose** in doing so.

• The different distribution scheme for the more immediately dangerous vaccine lots suggests that the vaccine manufacturers **knew** that those particular vaccine lots would imminently kill and hospitalize more people per lot over a broader area of the U.S.

• This is evidence of **premeditated intent to injure and kill** the public by distributing a dangerous vaccine broadly across the country that the vaccine makers knew would kill and hospitalize the recipients shortly after being vaccinated. It seems that their purpose was to spread the death and injury broadly to conceal the deliberate suffering caused by the vaccines that would be camouflaged by the many uninjured vaccine recipients.

The more deadly batches were being spread broadly over the country to disperse the adverse events more evenly. A concentration of adverse events in any given area would raise concerns. But a sprinkling of adverse events among those who had none could be explained away as unusual. The benign vaccine recipients could say that they received the COVID-19 vaccine with no adverse symptoms.

They could not have a concentration of persons receiving vaccines being hospitalized and dying all at once. So they sprinkled the "hot lots" broadly across the country.

The day after publication of the report by *The Expose*, Dr Mike Yeadon, former Vice-President of Pfizer, explained that the report has astounding implications. Dr. Yeadon stated:

> This information about different safety profiles of different "lots" (batches of finished product of covid19 vaccines) is completely without precedent.[1310]

Dr. Yeadon said that it is unimaginable that having batches of vaccines benign and others deadly could happen by mistake. He said:

> Errors made in the final steps of manufacturing which resulted in certain batches bring reasonably benign & others extraordinarily deadly. I just cannot imagine the kind of mistakes which could produce such radically different clinical profiles.[1311]

Dr. Yeadon's only rational conclusion is that there was intentional modification of the vaccines.

> At some point in manufacturing, someone or some entity actively modified what was being filled into vials, and it was this which resulted in extreme skew of clinical safety profile.[1312]

Dr. Yeadon said that it is possibly intentional conduct by the vaccine makers. Indeed, how could anyone conclude otherwise given the different distribution schemes for the immediately dangerous lots of vaccines? Dr. Yeadon concluded:

> There has been so much truly awful behaviour of "elites" that I'm simply not willing (as I would have historically) to dismiss the possibility that this has been done on purpose.[1313]

Dr. Yeadon called for all COVID-19 vaccinations to cease.

> What I do know, and this is a test of whether there's the slightest sign of integrity from these companies as well as the regulatory agencies, is that all use of the affected produce must immediately cease, all batches of drug substance & lots of drug product should cease.
>
> The materials should be recalled to a place of stable storage & an intense analytical investigation initiated.
>
> Unless factors are found which adequately explain the huge differences in clinical adverse event profiles, administration to humans must not restart.
>
> If the manufacturers do not exhibit sufficient control of drug product, the authorisation they hold from various regulatory authorities are utterly voided.
>
> Just when you thought this debacle couldn't possibly get any worse, it gets much worse.
>
> Expect to hear more about this.
>
> Meanwhile, who in their right mind would roll up their sleeve?[1314]

What I found interesting about Dr. Yeadon's review of *The Expose* report was that he only addressed the disparity in the deadliness of the vaccines. He did not address the elephant in the room. He did not mention that the drug makers distributed the immediately deadly vaccines entirely differently. That different distribution indicates that the drug makers knew which batches were deadly. Otherwise, they would not know which batches to distribute more broadly. That fact alone shows intent to harm and kill. Dr. Yeadon, Pfizer's former vice president, ignored the evidence implicating Pfizer and Moderna in premeditated criminal conduct.

Dr. Yeadon calls for a cessation of vaccination while a safety investigation is conducted. He should be calling for a cessation of vaccination while a criminal investigation is conducted.

Karl Denninger is a technology expert, businessman, and political activist who is credited with starting the Tea Party Movement. He runs a blog called The Market Ticker. On November 2, 2021, Karl Denninger posted an article that characterized the allegation that the vaccine makers were distributing certain bathes of COVID-19 vaccines to kill and injure people, a tinfoil hat conspiracy theory.[1315]

Denninger set out to disprove that theory and show just how ridiculous it was. But, as he used his software skills to mine the Vaccine Adverse Events Reporting System (VAERS) data, he came to a disturbing conclusion. He found that, indeed, the vaccine makers had created a certain small number of batches of vaccines that caused almost all of the deaths and adverse events. Denninger explained:

> What originally got my attention was the tinfoil hat crowd screaming about lots being intentionally distributed to certain people to kill them — in other words certain Covid-19 vaccine lots were for all intents and purposes poisoned. That was wildly unlikely so I set out to disprove it and apply some broom handles to the tinfoil hatters heads. What I found, however, was both interesting and deeply disturbing.[1316]

Denninger was flummoxed by his findings that a few lots

of COVID-19 vaccines were causing almost all of the deaths and hospitalizations. He was further mystified that the same activity was displayed by the makers of each of the three COVID-19 vaccines used in the U.S. Denninger found those facts very troubling. How could the same manufacturing anomaly happen across all three manufacturers unless it was part of a plan to do so?

Notice in the charts prepared by Denninger that all three of the COVID-19 vaccine manufactures did the same thing. They all manufactured a concentration of immediately deadly lots of COVID-19 vaccines. This phenomenon cannot be by chance. Denninger points out that these are independent companies; the concentration of deadly vaccines into a few batches by all companies "cannot be explained as random chance." It is a joint effort; the data shows a conspiracy to kill and injure.

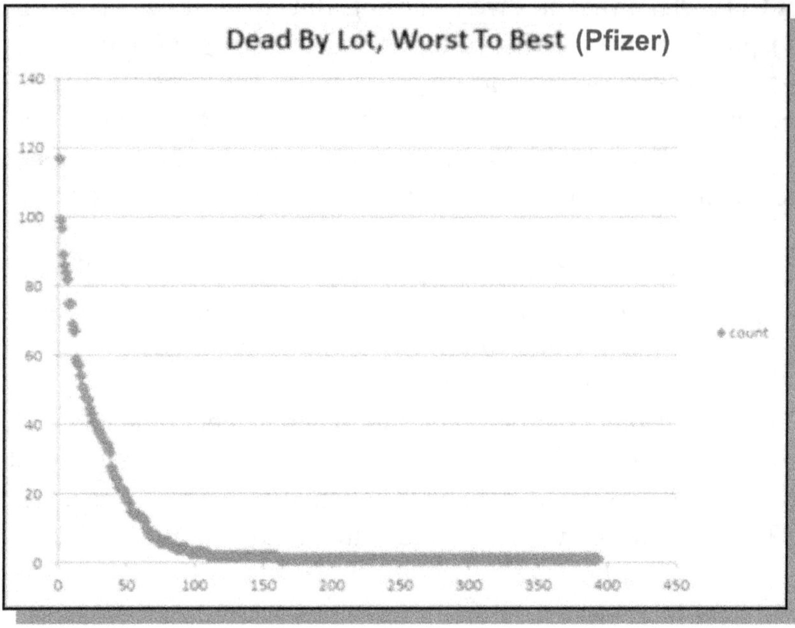
Dead By Lot, Worst To Best (Pfizer)
140
120
100
80
60
40
20
0
0
50
100
150
200
250
300
350
400
450
count

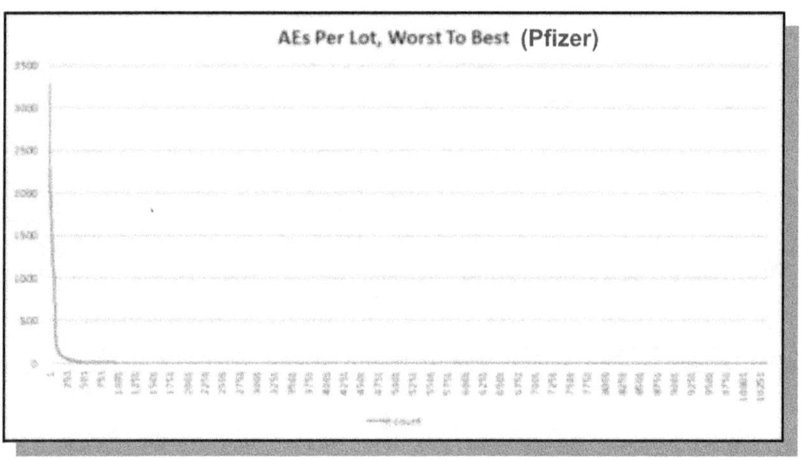
AEs Per Lot, Worst To Best (Pfizer)

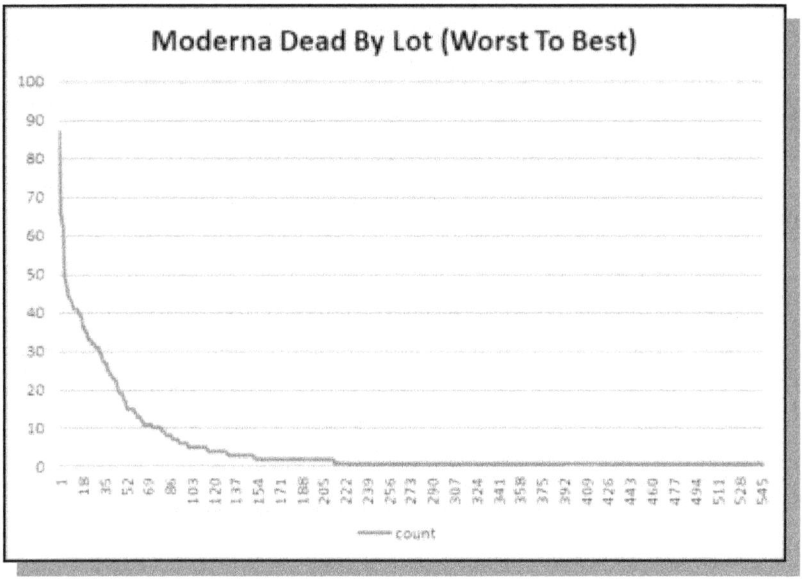
Moderna Dead By Lot (Worst To Best)
100
90
80
70
60
50
40
30
20
10
0
1 18 35 52 69 86 103 120 137 154 171 188 205 222 239 256 273 290 307 324 341 358 375 392 409 426 443 460 477 494 511 528 545
count

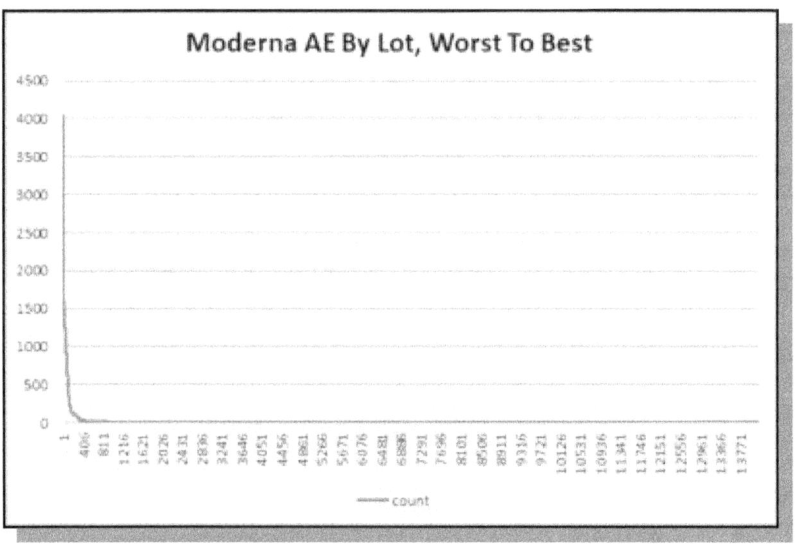
Moderna AE By Lot, Worst To Best
4500
4000
3500
3000
2500
2000
1500
1000
500
0
count

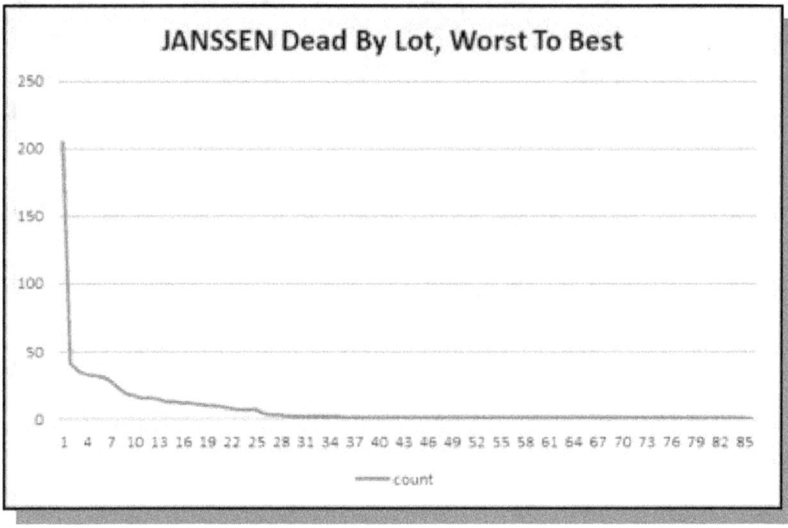
JANSSEN Dead By Lot, Worst To Best
count

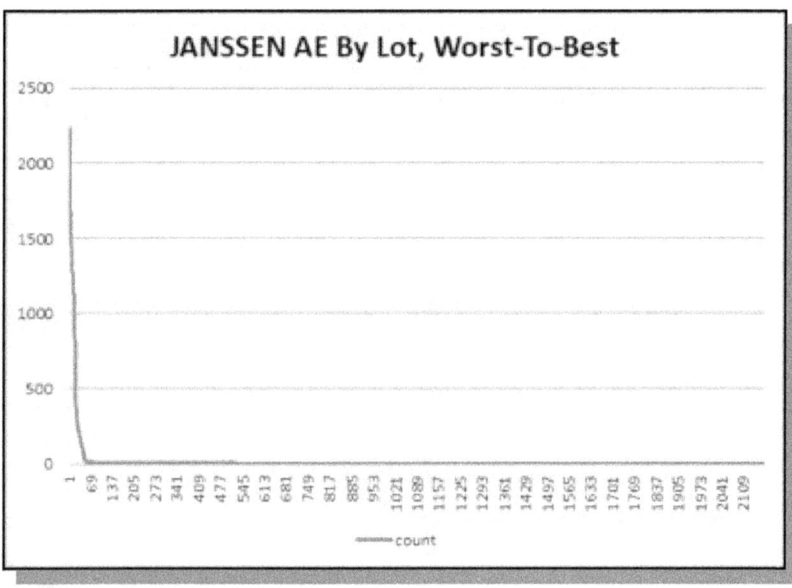
JANSSEN AE By Lot, Worst-To-Best
count

Denninger was also troubled that the CDC, which runs the VAERS system, knows about this. He deduced that the CDC is keeping it hidden from the public by configuring VAERS in such a way to make it very difficult for the public to find the information. Notably, neither the CDC nor the FDA is doing anything about it. Denninger explains:

> Something is very wrong here folks and the people running VAERS either aren't looking on purpose, know damn well its happening and are saying nothing about it on purpose — never mind segregating the data in such a fashion that casual perusal of their downloads won't find it — or saw it immediately and suppressed reporting on purpose.[1317]

As with Dr. Mike Yeadon, Karl Denninger does not examine the elephant in the room other than to notice it is there. Denninger states: "Oh if you're interested the nastiest lot was literally everywhere in terms of states reporting adverse events against it; no, they didn't concentrate them in one state or region either." That statement is meaningless without giving it context. Denninger fails to explore the implications that the more immediately dangerous COVID-19 vaccine lots were distributed over a broad geographic area. In contrast, the more immediately benign vaccines were concentrated in particular geographic areas of distribution. That unique treatment for the more deadly vaccines suggests prior knowledge of their deadliness and an intent to spread the harm over a broad area.

Dr. Russell Blaylock is the author of The Blaylock Wellness Report newsletter. He is a nationally recognized board-certified neurosurgeon, health practitioner, author, and lecturer. For 26 years, Dr. Blaylock practiced neurosurgery and had a nutritional practice. He recently retired from his neurosurgical duties to devote full attention to nutritional research.

He thinks the unusual manufacturing and distribution of the "hot lots" is purposeful and clear proof that the pharmaceutical companies are intentionally injuring and killing people with their vaccines.

> The incidence of deaths and serious complications among these "hot lots" varied from over 1000% to several thousand percent higher than comparable safer lots. If you think this was by accident—think again. This is not the first time "hot lots" were, in my opinion, purposefully manufactured and sent across the nation—usually vaccines designed for children. In one such scandal, "hot lots" of a vaccine ended up all in one state and the damage immediately became evident. What was the manufacture's response? It wasn't to remove the deadly batches of the vaccine. He ordered his company to scatter the hot lots across the nation so that authorities would not see the obvious deadly effect. ... In my opinion these examples strongly suggest an intentional alteration of the production of the "vaccine" to include deadly batches.[1318]

In a 20203 Danish study involving 10,793,766 Pfizer-BioNTech COVID-19 vaccine doses administered to 4,026,575 persons involving 52 different vaccine batches, it was found that 71% of adverse events were caused by only 4% of the vaccine batches.[1319] For comparison, one batch (EWG6126) caused an adverse event in one out of every 1,000 injections, while another batch (EJ6134) caused an adverse event in one of every 20 injections.[1320] That is quite a disparity.

Government Complicity

We now have proof that persons and entities within the federal government purposely planned to poison and kill the population through the COVID-19 vaccines. Documentation has been obtained that shows that the CDC contracted with General Dynamics to handle the reporting of the expected explosion of adverse events caused by the COVID-19 vaccines being reported in the Vaccine Adverse Event Reporting System (VAERS). The contract states that the CDC anticipated up to 1,000 reports per day would be filed after the rollout of the COVID-19 vaccines, with up to 40% of those reports serious. The following clause can be found on page 7 of the 47-page contract.

> IV. DESCRIPTION OF WORK:
> The contractor shall implement a staffing and operations plan focusing only on vaccine adverse event (VAE) reports after SARS-CoV-2 vaccines. The total number of reports received during periods of peak activity (which are not expected to reflect sustained activity) is expected to be 1,000 reports per day, with up to 40% of the reports serious in nature.

The contract was entered on August 27, 2020. At that time, there were no COVID-19 vaccines close to approval. Josh Guetzkow revealed that "the Pfizer/BioNTech vaccine trial phase 2/3 had only started a month earlier on July 27, [2020]."[1321] Guetzkow explains:

> This means that months before the EUA of any COVID vaccines, the CDC anticipated up to a 600% increase over the average annual number of VAERS reports in recent years with 8 times the rate of serious reports.[1322]

As shocking as that is, Guetzkow reveals something that confirms the death and disease from the vaccines were not just foreseen; they were intended. "There is no clause in the contract giving the CDC an option to cancel or suspend the contract in the event that vaccines would not be authorized."[1323] Guetzkow concluded, "[i]t certainly appears that by August 2020, the impending emergency use authorization of at least one COVID-19 vaccine was a foregone conclusion."

Indeed, the ultimate vaccine customer, the U.S. Government, agreed to pay billions of dollars to purchase vaccines before the passage of the EUA. The testing for safety and efficacy had not yet been completed on the vaccines when the government agreed to buy them. On July 22, 2020, Jared S. Hopkins and Chris Wack, writing for the Wall Street Journal, reported that "[t]he U.S. has agreed to pay Pfizer Inc. and BioNTech SE nearly $2 billion to secure 100 million doses of their experimental COVID-19 vaccine to provide to Americans free of charge."[1324]

The context for that announcement to pay $billions must be understood. As of that date, neither Pfizer nor BioNTech nor any other pharmaceutical company had yet proven that their proposed vaccines were safe or effective. It seems that the government and drug companies did not care. We were going to be vaccinated regardless. What do you think the chances were of the FDA not issuing an EUA for the experimental vaccines for which the U.S. Government had already paid $2 billion? The chances of the EUA not being allowed were slim to none, and slim has left town.

Hopkins and Wack revealed some important details. The U.S. Government had also agreed on or before July 2020 to acquire an additional 500 million vaccine doses. That is despite the fact, as reported by Hopkins and Wack at that date (July 22, 2020) "[n]o Covid-19 vaccine in development has proven to work safely yet, although dozens are being studied."[1325]

That means that the skids were greased for the emergency use authorization (EUA) for the vaccines to be granted. And the terms of the August 2020 contract mean that, in fact, both the government and the vaccine makers knew that the vaccines would be dangerous to the populace's health. It seems they planned that the COVID-19 vaccines would be dangerous.

The plan was in place for the COVID-19 vaccines to be granted EUA status, and they expected death and disease to soon follow. The contract expected 1,000 VAERS COIVD-19 vaccine reports to be filed daily, with "up to 40% of reports serious in nature." The contract with General Dynamics states that the government expects an explosion of VAERS reports from the COVID-19 vaccines. The agreement says that historically (2014-1018), there had been an annual average of 53,000 VAERS reports for all vaccines. But the contract states that the CDC expected six (6) times that rate from the COVID-19 vaccine alone.

The contract also reveals that typically 5% of reports from the U.S. were classified as serious. But the CDC expected that to shoot up to 40% for the COVID-19 vaccines. That is proof that the CDC knew the COVID-19 vaccines were dangerous before they were even authorized. The contract proves that the COVID-19 vaccines were not part of a plan that went awry; the vaccines did exactly what the government expected them to do: bring death and disease to an unsuspecting public.

Once the EUA was issued and the vaccines were administered, the news of the expected death and disease caused by the COVID-19 vaccines began to percolate within the populace. There was thus more resistance to the vaccine. President Biden noted this in his September 9, 2021 address announcing a federal worker vaccine mandate.

> This is a pandemic of the unvaccinated. And it's caused by the fact that despite America having an unprecedented and successful vaccination program, despite the fact that for almost five months free vaccines have been available in 80,000 different locations, we still have nearly 80 million Americans who have failed to get the shot.[1326]

The government responded to the increased public

resistance to the vaccines by instituting vaccine mandates. Biden stated: "As your President, I'm announcing tonight a new plan to require more Americans to be vaccinated, to combat those blocking public health." On September 9, 2021, Biden issued an order requiring all federal workers and contractors to be vaccinated with one of the COVID-19 vaccines. That was followed on November 4, 2021, by the federal government mandating through OSHA that employers who have 100 or more workers must require those workers to be vaccinated.[1327] In his September 9, 2021 announcement of his government employee vaccine mandate, he mischaracterized the COVID-19 vaccines as "safe, effective, and free." President Biden stated:

> If you want to work with the federal government and do business with us, get vaccinated. If you want to do business with the federal government, vaccinate your workforce.[1328]

Biden further stated that "the vaccines provide strong protections for the vaccinated." The rush to mandate vaccination was in the face of increasing evidence that the COVID-19 vaccines were dangerous and do not prevent infection or spread of COVID-19. Indeed, President Biden knows it is not true that a vaccinated person is protected from being infected and spreading COIVD-19. When announcing his Presidential Order, President Biden explained that he is mandating the vaccines to prevent unvaccinated persons from spreading COVID-19 to the vaccinated persons.

> The bottom line: We're going to protect vaccinated workers from unvaccinated co-workers. We're going to reduce the spread of COVID-19 by increasing the share of the workforce that is vaccinated in businesses all across America.[1329]

That statement makes no sense if the purpose of the

mandate is to prevent infection and spread of COVID-19. If the vaccines are effective, the vaccinated person should not be in danger of infection from an unvaccinated person. The whole objective of a vaccination is to protect the vaccine recipient from disease. But the President knows that the vaccines are not effective. President Biden impeaches his credibility and undermines his stated reason for the COVID-19 vaccination mandate of stopping the spread of the disease by admitting that the vaccines do not protect the vaccinated persons from COVID-19. He implicitly admits that his mandate will be ineffective in achieving its objective. But remember, Biden is using the power of the federal government to force people to be vaccinated. His stated reason is a lie. The real reason is to kill and injure people.

If one reads carefully the announcement requiring vaccinations for federal workers, President Biden acknowledged that he knows the vaccines do not prevent infection or spread of COVID-19. He follows the convention of calling those vaccinated persons who subsequently become ill with COVID-19 "breakthrough" cases. President Biden admits that he is instituting a mandatory vaccination program that only helps with the symptoms of COVID-19 for the vaccinated persons and will not stop its spread. The President of the United States announced a mandatory vaccination program to stop the spread of COVID-19 while acknowledging that the vaccines are ineffective in preventing the spread of the disease. A vaccinated person is just as likely to spread COVID-19 as an unvaccinated person. President Biden stated:

> I understand the anxiety about getting a “breakthrough” case. But as the science makes clear, if you’re fully vaccinated, you’re highly protected from severe illness, even if you get COVID-19.[1330]

President Biden further announced the need for a booster

shot program, which is an implicit admission that he knows the initial vaccination does not give lasting protection from the disease.

> As soon as they are authorized, those eligible will be able to get a booster right away in tens of thousands of site across the — sites across the country for most Americans, at your nearby drug store, and for free.[1331]

Both Biden's private sector and government vaccine mandates have been halted by court action.[1332] In light of the newly revealed VAERS contracts indicating that the COVID-19 vaccines were known to be dangerous, it is clear that the vaccine mandate attempts by the federal government were intended to force recalcitrant persons to be vaccinated so that more people would be killed and harmed.

The CDC knew within the first two months that the COVID-19 vaccines were killing people at a break-kneck speed never before seen from any other vaccine. By February 17, 2021, the VAERS mortality data from the CDC had shown that the COVID-19 vaccines were approximately 180 times (18,000%) more deadly than the flu vaccines.[1333] Yet, with that information in hand, the CDC kept hawking the vaccine. While bodies continued to pile up, the CDC's COVID-19 vaccine promotion continued unabated. Indeed, the government kept the accelerator to the floor and issued rules and orders mandating the dangerous vaccines. This shows a clear intent to kill. There is simply no other reasonable explanation.

The COVID-19 vaccines are dangerous and ineffective. After pushing millions to vaccinate, the CDC has now implicitly acknowledged that vaccines do not have any beneficial effect on preventing the infection or spread of COVID-19. On September 23, 2022, the CDC guidance was updated to note that "vaccination status is no longer used to inform source control, screening testing, or post-exposure recommendations."[1334]

50 The Emperor Has No Virus

The vaccine protocol is based on germ theory. Germ theory is the perfect scientific theory to control the masses. Many do not know that there is not a single study published in the history of medicine that has isolated a particle of virus that is capable of transmitting a disease from an ill person to a well person. The commonly accepted germ theory of illness spread by viruses is just a theory. It has never been proven. Indeed, there is significant evidence that it is wrong. The research paper written by Dr. Milton J. Rosenau, M.D., in 1919, stands as a refutation of the commonly accepted germ theory.[1335]

Most people, and even most doctors, are ignorant of Dr. Resonau's experiments. Dr. Resenau conducted experiments during the height of the Spanish Flu epidemic. He wanted to establish the means by which influenza was spread. He took 100 healthy volunteers who agreed to be exposed to the Spanish Flu. They were exposed to influenza under controlled conditions but none of them contracted the flu.

Dr. Rosenau explained that his medical team "proceeded rather cautiously at first by administering a pure culture of bacillus of influenza, Pfeiffer's bacillus, in a rather moderate amount, into the nostrils of a few of these volunteers." None of the volunteers came down with the flu.

He next obtained the extractions from the lungs of recently deceased flu victims. He then lined up 19 volunteers and used an atomizer to spray the suspensions of the flu extractions into the noses and into the eyes, and back into the throats of 19 volunteers. None of the volunteers contracted the flu.

Dr. Rosenau then obtained material and mucous secretions from the mouth and nose and throat and bronchi of live persons who had the Spanish Flu and transferred that to 10 volunteers by spraying the infected phlegm directly "into each nostril and into the throat, while inspiring, and on the eye." None of the volunteers got sick.

Next, Dr. Resenau's team used cotton swabs to transfer infected "material directly from nose to nose and from throat to throat, using a West tube for the throat culture, so as to get the material not only from the tonsils, but also from the posterior nasopharynx." None of the 19 volunteers who received the infected swabs got sick.

Dr. Rosenau explains that "[o]ur next experiment consisted in injections of blood. We took five donors, five cases of influenza in the febrile stage, some of them again quite early in the disease. We drew 20 'c.c. from the arm vein of each, making a total of 100 c.c, which was mixed and treated with 1 per cent, of sodium citrate. Ten c.c. of the citrated whole blood were injected into each of the ten volunteers. None of them took sick in any way."

Dr. Rosenau was not done. "Then we collected a lot of mucous material from the upper respiratory tract, and filtered it through Mandler filters. While these filters will hold back the bacteria of ordinary size, they will allow 'ultramicroscopic' organisms to pass. This filtrate was injected into ten volunteers, each one receiving 3.5 c.c. subcutaneously, and none of these took sick in any way."

Dr. Rosenau thought perhaps that influenza was passed by direct human contact. So he had 10 volunteers engage in social contact with persons known to be infected with influenza.

> The volunteer was led up to the bedside of the patient; he was introduced. He sat down alongside the bed of the patient. They shook hands, and. by instructions, he got as close as he conveniently could, and they talked· for five minutes. At the end of the five minutes, the patient breathed out as hard as he could, while the volunteer, muzzle to muzzle (in accordance with his instructions, about 2 inches between the two), received this expired -breath, and at the same time was breathing in as the patient breathed out. This they repeated five times, and they did it fairly faithfully in almost all of the instances. After they had done this for five times, the patient coughed directly into the face of the volunteer, face to face, five different times. ... After our volunteer had had this sort of contact with the patient, talking and chatting and shaking hands with him for five minutes, and receiving his breath five times, and then his cough five times directly in his face, he moved to the next patient whom we had selected, and repeated this, and so on, until this volunteer had had that sort of contact with ten different cases of influenza, in different stages of the disease, mostly fresh cases, none of them more than three days old.
>
> We will remember that each one of the ten volunteers had that sort of intimate contact with each one of the ten different influenza patients. They were watched carefully for seven days—and

none of them took sick in any way.[1336]

After failing to transmit influenza to any of the volunteers during his many experiments, Dr. Rosenau concluded that he did not know how influenza is contracted. "As a matter of fact, we entered the outbreak with a notion that we knew the cause of the disease, and were quite sure we knew how it was transmitted from person to person. Perhaps, if we have learned any thing, it is that we are not quite sure what we know about the disease."

Dr. Rosenau's experiments do not stand alone. Eleanor McBean reveals:

> Numerous experiments with germs conducted in the past have conclusively proven that bacteria does not and cannot produce disease in a healthy organism. Years ago, Dr. Pettenkofer, professor at the University of Vienna, came to the conclusion that germs alone do not produce pathology and for years defended his position from the lecture platform and in his writings. On more than one occasion he and his assistants swallowed the contents of glasses containing millions of living cholera germs. Dr. Thomas Powell of California, who is believed to have taken more germs than any other man, challenged his medical colleagues to produce a single disease by germ inoculation. He was inoculated with cholera germs, bubonic plague germs and bacteria of every description and which was fed to him in every kind of food, yet nothing happened. Read U.S. Government Bulletin "Hygienic Laboratory—Bulletin No. 123, Feb. 1921," for further proof on contagious diseases.[1337]

51 The Spanish Flu of 1918

If the Spanish Flu was not a contagious virus, how did it spread to kill 20 million people? In preparation for WWI, a massive military vaccination experiment involving several prior developed vaccines, one being an anti-meningitis vaccine, took place in Fort Riley, Kansas.[1338] It was no coincidence that the first "Spanish Flu" case was reported at Fort Riley, shortly after the first soldiers received their experimental vaccines. Dr. Sal Martingano, FICPA, explains:

> The fledgling pharmaceutical industry, sponsored by the 'Rockefeller Institute for Medical Research', had something they never had before – a large supply of human test subjects. Supplied by the U.S. military's first draft, the test pool of subjects ballooned to over 6 million men.
>
> Autopsies after the war proved that the 1918 flu was NOT a "FLU" at all. It was caused by random dosages of an experimental 'bacterial meningitis vaccine', which to this day, mimics flu-like symptoms. The massive, multiple assaults with additional vaccines on the unprepared immune systems of soldiers and civilians created a "killing

> field". Those that were not vaccinated were not affected.
>
> WWI U.S. soldiers were given 14 – 25 untested, experimental vaccines within days of each other, which triggered intensified cases of ALL the diseases at once. The doctors called it a new disease and proceeded to suppress the symptoms with additional drugs or vaccines.[1339]

Dr. Martingano reveals that when WW1 ended sooner than expected, it left huge quantities of unused experimental vaccines. A government campaign generated fear among the people that the returning soldiers would spread diseases to their families. The campaign was effective because the soldiers who were pumped full of the experimental toxic vaccines came home as weak invalids. Their illnesses were, in reality, symptoms of being poisoned by the vaccines. But the government convinced the public that the soldiers had contracted diseases from Europe. And for that reason, citizens should be vaccinated for their own health and safety. The U.S. citizens lined up to be vaccinated with the same vaccines that made the soldiers ill. As a result, millions of civilians died in the same manner as the soldiers. That is what caused the great "Spanish Flu of 1918."

Eleanor McBean, in her 1977 book, *Swine Flu Exposed*,[1340] gives her account of the "Spanish Flu."

> As has been stated before, all medical and non-medical authorities on vaccination agree that vaccines are designed to cause a mild case of the diseases they are supposed to prevent. But they also know and admit that there is no way whatsoever to predict whether the case will be mild or severe - even deadly. With this much uncertainty in dealing with the very lives of people,

it is very unscientific and extremely dangerous to use such a questionable procedure as vaccination.

Many vaccines also cause other diseases besides the one for which they are given. For instance, smallpox vaccine often causes syphilis, paralysis, leprosy, and cancer. (See the chapters on smallpox and plagues.) Polio shots, diphtheria toxin-antitoxin, typhoid vaccine, as well as measles, tetanus and all other shots often cause various other stages of disease such as post-vaccinal encephalitis (inflammation of the brain,) paralysis, spinal meningitis, blindness, cancer (sometimes within two years), tuberculosis, (two to twenty years after the shot,) arthritis, kidney disease, heart disease (heart failure sometimes within minutes after the shot and sometimes several hours later). Nerve damage and many other serious conditions also follow the injections.

When several shots are given (different vaccines) within a few days or a few weeks apart, they often trigger intensified cases of all the diseases at once, because the body cannot handle such a large amount of deadly poison being injected directly into the bloodstream. The doctors call it a new disease and proceed to suppress the symptoms.

When poison is taken by the mouth, the internal defense system has a chance to quickly eject some of it by vomiting, but when the poisons are shot directly into the body, bypassing all the natural safeguards, these dangerous poisons circulate immediately throughout the entire body in a matter of seconds and keep on circulating until all the cells are poisoned.

I heard that seven men dropped dead in a doctor's office after being vaccinated. This was in an army camp, so I wrote to the Government for verification. They sent me the report of U.S. Secretary of War, Henry L. Stimson. The report not only verified the report of the seven who dropped dead from the vaccines, but it stated that there had been 63 deaths and 28,585 cases of hepatitis as a direct result of the yellow fever vaccine during only 6 months of the war. That was only one of the 14 to 25 shots given the soldiers. We can imagine the damage that all these shots did to the men. (See the chapter on What Vaccinations Did to Our Soldiers.)

The first World War was of a short duration, so the vaccine makers were unable to use up all their vaccines. As they were (and still are) in business for profit, they decided to sell it to the rest of the population. So they drummed up the largest vaccination campaign in U.S. history. There were no epidemics to justify it so they used other tricks. Their propaganda claimed the soldiers were coming home from foreign countries with all kinds of diseases and that everyone must have all the shots on the market.

The people believed them because, first of all, they wanted to believe their doctors, and second, the returning soldiers certainly had been sick. They didn't know it was from doctor-made vaccine diseases, as the army doctors don't tell them things like that. Many of the returned soldiers were disabled for life by these drug-induced diseases.

Many were insane from postvaccinal encephalitis, but the doctors called it shell shock, even though many had never left American soil.

The conglomerate disease brought on by the many poison vaccines baffled the doctors, as they never had a vaccination spree before which used so many different vaccines. The new disease they had created had symptoms of all the diseases they had injected into the man. There was the high fever, extreme weakness, abdominal rash and intestinal disturbance characteristic of typhoid. The diphtheria vaccine caused lung congestion, chills and fever, swollen, sore throat clogged with the false membrane, and the choking suffocation because of difficulty in breathing followed by gasping and death, after which the body turned black from stagnant blood that had been deprived of oxygen in the suffocation stages. In early days they called it Black Death. The other vaccines cause their own reactions — paralysis, brain damage, lockjaw, etc.

When doctors had tried to suppress the symptoms of the typhoid with a stronger vaccine, it caused a worse form of typhoid which they named paratyphoid. But when they concocted a stronger and more dangerous vaccine to suppress that one, they created an even worse disease which they didn't have a name for. What should they call it? They didn't want to tell the people what it really was — their own Frankenstein monster which they had created with their vaccines and suppressive medicines. They wanted to direct the blame away from themselves, so they called it Spanish Influenza. It was certainly not of Spanish origin, and the Spanish people resented the implication that the world-wide scourge of that day should be blamed on them. But the name stuck and American medical doctors and vaccine makers were not suspected of the crime of this widespread devastation — the 1918 Flu Epidemic. It is only in recent years that researchers have been digging up the facts and laying the blame where it belongs.

Some of the soldiers may have been in Spain before coming home, but their diseases originated in their own home-based U.S. Army Camps. Our medical men still use that same dodge. When their own vaccines (required for travel) cause vaccine diseases abroad they use this as grounds for a scare campaign to stampede people into the vaccination centers. Do you remember the Hong Kong Flu and the Asian Flu and the London Flu scares? These were all medically-made epidemics mixed with the usual common colds which people have every year.

***

All the doctors and people who were living at the time of the 1918 Spanish Influenza epidemic say it was the most terrible disease the world has ever had. Strong men, hale and hearty, one day would be dead the next. The disease had the characteristics of the black death added to typhoid, diphtheria, pneumonia, smallpox, paralysis and all the diseases the people had been vaccinated with immediately following World War 1. Practically the entire population had been injected "seeded" with a dozen or more diseases — or toxic serums. When all those doctor-made diseases started breaking out all at once it was tragic.

That pandemic dragged on for two years, kept alive with the addition of more poison drugs administered by the doctors who tried to suppress the symptoms. As far as I could find out, the flu hit only the vaccinated. Those who had refused the shots escaped the flu. My family had refused all the vaccinations so we remained well all the time. We knew from the health teachings of Graham, Trail, Tilden and others, that people cannot contaminate the body with poisons without causing disease.

When the flu was at its peak, all the stores were closed as well as the schools, businesses — even the hospital, as the doctors and nurses had been vaccinated too and were down with the flu. No one was on the streets. It was like a ghost town. We [who didn't taken any vaccines] seemed to be the only family which didn't get the flu; so my parents went from house to house doing what they could to look after the sick, as it was impossible to get a doctor then. If it were possible for germs, bacteria, virus, or bacilli to cause disease, they had plenty of opportunity to attack my parents when they were spending many hours a day in the sick rooms. But they didn't get the flu and they didn't bring any germs home to attack us children and cause anything. None of our family had the flu — not even a sniffle— and it was in the winter with deep snow on the ground.

It has been said that the 1918 flu epidemic killed 20,000,000 people throughout the world. But, actually, the doctors killed them with their crude and deadly treatments and drugs. This is a harsh accusation but it is nevertheless true, judging by the success of the drugless doctors in comparison with that of the medical doctors.

While the medical men and medical hospitals were losing 33% of their flu cases, the non-medical hospitals such as BATTLE CREEK, KELLOGG and MACFADDEN'S HEALTH-RESTORIUM were getting almost 100% healings with their water cure, baths, enemas, etc., fasting and certain other simple healing methods, followed by carefully worked out diets of natural foods. One health doctor didn't lose a patient in eight years. The very successful health treatment of one of those drugless doctors who didn't lose any patients will be given in the other part of this book, titled VACCINATION CONDEMNED, to be published a little later.

If the medical doctors had been as advanced as the drugless doctors, there would not have been those 20 million deaths from the medical flu treatment.

There was seven times more disease among the vaccinated soldiers than among the unvaccinated civilians, and the diseases were those they had been vaccinated against. One soldier who had returned from overseas in 1912 told me that the army hospitals were filled with cases of infantile paralysis and he wondered why grown men should have an infant disease. Now, we know that paralysis is a common after-effect of vaccine poisoning. Those at home didn't get the paralysis until after the world-wide vaccination campaign in 1918.[1341]

52 SARS-CoV-2 Virus Has Never Been Isolated

With all of the worldwide fervor over the COVID-19 pandemic, one might think that, certainly, the SARS-Cov-2 virus that causes COVID-19 has been isolated. That is not the case at all. A little known fact is that the alleged SARS-CoV-2 virus has never been isolated.

Incidentally, the CDC distinguishes between SARS-CoV-2 and COVID-19. The CDC states that SARS-CoV-2 is the virus that causes the disease COVID-19. COVID-19 means "coronavirus disease 2019" whereas SARS-CoV-2 means "severe acute respiratory syndrome coronavirus 2." But that distinction between the two acronyms is not commonly made by the public or the medical community.[1342] Most equate SARS-CoV-2 and COVID-19 and use them interchangeably to describe the alleged infectious pathogen that is purported to be transmitted from one person to another.[1343] Thus, this author will use those terms interchangeably to refer to the alleged pathogen.

The alleged SARS-CoV-2 virus has never been proven even to exist. Claims by governments and researchers to the contrary are simply false; they try to redefine what it means to isolate a virus and use obfuscatory language to conceal the deception. Please understand that the reported infections for SARS-CoV-2 among both unvaccinated and vaccinated persons are based on tests that are returning false-positive results.

Christine Massey is a biostatistician. On April 24, 2024, Christine Massey sent a Freedom of Information (FOIA) request to the CDC asking for any studies providing scientific evidence of the isolation of the alleged hantavirus proving that it causes illnesses it is purported to cause.[1344] On May 10, 2024, Roger Andoh, acting as CDC/ATSDR FOIA Officer in the Office of the Chief Operating Officer, gave a sweeping response that the CDC has not conducted any controlled studies that purify and isolate the hantavirus or any other virus because the CDC does not perform such studies. Massey explains that "the 'experts' in the Division of High-Consequence Pathogens and Pathology have never obtained scientific evidence of purported 'viruses' existing in 'hosts' and causing the illness/symptoms that they are claimed to cause."[1345] The CDC has confessed that it has never isolated, and thus has never scientifically proven, the existence of any virus.

Furthermore, there is not a single study of the alleged SARS-CoV2 virus being isolated or purified.[1346] That can mean only one thing. Drs. Thomas Cowan and Andrew Kaufman succinctly concluded that "[t]he SARS-CoV2 virus does not exist."[1347] On November 30, 2021, Christine Massey submitted an affidavit in a Canadian Federal Court averring that she has received responses to freedom of information (FOI) requests from Canadian and U.S. government agencies. She further stated that she had obtained records from FOI requests made by others to more than 138 institutions from 28 countries worldwide. Astoundingly, no institution was "able to cite even one record describing the isolation and purification of SARS-CoV-2 [the alleged virus purported to cause COVID-19]."[1348] As of August 23, 2022, that number has expanded to 208 institutions in 35 countries. Yet still, none of the institutions "have provided or cited any record describing actual 'SARS-COV-2' isolation/purification."[1349] The very existence of the SARS-Cov-2 virus seems to be a myth.

So, why, then are people testing positive for a non-existent SARS-CoV-2? A group of 22 highly respected scientists led by Pieter Borger, MSc, Ph.D., demanded a retraction of the report by Christian Drosten and Victor Corman that established the PCR test used worldwide for the SARS-CoV-2 virus. They cited "10 major scientific flaws at the molecular and methodological level" in the research that produced the SARS-CoV-2 PCR test. The scientists predicted that those flaws would result in false positive results. The most notable shortcoming of the research by Corman/Drosten was that the resulting SARS-COV-2 PCR test was arrived at without isolating the SARS-CoV-2 (COVID-19). How can one test for something that has not first been isolated? The scientists stated:

> The first and major issue [with the Corman/Drosten report] is that the novel Coronavirus SARS-CoV-2 (in the publication named 2019-nCoV and in February 2020 named SARS-CoV-2 by an international consortium of virus experts) is based on in silico (theoretical) sequences, supplied by a laboratory in China, because at the time neither control material of infectious ("live") or inactivated SARS-CoV-2 nor isolated genomic RNA of the virus was available to the authors. To date no validation has been performed by the authorship based on isolated SARS-CoV-2 viruses or full length RNA thereof. According to Corman et al.:
>
> "We aimed to develop and deploy robust diagnostic methodology for use in public health laboratory settings without having virus material available."[1350] (endnotes deleted)

The alleged SARS-CoV-2 virus was identified in silico, meaning that it was created using a computer simulation. Essentially, the SARS-Cov-2 virus is a computer-generated theoretical virus that does not actually exist. The scientists concluded the obvious. A diagnostic test for SARS-CoV-2 is invalid if it is based on research without access to any actual virus material available on which to base the test.

Kary B Mullis invented the polymerase chain reaction (PCR) method, for which he won the 1993 Nobel Prize in Chemistry.[1351] He died suddenly in August 2019, four months before the January 2020 publication of the Corman-Droster PCR test paper that formed the basis for the SARS-CoV-2 PCR test. Before his death, Mullis explained that with enough amplification the PCR test could be used to find almost anything. He said that "with PCR, if you do it well, you can find almost anything in anybody."[1352] For that reason, Mullis cautioned that the PCR test should not be used to diagnose whether someone is ill. Mullis said that PCR is "a process that's used to make a whole lot of something out of something. That's what it is. It doesn't tell you that you're sick, and it doesn't tell you that the thing you ended up with really was going to hurt you or anything like that."[1353] Thus, the inventor of the PCR test is on record stating that it is improper to use a PCR test to diagnose if someone is ill or infected with a virus.

The PCR COVID-19 test is done using reagents to extract a sample of RNA. An enzyme called reverse transcriptase converts the RNA to a complementary sequence of DNA. That DNA (called a primer) is replicated (amplified) many times over so the particular targeted DNA sequence in it can be detected. The more stages of replication the more likely the targeted sequence will be detected. Each time the DNA in the sample is amplified it doubles the number of molecules. The doubling is exponential after each cycle of amplification. But the number of cycles can vary from laboratory to laboratory. The probability of testing positive increases as a function of the number of cycles. The PCR cycles for a SARS-CoV-2 test from most laboratories are set at 40 cycles.[1354]

Amandha Dawn Vollmer holds a Doctor of Naturopathic Medicine degree from the Canadian College of Naturopathic Medicine in Toronto and a Bachelor of Science in Agricultural Biotechnology. She has discovered that the test for SARS-CoV-2 is not actually testing for SARS-CoV-2. The polymerase chain reaction (PCR) test for SARS-CoV-2 is based on the research of German scientists Christian Drosten and Victor Corman who cobbled together the COVID-19 PCR test used worldwide to detect the SARS-CoV-2 virus. Amandha Vollmer discovered that the Corman/Drosten PCR test protocol adopted by the World Health Organization (WHO) to detect SARS-CoV-12 is actually testing for chromosome 8, which is present in everyone.[1355] One of the primer sequences in the PCR test for SARS-CoV-2 that is promoted by the WHO is found in all human DNA. Essentially, we are the virus. That is why there is a 97% false positive rate on the COVID-19 PCR test. People are testing positive for SARS-CoV-2 because they're human.

ctccctttgttgtgttgt = The DNA sequence for the PCR test for SARS-CoV-2.[1356]

ctccctttgttgtgttgt = Chromosome 8, which is present in all homo sapiens (humans).[1357]

The false positive error is compounded because of the high PCR threshold cycle rates employed. Each amplification level exponentially increases the likelihood of detecting the presence of chromosome 8. The PCR test amplifies the test sample as an exponent of the number of cycles. Each cycle doubles the prior cycle. For example, if you start with a penny and each day you double the amount of money you had on the previous day, at the end of 28 days (cycles) you would have more than a million dollars. If you continued to double your money each day past the 28th day, you would have more than five billion dollars after 40 days (cycles). That is the kind of amplification that the PCR test performs. The CDC has recommended 40 cycles for the PCR test.[1358] And most laboratories during the alleged pandemic were performing tests using that recommended 40-cycle standard. Anthony S. Fauci is the Director of the National Institute of Allergy and Infectious Diseases (NIAID). Dr. Fauci admitted that performing PCR tests to detect COVID-19 at 35 or more cycles will result in false-positives and the confidence in any such positive result for SARS-CoV-2 is "minuscule." Dr. Fauci stated:

> If you get a cycle threshold of 35 or more, the chances of it being replication-confident are minuscule...you almost never can culture virus from a 37 threshold cycle... someone does come in with 37, 38, even 36, you gotta say it's just dead nucleotides period.[1359]

"Any test with a cycle threshold above 35 is too sensitive, agreed Juliet Morrison, a virologist at the University of California, Riverside. 'I'm shocked that people would think that 40 could represent a positive,' she said."[1360]

Apoorva Mandavilli reported that experts with whom she conferred determined that "[i]n Massachusetts, from 85 to 90 percent of people who tested positive in July with a cycle threshold of 40 would have been deemed negative if the threshold were 30 cycles."[1361] Dr. Michael Mina, an epidemiologist at the Harvard T.H. Chan School of Public Health, said about the Massachusetts findings that "I would say that none of those people should be contact-traced, not one,"[1362]

The Portugal Court of Appeals in Lisbon agreed with the trial court, which granted a *writ of habeas corpus* on behalf of German tourists. The court of appeals ruled that German tourists were illegally detained by the Azores Regional Health Authority and ordered to be quarantined because the PCR test that was the basis of the detention is unreliable for detecting SARS-CoV-2. Peter Andrews reported that the Portuguese court cited a study conducted by "some of the leading European and world specialists," proving that the usual testing standard for a PCR test results in a SARS-CoV-2 false-positive result 97% of the time.[1363]

The Portugal Court of Appeals in Lisbon, based upon a study by some of the leading European and world specialists, concluded that "[t]his means that if a person has a positive PCR test at a cycle threshold of 35 or higher (as in most laboratories in the USA and Europe), the chances of a person being infected are less than 3%. The probability of a person receiving a false positive is 97% or higher."[1364]

The antigen tests are just as inaccurate and prone to false positives. Indeed, the FDA warned unequivocally that the antigen tests are inaccurate and give false positives. "The U.S. Food and Drug Administration (FDA) is alerting clinical laboratory staff and health care providers that false positive results can occur with antigen tests."[1365]

Indeed, the FDA has now admitted that "all tests," for COVID-19, antigen and PCR, are inaccurate. The FDA states:

> The FDA reminds clinical laboratory staff and health care providers about the risk of false positive results with all laboratory tests. Laboratories should expect some false positive results to occur even when very accurate tests are used for screening large populations with a low prevalence of infection.[1366]

Notice that the warning goes to "all laboratory tests," including both antigen and PCR tests. That astounding admission by the FDA has gone unreported by the major media outlets, even as many states, including Virginia, are issuing more draconian social distancing and masking orders based on those inaccurate false-positive COVID-19 test results.

The FDA explains the scope of the false positives using the antigen test. The following is guidance from the FDA:

> Remember that positive predictive value (PPV) varies with disease prevalence when interpreting results from diagnostic tests. PPV is the percent of positive test results that are true positives. **As disease prevalence decreases, the percent of test results that are false positives increase.**
>
> For example, a test with 98% specificity would have a PPV of just over 80% in a population with 10% prevalence, meaning 20 out of 100 positive results would be false positives.
>
> The same test would only have a PPV of approximately 30% in a population with 1% prevalence, meaning 70 out of 100 positive results would be false positives.
>
> This means that, in a population with 1% prevalence, only 30% of individuals with positive test results actually have the disease.[1367]
>
> At 0.1% prevalence, the PPV would only be 4%, meaning that 96 out of 100 positive results would be false positives.

That is why there was a push for testing asymptomatic persons. The government knew that many would falsely test positive for COVID-19. The lockdowns, social distancing, and mask mandates are all based on the premise that those with no symptoms of COVID-19 can still spread the disease. But research has proven that there is no asymptomatic transfer of SARS-Cov-2, the alleged virus purported to cause COIVD-19.[1368] The tyrannical overlords ignore such inconvenient studies. Once persons tested positive for COVID-19, they were tallied up as COVID-19 patients. Some who are ill with the flu may test positive for SARS-Cov-2.[1369] That is why the flu disappeared during the 2020-2021 flu season.[1370] All persons with the flu were counted not as flu cases but as COVID-19 cases.[1371] They then used the COVID-19 scam to push the poisonous COVID-19 vaccines on the population and begin the actual killing. Their objective from the beginning was to force the toxic vaccines on the world population.[1372]

53 The Lie of Asymptomatic Virus Spread

In the spring of 2020, a false premise was published far and wide that asymptomatic carriers of SARS-Cov-2, the alleged virus that purports to cause COVID-19, threatened to spread the alleged virus to others. Under that theory, someone who is not sick and feels no symptoms of illness could, nonetheless, spread the SARS-COV-2 virus to others. That was an unproven theory. But that theory was the basis upon which the world's governments shut down businesses and schools, mandated masks, required social distancing, and ultimately required mass COVID-19 vaccinations. The theory that a person could carry the SARS-CoV-2 virus without displaying symptoms and then spread it to others is now known to have been false.

The theory of the asymptomatic spread of SARS-CoV-2 was doubted by many. David Zweig explains that "[i]n June 2020, Dr. Maria Van Kerkhove, head of the World Health Organization's emerging diseases and zoonosis unit, said that transmission from asymptomatic people was 'very rare.'"[1373] Allyson M Pollock, professor of public health at Newcastle University, posted an article in the British Medical Journal, likening the rarety of asymptomatic transfer of SARS-CoV-2 to finding a needle in a haystack. Dr. Pollock stated that "[s]earching for people who are asymptomatic yet infectious is like searching for needles that appear and reappear transiently in haystacks, particularly when rates are falling."[1374] The governments of the world were well aware of the study conducted between May 14 and June 1, 2020, involving almost 10 million residents of Wuhan, China. That massive study found zero transmission of SARS-CoV-2 from asymptomatic carriers of the alleged virus.[1375]

Unbeknownst to the general public is that from the outset the CDC and state governments had available a test that could have been used to determine if someone who tested positive for SARS-CoV-2 in a PCR test could spread the alleged virus to others. The world's governments kept that test secret because it undermined their asymptomatic premise for their oppressive measures. David Zweig explains:

> [A]s early as May and June of 2020, a test existed that, if it had been rolled out in medical centers and regular labs nationwide, could have enabled people to know for certain whether they were infectious or not. ... This raises serious questions for those in charge of the CDC, NIH, and NIAID for why resources were not allocated toward making this test broadly available.[1376]

The federal and state governments knew about the test when they were locking down society. Indeed, in June 2021, the CDC published a study proving the efficacy of the new test for infectiousness.[1377] But if you are a government locking people down, shutting down businesses, and masking people, on a false pretense, the last thing you want is to have your pretense be proven false. And that is just what the test would have done. David Zweig reveals how:

> And what they found does not match the narrative about a common threat of people walking around

> without symptoms infecting others. For the majority of the pandemic only 4% of asymptomatic SARS-CoV-2 PCR-positive patients were shown to be infectious.[1378]

Dr. Ralph Tayyar, an infectious diseases fellow at Stanford, explained:

> "The probability of a kid in class who is not sick actually being infectious is very low," he said. Think about it this way: even if every single student in a school without symptoms was infected, 96 percent of them still weren't capable of transmitting to others. Yet, of course, most people without symptoms are not infected. Moreoer, just because 4 percent were technically capable of infecting others does not mean that in actuality they had sufficient amount of replicating virus to do so. We are talking about a subgroup of a subgroup of a subgroup.[1379]

It gets worse, as the false positive COVID-19 PCR test rate from the beginning has been estimated to be as high as 97%. So we have a 97% population of false positive PCR results. That means that we have potentially 3% of the positive PCR positive test being infected with SARS-CoV-2, with only 4% of that 3% theoretically being able to pass on the alleged virus. That leaves us with an actual risk of spread among asymptomatic persons testing positive for SARS-CoV-2 at 0.12%. The risk goes down even further because that 0.12% only tells you that the person can potentially spread the alleged virus. A much smaller percentage of those have sufficient replication of the alleged virus in their system to spread the alleged it. Ultimately, the chance of an asymptomatic person spreading SARS-CoV-2 is minuscule. It is like finding a needle in a haystack.

The asymptomatic spread theory and the concealment of its falsity were done to ensure the success of the vaccination propaganda campaign. The goal from the beginning was a mass-vaccination program. The vaccines were the end goal. The vaccines are bioweapons to injure and kill people. That is not hyperbole. Dr. Michael Yeadon is the former Vice-President of Pfizer's allergy and respiratory research unit. He left Pfizer to found the biotechnology company, Ziarco, where he served as CEO. Ziarco was later sold to Novartis for $325 million. Dr. Yeadon has 32 years of experience designing drugs. He has maintained many close ties with insiders at Pfizer. In a May 8, 2023, interview with CHD, Dr. Yeadon had this to say about the COVID-19 vaccines:

> We are facing something much worse than an alleged virus. At the very least, these things that people that are being injected with, the injuries to people from these [inaudible] vaccines, I'm afraid, I wish I could tell you it was accidental. But it wasn't accidental. I spent 32 years in rational drug design. I know, and I knew, and wrote it before any of them had emergency use authorization, that they were dangerous. And I am afraid, and I am convinced and would say with my hand on the Bible, in front of a court, a judge, that these injections have been made to injure people, to maim and kill.[1380]

Furthermore, Leading Reports reported on May 11, 2023, that Dr. Yeadon "claims that the COVID vaccines are bioweapons designed to kill billions of people as part of a depopulation agenda by the 'Deep State.'"[1381]

54 Exosomes

An often identified culprit for disease is bacteria. But many will be surprised to learn that there has never been proven that any bacteria has ever caused a disease. Indeed, the entire germ theory is based on unproven assumptions. Dr. Thomas Cowan explains that bacteria are microbial patsies.

> [B]acteria are found at the site of disease for the same reason that firemen are found at the site of fires. Bacteria are the cleanup crew tasked with digesting and getting rid of dead and diseased tissues. Claiming that bacteria cause a certain disease is no more reasonable than claiming that firemen cause fires, especially as experimental evidence shows this to be false. Likewise, maggots on a dead dog are there to clean up dead tissue—no one would accuse the maggots of killing the dog. In fact, one therapy for necrotic tissue is maggot therapy (applying maggots to the wound). The maggots kill only the dead tissue; when there is only live tissue left to eat, they die off.[1382]

The bacteria theory of disease had problems. Scientists

could not always find an offending bacterium for a disease. Louis Pasteur speculated that some pathogen was too small to be detected in a microscope. In the end, Pasteur admitted his germ theory of bacterial cause for disease was wrong. He acknowledged that his effort to prove his theory of bacterial contagion was a failure, He made a deathbed confession: "The germ is nothing; the terrain is everything." By terrain, he means the condition of a person who has been subjected to a stress or toxin in the environment causing the illness. A contemporary rival of Pasteur, Antoine Bechamp, advocated the terrain theory.

Dr. Cowen reveals that the eureka moment for scientists wedded to the germ theory came with the invention of the electron microscope;. The scientists could then see tiny "particles" at the disease site. They called these particles viruses, after the Latin word for toxin.

The concept of viruses causing diseases was just a hypothesis. You see, scientists only hypothesized that the "particles" they saw were disease causing viruses. The germ theory of diseases caused by viruses was based on that hypothesis. You might be surprised to learn that there has been no direct evidence of the existence of viruses. Derek M Yellon PhD, DSc, FRCP (Hon), FACC, FESC, FAHA, Professor of Molecular & Cellular Cardiology at University College London (UCL) explains:

> We already know that "viruses" began first as an idea in the early 1900's once it was discovered that bacteria were unable to be blamed for every disease and were also found regularly in healthy subjects. It was assumed that there must be something smaller than bacteria in the fluids causing disease. The concept of the "virus" came before there was ever any evidence submitted for the existence of this invisible entity. Over 100 years later, we still have no direct evidence as to the existence of

> "viruses," only indirect evidence used to infer their existence.[1383]

All studies, vaccines, and pharmaceuticals developed to fight viral infections are based on the assumption that viruses exist. Dr. Stefan Lanka explains that the theory that viruses cause disease has never been proven. Even more surprising is his revelation that there has never been the isolation of a virus in the history of medicine.

> The fact is and remains that a virus has never been isolated according to the meaning of the word isolation, and it has never been photographed and biochemically characterised as a whole unique structure. The electron micrographs of the alleged viruses, for example, really only show cellular particles from dying tissue and cells, and most photos show only a computer model (CGI – computer generated images). Because the involved parties BELIEVE that the dying tissue and cells transform themselves into viruses, their death is also regarded as propagation of the virus. The involved parties still believe this because the discoverer of this method was awarded the nobel Prize and his papers remain the reference papers on "viruses."[1384]

If the so-called viruses seen in diseased cells are not viruses, what are they? Dr. Thomas Cowan reveals that they are exosomes. Exosomes, like bacteria, have been renamed "viruses" and made the patsies. Their function is to package up and expel toxins from the body. They are not viruses; they are not bad guys; they are good guys. They are the garbage collectors. But they find themselves falsely accused simply becaue they have been found at the scene of the disease. Dr. Cowan explains:

> When a living organism is threatened in almost any way—through starvation, chemical poisoning, or electromagnetic effects—the cells and tissues have a mechanism for "packaging," "propagating" and releasing these poisons. Modern researchers have shown that exosomes have exactly the same attributes as "viruses." They are the same size, contain the same components, and act on the same receptors. HIV researcher James Hildreth, president and CEO of Meharry Medical College and former professor at Johns Hopkins, put it this way: "The virus is fully an exosome in every sense of the word." Exosomes are completely indistinguishable from what the virologists have been calling "viruses."[1385]

Dr. Cowan explains that Exosomes do not attack cells, as is theorized with viruses under the germ theory. Instead, exosomes are created by your cells and expelled by your cells as those cells try to rid themselves of an environmental toxin. The exosomes are containers of toxins ejected from your cells.

> Here's how exosomes work: let's say you have a poorly nourished organism, then you expose it to a common environmental toxin. The tissues and cells that are affected begin to produce, package, and secrete these poisons in the form of exosomes. This is a way of ridding the cells and tissues of substances that would do it great harm. The greater the exposure to toxic assaults, the more exosomes will be produced. Studies have shown that if one somehow stops the cells from producing and excreting these exosomes, then the cells and tissues, in fact the organism, will have a worse outcome. This research demonstrates that the production and excretion of exosomes is a crucial

detoxification function of all cells and tissues.[1386]

Exosomes also act as a warning system to the other cells. They send signals to the other cells that danger is afoot and they need to prepare for it. Exosomes are not a source of illness; they are a detoxification system. Dr. Cowan calls them "toxin gobbling messengers." Dr. Cowan likens them to "true firemen, obviously present in higher amounts in cases of disease, in which a higher burden of poisoning has occurred." But these beneficial exosomes have been made the bad guy, and called viruses because they contain toxins of which the body is trying to rid itself. Dr. Cowan concludes:

> The germ theory is wrong; the virus theory is wrong. Viruses are not here to kill us; in reality they are exosomes whose role is to provide the detoxification package and the communication system that allows us to live a full and healthy existence. A war on viruses is a war on life. It's clear that the misidentification of exosomes as viruses was a tragic mistake, one that it's about time we correct, once and for all.[1387]

Although the germ theory was shown to be bankrupt and its primary champion eschewed it on his deathbed, it has been the religious dogma of modern medicine for two centuries. Why would that be? Because the governments of the world saw in that theory a way of controlling their population. As we have experienced during the COVID-19 scam-demic, the governments used the threat of the contagious disease to justify draconian lockdowns, social distancing, masking, tracking and tracing, relocation camps, and mandatory vaccinations. It was all based on the discredited germ theory.

55 Relocation Camps

The germ theory is a gift to governments that keeps on giving. It provides the perfect excuse for governments to enact new freedom-stealing responses every time there is a new epidemic. It seems the quacks at the CDC just cannot stop themselves. The CDC is staffed by Orwellian Dr. Strangeloves. They are actually entertaining throwing people in concentrations camps. Oh, but don't you worry, it will be for your own good; to protect you from a contagious disease. In a document titled, *Interim Operational Considerations for Implementing the Shielding Approach to Prevent COVID-19 Infections in Humanitarian Settings,*[1388] the CDC proposes a plan implementing house arrest, neighborhood lockdowns, evictions and relocations, and internment in concentration camps. That is not hyperbole. The CDC has posted its strategy on its CDC website.[1389]

The strange thing is that this plan by the CDC is NOT a strategy of quarantining sick people. Instead, it is a strategy to prevent uninfected people that the CDC has determined are at risk of dying from disease. In essence, it is a backward strategy that calls for the quarantining of uninfected persons. In all of medical history, the strategy has always been to quarantine the sick. The CDC plans to quarantine the healthy to prevent them from getting sick. The tyranny resulting from such a strategy is obvious.

It is unscientific quackary and dystopian tyranny. The relocation proposed by the CDC, euphemistically called "shielding," is not based on infection. Thus, it goes beyond what is commonly thought to be quarantining because quarantining requires that the quarantined person be infected. Indeed, that seems to be why the CDC document does not even use the word quarantine.

Relocation proposed in the CDC document is based on the risk of death from infection. The CDC document cites to a publication from the London School of Hygiene and Tropical Medicine,[1390] The strategy outlined in that document is: **"The population targeted by the shielding approach consists of the individuals at high risk of death from SARSCoV-2 infection, mainly defined by age or presence of co-morbidities."**[1391] Thus, it is the risk of death from infection that determines the targets for relocation and shielding, not actual infection. That opens up this strategy to implementation virtually everywhere within the United States. The forced relocation of persons is euphemistically called being "relocated to safe or green zones."

> High-risk individuals would be temporarily relocated to safe or "green zones" established at the household, neighborhood, camp/sector or community level depending on the context and setting. They would have minimal contact with family members and other low-risk residents.

House Arrest

At the "household level," the green zone could be in the person's own home. The CDC relies on the strategy set forth in the publication from the London School of Hygiene and Tropical Medicine, which states:

> Green zone: a specific area (a room, or a shelter in

> case of multi-shelter compound) within the household.
>
> High-risk individuals are physically isolated from the other household members.
>
> Movement outside the green zone should be minimised (shower/latrines; if needed, a short walk during quiet hours when children are sleeping), and social distancing measures should be applied during such movements. Other household members should not enter the green zone.[1392]

The green zone is house arrest. Indeed, it is worse than house arrest because there is a green zone within the house. That green zone will have to be enforced, which means that a government official will need to reside in the house to oversee the green zone enforcement.

Neighborhood Lockdowns Evictions and Relocation

At the "neighborhood level," the CDC plans on enforcing whole neighborhood lockdowns, evictions and relocations. Persons will be evicted and relocated to different houses in the neighborhoods. The persons deemed to be at high risk for COVID-19 will be relocated to one sector of houses in a single area of the neighborhood. Those houses will be commandeered by the CDC. The persons living in those houses will be evicted and forced to leave their houses. The CDC will then take over control of the house. The former residents will then be "voluntarily" relocated to live with another family in the neighborhood. The plan calls for the following:

> Neighbouring households voluntarily 'house swap' and group their high-risk member in the green zone.[1393]

Notice that Block Level allows for house swapping voluntarily. That concept of voluntariness is mentioned a couple of times in the London School document. But it applies only after the persons have been "forcibly displaced." Thus, under the London School plan, the people will be forcibly moved to the camps against their will. Indeed, the London School provides the following definition for "camps or camp-like settings:"

> **Forcibly displaced population**, including refugees and internally displaced living in high density formal or unformal settlements, under collective or individual shelters.[1394]

It is only once the persons are forcibly moved to the camps that that the government asks for their voluntary cooperation. And it seems to only apply after the green zones have been forcibly set up and administered. Once the government sets up the camp area comprised of 5-10 households, it is then that high-risk persons in the green zone are allowed to house swap within that zone. But movement outside the green zone "should be minimized."

Concentration Camps

At the "sector level," the CDC plans on having concentration camps called "camp shelters" that are also euphemistically called "green zones." Among the rules is: "No movement outside the green zone."

> Green zone: a specific group of shelters within a camp sector (max 50 high-risk individuals per single green zone). High-risk individuals are physically isolated in the green zone.[1395]

Below is a graphic from the report from the London School of Hygiene and Tropical Medicine relied on by the CDC in their Orwellian three-part strategy of house arrest, neighborhood relocation, and concentration camps the CDC plans to use to oppress U.S. citizens.

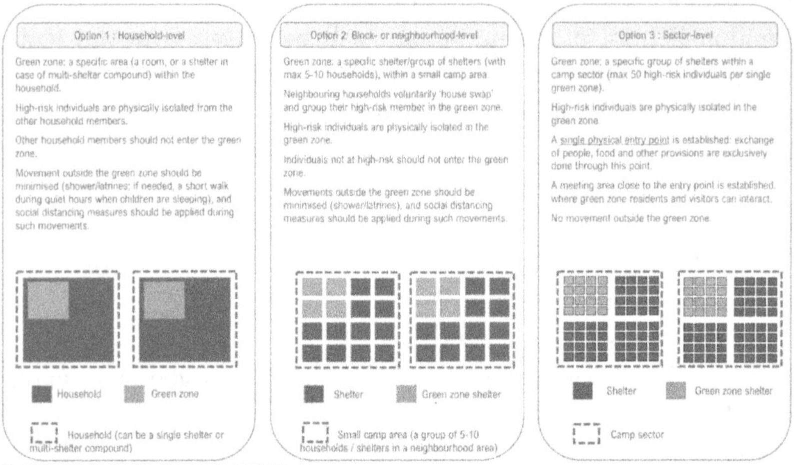

Figure 1: Representation of housing arrangements for each shielding option.

The most astounding thing about this strategy proposed by the CDC is that the CDC admits that "there is no empirical evidence whether this approach will increase, decrease or have no effect on morbidity and mortality during the COVID-19 epidemic in various humanitarian settings."[1396] The CDC is proposing an unconstitutional and inhumane scheme of relocation camps without knowing if it will work. Every employee in the CDC has taken an oath to support and defend the constitution. Yet, they propose a scheme that any liberty-loving American school child in a past era would recognize as violating the U.S. Constitution.

The CDC has no idea if the dystopian oppression that they plan on imposing will work in preventing the spread of COVID. So then, you might ask, why are they proposing it? Because this has nothing to do with preventing the spread of disease. It has everything to do with taking away your God-given rights to life, liberty, and property. COVID-19 is a propaganda cover for imposing communist oppression.

Federal Regulations Do Not Allow Shielding

While the CDC proposed plan does not use the word quarantine (which is strange in-and-of-itself), the plan is essentially a mass-quarantine strategy but without any actual infection. Thus, instead of using the word quarantine, the plan uses the word "shielding." That is significant because quarantine is something you do to someone who is ill. Whereas shielding, as used by the CDC, is a strategy to prevent someone deemed at risk of death from becoming ill. In the history of medicine, there has never been implemented a strategy of "shielding" uninfected persons. The medical strategy has always relied on the theory of quarantining sick people. The CDC strategy is backward. It is backward for a reason. It is the perfect strategy to strip a population of its freedom.

The federal regulations seem to allow quarantining someone who is not actually infected. But there must be some exposure to an infected person for the federal regulations to be operative. The regulations do not allow for shielding someone simply by virtue of their risk of dying from a disease.

42 C.F.R. § 70.1 states: "Quarantine means the separation of an individual or group reasonably believed to have been exposed to a quarantinable communicable disease, but who are not yet ill, from others who have not been so exposed, to prevent the possible spread of the quarantinable communicable disease."

You can be quarantined even though you are NOT ill. You can be quarantined if they reasonably believe that you have been exposed to a communicable disease. As broad as that is, it does not allow for "shielding" someone who is not infected from getting a disease that is deemed to be deadly to them.

Under 42 C.F.R. § 70.6, you only need to be in a "qualifying stage" of the disease to be quarantined. Qualifying stage includes: “The precommunicable stage of the quarantinable communicable disease, but only if the quarantinable communicable disease would be likely to cause a public health emergency if transmitted to other individuals.” 42 CFR § 70.1.

Under the 42 C.F.R. § 70.6, if you have a qualifying stage of exposure, which includes a “precommunicable stage of the quarantinable communicable disease” you can be quarantined. So, what does that mean? That means that you can be quarantined through apprehension and detention, while you are not ill, nor are even a threat to spread the disease, if they reasonably believe that you have been exposed to a person who has a quarantinable communicable disease.

The regulations are already on the books calling for the apprehension and detention of any person the CDC believes has been exposed to COVID-19, even if you are not ill.[1397]

42 C.F.R. § 70.6 authorizes the apprehension and detention of persons with (or even without) a quarantinable communicable disease if they have been exposed to someone who has had the disease. They will feed you and force you to receive “appropriate medical treatment” (i.e. vaccines) while you are detained.

> The Director will arrange for adequate food and water, appropriate accommodation, appropriate medical treatment, and means of necessary communication for individuals who are apprehended or held in quarantine or isolation under this part.[1398]

The director referenced in the regulations is the director of the CDC. Such autocratic powers are unconstitutional. Even as nonsensically broad, oppressive, and unconstitutional as those federal regulations are, they do not allow for shielding uninfected persons at risk of death from disease as proposed by the CDC.

56 Inflating COVID-19 Death Statistics

America's Frontline Doctors (AFLD) is a group of doctors who have joined to fight the government's medical oppression. AFLD has sued the U.S. Government, alleging that the COVID-19 emergency is a scam based upon inflated statistics of death and illness designed to bring about a medical tyranny to take away the freedoms of all Americans. The complaint states in pertinent part:

> [T]he Emergency Declaration upon which they are all based was unjustified. As Plaintiffs allege in detail and will show at trial with expert medical and scientific evidence, including the Defendants' own data and studies, **there is not now, and there never has been, a bona fide "public health emergency" due to the SARS-Cov-2 virus or the disease COVID-19.** Virtually all of the PCR tests were calibrated to produce false positive results, which has enabled the Defendants and their counterparts in state governments to publish daily reports containing seriously inflated COVID-19 "case" and "death" counts that grossly exaggerate the public health threat.[1399]

The false positive COVID-19 tests laid the foundation for creating a pandemic where there was none. Deborah Birx, M.D. revealed how the scheme worked. Dr. Birx was the U.S. Global Aids Coordinator & U.S. Special Representative for Global Health Diplomacy and Physician-Ambassador to the office of the Vice President and the U.S. Government Coronavirus Response Coordinator. During an April 7, 2020, task force press briefing, Dr. Birx was asked by a reporter about the allegations by many that the coronavirus deaths have been artificially inflated. The reporter asked: "Can you talk about your concerns about deaths being misreported by coronavirus because of either testing or standards for how they're characterized?"[1400] Dr. Birx then admitted that, in fact, that the COVID-19 deaths were being inflated. Dr. Birx explained that the United States has taken a "liberal approach" to reporting COVID-19 deaths. She stated that it is "straightforward." That "straightforward" approach is to report someone who dies "with" COVID-19 as a COVID-19 death. Implied in her statement is that any deceased person who tests positive for COVID-19 is recorded as dying "of" COVID-19, regardless of the actual cause of death. To put it more succinctly, every person who dies "with" COVID-19 is recorded as dying "of" COVID-19.

Dr. Birx distinguished the U.S. approach from other countries where, for example, if someone died of heart failure or kidney failure and they test positive for COVID-19, some other countries might report that as a kidney failure or heart failure death and not a COVID-19 death. Not so in the United States. The "liberal approach" taken in the U.S. is that if someone dies with COVID-19 they are added to the COVID-19 death total even though they actually died of kidney failure or heart failure. Dr. Birx answered the reporter's question as follows:

> So, I think, in this country, we've taken a very liberal approach to mortality, and I think the reporting here has been pretty straightforward over the last five to six weeks. Prior to that, when there

wasn't testing in January and February, that's a very different situation and unknown.

There are other countries that if you had a pre-existing condition and let's say the virus caused you to go to the ICU and then have a heart or kidney problem — some countries are recording that as a heart issue or a kidney issue and not a COVID-19 death.

Right now, we're still recording it, and we'll — I mean, the great thing about having forms that come in and a form that has the ability to mark it as COVID-19 infection — the intent is, right now, that those — **if someone dies with COVID-19, we are counting that as a COVID-19 death.**[1401] (emphasis added)

Illinois Department of Public Health Director Dr. Ngozi Ezike followed the guidance from the CDC and admitted that the State of Illinois was recording persons who died with COVID-19 as having died from COVID-19, regardless of whether COVID-19 was the actual cause of the deaths. Health Director Ezike stated:

I just want to be clear in terms of the definition of people dying of COVID. The case definition is very simplistic. It means at the time of death it was a COVID positive diagnosis. ... It means, technically, even if you died from a clear alternate cause, but you had COVID at the same time, it is still listed as a COVID death. So. everyone who is listed as a COVID death, doesn't mean that was the cause of the death, but they had COVID at the time of death.[1402]

That reporting scheme of the State of Illinois was per the

guidance given by the CDC. The CDC was beating the bushes, so to speak, to generate the inflated COVID-19 statistics. The CDC issued guidance to the state health commissioners to alter how they report COVID-19 deaths in order to artificially inflate the deaths from COVID-19.

The CDC data manipulation was planned. And it had a purpose. To create a COVID-19 pandemic where none really existed. It was a massive statistical lie campaign. And it constituted a federal crime. Oregon State Senators Kim Thatcher and Dennis Linthicum petitioned U.S. Attorney Scott Asphaug to approve a grand jury investigation into the criminality of the CDC and FDA.[1403] They based their allegations on information and data from a large team of world-renowned doctors, epidemiologists, virologists, and attorneys.[1404] The Senators averred that in the March 2020 alert, the CDC illegally changed the National Vital Statistics System so that mortality data compilers could massage data to falsely report COVID-19 as the "cause" of death. This new set of rules, which only applied to COVID-19, departed from the standard procedures that had been in effect for the prior 17 years.

The CDC statistics reported deaths as being from COVID-19 when the deaths were actually from something else. Comorbidity is defined as the simultaneous presence of two or more chronic diseases or conditions in a patient. The CDC has reported that 94% percent of people they have reported who have died of COVID-19 in the U.S. were suffering from an average of 2.5 chronic diseases or conditions in addition to COVID-19.[1405] Thus, the statistical total of 161,392 deaths (as of August 22, 2020) from COVID-19 reported by the CDC does not mean that the decedents making up that total actually died from COVID-19. The reported people dying "with" COVID-19 are being misrepresented as people who died "from" COVID-19. This inflated the COVID-19 deaths and created a false sense of danger among the public.

The CDC reports that as of August 22, 2020, only 6% of the 161,392 reported COVID-19 deaths were from COVID-19 alone. The remaining 151,708 of persons who died while testing positive for COVID-19 died from some cause (i.e., a comorbidity) in addition to COVID-19. The astounding thing is that each of those 151,708 persons who died had 2.5 comorbidities in addition to COVID-19. That means that 94% of the persons reported dying of COVID-19 actually died from a combination of diseases and injuries, which may or may not be COVID-19.

With this surreal definition of what is a COVID-19 death being pushed by the CDC, the local health officials are only limited by their creativity when deciding that a death is from COVID-19. The Orange County (Florida) Health Officer Dr. Raul Pino did not seem to think it was unusual that a man who died from a motorcycle accident was misrepresented as having died of COVID-19. Dr. Raul Pino even tried to make the irrational argument that it is okay to report a person who died in a motorcycle accident as having died from COVID-19 because "it could have been the COVID-19 that caused him to crash."[1406]

Daniella Lama reporting for Fox 35 News in Orlando discovered that the Florida Department of Health has decided that all persons who test positive for COVID-19 in Florida are automatically listed as COVID-19 deaths if they subsequently die unless there is an extra step taken by the reporting agency to exclude them from the COVID-19 death statistics.[1407] That extra step to exclude the motorcycle decedent was not done, which is why he was listed automatically as a COVID-19 death. Obviously, the statistical system is rigged to capture all persons who have ever tested positive with COVID-19 as a COVID-19 death if they subsequently die. If the extra step is not taken to exclude them from the statistical count then they will be listed as a COVID-19 death. With the fear of the disease ramped up by these artificially inflated COVID-19 death statistics, the public was primed to accept the emergency use authorized COVID-19 vaccines.

Why would county health officials and hospitals go along with this scam? Because there is money in it. "For the love of money is the root of all evil." 1 Timothy 6:19. Minnesota State Senator and Dr. Scott Jensen, M.D., revealed that hospital administrations are incentivized to diagnose and treat a person for COVID-19.[1408] The system is financially skewed toward diagnosing and treating COVID-19 even though the patient may not actually be ill from COVID-19. The patients may be in the hospital for an entirely different reason, but if they test positive for COVID-19 or they are diagnosed as having COVID-19, then the hospital hits the financial jackpot and can begin raking in the financial windfall from the federal government through the Coronavirus Aid, Relief and Economic Security Act (CARES Act).

The CDC and NIH are fanning the hysteria of a health emergency that does not really exist. It is doing so by artificially inflating the COVID-19 numbers in order to portray a false sense of emergency to justify its own draconian COVID-19 orders.

Dr. Kristin Held is the President of the Association of American Physicians and Surgeons (AAPS). On July 20, 2020, she explained in a post the trickery used by the CDC and the State Boards of Health to inflate the COVID-19 infection and death rates.

Dr. Held revealed a little-known fact that "[t]he Council of State and Territorial Epidemiologists (CSTE) adopted new definitions of COVID-19 cases and COVID-related deaths in April [2020] that were adopted by the Centers for Disease Control and Prevention (CDC) in May. The states were then encouraged to adopt the new definitions."

These new definitions had the direct effect of artificially inflating the COVID-19 case and death statistics. Dr. Held reveals that under the new criteria "COVID-related deaths can include anyone who has COVID-19 listed on their death certificate as one of the causes of death- it doesn't have to be the first or second cause, and no COVID-19 testing is required."[1409]

There is a political motivation to increase COVID-19 case and death statistics. Dr. Held reveals that the Federal Government is handsomely compensating the hospitals that go along with that political program. She explains:

> Why would someone want to inflate case counts, and what are the risks and benefits of doing so? As reported in Modern Healthcare, July 17, 2020, "HHS to send $10 billion in round two of relief grants to COVID-19 hot spots." Modern Healthcare reports, "Hospitals that had more than 161 COVID-19 admissions between January 1 and June 10 will be paid $50,000 for each COVID-19 admission. HHS asked hospitals to start submitting COVID-19 admission data on June 8."
>
> Hospitals that use the new CDC definition stand to make millions of dollars. The first round of HHS grants was $12 billion and paid $76,975 per admission to hospitals that had more than 100 COVID-19 admissions from January 1 through April 1. Clearly, states hit early got tons of money- Illinois got $740 M, New York got $684 M, and Pennsylvania got $655 M alone. Additionally, Medicaid will pay out $15 billion in relief funds- hospitals must apply by August, so the more cases the better the return.
>
> ***
>
> Remember, this is on top of the extra money commercial insurers and the extra 20% Medicare

> pay the hospitals for patients hospitalized "with COVID-19." The hospitals reporting the most cases get the most money. In addition to expanding the definition of a New COVID-19 case to include exposure to a COVID-19 positive patient and a self-reported fever, lowering admission thresholds, and requiring testing on every admission, the ability to code a hospital admission as "with-COVID" is easy and becomes a very lucrative business model.

Dr. Held concludes:

> Clearly, hospitals are financially incentivized to code more COVID cases and deaths. Definitions matter. Another sad consequence is that we are losing freedoms and destroying our state and country based on the inflated numbers. Our reopenings are based on these numbers –we have lost our ability to congregate in groups of 10 or more, go to church, school, weddings, funerals, sporting events, concerts, or go anywhere without a mask, or hug our parents, grandparents, children, grandchildren, and the lonely.[1410]

It took time for the states to implement the CDC's new definition for COVID-19. But eventually, that new definition bore the sour fruit planned by the CDC. As the states began implementing the new CDC guidance, we found a spike in COVID-19 cases. In the middle of June 2020, the U.S. COVID-19 cases steadily increased from approximately 20,000 reported cases per day to 300,000 reported cases per day by the beginning of January 2021.[1411] That suspicious spike in numbers came on the heels of the new reporting criteria for cases instituted by the CDC. Dr. Held wonders about that spike.

> We must answer the question, what happened June 14-16, because something did when you look at the stats. (Did redefining what constitutes a COVID-19 case, hospitalization, or death change the numbers? Did federal financial aid to hospitals change admitting thresholds and practices? Did the FDA withdrawing its Emergency Use Authorization (EUA) for Hydroxychloroquine (HCQ) alter outpatient treatment resulting in COVID-surging? Was it the Riots? Or what?)[1412]

Dr. Held was writing her suspicions on July 20, 2020, when the spike had only reached approximately 75,000 cases per day. Dr. Held thought that was somewhat suspicious. But the daily increase in COVID-19 cases continued until it reached 300,000 cases per day by January 2021. It seems that the "second wave" predicted by Dr. Fauci and others was something they planned to happen by rigging the COVID-19 numbers. It coincided perfectly with the flu season. Interesting that influenza all but disappeared in the fall and winter of 2020. They just redefined all influenza cases as COVID-19 cases.

Dr. (and Minnesota State Senator) Scott Jensen reveals that the guidance by the CDC is to put COVID-19 down as the cause of death even though the death actually resulted from something else. Indeed, the CDC is advising that COVID-19 is to be considered not on testing and a diagnosis that COVID-19 is the cause of death but rather based upon it being "suspected or likely." Health officials and doctors are being asked to put on the death certificate "probable" or "presumed" death from COVID-19 based upon a clinical judgment (i.e., a guess) without any actual scientific test or diagnosis.[1413] In his expert opinion, Dr. Jensen concluded that COVID-19 death statistics are being gamed to inflate the death rate.

Dr. Scott Jensen was named Minnesota Family Doctor of

the Year seven years ago. Now he finds himself and his pristine record and reputation under attack after he exposed the dirty secret that the threat from COVID-19 is not real and the states are deceptively inflating the COVID-19 deaths. The Minnesota Board of Medical Practice has now notified Dr. Jensen that they are investigating him on alleged charges of improper medical practice. Among the charges are that he spread disinformation by "advising against vaccines and masks."[1414] Further, the medical board alleged that Dr. Jensen "promoted conspiracy theories that the Minnesota Department of Health instructed providers to falsify death certificates to list COVID-19."[1415] The Orwellian medical board characterizes good medical advice as "disinformation" and true statements as "conspiracy theories." The pharmaceutical cartel is moving against Dr. Jensen as an object lesson to frighten any doctor who would dare to speak up against their medical tyranny and quackery.

The CDC guidance referenced by Dr. Jensen states in pertinent part:

> In cases where a definite diagnosis of COVID–19 cannot be made, but it is suspected or likely (e.g., the circumstances are compelling within a reasonable degree of certainty), it is acceptable to report COVID–19 on a death certificate as "probable" or "presumed." In these instances, certifiers should use their best clinical judgement in determining if a COVID–19 infection was likely. However, please note that testing for COVID–19 should be conducted whenever possible.[1416]

The CDC states that testing for COVID-19 is ideal but not necessary in order to categorize a death as being COVID-19 as long as the "circumstances are compelling within a reasonable degree of certainty." Basically, that means whatever a particular doctor wants it to mean. The CDC instructions for filling out death certificates are contrary to the traditional method of only putting down the scientific finding for a "cause of death." The CDC guidance opens the door for a doctor to opine under a "reasonable degree of certainty" standard that virtually any death is a COVID-19 death. And that is precisely what the CDC wants. The CDC guidance states:

> Ideally, testing for COVID–19 should be conducted, but it is acceptable to report COVID–19 on a death certificate without this confirmation if the circumstances are compelling within a reasonable degree of certainty.[1417]

Below is the scenario on page 6 of the CDC Guidance for Certifying Deaths Due to COVID-19. Please read it carefully. You do not need to be a doctor to understand that the CDC instructs doctors to lie on death certificates. They are trying to inflate the death statistics. Why else would the CDC give specific instructions in filling out death certificates regarding how to characterize a decedent as having died from COVID-19?

The CDC is interested in ensuring that every possible COVID-19 death is caught. And they have an interest in turning deaths with only inferential COVID-19 evidence into COVID-19 deaths. Why are the instructions contrary to all standard medical procedures for filling out death certificates?

The CDC is instructing Doctors to mark down that a patient died of COVID-19 even without any scientific tests to indicate that the patient had COVID-19 at the time of death. The new standard is now simply an inference that it was "likely" that the patient died of COVID-19. In the scenario presented by the CDC, that likelihood is based on the decedent being exposed five days before her death to a person subsequently diagnosed with COVID-19. The CDC scenario presented on page 6 of the CDC death certificate guidance is as follows:

An 86-year-old female passed away at home. Her husband reported that she was nonambulatory after suffering an ischemic stroke 3 years ago. He stated that 5 days prior, she developed a high fever and severe cough after being exposed to an ill family member who subsequently was diagnosed with COVID–19. Despite his urging, she refused to go to the hospital, even when her breathing became more labored and temperature escalated. She was unresponsive that morning and her husband phoned emergency medical services (EMS). Upon EMS arrival, the patient was pulseless and apneic. Her husband stated that he and his wife had advanced directives and that she was not to be resuscitated. After consulting with medical command, she was pronounced dead and the coroner was notified.

Comment: Although no testing was done, the coroner determined that the likely UCOD [Underlying Cause of Death] was COVID–19 given the patient's symptoms and exposure to an infected individual. Therefore, COVID–19 was reported on the lowest line used in Part I. Her ischemic stroke was considered a factor that contributed to her death but was not a part of the direct causal sequence in Part I, so it was reported in Part II.[1418]

With those standards in mind, state health officials have been able to classify virtually any death where a person tests positive for COVID-19 as a COVID-19 death, regardless of the actual cause of death, and they are doing so. The vast majority of the deaths being counted as "probable cases" are actually of people who may have had COVID-19 but died from something else. For example, on July 23, 2020, Danielle Waugh from CBS 12 News investigated evidence that only 169 of the 581 reported deaths in

Palm Beach County were of persons who allegedly had COVID-19 without any contributing illness.[1419] That calls into question the legitimacy of more than 70% of the reported deaths from COVID-19.

Early on, the states adopted the new CDC guidelines. For example, Virginia Department of Health (VDH) states that "VDH adopted the updated CDC confirmed and probable surveillance case definitions on August 27, 2020."[1420] Indeed, the VDH provided a link directly to the CDC website defining confirmed and probable cases.[1421]

The VDH is like most state health departments who follow the new guidance for reporting COVID-19 cases and deaths. The VDH acknowledges that when it reports COVID-19 cases they are not based on a medical diagnosis of COVID-19. Thus, a person does not need to actually have COVID-19 to be included in the Virginia COVID-19 statistics. The VDH explains:

> Public health uses standardized case definitions to count cases. These case definitions make it easier to compare data over time, across states, or even between different counties. A case definition is different from a diagnosis, and is used for a different purpose. A diagnosis is helpful for treatment and medical billing while a case definition is used for public health surveillance. For COVID-19, Virginia uses the CDC COVID-19 confirmed and probable case definitions. These definitions suggests [*sic*] that we report two case statuses:
>
> Confirmed cases – Confirmed cases include anyone who tests positive for SARS-CoV-2 RNA in a clinical or autopsy specimen using a molecular amplification test.

> Probable cases – There are a few ways to identify a probable case. In Virginia, anyone who is positive using an approved antigen test or anyone who displays a specific set of symptoms and has an epidemiologic linkage (contact with another confirmed or probable case or part of a risk cohort), or anyone whose death certificate mentions COVID-19 or SARS-CoV-2 without a positive lab result counts as a probable case.[1422]

The VDH further acknowledges that the COVID-19 statistics received from hospitals overstate the COVID-19 risk. The hospitalization statistics include "those who have [COVID-19] tests pending" but who have not actually tested positive for COVID-19. The VIDH explains that "[t]hese data do not have the same kind of rigorous case definition that epidemiologic case data do because they are not intended for the same purpose. For healthcare system preparation, an overestimation is better than an underestimation."[1423]

The VDH explains that in order to be consistent, it must use that same overstatement across the board when reporting COVID-19 statistics. "For our purposes, it's important that the same case definition be applied to the numerator (the number of cases that result in hospitalization) and the denominator (the total number of cases)."[1424]

Virginia went beyond the CDC guidance and artificially goosed up its COVID-19 case statistics even more. On or before June 19, 2020, NBC News reported that the State of Virginia would start reporting the number of positive COVID-19 tests as COVID-19 cases rather than the number of persons who tested positive. Thus, a person who receives a positive COVID-19 test result one day and two days later tests positive again would be counted as two confirmed COVID-19 cases rather than one case. Since almost all who tested positive for COVID-19 would repeatedly get tested to determine if they were no longer infected, there could be several positive COVID-19 tests per patient before they tested negative. This inevitably would artificially inflate the COVID-19 cases in Virginia. That is the only thing that such a contrivance would achieve. NBC reported:

> The Virginia Department of Health announced it will now count the number of positive virus tests instead of the number of people who test positive.
>
> That means if one person is tested three-times and all three tests come back positive, it counts as three instead of how the numbers were being counted before, which would have only been one because it was a single patient.[1425]

The only reason to count the number of tests is to deceptively inflate the number of COVID-19 cases in Virginia. There is no way around it. That is out-and-out chicanery.

The inflated COVID-19 numbers can be explained in part by the built-in financial incentive for medical professionals to diagnose a patient with COVID-19. USA TODAY revealed that "[t]he coronavirus relief legislation created a 20% premium, or add-on, for COVID-19 Medicare patients."[1426] There are financial incentives in addition to the 20% premium. Dr. Jensen explained the additional financial incentive for hospitals to make a diagnosis of COVID-19:

> Hospital administrators might well want to see COVID-19 attached to a discharge summary or a death certificate. Why? Because if it's a straightforward, garden-variety pneumonia that a person is admitted to the hospital for – if they're Medicare – typically, the diagnosis-related group lump sum payment would be $5,000. But if it's

> COVID-19 pneumonia, then it's $13,000, and if that COVID-19 pneumonia patient ends up on a ventilator, it goes up to $39,000.[1427]

USA TODAY checked out the claim by Dr. Jensen. "USA TODAY reached out to Marty Makary, a surgeon and professor of health policy and management at Johns Hopkins Bloomberg School of Public Health, about the claim. Makary said in an email April 21 that 'what Scott Jensen said sounds right to me.'"[1428] USA TODAY determined that Dr. Jensen's claim was accurate.[1429]

Andrew Mark Miller, reporting for the Washington Examiner, revealed that because U.S. hospitals are reimbursed 13,000 for every COVID-19 diagnosis and 39,000 for every COVID-19 patient put on a ventilator, "U.S. Centers for Disease Control and Prevention Director Robert Redfield agreed that some hospitals have a monetary incentive to overcount coronavirus deaths."[1430] Dr. Redfield expressed that opinion while testifying before a U.S. House of Representatives Panel. Dr. Redfield acknowledged that the federal reimbursement scheme creates a perverse monetary incentive for U.S. hospitals to inflate the COVID-19 infection rate. Dr. Redfield explained that "when it comes to hospital reimbursement issues or individuals that get discharged, there could be some play in that for sure."[1431]

Edwin Mora, reported for *Breitbart* that "[a]ccording to Congressman [Blaine] Luetkemeyer, Adm. Brett Giroir from the U.S. Health and Human Services (HHS) Department has conceded that there is an economic incentive for hospitals to inflate their coronavirus fatalities. Giroir 'acknowledged that the statistics he is getting from the states are over-inflated,' the Republican lawmakers said."[1432]

According to Becker's Healthcare, as of April 2020, Virginia hospitals received from HHS $201,000 reimbursement per COVID-19 case. That figure was obtained from Kaiser Health

News, which "used a state breakdown provided to the House Ways and Means Committee by HHS along with COVID-19 cases tabulated by The New York Times for its analysis."[1433]

Despite the over reporting, the VDH nonetheless claims that the "the number of cases we have on record is an underrepresentation of the true burden."[1434] That nonsensical statement is based in part on the premise that there are people walking around with COVID-19 who show no symptoms. But that statement is based on the disproven premise of asymptomatic spread of SARS-CoV-2. The asymptomatic carrier theory was born from the fact that the PCR test for SARS-CoV-2 has potentially up to a 97% false positive rate. The medical authorities came up with a way to explain how people who are not sick with COVID-19 nonetheless test positive for the disease. They argue that the well-person tests positive for the disease because he is an "asymptomatic" carrier of SARS-CoV-2. Thus, the false-positive test problem is solved.

The asymptomatic spread theory is a fantastical fraud. That foundational lie underlies the government strategy against the mythical COVID-19 pandemic. In a court action for a preliminary injunction, America's Frontline Doctors (AFLD) averred that the government floated the false asymptomatic spread theory to justify lockdowns, masking, and social distancing measures designed to take away our liberties. The AFLD court filing states in pertinent part:

> **[I]t appears that these Defendants either did lie about asymptomatic spread, or were simply wrong about the science.** The theory of asymptomatic transmission – used as the justification for the lockdown and masking of the healthy – was based solely upon mathematical modeling. This theory had no actual study participants, and no peer review. The authors made

> the unfounded assumption that asymptomatic persons were "75% as infectious" as symptomatic persons. But in the real world, healthy false positives turned out to be merely healthy, and were never shown to be "asymptomatic" carriers of anything. Studies have shown that PCR test-positive asymptomatic individuals do not induce clinical COVID-19 disease, not even in a family member with whom they share a home and extended proximity. An enormous study of nearly ten million people in Wuhan, China showed that asymptomatic individuals testing positive for COVID-19 never infected others. Since asymptomatic individuals do not spread COVID-19, they do not need to be vaccinated.[1435]

Researchers Torsten Engelbrecht and Konstantin Demeter concluded:

> Lockdowns and hygienic measures around the world are based on numbers of cases and mortality rates created by the so-called SARS-CoV-2 RT-PCR tests used to identify "positive" patients, whereby "positive" is usually equated with "infected."
>
> But looking closely at the facts, the conclusion is that these PCR tests are meaningless as a diagnostic tool to determine an alleged infection by a supposedly new virus called SARS-CoV-2.[1436]

The researchers concluded that the RT-PCR test used to detect COVID-19 is so inaccurate that there may be between 22% and 78% false positives. But there is no way to be sure because there is no gold standard against which to verify the accuracy of the tests.

One study gives an example of the test's inaccuracy. "[A] study from Singapore in which tests were carried out almost daily on 18 patients and the majority went from 'positive' to 'negative' back to 'positive' at least once, and up to five times in one patient."[1437]

The apparent preponderance of false positives for asymptomatic subjects means that the people are asymptomatic because they do not have COVID-19. The asymptomatic carrier model that is being sold to the public is a myth. The positive tests are bogus results. The COVID-19 "outbreaks" and "hotspots" are really not "outbreaks" or "hotspots" at all.

Word has gotten out about the inaccuracies of the PCR test, and so the CDC's hand was forced to stop using it. On July 21, 2021, the CDC announced that laboratories should cease using the PCR to test for COVID-19 beginning on December 31, 2021.[1438] If the PCR test is so inaccurate as to cause the CDC to recommend against using it, why is the CDC waiting until December 31, 2021, to transition to a more accurate test? It seems that the CDC is not at all concerned about the accuracy of its COVID-19 testing. The PCR test will be replaced with the antigen test, which the FDA acknowledges is also inaccurate.

It must be understood that most states report Total COVID-19 Deaths as being the number of confirmed and probable COVID-19 deaths. Virginia is one example. The Total Deaths number for Virginia from COVID-19 is a scam on two levels. First, a probable case does not require that the person test positive for COVID-19. In the written guidance, the CDC has told local officials to put on the death certificate "probable" or "presumed" death from COVID-19 based upon a clinical judgment (i.e., a guess) without any actual scientific test or diagnosis.

It does not take much to be a probable case of COVID-19. One could have a headache and have recently been within 6 feet for at least 15 minutes of someone who is himself a probable case of COVID-19 or a member of a risk cohort for COVID-19 as defined by public health authorities during an outbreak. Thus, neither the person who is supposed to be the spreader of the disease nor the person supposed to have gotten COVID-19 needs to have COVID-19 to be included in the statistics for COVID-19 Total Cases or Total Deaths.

It gets worse. The confirmed cases of deaths from COVID-19 are not what you would think they are. A confirmed COVID-19 death does not mean that the person died *from* COVID-19. It means that the person died *with* COVID-19.

A close reading of the Virginia Department of Health (VDH) rules for reported deaths reveals that the "VDH is counting any death that occurs in a person who was reported to the health department as having COVID-19."[1439]

Thus, the VDH is not reporting only those people who died *from* COVID-19. They are artificially inflating the numbers by including the numbers of people who died from some other cause and tested positive for COVID-19 prior to their death. The VDH death statistics include both those who died *from* COVID-19 and those who died *with* COVID-19, even though those who died *with* COVID-19 actually died from some cause other than COVID-19. The department of health states that it will not include those who died from "an injury or accident" among the COVID-19 deaths. But that is the only exclusion. All other people who die *with* COVID-19 from some cause other than injury or accident are listed by the VDH as a COVID-19 death.

The VDH exclusion criteria only excludes from the COVID-19 statistics deaths due to "injury or accident." What about non-traumatic causes of death like cancer, diabetes, emphysema, heart disease, or stroke? Is someone who dies of any of those illnesses listed, nonetheless, as a COVId-19 death?

Apparently so. Thus, if someone dies of cancer but tests positive for COVID-19 he will be listed as a COVID-19 death.

How inflated are the death statistics? The CDC offers an answer. That answer is that only 6% of reported COVID-19 deaths died only from COVID-19. All other reported deaths are people who had comorbidities. The CDC explains that its reported statistics show "health conditions and contributing causes mentioned in conjunction with deaths involving coronavirus disease 2019 (COVID-19). For 6% of the deaths, COVID-19 was the only cause mentioned. For deaths with conditions or causes in addition to COVID-19, on average, there were 2.6 additional conditions or causes per death."[1440]

Some of the comorbidities listed by the CDC include cardiac arrest, diabetes, Alzheimer disease, renal failure, injury (intentional, unintentional, poisoning, and other adverse events), malignant neoplasms (a.k.a. cancerous tumors). In that partial list, the only comorbidity that is not reported as a COVID-19 death in Virginia by the VDH are those who die from "an injury or accident."

The Colorado Department of Public Health and Environment (CDPHE) has also followed CDC guidelines to inflate COVID-19 numbers. The CDPHE told NBC News 9 Denver that "[w]e classify a death as confirmed when there was a case who had a positive SARS-CoV-2 (COVID-19) laboratory test and then died."[1441] Thus, if a person dies from some cause other than COVID-19, he would still be listed as a COVID-19 death if he tests positive for COVID-19. The CDPHE further explained that simply because there is no test does not mean a person will not be listed as a COVID-19 death. The CDPHE stated: "We also classify some deaths as probable."[1442]

With those standards in mind, they are able to classify virtually any death where a person tests positive for COVID-19 as a COVID-19 death, regardless of the actual cause of death, and they are doing so. A case in Montezuma County in Colorado illustrates that point.

> The coroner of Montezuma County in southwestern Colorado couldn't believe it when the state's health department concluded a May 4 death in his county was the result of COVID-19.
>
> "I know it's not correct," George Deavers told 9Wants to Know Thursday. "Nowhere on the death certificate is COVID even listed. It had nothing to do with his death."
>
> Deavers ought to know. The death certificate he signed just this week lists the official cause of death for the 35-year old man as "ethanol toxicity."
>
> In other words, Deavers said, he died because he drank too much alcohol.
>
> "We did blood work. The blood work came back at 550 [mg/dL]. Anything over 300 is lethal," he said. To be clear, Deavers did test the body for COVID after he received word that the man might have had recent contact with someone with the virus. That test showed the man did, in fact, have COVID-19, but Deavers said he's "99.9% certain" the virus did not cause the man's death.[1443]

The death certificate indicated the cause of death as ethanol toxicity. There was no mention of COVID-19 as even a contributing factor, yet the state of Colorado reported the man as having died of COVID-19 simply because he had tested positive for COVID-19.

The Colorado Department of Public Health and Environment (CDPHE) disagreed with the coroner who filled out the death certificate. The CDPHE continued to list the death from alcohol poisoning as a COVID-19 death despite the coroner's objection. Indeed, the CDPHE refused to even return the coroner's calls.

Why would they do that? Because the state did not want to give Montezuma County a variance from the state COVID-19 emergency business closure restrictions. The state wanted to artificially pump up the death rate in the county from COVID-19 as an excuse to continue with the business closures in that county. NBC News 9 Denver reported:

> In a letter sent Monday to the Montezuma County Administrator, CDPHE's Executive Director Jill Hunsaker Ryan said, "Our reviewers have some concerns about vulnerabilities in Montezuma County and want to monitor the situation further before considering a variance."[1444]

Indeed, the fraud has gotten so bad in Colorado that State Representative Mark Baisley has sent a formal letter requesting 18th Judicial District Attorney George Brauchler to investigate and criminally prosecute the Executive Director of the Colorado Department of Public Health and Environment (CDPHE), Jill Hunsaker Ryan. Baisley, in the letter, accused Ryan of fraudulently overruling death findings by attending physicians in cases where patients also tested positive for COVID-19 in order to artificially inflate the number of COVID-19-related deaths.[1445]

The Colorado Governor has dismissed any notion of a criminal investigation of the Director of the CDPHE. Of course he would; the director is his subordinate and is acting at his direction. So, how has Colorado Governor Jared Polis addressed the issue? "In a conference call with reporters Friday afternoon, CDPHE officials revealed they would be announcing two numbers concerning deaths among COVID-19 patients going forward. One number would show the total number of people who died while sick with COVID-19. The other number would be how many people had died as a result of COVID-19."

You read that correctly, the State of Colorado has decided to keep two books, just like all crooked businesses do. One book will report the actual deaths allegedly caused by COVID-19. The other book will register the phony "total" number of people who died with COVID-19, which means they only tested positive for COVID-19 and have died from some other cause.

So when you hear the total number of deaths from COVID-19 in Colorado, you cannot be sure you are not hearing the inflated number. The public will not know that the "total" number being reported may only mean the decedent had COVID-19 and could have died from something else. The only reason the governor went from out-and-out lying by reporting all persons dying with COVID-19 as "COVID-19 deaths" to now keeping two sets of books is that he was embarrassed when he got caught fraudulently reporting a death from alcohol poisoning as a COVID-19 death only because the decedent also tested positive for COVID-19.

The CDC scheme made no sense to the electorate, so the governor changed course to cover the fraud. But he still wants to have his cake and eat it too. He wants to keep getting federal money by adding in those who die with COVID-19 to those who allegedly die from COVID-19. That way, the state can get more federal money. The federal government is paying the states a lot to play this deceptive game of hyping the COVID-19 scare, locking us down, masking us, and forcibly vaccinating us. It is what the federal government asked for, and it is paying the states a lot of money to do it. COVID-19 is not a threat to public health but a phantom virus to scare citizens into slavery. It is about tyranny.

Indeed, the State of Colorado brought in more than $360 million from the first $30 billion installment sent from the federal government's CARES Act Public Health and Social Services Emergency Fund to the states.[1446] Those funds were sent to the states to encourage the states to enforce the draconian measures necessary to investigate and inflate case statistics, engage in contact tracing, testing services, personal protective equipment, and emergency preparedness and response.[1447] More COVID-19 cases extended the emergency and ensured federal money would flow. The more tyranny imposed by the states meant more money was sent to the states.

Dr. Anthony Fauci is the Director of the National Institute of Allergy and Infectious Diseases (NIAID), an agency in the National Institute of Health (NIH). The CDC and the NIH are both operational agencies in the Department of Health and Human Services. Anthony Fauci is portrayed as the nation's top infectious disease expert. He is a member of the White House coronavirus task force. Dr. Fauci does not realize it, but he has confirmed that the fraud by the CDC is knowing and intentional. He did this by trying to explain the acknowledged fact that 94% of COVID-19 decedents had on average 2.5 comorbidities. Dr. Fauci did not dispute that fact. He accepted that fact as true. But how he characterized that fact was breathtaking in its incredulity. Dr. Fauci told an ABC News interviewer on September 1, 2020, that it "does not mean that someone who has hypertension or diabetes who dies of COVID didn't die of COVID-19. They did." Dr. Fauci further stated that "it's not 9,000 deaths from COVID-19, it's 180-plus-thousand deaths."[1448]

That statement by Dr. Fauci is telling. Dr. Fauci is stating a hypothetical case, but he is perfectly comfortable to say that someone (anyone) who is listed in the CDC COVID-19 death list who died with 1) hypertension (i.e., high blood pressure), or 2) diabetes, and 3) COVID-19 most definitely died of COVID-19. Dr. Fauci picks one of the three illnesses (COVID-19), and without even knowing the facts or the patient, he is able to divine that every decedent with those simultaneous illnesses always dies from COVID-19.

Dr. Fauci did not equivocate. He emphatically stated that all the diabetics and people with high blood pressure listed by the CDC as having died of COVID-19, in fact died of COVID-19 regardless of the seriousness of their hypertension or diabetes. No, ifs, ands, or buts about it. He stated emphatically that every person listed by the CDC as a COVID-19 death actually died "from" COVID-19 regardless of the comorbidity. Dr. Fauci was forcible and clear: "So the numbers you've been hearing — there are 180,000-plus deaths [as of September 1, 2020]— are real deaths from COVID-19. Let (there) not be any confusion about that."[1449]

Not only is Dr. Fauci's statement incredible on its face. It is contrary to the known facts. States are reporting persons *with* COVID-19 as being COVID-19 deaths, regardless of their comorbidities that could be the real cause of the deaths. The states are doing that under the specific guidance from the CDC. The CDC is receiving that data from the states that they requested the states to send them. Indeed, an Illinois State Health Official announced during a press conference: "Technically, even if you died from a clear alternate cause but you had COVID at the same time, it is still listed as a COVID death."[1450]

In a Johns Hopkins News-Letter dated November 22, 2020, (later retracted) "Genevieve Briand, assistant program director of the Applied Economics master's degree program at Hopkins, critically analyzed the effect of COVID-19 on U.S. deaths using data from the Centers for Disease Control and Prevention (CDC)."[1451] She found that there was zero increase in deaths across the United States between 2018 and 2020. She determined that "the percentages of deaths among all age groups remain relatively the same." She thus concluded that COVID-19 "has relatively no effect on deaths in the United States."[1452] Briand was puzzled because the CDC had reported a sudden increase in deaths due to COVID-19. There should have been an increase in total deaths reported to the CDC by approximately 267,000. But there was no such increase. When Briand examined the death statistics from the CDC, she made the disturbing discovery that deaths from heart disease, respiratory disease, influenza, and pneumonia dropped during the COVID-19 outbreak. She saw in the statistics that deaths were being shifted from those other categories to COVID-19. "Briand believes that deaths due to heart diseases, respiratory diseases, influenza and pneumonia may instead be recategorized as being due to COVID-19."[1453]

The Briand article was retracted for the reason that Johns Hopkins was concerned that the article "has been used to support dangerous inaccuracies that minimize the impact of the pandemic."[1454] But in the retraction notice, Johns Hopkins actually acknowledged the principal finding made by Briand that the number of deaths due to heart diseases, respiratory diseases, influenza and pneumonia had been shifted to the COVID-19 list of deaths. The retraction states that "Briand also claimed in her analysis that deaths due to heart diseases, respiratory diseases, influenza and pneumonia may be incorrectly categorized as COVID-19-related deaths. However, COVID-19 disproportionately affects those with preexisting conditions, so those with those underlying conditions are statistically more likely to be severely affected and die from the virus."[1455] Notice that the retraction does not dispute Briand's finding, but rather tries to explain it as being caused by the fact that "those with those underlying conditions are statistically more likely to be severely affected and die from the virus."[1456] The retraction notice did not contradict the conclusion of Briand's study that the COVID-19 death statistic is a statistic that lists those who die "with" COVID-19 and not necessarily those who die "from" COVID-19.[1457]

The artificial inflation of COVID-19 deaths is a worldwide phenomenon. On July 16, 2020, Dr. Yoon K Loke and Dr. Carl

Heneghan studied the death statistics in England and discovered that they were being artificially inflated.[1458] Dr. Yoon K Loke is Professor of Medicine and Pharmacology, Norwich Medical School, University of East Anglia, UK. Dr. Carl Heneghan is Professor of Evidence-Based Medicine and Director of Studies for the Evidence-Based Health Care Programmes at the University of Oxford. Dr. Heneghan set up and directs the Oxford COVID Evidence Service.

According to the definitions used by the National Health Service (NHS) and Public Health England (PHE) for a COVID-19 death, nobody who tests positive for COVID-19 could ever recover from that disease. Drs. Loke and Heneghan reported that "[a] patient who has tested positive, but successfully treated and discharged from hospital, will still be counted as a COVID death even if they had a heart attack or were run over by a bus three months later."[1459]

The Department of Health uses the PHE statistics to announce COVID-19 deaths. As of July 3, 2020, the PHE has reported 45,199 COVID-19 deaths.[1460] The recent study by Drs. Loke and Heneghan calls into question the accuracy of that death tally. Now, it is not clear how many of those people actually died of COVID-19. "It turns out you could have been tested positive in February, recovered, then hit by a bus in July and you'd be recorded as a Covid death."[1461]

The doctors who did the study calculated that "if the counting method is not changed it would mean all 290,000 people who have tested positive for coronavirus would eventually be added to the death toll, regardless of when and how they died."[1462] That is a real problem because most of the people who are hospitalized for COVID-19 are elderly people who have many comorbidities. When they recover from COVID-19 and are released from the hospital, they are more likely to die in the ordinary course of old age from one of their many comorbidities.

And so, the elderly who die from some other illness will be counted as COVID-19 deaths, although they did not actually die from COVID-19.

What is the danger from COVID-19? Anthony S. Fauci is the Director of the National Institute of Allergy and Infectious Diseases (NIAID). He is in charge of the federal response to the COVID-19 threat. On March 4, 2020, Dr. Anthony Fauci testified in a public hearing before the U.S. Congress. During his testimony, Dr. Fauci stated ominously that "the mortality for seasonal flu is point one percent (0.1%). So even if it [the mortality rate for COVID-19] goes down to one percent, it's still 10 times more fatal [than the seasonal flu]."[1463] On March 11, 2020, Dr. Fauci repeated that statistic in testimony before the U.S. Congress. "I think if you count all the cases of minimally symptomatic or asymptomatic infection, that probably brings the mortality rate down to somewhere around one percent, which means it is 10 times more lethal than the seasonal flu."[1464]

Yet, when Dr. Fauci is talking to doctors, he changes his tune. The New England Journal of Medicine is typically only read by doctors and scientific researchers. And so, what did Dr. Fauci say about the COVID-19 virus when writing to doctors? In a March 26, 2020 article in the New England Journal of Medicine, Dr. Fauci stated that "the overall clinical consequences of COVID-19 may ultimately be more akin to those of a severe seasonal influenza (which has a case fatality rate of approximately 0.1%)."[1465]

Keep in mind that statement in the New England Journal of Medicine by Dr. Fauci was made in the midst of medical emergencies being announced in many states that included school and business closures, recommendations of social distancing, and state government-mandated limits on public gatherings. All of these measures were recommended by Dr. Fauci, who had fanned the flames of hysteria over the medical danger of COVID-19 among the public. But while Dr. Fauci was telling the public that COVID-19 was ten (10) times more deadly than the flu, he was telling doctors and scientists that "the overall clinical consequences of COVID-19 may ultimately be more akin to those of a severe seasonal influenza (which has a case fatality rate of approximately 0.1%)."

By the way, Dr. Fauci was joined in that article by his co-author, Robert R. Redfield, who is the Director of the U.S. Center for Disease Control (CDC). Basically, the U.S. health czars are on record admitting that what they continue to tell the public is a deadly virus is not really deadly at all. The COVID-19 scare is a scam. Fauci and Redfield confessed that COVID-19 is no more deadly than the ordinary flu in the middle of the hysteria they created.

In early March, 2020, Dr. Fauci told the public that the COVID-19 is ten (10) times more deadly than the ordinary flu. After that, on March 26, 2020, Dr. Fauci writes to doctors in the New England Journal of Medicine that "the overall clinical consequences of Covid-19 may ultimately be more akin to those of a severe seasonal influenza (which has a case fatality rate of approximately 0.1%)." Then after he writes that statement, he continues to tell the public that COVID-19 is one of the worst pandemics in history and warns against lifting the draconian restrictions on social gathering and mask-wearing.

How was Dr. Fauci able to pull off that statistical sleight of hand, trick Congress, and bring about the hysteria that COVID-19 was ten times more deadly than the common flu? Dr. Ronald B. Brown of the School of Public Health and Health Systems at the University of Waterloo explains that when Dr. Fauci testified before Congress, he compared apples with oranges. Dr. Brown reveals that Dr. Fauci misleadingly compared the Infection Fatality Rate (IFR) for the seasonal flu with the Case Fatality Rate (CFR) for COVID-19.[1466] That resulted in the incorrect conclusion that the novel coronavirus was ten times deadlier than the average flu.

Both the CFR and IFR report in the numerator those who die from the disease. But they each have different denominators. The difference is that a Case Fatality Rate (CFR) only includes in the denominator those who actually are diagnosed with and have symptoms of the disease, whereas the Infection Fatality Rate (IFR) includes in the denominator cases and undiagnosed, asymptomatic, and mild infections. CFR is a subset of IFR. All cases are infections, but not all infections are cases. Thus, there is a greater population of infections than cases. That means that the CFR ratio will always be a larger percentage than the IFR ratio. The graphic below is from Brown's report and illustrates the difference between the CFR and the IFR.

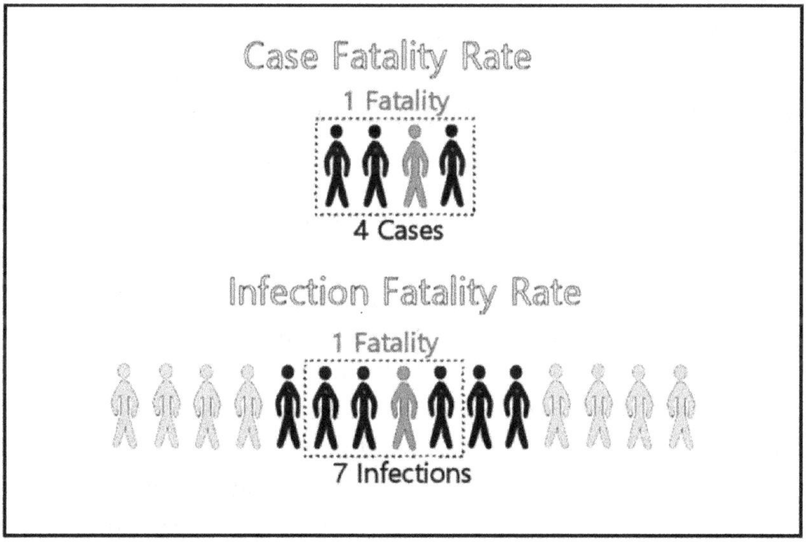

Four (4) cases with one (1) fatality = 25% CFR. Seven (7) infections with one (1) fatality = 14.28% IFR.

Dr. Fauci erroneously reported the CFR for the seasonal flu

as being 0.1%. He then stated that the CFR for COVID-19 was 1%. He ominously testified before Congress that simple math reveals that COVID-19 is ten (10) times deadlier than the flu. It turns out that Dr. Fauci was reporting the IFR for the seasonal flu and misrepresenting it as the CFR for the seasonal flu. The actual CFR for the seasonal flu is 1%. That is virtually the same as the CFR for COVID-19. Thus, the lethality of COVID-19 is about the same as the seasonal flu. Dr. Fauci's testimony that COVID-19 is ten (10) times more deadly than the flu was wrong.

When Dr. Anthony Fauci testified in a public hearing before the U.S. Congress on March 4, 2020, and ominously said that "the mortality for seasonal flu is point one percent (0.1%). So even if it [the mortality rate for COVID-19] goes down to one percent, it's still 10 times more fatal [than the seasonal flu],"[1467] he knew that was not true because in a March 26, 2020 article in the New England Journal of Medicine, Dr. Fauci stated that "the overall clinical consequences of Covid-19 may ultimately be more akin to those of a severe seasonal influenza (which has a case fatality rate of approximately 0.1%)."[1468]

At no time did Dr. Fauci ever retract his misleading public pronouncement that COVID-19 is ten-times more deadly than the flu. Indeed, he doubled down. On July 29, 2020, ABC News reported that Dr. Fauci upped the hysteria another notch when Dr. Fauci "suggested Wednesday that Americans should consider wearing goggles or a face shield in order to prevent spreading or catching COVID-19."[1469] On that same day (July 29, 2020) in an interview with ABC News commentator Dr. Jen Ashton, Dr. Fauci ominously states: "Look at the number of deaths—that's the worst we've had in respiratory outbreak in over 100 years, since the 1918 outbreak of the Spanish Flu. And we still have a ways to go."[1470]

It turns out that the evidence is beginning to show that the actual mortality rate for COVID-19 is indeed more akin to the seasonal flu, just as Dr. Fauci admitted in his New England Journal of Medicine article. Dr. John Ioannidis, who is a professor of medicine and epidemiology at Stanford University, has looked at the worldwide COVID-19 mortality data and concluded that "[a]t a very broad, bird's eye view level, worldwide the IFR [infection fatality rate] of COVID-19 this season may be in the same ballpark as the IFR of influenza."[1471]

Deborah Birx, M.D. is U.S. Global Aids Coordinator & U.S. Special Representative for Global Health Diplomacy and Physician-Ambassador to the office of the Vice President and the U.S. Government Coronavirus Response Coordinator. She stated during a March 23, 2020, White House press conference: "99% of all the mortality coming out of Europe in general is over 50 and pre-existing conditions. The pre-existing condition piece still holds in Italy, with the majority of the mortality having three or more pre-existing conditions. ... Death rates escalate with age and pre-existing conditions. So I really want to be clear that although it may be very low if you're under 40 or very low if you're under 50 or very low if you're under 70, there is an inflection curve. The average age of the person is dying in Italy is in the mid-80s. So there is really a significant issue in our older generation."[1472]

Recall that early in the alleged COVID-19 pandemic, Italy was in the news as being struck by the disease. That was the function of the very large elderly population in Italy. Thus, they had more people dying because they had more older people. "The average life expectancy in Western Europe was 79 years for males and 84 years for females in 2019."[1473] So we know that, in Italy, the people allegedly dying from COVID-19 were dying at the age of the average mortality rate for older people. Furthermore, Italian authorities revealed in March 2020 that 99% of all coronavirus deaths were from people with pre-existing conditions.[1474]

So the people that were trumpeted as dying from COVID-19 early in the purported pandemic were the older sick people. That is the group of people one would expect to die daily.

Putting those statistics together, we find the COVID-19 virus is no more deadly than the ordinary flu. And the people threatened by COVID-19 are the same as those threatened by the seasonal flu: older people with pre-existing health infirmities. But the media publicized those deaths as though they were something unusual. The COVID-19 pandemic was just theater. It was false propaganda.

Dr. Ionnidis stated that the fatality rate for COVID-19 could be as low as 0.2%, but no higher than 0.4%. That higher number (0.4%) was gathered from infections among elderly patients and healthcare workers. The more likely 0.2% rate is much lower than the 1-3% range of figures often bandied about by the government fear-mongers. Keep in mind that Dr. Ionnidis is using government-reported figures, which have been proven to be inflated anyway.[1475] Incidentally, the mortality rate in the United States from all causes is approximately 1%.[1476]

Please recall, as explained above, that the statistics include all deaths "involving" COVID-19 not deaths "from" COVID-19. That means that the persons could have died from some other cause, but the decedent was determined to have COVID-19 at the time of death. Thus they are reported as a death "involving" COVID-19.[1477]

The CDC admits that they double count deaths. "Deaths involving more than one condition (e.g., deaths involving both diabetes and respiratory arrest) were counted in both totals."[1478] That means that a person who is murdered but tests positive for COVID-19 is tallied as both a murder death and a COVID-19 death. It is for that reason that the CDC advises: "To avoid counting the same death multiple times, the numbers for different conditions should not be summated."[1479]

Furthermore, the CDC admits that its statistics of COVID-19 deaths are not confirmed to have COVID-19. The

COVID-19 statistics include both "[d]eaths with confirmed or presumed COVID-19."

On February 1, 2021, Patrick Howley, writing for National File, reported that an investigation by the Public Health Policy Initiative uncovered evidence that the Centers for Disease Control and Prevention (CDC) violated federal law by fraudulently inflating COVID-19 fatality numbers.[1480] Howley reported that the investigation revealed that the "CDC illegally inflated the COVID fatality number by at least 1,600 percent."[1481] Howley explained how that was done:

> On March 24th the CDC published the NVSS COVID-19 Alert No. 2 document instructing medical examiners, coroners and physicians to deemphasize underlying causes of death, also referred to as pre-existing conditions or comorbidities, by recording them in Part II rather than Part I of death certificates as "…the underlying cause of death are expected to result in COVID-19 being the underlying cause of death more often than not." This was a major rule change for death certificate reporting from the CDC's 2003 Coroners' Handbook on Death Registration and Fetal Death Reporting and Physicians' Handbook on Medical Certification of Death, which have instructed death reporting professionals nationwide to report underlying conditions in Part I for the previous 17 years. This single change resulted in a significant inflation of COVID-19 fatalities by instructing that COVID-19 be listed in Part I of death certificates as a definitive cause of death regardless of confirmatory evidence, rather than listed in Part II as a contributor to death in the presence of pre-existing conditions, as would have been done using the 2003 guidelines. The research

> draws attention to this key distinction as it has led to a significant inflation in COVID fatality totals. By the researcher's estimates, COVID-19 recorded fatalities are inflated nationwide by as much as 1600% above what they would be had the CDC used the 2003 handbooks.[1482]

The graph below is from the Public Health Policy Initiative report and represents the actual deaths due to COVID-19 if those deaths had been reported according to the traditional CDC rules that were listed in the 2003 CDC Medical Examiner's and Coroner's Handbook on Death Registration,[1483] which were in effect until the CDC issued the new COVID-19 reporting rules on March 24, 2020. The new reporting rules only apply to COVID-19. All other causes of death still follow the traditional rules set forth in the 2003 CDC Handbook.[1484] Notice how the new CDC guidance for reporting COVID-19 deaths initiated in the March 24, 2020 COVID-19 Alert No. 2[1485] artificially inflated the number of deaths from COVID-19 1600%.

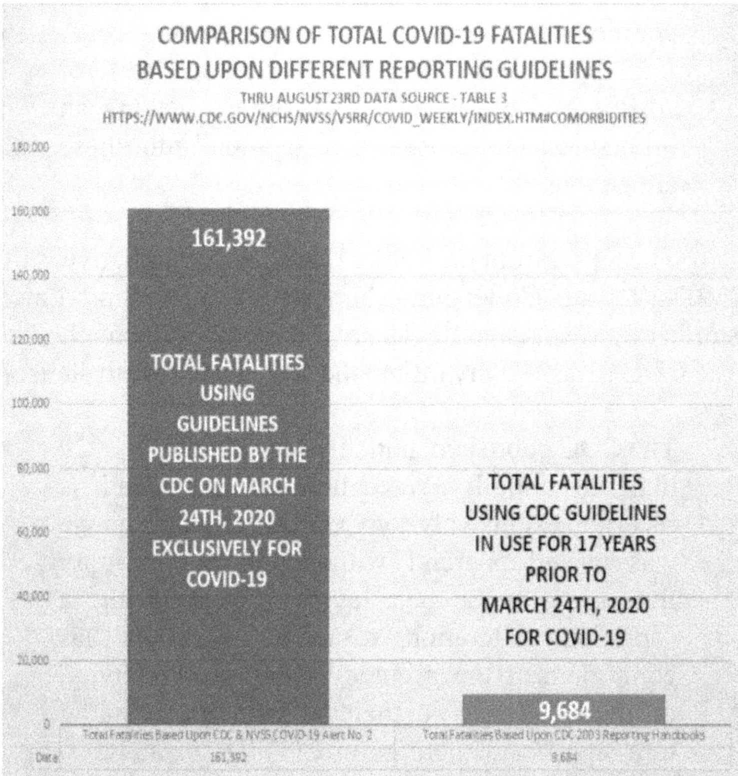

Figure 9. COVID-19 Using the March 24 Exclusive Guidelines vs Using the 2003 Guidelines. Had the CDC used the 2003 guidelines, the total **COVID-19** be approximately 16.7 times lower than is currently being reported. [1][30][State & Territory Health Departments]

Howley explains the effect of the CDC fraud and what should be done about it:

> By enacting these new rules exclusively for COVID-19 in violation of federal law, the research alleges that the CDC significantly inflated data that has been used by elected officials and public health officials, in conjunction with unproven projection models from the Institute for Health Metrics and Evaluation (IHME), to justify extended closures for schools, places of worship, entertainment, and

> small businesses leading to unprecedented emotional and economic hardships nationwide. A formal petition has been sent to the Department of Justice as well as all US Attorneys seeking an immediate grand jury investigation into these allegations.[1486]

The report from the Public Health Policy Initiative is titled COVID-19 Data Collection, Comorbidity & Federal Law: A Historical Retrospective.[1487] The report explains the method used by the CDC to artificially inflate the COVID-19 death statistics.

> The CDC published guidelines on March 24, 2020 that substantially altered how cause of death is recorded exclusively for COVID-19. This change was enacted apparently without public opportunity for comment or peer-review. As a result, a capricious alteration to data collection has compromised the accuracy, quality, objectivity, utility, and integrity of their published data, leading to a significant increase in COVID-19 fatalities. This decision by the CDC may have subverted the legal oversight of the OMB as Congressionally authorized by the PRA & IQA as well.[1488]

The Public Health Policy Initiative report explains that under this newly adopted CDC reporting scheme, "COVID-19 became emphasized as a cause of death as frequently as possible, while comorbidity was simultaneously deemphasized as causes of death."[1489] The CDC's new rules for reporting COVID-19 deaths had the effect of inflating the reported COVID-19 deaths.

The March 24, 2020 COVID-19 Alert No. 2[1490] from the CDC referred to additional documents providing further guidance, which seemed to be a reference to a March 4, 2020 CDC document titled Guidance for Certifying COVID-19 Deaths,[1491] which explained how to list COVID-19 in Part I of the Death Certificate to show how to list COVID-19 as the "underlying cause" of death. Since the new rules were such a clear departure from the prior practice, it was necessary for the CDC to elaborate with further guidance in April 2020.[1492] But that further guidance did not change the original March 24, 2020, Alert No. 2, which explicitly stated that **"the [new] rules for coding and selection of the underlying cause of death are expected to result in COVID-19 being the underlying cause more often than not."**[1493]

State officials have used the CDC guidance as a license to commit fraud. Officials put on a public facade that they are honestly portraying the death figures as they follow the lead of the CDC in its waltz of deception. But some state officials don't just go along with the flow; they jump on board, give it their all and enthusiastically jimmy up the numbers. For example, Washington State officials have been caught red-handed lying about the COVID-19 deaths in their state. They are engaging in outright fraud to inflate their COVID-19 fatality numbers. Below is a December 16, 2020, press release from the Freedom Foundation:[1494]

> (OLYMPIA, Wash.) — Seven months after a Freedom Foundation investigation showed [the State of Washington government] was inflating the number of COVID-19 fatalities in Washington state and promising to fix its flawed reporting procedures, further research[1495] indicates the state's Department of Health (DOH) is still over-reporting the totals by potentially hundreds of deaths.

The Freedom Foundation found that the government of Washington State was artificially inflating the reported COVID-19 deaths. The Freedom Foundation began investigating the state's shenanigans in May 2020. The Freedom Foundation found at that time that the Washington "DOH was attributing to COVID-19 every death in which the deceased previously tested positive for the virus." That means that if someone had ever tested positive for COVID-19 at any time in his life and subsequently died, the State of Washington would count that person as having died from COVID-19, regardless of the actual cause of death. That is fraud. The Freedom Foundation determined:

> Washington's data was riddled with cases — as much as 13 percent of the total — in which the death certificate made no reference to COVID-19 as a cause of death. In several cases, even gunshot deaths were chalked up to the virus.[1496]

Governor Jay Inslee dismissed the May 21, 2020 findings of the Freedom Foundation as "dangerous," "disgusting" and "malarkey." He further accused the Freedom Foundation of "fanning these conspiracy claims from the planet Pluto" and not caring about the lives lost to COVID-19.[1497] But his subordinates undermined his claims by acknowledging that the Freedom Foundation was correct. A DOH health statistics manager admitted that the Washington DOH COVID-19 death statistics include deaths of all persons who tested positive for COVID-19 in its totals, even if the victims died from other causes, such as gunshot wounds. She explained that "[o]ur (DOH COVID-19) dashboard numbers do include any deaths to a person that has tested positive to COVID-19."[1498]

Since the Freedom Foundation has been proven correct, Governor Inslee's opinion, in his official capacity as Governor of Washington, is that the way Washington State was reporting COVID-19 deaths before May 21, 2020, was "dangerous, disgusting, malarkey" and "from the planet Pluto." And since it has been proven that they are still doing it. That makes the Washington officials providing those phony death statistics dangerous, disgusting, and full of malarkey. Those are Governor Inslee's words, not mine.

After having been caught, state officials promised to correct the misreporting. But the Freedom Foundation determined that Washington State officials did not fix anything and continued with the fraud.

> "Make no mistake. This isn't an innocent accounting error we're talking about", said Aaron Withe, Freedom Foundation National Director. "This is a state agency under the authority of Gov. Jay Inslee that continues to misrepresent the number of people who have died of COVID even after it was already caught doing the same thing."
>
> Withe continued, "It's a nakedly political act intended to scare the public into letting him continue to abuse the almost unlimited "emergency powers" that have needlessly bankrupted thousands of Washington businesses and thrown tens of thousands of its residents out of work."[1499]

The follow-up December 2020 probe[1500] by the Freedom Foundation found that "170 death certificates contained no reference whatsoever to COVID-19. Another 171 only referenced COVID-19 as a 'contributing factor' and not part of the causal chain of events leading to death."[1501] Now, that is dangerous, disgusting, malarkey by state officials.

The deceptive practice of artificially inflating the COVID-19 death statistics was worldwide. For example, a UK National Health Service (NHS) Director revealed in a Twitter thread how UK hospitals lied about COVID-19 being the cause of death to create the false illusion of a COVID-19 pandemic. Unsurprisingly, that Twitter thread has since been censored by redacting the most damning information.[1502] But *The Expose* has preserved the original thread.[1503]

The NHS Director explained how in 2016 a strange change began to be instituted that changed how deaths were certified across the UK. Instead of a death being certified by medical professionals who treated the decedent, the certification was to be assigned to a single Medical Examiner at the hospital. Once the NHS Director saw how people who died from causes other than COVID-19 were being classified as COVID-19 deaths, he realized that the 2016 change was part of a plan to create the false impression of a COVID-19 pandemic where there was none. He concluded:

> I have no doubt in my mind, that the Government has planned the entire pandemic since 2016 when they first proposed the change to medical death certification.[1504]

Once the death certification was centralized in a single officer in the hospital, it was not hard to falsify the deaths as COVID-19 deaths with the simple trick of false-positive PCR tests. The NHS Director explained:

> If a patient tests positive for COVID-19 with a PCR Test, this doesn't mean they are infected. If tested again, they may well turn out with a negative test. However, in the NHS, patients are only tested once and this stays on their record throughout their admission. Hospital policies were changed alongside the implementation of the Medical Examiner System, to ensure that any patient who died within 30 days of a positive test, would have to have COVID-19 as their primary cause of death. This was regulated by the Medical Examiner.[1505]

Persons who died from a myriad of causes were suddenly deemed COVID-19 deaths with a stroke of the pen by the hospital assigned Medical Examiner. The NHS Director explains:

> The highest cause of death at every hospital per annum pre COVID-19 is Pneumonia. Pneumonia is a respiratory disease like COVID-19. Pneumonia can be broken down into 4 different causes of death: Bronchopneumonia, spiration Pneumonia, Community-Acquired Pneumonia and Hospital Acquired Pneumonia. These four causes when added together kill the largest number of people on an annual basis prior to the pandemic. The Medical Examiner (one individual in each hospital), was certifying all these pneumonia deaths as COVID-19 deaths. When four different diseases [are] grouped and now being called COVID-19, you will inevitably see COVID-19 with a huge death rate. The mainstream media was reporting on this huge increase in COVID-19 deaths due to the Medical Examiner System being in place.. Patients being admitted and dying with very common conditions such as old age, myocardial infarctions, end-stage kidney failure, haemorrhages, strokes, COPD and cancer etc. were all now being certified as COVID-19 via the Medical Examiner System.[1506]

The entire system was incentivized by money. The NHS Director stated that "[h]ospitals were incentivised to report COVID-19 deaths over normal deaths, as the government was paying hospitals additional money for every COVID-19 death that was being reported. The Medical Examiner system ensured that COVID-19 was being put down as the cause of death."[1507] Doctors who knew what was going on dared not say anything because they knew it would mean an end to their medical careers.

> Any doctor who argued against COVID-19 as a cause of death was bullied and vilified. The General Medical Council ("GMC") maintains a

> register of all doctors within the UK. This ensures that there is a fear of being struck off for speaking out against an agenda. The GMC effectively controls all doctors in the UK. Even if a doctor realises what is going on and wants to speak out. They will think twice about talking, as they would be risking their entire career and everything that they've worked so hard for. Doctors essentially have their hands tied, many have families, kids, mortgages and mouths to feed. If I was in their situation, I would think twice about speaking out, for fear of being struck off by the GMC and losing everything.[1508]

The NHS Directors saw clinical decisions in treating patients designed to hasten death.

> The NHS treatment pathway [for CIVD-19] involved patients being placed onto ventilators. There is a 50% chance of death from this clinical decision alone. How many innocent people have died from the clinical decision to place them on a ventilator.[1509]

The NHS Director also saw the strange behavior of doctors promoting the experimental COVID-19 vaccines, which seemed to be the objective of the pandemic hoax.

> In my 12 years of NHS service, never has a doctor pushed or influenced the public to take a vaccine. Yet on social media, I was seeing close friends who were doctors, starting to post on social media that they have taken the vaccine and that the public should. I wouldn't be surprised if doctors were being forced to promote the vaccine by their superiors or if they were receiving monetary gain in

doing so.[1510]

The HHS Director saw first-hand the devastation caused by the COVID-19 vaccines.

> During board rounds (where every admitted patient is discussed), we were seeing patients on a daily basis being admitted due to suffering from adverse effects of taking the vaccine. Patients were blacking out after taking the vaccine or suffering from clots or strokes.[1511]

57 Closing Down Schools For No Good Reason

On May 7, 2020, Nicole Chavez and Artemis Moshtaghian reported for CNN that "Officials in 48 US states, as well as Washington DC, have ordered or recommended school closures for the rest of the school year."[1512] The CNN report revealed that "[s]chools in all five US territories — American Samoa, Guam, Northern Mariana Islands, Puerto Rico, and US Virgin Islands — also are closed for the remainder of the school year." The closures included almost all colleges.[1513] The CNN article explains that the draconian school shutdowns were to "reduce the spread of the novel coronavirus."

That nonsense was not based on reality. It was a well-orchestrated shutdown of society based on irrational hysteria mixed with cunning malevolence. While many schools reopened for the fall semester of 2020, many other schools remained closed during the remainder of the 2020 school year. As of September 2020, only four U.S. states (Texas, Florida, Arkansas, and Iowa) required the schools to open statewide for in-person student instruction.

States had a myriad of different plans involving remote learning, restrictions by region, opening according to the discretion of the local school district, hybrid remote/in-person instruction, etc.

President Trump was roundly criticized in August 2020 for defending "his call to reopen schools this fall by claiming children are 'virtually immune' from COVID-19 and that the coronavirus will 'go away" soon.'"[1514]

It turns out that President Trump was more correct than he was wrong. It is fair to say that COVID-19 poses no real health risk to school-aged children. The clamor to shut down schools was not based on the evidence.

John Cullen, who is a software engineer and statistician, has discovered an astounding truth that has been hiding in plain sight. In an interview with Jason Goodman, Cullen revealed that the threat to school-aged children by COVID-19 is virtually nill.[1515]

Cullen analyzed the CDC statistics and discovered that the total deaths of children with COVID-19 across the entire United States for the period of February 1, 2020, to September 19, 2020, for school-aged children between the ages of 5 years old and 14 years old was 31. Over a seven-month period, during the heat of the alleged COVID-19 pandemic, 31 children died with COVID-19.

Table 1. Deaths involving coronavirus disease 2019 (COVID-19), pneumonia, and influenza reported to NCHS by sex and age group. United States. Week ending 2/1/2020 to 9/19/2020

Updated September 23, 2020

Sex	Age group	All Deaths involving COVID-19 (U07.1)[1]	Deaths from All Causes	Deaths involving Pneumonia, with or without COVID-19, excluding Influenza deaths (J12.0–J18.9)[2]	Deaths involving COVID-19 and Pneumonia, excluding Influenza (U07.1 and J12.0–J18.9)[2]	All Deaths involving Influenza, with or without COVID-19 or Pneumonia (J09–J11)[3]
Total						
	All ages	**188,470**	2,022,937	192,312	84,930	6,699
	Under 1 year	**20**	11,313	105	3	16
	1–4 years	**15**	2,158	73	2	42
	5–14 years	**31**	3,356	102	8	52
	15–24 years	**353**	21,615	438	128	53
	25–34 years	**1,457**	44,521	1,610	651	151
	35–44 years	**3,809**	62,852	3,643	1,693	250
	45–54 years	**10,057**	115,528	9,425	4,698	577
	55–64 years	**23,991**	264,573	25,205	11,661	1,240
	65–74 years	**40,613**	401,024	42,712	19,609	1,453
	75–84 years	**49,871**	489,060	52,492	23,175	1,478
	85 years and over	**58,253**	606,937	56,507	23,302	1,387

CDC Table Showing Deaths "Involving" COVID-19 by Age Bracket

Please be aware that the statistics include all deaths "involving" COVID-19 not deaths "from" COVID-19. Thus, the persons listed as deaths "Involving COVID-19" probably died from another cause. Being in the "Involving COVID-19" death column only means that the person was thought to have COVID-19 at the time of death. The CDC explained that during the reporting period, 94% percent of people reported to have died "Involving COVID-19" in the U.S. suffered from an average of 2.5 chronic diseases or conditions in addition to COVID-19.[1516]

The CDC admits that they are giving duplicate counts of the deaths. Thus, a decedent who dies from more than one medical condition would be duplicate counted in the columns for each condition. Under that rubric, a person who dies of heart failure and is also presumed to have COVID-19 would be counted as both a death by heart failure and a COVID-19 death. Even more astounding, the COVID-19 death statistics include those who have only been presumed to have COVID-19. There is no scientific verification of the COVID-19 diagnosis. The COVID-19 death statistics are being artifically inflated.

Even assuming that every one of the 31 children died "from" COVID-19 (which is to assume something that the CDC admits is not the case) there is simply no way that an illness that accounts for the deaths of only 31 children nationwide can justify closing virtually every elementary and middle school in the United States.

But if we extrapolate from the fact that 94% of all CDC reported COVID-19 deaths have an average of 2.5 chronic diseases in addition to COVID-19, we find that only 6% of the 31 children between the ages of 5 and 14 years old died exclusively "from" COVID-19. Thus, we find that only two (2) children between the ages of 5 and 14 years old died exclusively from COVID-19. That shockingly low number of deaths from COVID–19 for the entire United States is no justification for closing down virtually every elementary and middle school in the United States. It is even more irrational to shut down schools when you consider that even that low extrapolated number of deaths "from" COVID-19 is inflated because the COVID-19 starting numbers included those presumed (i.e., guessed) to have COVID-19.

Another notable fact about the CDC statistics is that of all persons in the United States between the ages of 15 years old and 24 years old, only 353 people died with COVID-19 between February 1, 2020, to September 19, 2020. Again, those persons are reported as deaths "involving" COVID-19, not deaths from COVID-19. But the number of deaths does not justify closing down virtually every high school and college in the country.

If we take the CDC at its word that only 6% of all reported COVID-19 deaths died only "from" COVID-19, we find only 21 persons between the ages of 15 and 24 died exclusively "from" COVID-19. That extremely low number of deaths exclusively from COVID–19 across the entire United States for persons 15-24 years of age is no justification for closing down virtually every high school and college in the United States. Remember that even the extrapolated 21 deaths "from" COVID-19 is still inflated because it is only a guess. That is because the COVID-19 numbers included those presumed (i.e., guessed) to have COVID-19.

With that evidence that COVID-19 poses little to no threat to children. What did the CDC do? In October 2022, the CDC Advisory Committee on Immunization Practices (ACIP) voted 15-0 to add the COVID-19 vaccine to the childhood immunization schedule. Why would they do that? The vaccine is not needed. COVID-19 is not a threat to children. It is all about the money and protecting pharmaceutical companies from liability. With the vaccine added to the childhood vaccine schedule, vaccine makers can now manufacture fully "approved" vaccines and have complete liability protection forever after the EUA for the COVID-19 vaccines expires.

58 None Dare Call It Conspiracy

Conspiracy is a concept that has been propagandized into disfavor, much to the delight of Satan and his minions, who are only too happy to push the idea that if one believes there is a world conspiracy against Jesus Christ and his followers, he must be a radical on the fringe of society or worse. Most people are afraid of being marginalized and thus avoid speaking of conspiracies. People instead try to construe events as coincidental when actually they can only be explained as the product of prior agreements of conspirators who have combined in coordinated actions.

This conspiracy against the LORD and his anointed has been festering since the fall of man in the garden of Eden and involves the kings and rulers of the earth.

> Why do the heathen rage, and the people imagine a vain thing? **The kings of the earth set themselves, and the rulers take counsel together, against the LORD, and against his anointed,** ***saying*****, Let us break their bands asunder, and cast away their cords from us**. He that sitteth in the heavens shall laugh: the Lord shall have them in derision. (Psalms 2:1-4)

This monstrous conspiracy, while it involves men, it is not headed by a man. "For we wrestle not against flesh and blood, but against principalities, against powers, against the rulers of the darkness of this world, against spiritual wickedness in high *places*." (Ephesians 6:12) The kingpin of this diabolical conspiracy is that terrible dragon, Satan. He is the adversary of Almighty God. He is also an adversary to all of God's creation. Satan tried to tempt Jesus into worshiping him, but Jesus quoted from God's word and told Satan that one should only worship God.

> Again, the devil taketh him up into an exceeding high mountain, and sheweth him all the kingdoms of the world, and the glory of them; And saith unto him, All these things will I give thee, if thou wilt fall down and worship me. Then saith Jesus unto him, Get thee hence, Satan: for it is written, Thou shalt worship the Lord thy God, and him only shalt thou serve. (Matthew 4:8-10)

If you are a disciple of God's perfect and holy Son Jesus Christ, then Satan and his antichrist hate you. "Be sober, be vigilant; because your adversary the devil, as a roaring lion, walketh about, seeking whom he may devour." (1 Peter 5:8) God, however, has a means by which one can avoid becoming the prey of Satan: "Submit yourselves therefore to God. Resist the devil, and he will flee from you." (James 4:7) In order to resist the devil one must first know his plans and methods.

Event 201, a Global Pandemic Exercise, was held on October 18, 2019. The Johns Hopkins Center for Health Security, in partnership with the World Economic Forum and the Bill and Melinda Gates Foundation, hosted Event 201, a high-level pandemic exercise involving a select invitation-only group of almost 130 people, at the luxurious Pierre Hotel in New York, NY.[1517] The exercise illustrated areas where public/private partnerships will be necessary to respond to a severe pandemic to diminish large-scale economic and societal consequences.

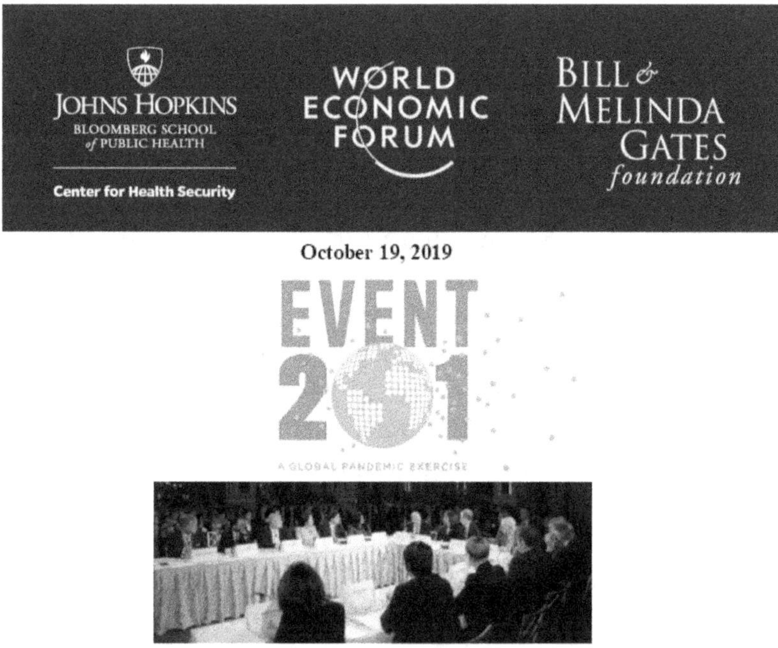

The sponsors of Event 201 explained:

> **Event 201** simulates an outbreak of a **novel zoonotic coronavirus** transmitted from bats to pigs to people that eventually becomes efficiently transmissible from person to person, leading to a severe pandemic. The pathogen and the disease it causes are **modeled largely on SARS**, but it is more transmissible in the community setting by people with mild symptoms.[1518]

The pathogen in the fictional exercise was described as follows:

> Coronavirus Acute Pulmonary Syndrome (CAPS) is an acute respiratory infection that can progress to pneumonia and acute respiratory distress syndrome. It is caused by a swine-origin coronavirus (CAPS virus).[1519]

Notice how similar "Coronavirus Acute Pulmonary Syndrome (CAPS)" is to the real "Severe Acute Respiratory Syndrome (SARS), and Severe Acute Respiratory Syndrome Coronavirus (SARS-Cov), and SARS-Cov 2 which is alleged to cause the Coronavirus Disease of 2019 (COVID-19). The exercise mentioned the development of a vaccine. The exercise document describing CAPS states that "[t]here is no licensed vaccine for any coronavirus, although some are in development for SARS and MERS."[1520] Other Event 201 materials state that "[t]here is no possibility of a vaccine being available in the first year."[1521] That was precisely what happened with COVID-19. It was not until December 11, 2020 that the first COVID-19 vaccine was given emergency use authorization (EUA).

The outcome of the CAPS pandemic in Event 201 was catastrophic: 65 million people died in the first 18 months.[1522] That is many more than the reported 6 million COVID deaths. One of the goals of the exercise was to propagandize the population.[1523] One of the concerns of the exercise was how to ensure that "reliable information" gets to the public and how to best prevent the public from being swayed by "damaging false information." They discussed how to control the flow of information to the public. One participant considered it important that they had the ability to **"flood the zone" with information.**

Senator Joseph McCarthy was not wrong. Communists have infiltrated the CIA. It is an intelligence agency that works to undermine the God-given liberties of the American people. During Event 201, we find Avril Haines in attendance.[1524] Haines was the Former Deputy Director Central Intelligence Agency and Former

Deputy National Security Advisor, who, on January 21, 2021, was sworn in as the Director of National Intelligence. At Event 201, we find Haines sitting alongside George Gao, the Director-General of the Chinese Center for Disease Control and Prevention (China CDC).[1525] It is no surprise then that we find social distancing introduced as a response to COVID-19. Social distancing is simply the Western term for the Chinese Communist party's feudal practice of lockdowns. Gao used fraudulent science to advocate wearing ineffective and unsafe masks to purportedly prevent the spread of COVID-19.[1526] The U.S. Government acted in lockstep with the Chinese Government's tyrannical response to COVID-19.[1527] It was planned that way during Event 201. And they are not done. This is a conspiracy against God and man.

One participant in the Event 201 exercise, Matthew Harrington, was the global chief operating officer at Edelman, an industry-leading communications firm. Harrington said that pressure should be put on social media companies to use their platforms to become advocates for the orthodox script given to them from the science and health communities.

> I would marry the business leadership of the employer with business leadership organizations, such as the BRT and like enterprises around the globe. But I also think we're at a moment where the **social media platforms** have to step forward and recognize the moment to assert that they're a technology platform and not a broadcaster is over. **They in fact have to be a participant in broadcasting accurate information and partnering with the scientific and health communities to counterweight, if not flood the zone**, of accurate information. Because to try to put the genie back in the bottle of the misinformation and disinformation is not impossible.[1528]

Kevin McAleese, who is the communications officer for Bill Gates funded agricultural projects, took part in the Event 201 exercise. He said that the governments need to manage the private media companies. Further the governments need to identify "every bad actor" who is disseminating "disinformation."

> To me, it is clear **countries** need to make strong efforts to manage both **mis- and disinformation**. We know **social media companies are working around the clock to combat these disinformation campaigns**. The task of identifying every bad actor is immense. Experts agree that new disinformation campaigns are being generated every day. This is a huge problem that's going to keep us from ending the pandemic.[1529]

Tom Inglesby, who is the director of Bloomberg's Johns Hopkins Center for Health Security asked whether the governments should force media companies to push the government propaganda. "In this case, do you think governments are at the point where they need to require social media companies to operate in a certain way?"[1530] Lavan Thiru, Singapore's Finance Minister suggests that the government might make examples of dissidents with **"government or enforcement actions against fake news.**"[1531]

Lo and behold, within a month of Event 201, on November 17, 2019, the first person was reportedly infected in Wuhan, China, with what became later known as SARS-CoV-2.[1532] And on December 10, 2019, the first Wuhan patients were hospitalized. The CDC puts the date of the first "cluster of patients" in Wuhan at December 12, 2019.[1533]

On November 12, 2019, the US Department of Defense awarded a contract to Labyrinth Global Health for "COVID 19 Research" in Ukraine.[1534] The Department of Defense has funded approximately 16 bio-labs in Ukraine. The November 12, 2019, contract is quite incriminating because it describes "COVID 19 Research." It proves that the COVID-19 pandemic was planned ahead of time. We know that because on the date of the contract, November 12, 2019, there was no such thing as "COVID-19." That acronym had not been coined for public dissemination at that time. Indeed, the alleged SARS-CoV-2 virus, which purportedly caused what later became known as "COVID-19," had not even been identified before November 12, 2019.

The first person alleged to have contracted SARS-CoV-2, which allegedly caused the illness that later became known as "COVID-19" was a 55-year-old man from Hubei Province in China on November 17, 2019.[1535] It was not until February 2020 that the alleged Wuhan, China virus that caused the disease that later became known as "COVID-19." So, the November 12, 2019, contract awarded by the Department of Defense was based on payment for research into a virus that did not officially exist. It was not until three months later that the world was introduced to the acronym "COVID-19."

Even more suspicious is that Labyrinth Global Health has a close working relationship with Peter Daszak's EcoHealth Alliance, which in turn is listed as a strategic partner of the Wuhan Institute of Virology, which has been a central player in the COVID-19 scamdemic.

As soon as the lockdowns, masking, and social distancing began, so did the censorship. It was as though they were following the Event 201 script. Indeed, the censorship has continued through the emergency authorization of the vaccines and the vaccine mandates. There is proof of collusion between the government and the social media companies. On October 10, 2022, Jeff Mordock reported for the Washington Times that according to a lawsuit filed by state attorneys general "[m]ore than 50 government officials across 13 agencies "threatened, cajoled and colluded" with social media companies to silence online speech about topics the Biden administration disliked."[1536]

The State of Missouri, through its Attorney General, and the State of Louisiana, through its Attorney General, have jointly filed suit against Joe Biden in his official capacity as President of the United States. The complaint alleges that federal government executive branch officials have violated the First Amendment to the U.S. Constitution, various federal statutes, and the administrative procedures act by censoring protected speech.[1537]

The States of Missouri and Louisiana have uncovered evidence proving that high federal officials have reached out to major electronic media firms to prod, prompt, cajole, threaten, and order them to censor information they labeled "misinformation." That "misinformation" included but was not limited to information about inflated COVID-19 dangers, the inefficacy of masks and COVID-19 lockdowns, information indicating that the COVID-19 vaccines are unsafe and ineffective, information about election fraud, and revelations about the Hunter Biden laptop prior to the 2020 Presidential election.[1538]

A court filing by Missouri and Louisiana reveals:

> Secretary Mayorkas of DHS commented that the federal Government's efforts to police private speech on social media are occurring "across the federal enterprise." Doc. 45, ¶ 233. It turns out that this statement is true, on a scale beyond what Plaintiffs could ever have anticipated. The limited discovery produced so far provides a tantalizing snapshot into a massive, sprawling federal "Censorship Enterprise," which includes dozens of federal officials across at least eleven federal agencies and components identified so far, who communicate with social-media platforms about

> misinformation, disinformation, and the suppression of private speech on social media—all with the intent and effect of pressuring social-media platforms to censor and suppress private speech that federal officials disfavor. The discovery provided so far demonstrates that this Censorship Enterprise is extremely broad, including officials in the White House, HHS [Health and Human Services], DHS [Department of Homeland Security], CISA [Cybersecurity & Infrastructure Security Agency], the CDC [Centers for Disease Control and Prevention], NIAID [National Institute of Allergy and Infectious Diseases], and the Office of the Surgeon General; and evidently other agencies as well, such as the Census Bureau, the FDA [Food and Drug Administration], the FBI [Federal Bureau of Investigation], the State Department, the Treasury Department, and the U.S. Election Assistance Commission. And it rises to the highest levels of the U.S. Government, including numerous White House officials. the breadth and extent of the federal Defendants' censorship activities is massive.[1539]

Missouri and Louisiana reveal specific instances where a team of federal officials were in direct contact with electronic social media firms.

> Meta, for example, has disclosed that at least 32 federal officials—including senior officials at the FDA, the U.S. Election Assistance Commission, and the White House—have communicated with Meta about content moderation on its platforms. ... [T]hese federal censorship activities include very senior officials within the U.S. Government, i.e.,

> "members of our senior staff," in Jen Psaki's words.[1540]

The electronic media seemed anxious to appease federal authorities.

> [O]n July 23, 2021, that senior Meta executive sent an email to Surgeon General Murthy stating, "I wanted to make sure you saw the steps we took just this past week to adjust policies on what we are removing with respect to misinformation, as well as steps taken to further address the 'disinfo dozen': we removed 17 additional Pages, Groups, and Instagram accounts tied to the disinfo dozen...." Ex. 3, at 2. Again, on August 20, 2021, the same Meta executive emailed Murthy to assure him that Facebook "will shortly be expanding our COVID policies to further reduce the spread of potentially harmful content on our platform. These changes will apply across Facebook and Instagram," and they included "increasing the strength of our demotions for COVID and vaccine-related content," and "making it easier to have Pages/Groups/Accounts demoted for sharing COVID and vaccine-related misinformation." Ex. 4, at 3. In addition, that senior Meta executive sent a "Facebook bi-weekly covid content report" to Surgeon General Murthy to White House official Andrew Slavitt, evidently to reassure these federal officials that Facebook's suppression of COVID-19 "misinformation" was aggressive enough for their preferences. Ex. 4, at 6-19.[1541]

Missouri and Louisiana uncovered evidence of White House officials pressuring Twitter to censor and deplatform an influential vaccine critic.

> [S]senior "WH" officials including Andrew Slavitt specifically pressured Twitter to deplatform Berenson, an influential vaccine critic—which Twitter did. Doc. 45, ¶¶ 187, 309. This pressure to deplatform Berenson appears to have occurred on April 21, 2021, when four Twitter employees participated in a Zoom meeting with at least three White House officials and one HHS official intended to allow the White House to "partner" with Twitter in censoring COVID-related "misinfo."[1542]

Missouri and Louisiana found that "such pressures from government officials on social-media companies, along with the many public statements alleged in the Complaint, have succeeded on a grand scale."[1543]

The evidence suggests a deep conspiracy between the federal government and social media giants.

> These federal bureaucrats are deeply embedded in a joint enterprise with social-media companies to procure the censorship of social-media speech. Officials at HHS routinely flag content for censorship, for example, by organizing weekly "Be On The Lookout" meetings to flag disfavored content, Ex. 6; sending lengthy lists of examples of disfavored posts to be censored, Ex. 6, at 21-22; serving as privileged "fact checkers" whom social-media platforms consult about censoring private speech, Ex. 7; and receiving detailed reports from social-media companies about so-called "misinformation" and "disinformation" activities online, Ex. 4; among others.[1544]

Efforts were made to keep these communications

undiscoverable by opening secret back-channels between the electronic social media giants and the federal government.

> Moreover, many of these substantive communications from federal officials flagging specific posts and content for censorship seem to occur through alternative channels of communication that Plaintiffs have not yet obtained (as the third-party social-media platforms contend they are shielded from discovery by the Stored Communications Act). For example, Facebook trained CDC and Census Bureau officials on how to use a "Facebook misinfo reporting channel." Ex. 9. Twitter offered federal officials a privileged channel for flagging misinformation through a "Partner Support Portal." Ex. 9, at 69. YouTube has disclosed that it granted "trusted flagger" status to Census Bureau officials, which allows privileged and expedited consideration of their claims that content should be censored.[1545]

The Biden Administration, with its brazen graft and corruption, is like a modern-day Tammany Hall. It is, in the truest sense, an organized crime syndicate. The bumbling and incompetent Biden is the perfect figurehead to do the bidding of his criminal handlers. Joe Biden tries to convince others that he is in control. In doing so, he talks like a degenerate crime boss. He was recently heard to say "nobody f**ks with Biden."

Looking at the social media policies, the cooperation with the medical orthodoxy and government propaganda is obvious. For example, "YouTube doesn't allow content that spreads medical misinformation that **contradicts local health authorities' (LHA) or the World Health Organization's (WHO)** medical information about COVID-19. This is limited to content that contradicts WHO or local health authorities' guidance on: Treatment, Prevention, Diagnosis, Transmission, The existence of COVID-19"[1546]

YouTube further warns:

> Don't post content on YouTube if it includes any of the following:
>
> Content that recommends use of **Ivermectin** or **Hydroxychloroquine** for the treatment of COVID-19
>
> Claims that COVID-19 **vaccines** do not reduce risk of serious illness or death
>
> Claims that an approved COVID-19 **vaccine** will cause **death**, infertility, miscarriage, autism, or contraction of other infectious diseases
>
> Claims that an approved COVID-19 **vaccine** will contain **substances** that are not on the vaccine ingredient list, such as **biological matter from fetuses** (e.g. fetal tissue, fetal cell lines) or animal products[1547]
>
> Claims that approved COVID-19 **tests** cannot diagnose COVID-19
>
> Denial that COVID-19 exists
>
> Claims that COVID-19 is caused by radiation from **5G** networks
>
> Claims that achieving herd **immunity** through **natural infection** is safer than vaccinating the

population

That does not include the outright deplatforming of persons who disagree with the medical orthodoxy. For example, on or about March 2021, Facebook deplatformed Robert Kennedy Jr.for having the temerity to point out that the COVID-19 vaccines are unsafe and ineffective and exposing regulatory corruption and authoritarian public health policies.

So suspicious was the COVID-19 alleged pandemic following closely on the heels of the Event 201 exercise, the sponsors of Event 201, the Johns Hopkins Center for Health Security, the World Economic Forum, and the Bill & Melinda Gates Foundation found it necessary to disavow any connection to the COVID-19 pandemic. They posted a notice claiming they "did not make a prediction" about the COVID-19 pandemic. But it is doubtful there was a question about predicting the COVID-19 pandemic. The real question was probably whether the exercise was a planning session for the COVID-19 draconian lockdowns and media censorship. The Event 201 sponsors claimed that "[a]lthough our tabletop exercise included a mock novel coronavirus, the inputs we used for modeling the potential impact of that fictional virus are not similar to nCoV-2019."[1548]

When this author went to the Event 201 webpage, I was met with a popup that requested me to "[s]ign up to receive updates on COVID-19 from our experts. We provide analysis of trends, new evidence and important news." How could they now claim to be experts who can provide unique "trends, new evidence and important news" about COVID-19, which they claim is a virus that is not similar to the fictional virus in their exercise? Below is a screen shot of that popup notice.

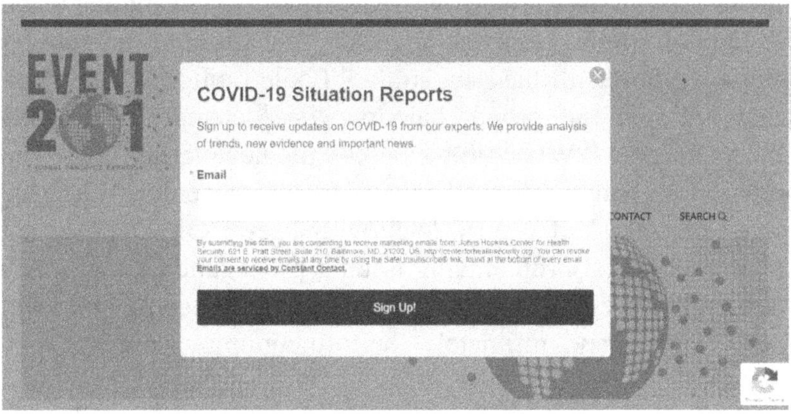

Indeed, the event's sponsors played key roles in responding to the COVID-19 pandemic. So they turned out to be experts after all. But not in a good way. Particularly notable were the actions of Bill Gates in pushing for mandatory vaccinations, from which he makes billions of dollars, and the World Economic Forum clamoring for massive economic shutdowns during the pandemic, which it euphemistically called "The Great Reset." Professor Klaus Schwab, Founder and Executive Chairman of the World Economic Forum, proudly proclaimed that "[t]he pandemic represents a rare but narrow window of opportunity to reflect, reimagine, and reset our world"[1549]

A document leak has given us a window into one part of this world conspiracy. Former UK Health Secretary Matt Hancock gave his WhatsApp encrypted messages to journalist Isabel Oakeshott to use as source material for her to co-write a book with Hancock called "Pandemic Diaries." What Oakeshott saw in those messages shocked her. So, she leaked the messages to a British Newspaper, *The Telegraph*.

The text messages reveal that the COVID-19 pandemic was a scam. *Russia Today* reported that Hancock conversed with Cabinet Secretary Simon Case on January 2021 in a text message and stated "that 'fear' would be a 'vital' factor in ensuring UK citizens' compliance with Covid restrictions."[1550] In another text to aid Damon Poole, Hancock advised: "We frighten the pants of [sic] everyone with the new strain." Poole replied: "Yep, that's what will get the proper bahviour [sic] change." To which Hancock asked: "When do we deploy the new variant"?[1551] That series of messages were allegedly sent on December 13, 2020. Notice that he asked when to "deploy" the new COVID-19 variant. He was obviously referencing issuing propaganda about a new "fictional" COVID-19 variant to scare people into compliance with the lockdowns and, ultimately, the forthcoming vaccines.

In another series of texts, Poole explained that he was trying to get Bill Gates' endorsement of the New Variant Assessment Platform (NVAP) - a service offering the UK's expertise in detecting new virus variants. Hancock replied: 'Tell him that considering how many people I'm getting his chips injected into, he owes me one!"[1552] That statement referenced the electromagnetic-sensitive graphene hydroxide detected in the COVID-19 vaccines. It seems that Hancock was acknowledging that the graphene hydroxide is designed to act somehow like computer chips.

The *Daily Mail* newspaper reported the leaked text messages but spun them to make it seem Hancock was only joking about chips in the vaccine.[1553] But there was nothing in the context of the text messages from which to draw that conclusion. The Daily Mail was trying to run interference and doing damage control. Under no circumstances could the public become informed that they were being contaminated with nano-particles capable of interacting with electromagnetic waves. And so the Daily Mail did its job of falsely spinning the statement as a joke.

59 Anthony Fauci Predicts the Pandemic

On January 10, 2017, Anthony Fauci predicted in a speech: "There is no question that there will be a challenge to the coming administration in the arena of infectious diseases, both chronic infectious diseases in the sense of already ongoing disease, and we have certainly a large burden of that, but also there will be a surprise outbreak. … the thing we're extraordinarily confident about is that we're going to see this in the next few years."[1554]

Dr. Fauci made the above statements in his keynote address at the Georgetown Medical Center at an event titled Pandemic Preparedness in the Next Administration.[1555] The conference was organized by the Center for Global Health Science and Security (GHSS)[1556] in partnership with the Harvard Global Health Institute. It is notable how the event was described by Kat Zamban of Georgetown University in the title to her January 12, 2020, article: Global Health Experts Advise Advance Planning for Inevitable Pandemic.[1557] Notice that the pandemic the experts would discuss was an "inevitable pandemic."

I want you, dear reader, to ponder that statement made by Dr. Fauci in his speech. As you do that, let us put it in context.

During the speech, Dr. Fauci bragged about his 32 years of experience studying infectious diseases as the Director of the National Institute of Allergy and Infectious Diseases (NIAID). Once he framed his expertise, he pronounced, based on that deep experience, that the Trump administration would be faced with an outbreak of an infectious disease. But let us look closer at that statement. It is very telling. In that statement, Dr. Fauci has given us a window into his mind and his involvement in the outbreak that he predicted.

You see, Dr. Fauci did not just guess that there would be an outbreak of an infectious disease; he was emphatic that "there is no question there will be a challenge" of a surprise outbreak of an infectious disease. In addition, Dr. Fauci punctuated his emphatic prediction of a disease outbreak with a closing statement that "the thing we're extraordinarily confident about is that we're going to see this in the next few years."

So, Fauci emphatically predicts an outbreak of an infectious disease during the upcoming Trump administration. He then gives a timetable. He states that the disease outbreak will happen in the next few years. Sure enough, at the end of 2019, we were greeted with the purported COVID-19 outbreak in Wuhan, China. Within months, it allegedly spread throughout the world and into the U.S.

But our analysis does not end there. You see, Dr. Fauci identified the infectious disease that he was predicting as a "surprise outbreak." Think about it. If the outbreak of the disease is a surprise, by definition, it cannot be foreseen. If a disease cannot be foreseen, it cannot be predicted. How could Dr. Fauci predict something that is a surprise to him? He cannot. By definition, he cannot have foreknowledge of an event that would surprise him. He can only predict a surprise to someone else. And the only way to predict a surprise to someone else is if he had advance knowledge of that surprising event.

Dr. Fauci is describing something that he knew would happen. It was only a surprise to the public. Premeditated murder is only a surprise to the murder victim. It is not a surprise to the perpetrator of the murder. The perpetrator of the murder can predict the murder. The perpetrator can describe the murder in advance as a surprise attack, but his meaning is that it will surprise the victim. Dr. Fauci was predicting the pandemic with emphatic certainty; there was "no question" in his mind, and he was "extraordinarily confident" that there would be a pandemic outbreak within a few years. And sure enough, the COVID-19 pandemic happened when he said it would happen.

But Dr. Fauci said the outbreak would be a surprise. If someone predicts a surprising event, that means that person had foreknowledge of the event because, by its very nature, a surprising event is something unexpected and thus not predictable. An accessory to a crime would certainly have foreknowledge. The surprise was on us, not Dr. Fauci. And it certainly was a surprise. Dr. Fauci was right about that.

If the pandemic were a surprise to Dr. Fauci, he could not have predicted it. But it happened just as he predicted it would happen. He called it a surprise, and it was. The only logical way that Dr. Fauci could have known there would be a surprise pandemic is if he was an accomplice in the plan to bring it about.

Dr. Fauci's subsequent leadership in the U.S. response to the very plan-demic he predicted only serves to further implicate him in the planning of it. Imagine, if you will, a fireman predicting that a large building will burn down, and that building is found ablaze as the target of a team of arsonists, just as predicted by the fireman. And leading the fire brigade called to put out the fire, we find the very fireman who predicted the demise of the building. Suppose that fireman is found giving orders that only served to hamper the effort to extinguish the fire, which resulted in the building being burned to the ground. Wouldn't that fireman be a suspect in that arson? Dr. Fauci is a criminal who has, by his slip of the tongue, revealed himself as an evil technocrat at the operational level of a worldwide conspiracy against God and man.

60 5G Radiation Sickness

If the planners of Event 201 were the planners of the COVID-19 pandemic, how could they have such control of events as to ensure the spread of a virus throughout the world to justify their draconian response? The answer is simple; they did not spread anything. The SARS-CoV-2 virus that allegedly causes COVID-19 does not exist. It was a scam from the beginning. They kicked off the scam-demic by using the trick of 5G microwave radiation. When subjects are exposed to 5G radiation, they suffer an illness strikingly similar to a bad flu (i.e., COVID-19). Extreme exposure causes persons to pass out and need hospitalization. They followed up the 5G trick by padding the COVID-19 statistics with influenza cases.

Notably, YouTube considers it disinformation to post "[c]laims that COVID-19 is caused by radiation from 5G networks."[1558] It is simply not something that the social media giants will tolerate. They are doing precisely what the planners of Event 201 suggested should be done. They are censoring information. Why? Because 5G radiation reveals, in part, what is really happening.

Exposure to electrical fields and radio frequency has a detrimental effect on health. Arthur Firstenberg explains:

> “Anxiety disorder,” afflicting one-sixth of humanity, did not exist before the 1860's, when telegraph wires first encircled the earth. No hint of it appears in the medical literature before 1866. Influenza, in its present form, was invented in 1889, along with alternating current.[1559]

We see a similar pattern today with advances in radio frequency communications.

> 2002-2003: 3G introduced to the world[1560]
> 2002-2003: SARS-CoV-1 (SARS) outbreak[1561]
>
> 2009: 4G introduced to the world[1562]
> 2009: H1N1 flu (Swine Flu) outbreak[1563]
>
> 2019-2020: 5G introduced to the world[1564]
> 2019-2020: SARS-CoV-2 (COVID-19) outbreak[1565]

Indeed, research has shown a correlation between 5G radiation and disease suffered by lab animals.

> The health studies conducted in animals revealed that millimeter waves which are used in 5G system, caused change in the body, manifested in structural alteration, suppression of all functions of the organism, the nervous, cardiovascular, immune, blood and other systems with the development complex symptoms. Based on evidence from studied carried out up to today by USA National Toxicology program, Italian Ramazzini study EU Reflex study and a growing number of several scientists say EMW is a "human carcinogen."[1566]

That study is not alone. Many studies show the detrimental

effects of radio frequencies on health. "In May, 2011 the International Agency for Research on Cancer (IARC) concluded that radiofrequency (RF) radiation in the frequency range 30 kHz-300 GHz is a 'possible' human carcinogen."[1567] The 30 kHz-300 GHz range encompasses the frequency range for both 4G and 5G cellular phones.

Dr. Tom Cowan explains that when one is exposed to 5G background radio frequencies, the millimeter waves degrade the oxygen in the atmosphere.[1568] It is as though the person is in a low-oxygen environment at the top of a mountain. Oxygen starvation interferes with certain pathways in your mitochondria, which are organelles in your tissues that use oxygen to make fuel.[1569] The person will suffer hypoxia and come down with all of the symptoms consistent with altitude sickness.

Dr. Cowan explains that "this causes "a hyper-inflammatory response, otherwise known as a cytokine storm, which is the body's way of getting rid of diseased tissue."[1570] That is precisely what we see with the sudden onset of COVID-19 illnesses in areas blanketed with 5G. Dr. Cowan opines that people are dying from hypoxia and an over-enthusiastic inflammatory response, which fits with the misdiagnosis of COVID-19; it is actually sickness from 5G millimeter waves.

On February 5, 2020. Japanese health officials boarded the Diamond Princess at port Yokohama in Tokyo Bay. Those health officials pronounced that 10 persons on board were diagnosed as having coronavirus, later known as SARS-CoV-2 (alleged to cause COVID-19). The ship was ordered quarantined for 14 days. Nobody could leave the ship during the quarantine period. Within three days, another 125 passengers were diagnosed with COVID-19. By February 13, 2020, a total of 218 people were diagnosed with COVID-19.[1571]

A little-known fact is that the Diamond Princess was

sporting some new high-tech 5G towers. An earlier news release explained that "Princess Cruises has announced a new dimension in its connectivity partnership with SES and will become the first global cruise ship fleet with early access to SES's O3b mPOWER network augmenting the Princess Medallion Class experience as it scales across the fleet, according to a press release."[1572]

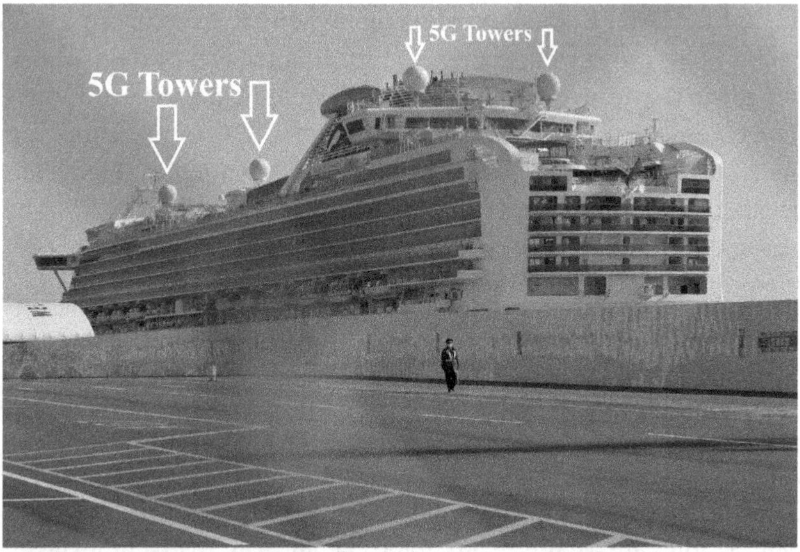

Figure 72: Diamond Princess on or about February 5, 2020, Docked at Tokyo Bay During Its COVID-19 Quarantine (Photograph: Philip Fong/Getty Images)

Is there a connection between the newly installed 5G network on the ship and the passengers being struck ill with coronavirus? It should be noted that only the Princess cruise line that had installed the 5G had outbreaks of COVID-19. In March 2020, the Grand Princess had outbreaks of COVID-19 before docking in San Francisco. The Ruby Princess was reported to have had an outbreak of COVID-19 involving 600 passengers prior to docking on March 19, 2020, in Sydney, Australia. All those ships are Medallion Class ships with the new 5G tower connectivity from SES's O3b mPOWER.

SES explains on its website that the O3b mPOWER is a next-generation 5G satellite signal system.

> Together with key stakeholders and technology partners, SES Networks is advancing satellite integration into 5G through standardization, technology development and demonstrations.
>
> ***
>
> SES Networks is advancing satellite integration into 5G through standardization, technology development and demonstrations.
>
> ***
>
> We've also invested in the revolutionary O3b mPOWER next-generation satellite system, which will augment our existing MEO assets with terabit-scale capabilities.[1573]

Connection Between 5G and COVID-19 Symptoms

What is the effect of 5G on humans? Dr. Magda Havas, Ph.D, sought to answer that question. Dr. Havas "compared the average number of cases, deaths, and tests for COVID-19 per million population in states with and without 5G."[1574]

Dr. Havas found that the standardized testing for states with and without 5G was similar. But he discovered a real difference in COVID-19 cases per million population for those states that deployed 5G. Dr. Havas found that "Covid-19 cases per million are 95% higher and covid-19 deaths per million are 126% higher in states with 5G."[1575]

	Total Cases per 1 million	Total Deaths per 1 million	Total Tests per 1 million	% Cases/Tests	% Deaths/Tests	n
Mean for States with mmWave 5G	2,566	128	14,629	15.64%	0.724%	33
Mean for States without mmWave 5G	1,288	55	14,324	8.82%	0.364%	18
with vs. without mmWave 5G	99%	131%	2%	77%	99%	
p-value for 1 tailed T-test	**0.0199**	**0.0455**	0.8	**0.00345**	**0.0191**	
Correlation to Population Density	0.269	0.169	0.245	0.233	0.154	
Correlation to Pop. Density (excl. outlier Wash DC)	**0.723**	**0.577**	0.496	**0.701**	**0.600**	
Correlation to Air Quality Index	0.110	0.0553	-0.104	0.291	0.187	

A Spanish study proved that countries with 5G had 220% more COVID-19 infections than countries that had not deployed 5G.[1576]

> The results obtained demonstrate a clear and close relationship between the rate of coronavirus infections and 5G antenna location.[1577]
>
> The case of San Marino is particularly significant. It was the first state in the world to install 5G and therefore, the state whose citizens have been exposed to 5G radiation the longest, and suspiciously, the first state in the world with infections. The probability of this happening is 1 in 37,636.[1578]

Indeed, San Marino is truly a stark indicator of 5G culpability for COVID-19. It was the first European state to adopt 5G technology and had virtually no regulations on its use. Notably, San Marino has the highest incidence per 1,000 population of COVID-19 in Europe. Indeed, its rate is a whopping 27 times greater than the infection rate in Croatia. Why such a stark difference between San Marino and Croatia? The reason is that Croatia does not have 5G.

5G Explains Cruise Ship COVID-19 Outbreak

Does 5G explain the COVID-19 outbreak on the Princess

cruise ships? A researcher has studied the COVID-19 outbreak aboard the Diamond Princess, and he concluded the following:

> When the Diamond Princess data was compared to the controls, it's clear that the death and infection rates of the Diamond Princess significantly surpass the death and infection rates of all the control data. Ongoing use of 5G can result in potential harm to populations. For the above reasons, this paper concludes that 5G wireless technology radiation is a probable factor for causing Covid-19 outbreaks, but still identifies other causes that still need to be tested. Governments are recommended to impose a moratorium on 5G wireless technology until it can be proven that this technology is safe for humans and the environment.[1579]

Wuhan is China's Experimental City For 5G

China has one of the largest 5G networks in the world.[1580] In November 2019, the Chinese government announced plans to blanket China with more than 130,000 5G base stations.

Wuhan, China, which started the entire alleged COVID-19 pandemic, was, interestingly enough, one of the first cities in China to be blanketed with 5G technology.[1581] In April 2018, the Chinese government announced that "[b]y 2020, 5G network will cover every corner of the city."

Sure enough, right on cue, as soon as the 5G network was fired up in Wuhan, the citizens started dropping like flies with symptoms that exactly mirrored the symptoms associated with COVID-19.

Indeed, the same hospital that treated most of the Wuhan COVID-19 patients was bathed in 5G electromagnetic radiation.

CGTN reported:

> In the battle against the novel coronavirus disease (COVID-19), China's leading network service provider, Huawei, built a 5G network at Huoshenshan Hospital in Wuhan, which has played a crucial role in treating coronavirus patients.[1582]

One might wonder why there is not a perpetual illness after an environmental radio frequency innovation. It may be that the exosomes that the body is excreting are in some way also helping to bring equilibrium to the body.[1583] That means the body adapts to the new environment and finds some balance after being exposed to the new technology. But before that point, the initial phase of disruption, there is a spike in death and disease. The world's governments have learned to know what the innovation will do (in this case, 5G) and prepare to use the technology rollout to strip us of some portion of our freedom by characterizing the expected illnesses as a viral pandemic requiring lockdowns, masking, social distancing, relocation camps, and mandatory vaccinations.

61 The Disappearing Flu

5G was good enough to kick-start the fake pandemic. But they knew that they could not irradiate enough people to keep that charade going, so according to plan, they started diagnosing influenza cases as COVID-19. Some who are ill with the flu may test positive for SARS-CoV-12 (alleged to cause COVID-19). That is why the flu disappeared during the 2020-2021 flu season. All persons with the flu were counted not as flu cases but as COVID-19 cases. They then used the COVID-19 scam to push the poisonous COVID-19 vaccines on the population and begin the actual killing. Their objective from the beginning was to force toxic vaccines on the world population.

Statistician John Cullen discovered that the World Health Organization (WHO) influenza data reveals that the COVID-19 statistics are being padded by falsely reporting influenza cases as COVID-19 cases.[1584] But to suggest that influenza cases are being misrepresented as COVID-19 cases is simply not allowed to be mentioned in the mainstream media. The charts below are annotated from the World Health Organization. They reveal that the COVID-19 statistics are being padded by falsely reporting influenza cases as COVID-19 cases.[1585] To suggest that influenza cases are being misrepresented as COVID-19 cases is simply not allowed to be mentioned in the mainstream media.

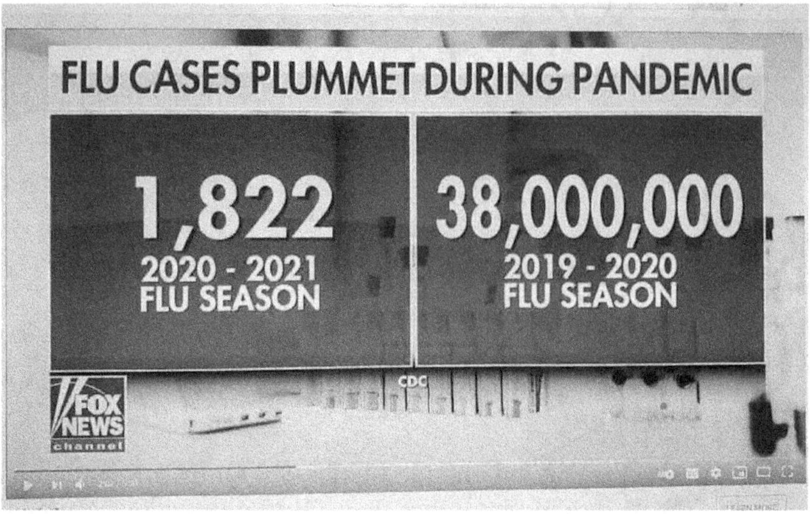

Peter Andrews, writing for Russia Today, reveals that there has been a 98% plummet in flu infections. He then reveals it is impolite within the scientific community to suggest that doctors are misclassifying influenza cases as COVID-19 cases. Andrews explains that "it only seems like the flu has disappeared because doctors and scientists have been wrongly classing other respiratory diseases as Covid. Please note that the boffins are already treating this suggestion as something akin to flat-Earth theory."[1586]

Andrews reveals that "Australia essentially 'skipped' their flu season this year, with not a single case reported since July (their peak). In fact, flu has more or less vanished throughout the Southern Hemisphere." Andrews was writing on October 26, 2020. The Southern Hemisphere had emerged from what should have been their fall and winter flu season. But they had none. And the Northern Hemisphere since followed suit with a collapse in reported flu cases. Jo MacFarlane reporting for The Daily Mail concluded from the WHO data that "flu, it seems, has all but vanished."[1587]

MacFarlane published his article on October 24, 2020, which was the beginning of what is supposed to be the fall and winter flu season in the Northern Hemisphere. MacFarlane could already see from the data that the expected seasonal flu epidemic was not making its appearance. The reported flu cases in the UK were down approximately 90%. He saw the disappearance of the flu revealed by "the figures provide a startling insight into what has become a creeping trend across the world."

Of course, MacFarlane states the obvious. "There are those who claim flu cases haven't vanished at all, but are instead being recorded as Covid-19." But after making that common-sense statement, MacFarlane quickly dismisses the thought. So, what is the explanation he announces for the disappearance of the flu in the midst of the alleged COVID-19 pandemic? It is the theory of … wait for it … "viral interference."

MacFarlane explains that "[w]hen an individual is infected with one virus, they are less likely to be infected by another during that time due to something called 'viral interference'." MacFarlane quotes Dr. Elisabetta Groppelli who claims that "[v]iruses are parasites. Once they enter a cell, they don't want other viruses to compete with. So the virus already in the body will effectively kick the other parasite out." It sounds good, but it is not true. Indeed, when one's immune system is focused on fighting off one particular pathogen, the body's immune resources are focused on that pathogen. With all of the body's immune resources focused on that one pathogen, the person does not have the reserves to fight an unrelated pathogen and is thus is more susceptible to an unrelated pathogen.

That is why the flu vaccine only works for the particular strain of the flu virus that is in the vaccine and no others. Often, persons who receive the flu vaccine end up getting the flu, but it is a different strain of the flu for which they have no protection. Under the theory of 'viral interference' the patient getting a flu shot should be protected from all strains of flu and not just the strain in the vaccine.

The phenomenon of a vaccinated person being more susceptible to an unrelated pathogen is known as pathogenic priming. Vaccines cause pathogenic priming, which injures a person's immune system such that the person is 4.4 times more likely to become ill from some other pathogen. For example, at least six major studies have shown that a person who gets the flu shot has had their immune system pathogenically primed to be more likely to become infected from coronavirus.

The charts below reveal a complete collapse in worldwide cases of influenza after COVID-19 made its appearance in the spring of 2020. Notice the complete disappearance of the flu during the 2020-2021 fall and winter seasonal flu period. That disappearance of flu correlates directly with the reported second-wave of COVID-19 cases and suggests that flu cases are being misreported as COVID-19 second-wave cases.

United States Influenza Cases

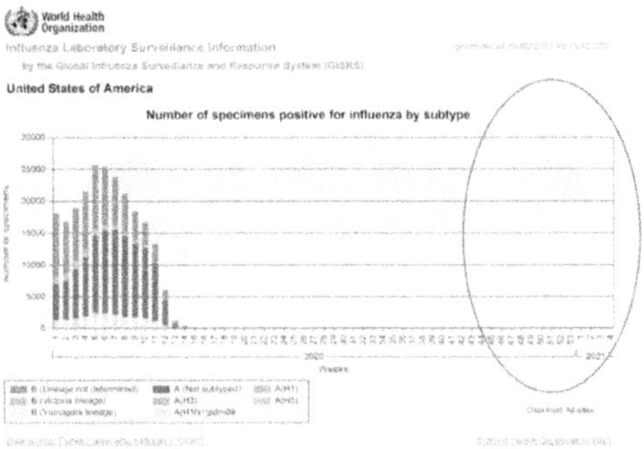

Flu disappears during the 2020-2021 Fall and Winter Flu Season in Direct Correlation with the Alleged COVID-19 Second Wave

The above World Health Organization (WHO) chart shows the number of people infected by influenza in the United States. Each Bar represents the number of infections in the United States for each week of 2020 through week number 4 of 2021. Notice that the influenza infections disappeared in the United States during week 15 of 2020. This correlates very closely with the emergence of COVID-19.

For comparison, below is a WHO chart that shows the number of people infected by influenza in the United States for the entire year of 2019 and the first 4 weeks of 2020. Each Bar represents the number of people infected in the United States for each week of 2019 through week 4 of 2021. Notice the difference from the chart above. This suggests that the disappearance of the influenza in week 15 of 2020 through week 4 of 2021 is because Influenza is being reported as COVID-19 infections. The complete disappearance of the flu during the fall and winter flu season of 2020-2021 suggests that the second wave of COVID-19 cases reported during that period are actually flu cases being falsely reported as COVID-19 cases.

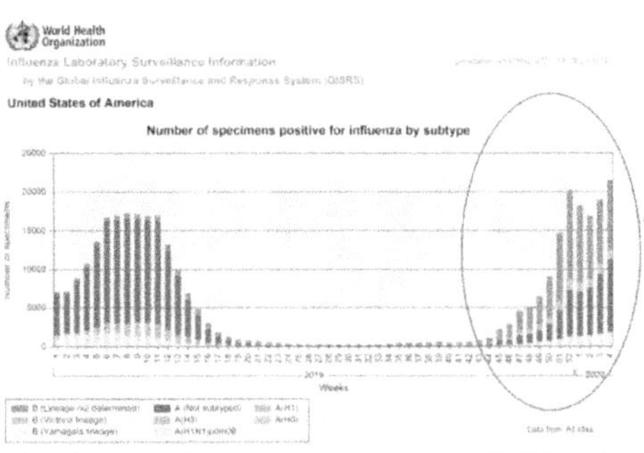

2019-2020 Fall and Winter Flu Season

Worldwide Influenza Cases

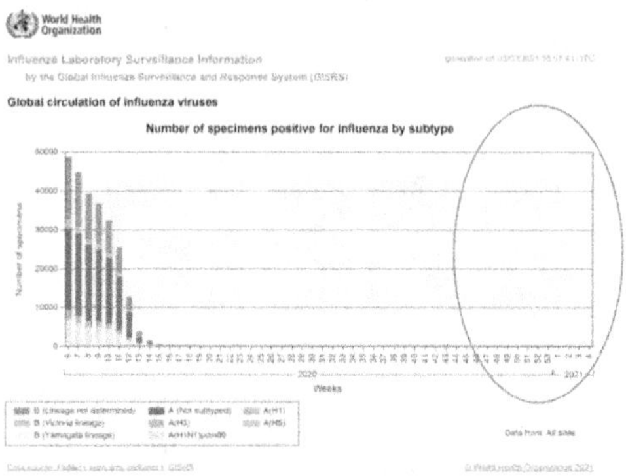

Flu disappears during the 2020-2021 Fall and Winter Flu Season in Direct Correlation with the Alleged COVID-19 Second Wave

The above World Health Organization (WHO) chart shows the number of people infected by influenza in the world. Each Bar represents the number of infections in the world for each week of 2020 through week number 4 of 2021. Notice that the influenza infections disappeared in the world during week 15 of 2020. This correlates very closely with the emergence of COVID-19.

For comparison, below is a WHO chart that shows the number of people infected by influenza in the world for the entire year of 2019 and the first 4 weeks of 2020. Each Bar represents the number of people infected in the world for each week of 2019 through week 4 of 2021. Notice the difference from the chart above. This suggests that the disappearance of the influenza in week 15 of 2020 through week 4 of 2021 is because Influenza is being reported as COVID-19 infections. The complete disappearance of the flu during the fall and winter flu season of 2020-2021 suggests that the second wave of COVID-19 cases reported during that period are actually flu cases

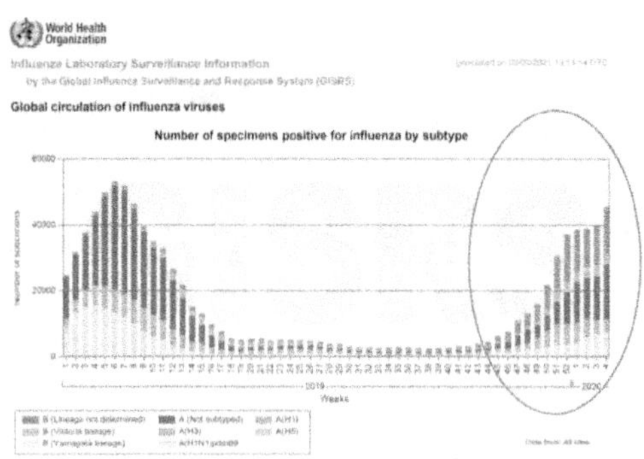

2019-2020 Fall and Winter Flu Season

This author knows someone who was in the ICU with her son at St. Joseph's hospital in Phoenix on August 29, 2020. She spent the day with her son in the ICU and spoke with the nurses. She was told by the nurses that none of the patients in the ICU were COVID-19 patients. Later, she was watching the local news, and it reported that the ICUs in the Phoenix hospitals were filled to 83% capacity with COVID-19 patients. St. Joseph's Hospital is one of the largest hospitals in Phoenix. It is a medical center with more than 500 beds. The local news channel was asked about the discrepancy, and they said they got their information from the local health authorities. The news report was deceptive propaganda. Incidentally, she was with her son in another hospital ICU earlier in the week outside of Phoenix, and there were no COVID-19 patients in that ICU at that time either.

Dr. Vernon Coleman is a general practitioner and a former Professor of Holistic Medical Sciences.[1588] Dr. Coleman is a Sunday Times best-selling author, who has written more than 100 books, selling over 2 million copies in the UK alone. Many of Dr. Coleman's books have been on bestseller lists worldwide. Dr. Coleman summarizes the COVID-19 pandemic scam:

> Covid-19 was, as I have been saying now for three years, nothing more than the rebranded flu. I proved this time and time again. But here, again, are some of the statistics I have used in the past which prove that covid-19 was no more deadly than the flu – because it was the flu. The pandemic myth has been deliberately sustained by the Government, their advisors and the media. But there were no more deaths in 2020 than most other years. Figures from the Office of National Statistics in the UK show that the number of deaths in 2020 was lower than the average for the last 30 years. In 2020 the age-standardised mortality rate per 100,000 people in England and Wales was 1,043.

But the average age-standardised mortality rate for the last 30 years was 1,161 per 100,000. So, there were fewer than average deaths in 2020. Some pandemic, eh? The same is true of every country in the world. Governments and doctors lied. There was no pandemic. It was a gargantuan hoax. And the minute I exposed the hoax I was attacked, vilified and lied about.[1589]

62 Veklury® (Remdesivir)

The medical establishment aims to increase deaths they can attribute to COVID-19. They are not limited to statistical shenanigans. They are ready, willing, and able to kill patients to add to the COVID-19 body count as long as they can conceal it under the cover of medical care. That is not hyperbole or a wild conspiracy theory.

Once the flu victims are hospitalized, and they test positive for COVID-19 using the rigged PCR tests, the killing starts. In order to ramp up the deaths, they are administered the toxic drug, remdesivir. After knocking out the inexpensive, safe, and effective hydroxychloroquine and ivermectin as treatments for COVID-19 the FDA decided that it would be a good thing to recommend instead an expensive, unsafe, and ineffective drug, remdesivir. One cannot understand the malfeasance and depravity of the FDA until you find out about remdesivir.

Dr. Bryan Ardis makes an astounding revelation. He states that Dr. Fauci pushed the use of Veklury® (remdesivir) as a treatment for COVID-19 knowing that it would be unsafe and ineffective for patients. Veklury® (remdesivir) is a nucleotide analogue RNA polymerase inhibitor. Dr. Ardis reveals that the symptoms of lungs filling with fluid and the other alleged

COVID-19 symptoms were actually side effects of kidney poisoning and other organ damage that are known side-effects of Veklury® (remdesivir). Dr. Ardis alleges that the devastating health toll allegedly caused by COVID-19 was actually caused by the National Institute of Health (NIH) recommended treatment of Veklury® (remdesivir).

Dr. Ardis states that the NIH even cited two studies on its website that showed that Veklury® (remdesivir) was ineffective and unsafe to patients. It seems that many doctors just blindly followed the recommendation of the NIH to use Veklury® (remdesivir) without actually reading the cited studies. This author tracked down those studies and read them.

NIH Recommends Remdesivir

On May 12, 2020, the NIH recommended the use of Veklury® (remdesivir) for severe cases of COVID-19.[1590] At that time, Veklury® (remdesivir) was an unapproved experimental drug made by Gilead Sciences. It was authorized by the FDA for emergency use treatment of COVID-19.

Conflicts of Interest

The May 12, 2020 recommendation from the NIH to use Veklury® (remdesivir) to treat COVID-19 came from the NIH Panel on COVID-19 Treatment Guidelines. There were nine (9) people on the NIH Panel on COVID-19 Treatment Guidelines with financial ties to Gilead Sciences, the maker of Veklury® (remdesivir). The following is a list of those people on the NIH Panel on COVID-19 Treatment Guidelines who had financial ties to Gilead Sciences, the manufacturer of Veklury® (remdesivir):[1591]

Rajesh Gandhi is on the advisory board of Gilead Sciences.

> David Glidden is a consultant for Gilead Sciences.
>
> Adaora Adimora is a consultant for Gilead Sciences and received research support from Gilead Sciences.
>
> Eric Daar is a consultant for Gilead Sciences and recieves research support from Gilead Sciences.
>
> Judith Aberg received research support from Gilead Sciences.
>
> Jason Baker received research support from Gilead Sciences.
>
> Susanna Naggie received research support from Gilead Sciences.
>
> Pablo Tebas received research support from Gilead Sciences.
>
> Roger Bedimo received an honoraria from Gilead Sciences.

The panel tried to steer doctors away from Hydroxychloroquine, by stating that "[t]here are insufficient clinical data to recommend either for or against using chloroquine or hydroxychloroquine for the treatment of COVID."[1592]

The panel, of course, had an interest in undermining inexpensive and effective treatments: "[T]he Panel recommends against the use of the following drugs for the treatment of COVID-19: The combination of hydroxychloroquine plus azithromycin because of the potential for toxicities." That was not true. Indeed, many subsequent studies have shown that the hydroxychloroquine plus azithromycin "combination is safe and may avoid worsening, virus persistence, and subsequent contagiosity."

In a previous chapter, this author explained the extreme efforts to discredit hydroxychloroquine. Doctors conducting studies purposely administered toxic levels of hydroxychlorquine to falsely show that it was dangerous to patients.[1593]

Remdesivir Adverse Events

Many of the studies cited in support of NIH's recommendation to use Veklury® (remdesivir) were in vitro studies or animal studies. A couple of the human studies were at best a mixed bag. Two of the most authoritative studies showed Veklury® (remdesivir) to be ineffective and unsafe.

On or about May 12, 2020, the FDA reported the following summary for study GS-US-5773:[1594]

> In a randomized, open-label clinical trial (Study GS-US-540-5773) of remdesivir in 397 subjects with severe COVID-19 treated with remdesivir for 5 (n=200) or 10 days (n=197), adverse events were reported in 71% and 74% of subjects, respectively, serious adverse events were reported in 21% and 35% of subjects, respectively, and Grade=3 adverse events were reported in 31% and 43% of subjects, respectively. Nine (5%) subjects in the 5-day group and 20 (10%) subjects in the 10-day group discontinued treatment due to an adverse event. All cause mortality at Day 28 was 10% vs 13% in the 5- and 10-day treatment groups, respectively.[1595]

Please do not miss the fact that there were reported 71% adverse events in the 5-day study and 74% adverse events in the 10-day study for patients taking Veklury® (remdesivir). 21%

suffered serious adverse events in the 5 day study, and 35% of the patients suffered serious adverse events in the 10-day study. Below is the chart of adverse events published in the study.[1596]

Table 3. **Summary of Adverse Events According to Remdesivir Treatment Group.***

Event or Abnormality	5-Day Group (N=200)	10-Day Group (N=197)
Any adverse event — no. of patients (%)	141 (70)	145 (74)
Nausea	20 (10)	17 (9)
Acute respiratory failure	12 (6)	21 (11)
Alanine aminotransferase increased	11 (6)	15 (8)
Constipation	13 (6)	13 (7)
Aspartate aminotransferase increased	10 (5)	13 (7)
Hypokalemia	10 (5)	12 (6)
Hypotension	9 (4)	12 (6)
Respiratory failure	7 (4)	14 (7)
Insomnia	10 (5)	11 (6)
Acute kidney injury	4 (2)	15 (8)
Adverse event leading to discontinuation of treatment — no. of patients (%)	9 (4)	20 (10)
Any serious adverse event	42 (21)	68 (35)
Acute respiratory failure	10 (5)	18 (9)
Respiratory failure	5 (2)	10 (5)
Septic shock	2 (1)	5 (3)
Acute respiratory distress syndrome	1 (<1)	5 (3)
Hypoxia	2 (1)	4 (2)
Respiratory distress	3 (2)	4 (2)
Dyspnea	4 (2)	1 (1)
Pneumothorax	2 (1)	3 (2)
Viral pneumonia	3 (2)	2 (1)
Aminotransferase levels increased	3 (2)	2 (1)
Any grade ≥3 laboratory abnormality — no. of patients/total no. (%)	53/195 (27)	64/191 (34)
Selected grade ≥3 laboratory abnormalities — no. of patients/total no. (%)		
Creatinine clearance decreased		
Grade 3	13/193 (7)	13/188 (7)
Grade 4	5/193 (3)	23/198 (12)
ALT elevation		
Grade 3	8/194 (4)	11/191 (6)
Grade 4	4/194 (2)	5/191 (3)
AST elevation		
Grade 3	11/194 (6)	7/190 (4)
Grade 4	3/194 (2)	4/190 (2)
Bilirubin increased		
Grade 3	1/193 (1)	3/190 (2)
Grade 4	0	1/190 (1)

* Adverse events listed are those that occurred in at least 5% of patients in either treatment group, and serious adverse events listed are those that occurred in 5 or more patients.

Hiding Remdesivir Adverse Events

This is where it gets deceptive. In a later published fact sheet dated October 2020, the FDA provided the following summary of that same study:[1597]

> Study GS-US-540-5773 was a randomized, open-label clinical trial in hospitalized adult subjects with severe COVID-19 treated with VEKLURY 200 mg on Day 1 and 100 mg once daily for 5 (n=200) or 10 days (n=197). Adverse reactions were reported in 33 (17%) subjects in the 5-day group and 40 (20%) subjects in the 10-day group. The most common adverse reactions occurring in at least 5% of subjects in either the VEKLURY 5-day or 10-day group, respectively, were nausea (5% vs 3%), AST increased (3% vs 6%), and ALT increased (2% vs 7%). Rates of any adverse reaction, serious adverse reactions, and adverse reactions leading to treatment discontinuation are presented in Table 6. [Chart 6 indicated that 3% of the 5 day group and 5% of the 10 day group had treatment discontinued due to adverse reactions.][1598]

After August 7, 2021, when this author published an analysis[1599] of the deception revealed by the October 2020 fact sheet, that fact sheet was given a watermark across it indicating it was "REVOKED." There was no explanation given for the revocation.[1600]

Notice the differences in reporting. The May 2020 report describes adverse events, whereas the October 2020 report changes the reporting to adverse reactions. The difference is that an adverse reaction denotes a causal relationship and an adverse event is an event that may or may not be causally related. A reaction is sometimes defined as the response to a medication where that response is at least reasonably possible to have been caused by the medication.[1601] By concealing the adverse events and only reporting adverse reactions, the October 2020 FDA report conceals the real danger from Veklury® (remdesivir). Keep in mind that an adverse reaction must be established by a reasonable possibility. Such nebulous standards for distinguishing adverse events from adverse reactions are ripe for abuse. An adverse event could be causally related but the reviewer may just decide it is not reasonable to infer it is causally linked, and thus it would not be called an adverse reaction.

May 2020 FDA Publication: "397 subjects with severe COVID-19 treated with remdesivir for 5 (n=200) or 10 days (n=197), **adverse events** were reported in 71% and 74% of subjects"

October 2020 FDA Publication: "**Adverse reactions** were reported in 33 (17%) of subjects in the 5-day group and 40 (20%) of subjects in the 10-day group."

May 2020 FDA Publication: Nine (5%) of subjects in the 5-day group and 20 (10%) of subjects in the 10-day group discontinued treatment due to an **adverse event**.

October 2020 FDA Publication: 3% of the 5 day group and 5% of the 10 day group discontinued treatment due to an **adverse reaction**.

May 2020 FDA Publication: **Serious adverse events** were reported in 21% and 35% of subjects, [in the 5 day and 10 day groups] respectively.

October 2020 FDA Publication: **Serious adverse reactions** were reported in 2% and 2% of subjects in the 5 day and 10 groups respectively.

This is where the deception becomes obvious. The study did not measure adverse reactions! The study protocols for GS-US-540-5773 published by Gilead states that they were only going to measure adverse events.[1602] There is no mention of any plan to measure adverse reactions.

Indeed, when one reads the data from the Gilead study (GS-US-540-5773) there is only a recording of adverse events.[1603] There is no measure or memorialization of adverse reactions. So, the question is, if Gilead did not plan to measure adverse reactions and there is no record of such measures, where did the adverse reaction figures come from?

It seems that the FDA has been caught in a deception, which explains why the October 2020 fact sheet was "REVOKED" without explanation.

Majority of Patients on Remdesivir Suffer Liver Damage

Amazingly, the May 2020 FDA publication indicated that a majority of the participants in the several remdesivir studies conducted have suffered liver damage.

> Transaminase elevations have been observed in the remdesivir clinical development program, including in healthy volunteers and patients with COVID19. In healthy volunteers who received up to 150 mg daily for 14 days, alanine aminotransferase (ALT) elevations were observed in the majority of patients, including elevations to up to 10 times baseline values in one subject without evidence of clinical hepatitis.

The FDA report stated that in the GS-US-540-5773 study 5% of the patients suffered moderate to severe liver damage. Whereas, 2% of the study patients suffered severe liver damage.

Kidney Damage From Remdesivir is Foreseeable

Another foreseeable side effect of Veklury® (remdesivir) is kidney damage. The FDA publication reveals that "[i]ntravenous administration (slow bolus) of remdesivir to rats at dosage levels of =3 mg/kg/day for up to 4 weeks resulted in findings indicative of kidney injury and/or dysfunction."

Invasive Mechanical Ventilation Required

In another later published study (ACTT-1, NCT04280705) reported in the October 10, 2020 FDA emergency use authorization fact sheet that alleged to show the benefits of Veklury® (remdesivir), 27% of the patients taking Veklury® (remdesivir) "were on invasive mechanical ventilation."[1604] There was no control group in that study. It seems that the ventilation was the result of Veklury® (remdesivir) because the study revealed that "[s]ubjects on mechanical ventilation at screening were excluded" from the study.

Early Study Termination Due to Adverse Events

In another human study conducted in China, 12% of the Veklury® (remdesivir) group participants had to discontinue therapy with Veklury® (remdesivir) due to adverse side effects. That compared to 5% in the control group.

Keep in mind that the control group in the chineses study was not truly a placebo group and the Veklury® (remdesivir) group was not truly a Veklury® (remdesivir) group. Both the control group and the Veklury® (remdesivir) group recieved corticosteroids, lopinavir/ritonavir, and interferon alfa-2b. The study was terminated early without any conclusions. The NIH admitted that "[t]he use of concomitant medications (corticosteroids, lopinavir/ritonavir, interferon) may have obscured the effects of remdesivir."

Another human study cited did not have a control group, and the NIH, therefore, admitted that "it is not possible to assess whether the use of remdesivir led to the improvement."

Remdesivir Proven Ineffective in Ebola Study

There was only one other human study cited, and the results were devastating for the patients in that study who were administered Veklury® (remdesivir).[1605] In that study, Veklury® (remdesivir) was compared to three other treatments for Ebola. The control group was not actually a placebo group. The group was administered a medicine identified as ZMapp (a triple monoclonal antibody agent).

There was something strange about the trial. In another trial study 22% of the study patients died within 28 days using ZMapp on patients with Ebola. But in the comparative study with Veklury® (remdesivir) the motrality rate for the control group using ZMapp shot up to 49.7% during the 28 day study.

The study administrators could only guess as to why their study patients were dropping like flies. They said: "The reason that mortality among patients who received ZMapp was 22% in the PREVAIL II trial (conducted during the outbreak in West Africa) and 50% in our trial (conducted during the current outbreak in the DRC) is unclear."

It should be noted that the World Health Organization (WHO) reports that "the average [Ebola virus disease] EVD case fatality rate is around 50%."[1606]

One thing that was clear was that the significantly higher mortality for ZMapp brought the control group closer to the 53.1% mortality rate of the Veklury® (remdesivir) group with the effect that Veklury® (remdesivir) was shown to be merely less effective rather than extremely deleterious. That higher mortality of 49.7%

for ZMapp also had the effect of showing that the other two treatment modalities were effective as compared to the control.

In any event, as the chart published in the study below reveals, Veklury® (remdesivir) had the highest mortality of any of the treatment modalities with 53.1% of the Ebola patients who were administered Veklury® (remdesivir) dying within 28 days.

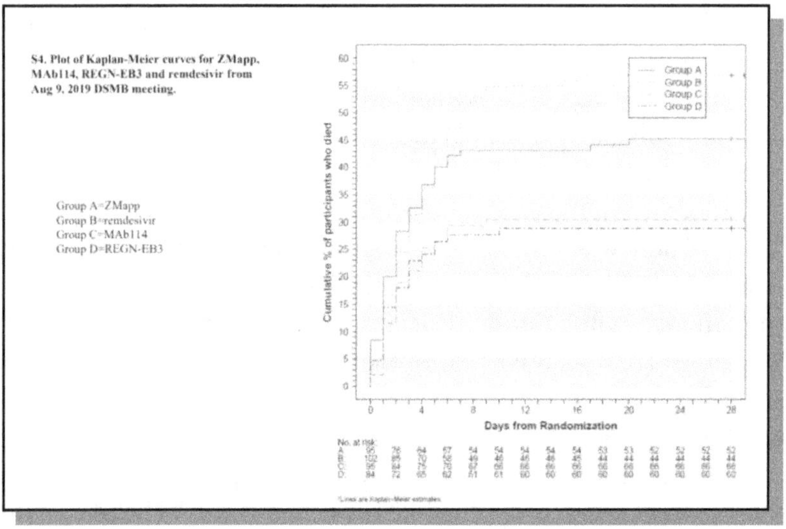

Yet, with those studies showing the Veklury® (remdesivir) is unsafe and ineffective, the NIH recommended Veklury® (remdesivir) as the treatment for COVID-19. The results were foreseeable. Its use to treat patients with COVID-19 were predictably ineffective and unsafe.

It seemed that nothing was going to stop the FDA's approval of remdesivir. On October 22, 2020, the FDA approved Veklury® (remdesivir) for use in adult and pediatric patients 12 years of age and older and weighing at least 40 kilograms (about 88 pounds) for the treatment of COVID-19 requiring hospitalization. That was notable because it was the first official

FDA approved treatment for COVID-19.[1607]

On January 21, 2022, the U.S. Food and Drug Administration (FDA) granted expedited approval of a supplemental new drug application (sNDA) for Veklury® (remdesivir) for the treatment of non-hospitalized adult and adolescent patients who are at high risk of progression to severe COVID-19.[1608] The FDA further expanded the emergency use authorization for Remdesivir to include treatment of non-hospitalized pediatric patients at high risk.

Below is a January 29, 2022 report by Faye Higbee of the RAIR Foundation USA. She concludes that the only rational conclusion from the government's action is that those holding the reigns of government are using remdesivir to kill us.[1609] Higbe writes:

> Remdesivir is a highly toxic drug that medical officials advocate in the fight against Covid. But what is it, and why do the same officials ferociously defend it when there are known side effects that are deadly? The FDA approved it under the name Veklury for IVs in non-hospitalized outpatient treatment on January 27, 2022. They also terminated approval of two monoclonal antibody drugs, saying they "didn't work" for the Omicron variant. Those two drugs had known life-extending properties for Covid patients. Let's have a look at the controversy and why there may be more to this than meets the eye.
>
> **Failed Drug**
>
> Remdesivir was developed in 2009 by Gilead Sciences to treat hepatitis C and respiratory syncytial virus (RSV), but it didn't work against

those diseases.[1610] So they "repurposed" it for Ebola and Marburg viruses in 2014. It wasn't effective in stopping the replication of those viruses either. Now it has once again been "repurposed" for Covid. But the narrative of the NIH is that it does stop the replication of the SARS-Cov-2 virus. It is not recommended for treating Covid patients, but that hasn't stopped the 'powers that be.'

RAIR Foundation USA spoke to an infectious diseases physician for this article involved in early clinical trials for Remdesivir at the beginning of the pandemic. She told us that Remdesivir was not effective for patients severely afflicted with Covid. They actually stopped the trials when they saw that patients' kidney and/or liver functions were elevating. In medical terminology, this is called: increased alanine transaminase or aspartate transaminase – these are the enzymes secreted by the liver or kidneys that can shut down during an IV of Remdesivir.

So why in the world would the FDA approve a drug that must be monitored for kidney/liver failure? The FDA now approves the drug to treat "non-hospitalized patients." The drug is administered through an IV, and patients must be closely monitored. But non-hospitalized?

Doctors have sounded the alarm for months, but their voices have fallen on deaf ears.[1611]

In this strange situation, we have the FDA revoking approval of the known life-extending drugs containing monoclonal antibodies, Regeneron being one of the two that were revoked. They say the drugs do nothing for the Omicron variant, which they claim is 99% of current cases. Omicron is the least dangerous of the variants. Take an aspirin and a cup of hot lemon tea and skip it. The only monoclonal antibody drug they left for use is Sotrovimab. Our doctor told us that there are two therapeutics she has used that work: Dexamethasone (a steroid that reduces inflammation) and monoclonal antibodies like Sotrovimab. But why revoke the antibody drugs and leave the known bad drug?

Dr. Death – the Fauci connection

Remember the problem of overuse of antibiotics? Use them too long, and the bacteria find a way to mutate around them. The same principle applies to antiviral medicines, which is one reason variants continue to emerge. Remdesivir is also a failed drug – even during Ebola studies, it was found to do little for patients afflicted with the virus and was actually highly toxic.

Monoclonal antibodies, which mimic the body's creation of antibodies against disease, were more effective then, as they are now." Remdesivir had a 53% death rate which is considerably higher than that of Covid, as opposed to the lowest death rate of the monoclonal antibody drug Regeneron. With Covid, Remdesivir statistics from 2,058 deaths on CMS data (Medicare) revealed a death rate of 26%, and 46% of those died within 14 days of treatment.[1612] The mortality rate from Covid is around 1%, depending on the country.

Dr. Anthony Fauci advocated for Remdesivir therapy in April of 2020. In his own citation of the Gilead study, 53 people from the US, Canada, Europe, and Japan, reported 60% adverse events – from renal failure to liver problems to multiple organ failure. The NIH even now warns about renal failure and liver toxicity from Remdesivir. The World Health Organization (WHO) – does not recommend it for use in Covid patients.[1613] Fauci does.

WHO has issued a conditional recommendation against the use of remdesivir in hospitalized patients, regardless of disease severity, as there is currently no evidence that remdesivir improves survival and other outcomes in these patients." World Health Organization

So we have a so-called "expert" doctor who advocates for a treatment that is known to kill and is not effective against the Covid virus. We have a Federal Agency that is also advocating it be used for Covid patients knowing full well that it can kill. That same agency pulled the life-saving monoclonal antibody treatments known to save lives. In the face of all the information against Remdesivir, it appears the Federal government and its experts are not "listening to the science" at all.

Dr. Bryan Ardis told podcast host Dr. Peter Breggin on January 25 that Fauci and his cronies are trying to kill us, and Covid is just the excuse. What do you think?[1614]

Dr. Peterson Pierre, M.D., alleges that the hospitals are financially incentivized to administer the toxic drug, remdesivir.

Upon checking the Centers for Medicare and Medicaid services, this author found that Dr. Pierre's allegation is true. Hospitals are given a "20% add-on payment under Section 3710 of the CARES Act" if they administer remdesivir to a patient diagnosed with COVID-19.[1615]

The ICD-10-PCS billing codes for the CARES Act add-on payment for remdesivir are XW033E5 (peripheral vein introduction) and XW043E5 (central vein introduction).

Adding to the financial incentives to administer remdesivir is the fact that the FDA has blocked the administration of safe and effective treatments like ivermectin. The FDA has ruled:

> The FDA has not authorized or approved ivermectin for the treatment or prevention of COVID-19 in people or animals. Ivermectin has not been shown to be safe or effective for these indications.[1616]

That statement by the FDA is not true. There have been 63 studies of the safety and effectiveness of ivermectin in treating COVID-19.[1617] Meta-analysis of those studies found an average of 69% improvement for early treatment and 86% improvement for prophylaxis. Those numbers are probably conservative because researchers found a negative bias against ivermectin in a review of the studies. The researchers determined that the statistical probability for the studies to falsely portray a positive outcome for ivermectin is one in one trillion.

Coquin de Chien posted the following chart in the October 20, 2022 edition of his newsletter.[1618]

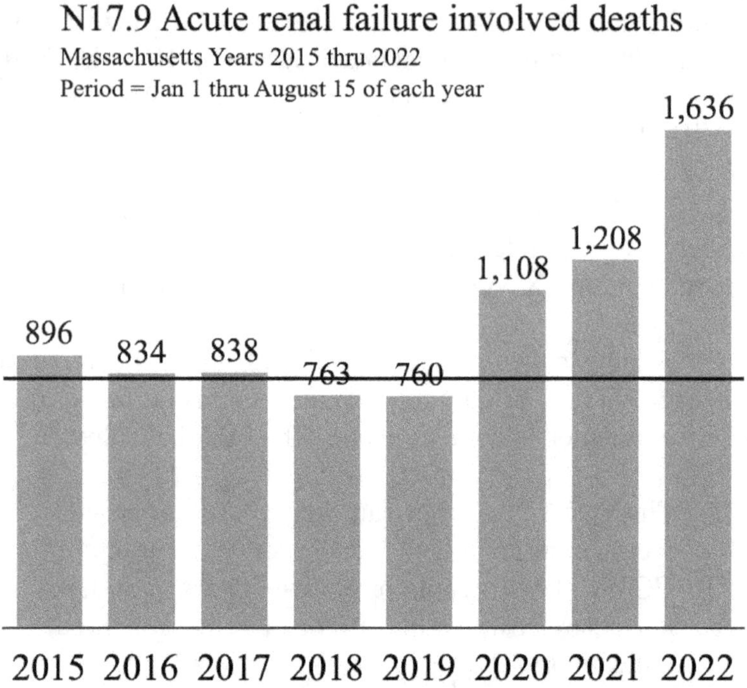

He explains that the chart shows the incidence of acute renal [kidney] failure in Massachusetts. He attributes the increase in renal failure beginning in 2020 to the administration of the drug Veklury® (remdesivir) as a treatment for COVID-19. His research drew him to the following conclusion:

> I don't know what else to write here. I cannot stress enough how much of an emergency this is. Everyone reading this article should write a letter to the governor, public health commissioner, state attorney general, and your local FBI office to report mass murder that demands criminal investigation. I wrote "criminal" investigation because there is no doubt what is happening here; and it is murder. The health industry will not investigate itself. There are doctors and nurses knowingly involved in the acts

> of hooking people up with "medicine" they know has a high kill rate.
>
> ***
>
> They are killing people. And they don't care. If you care, please do something. Demand investigation and prosecution. Remdesivir is on EUA. They think they are immune. But that immunity does not stand up because of the willful misconduct exception in the PREP Act; and because there is no immunity for murder. This is nothing less than murder. It is not manslaughter. They know. Scienter is apparent.[1619]

Coquin de Chien is making some serious charges. He claims that medical professionals, in collusion with the FDA and NIH, are intentionally killing patients by eschewing safe and effective treatments and instead treating them with the deadly drug Veklury® (remdesivir).

> For the love of money is the root of all evil: which while some coveted after, they have erred from the faith, and pierced themselves through with many sorrows. 1 Timothy 6:10.

63 Ventilators

Dr. Peterson Pierre, M.D., confirms what Minnesota State Senator and Dr. Scott Jensen, M.D., revealed. Senator Jensen explains that hospital administrations have an incentive to diagnose and treat a person for COVID-19.[1620] The system is financially skewed toward diagnosing and treating COVID-19 even though the patient may not actually be ill from COVID-19. The patients may be in the hospital for an entirely different reason, but if they test positive for COVID-19 or they are diagnosed as having COVID-19 then the hospital hits the financial jackpot and can begin raking in the financial windfall from the federal government through the Coronavirus Aid, Relief and Economic Security Act (CARES Act).

For example, a hospital is reimbursed $5,000 for ordinary pneumonia under Medicare. But under the CARES Act, the hospital can charge the federal government $13,000 if that same person tests positive for SARS-CoV-2 (the alleged viruse thought to cause COVID-19) or is diagnosed as having COVID-19. Although the patient is being treated for pneumonia, he is put on the COVID-19 billing rolls. If the patient is subsequently put on a ventilator, the payment from the federal government through the CARES Act goes up to $39,000.

Please understand that mechanical ventilation is a dangerous last-resort treatment. Studies have shown that between 66% and 86% of COVID-19 patients placed under mechanical ventilation die.[1621] One study reported that 31 of 32 (97%) mechanically ventilated COVID-19 patients died.[1622]

An April 22, 2020 study published by the Journal of the American Medical Association (JAMA) of COVID-19 patients hospitalized in New York City found the following:

> Mortality rates for those who received mechanical ventilation in the 18-to-65 and older-than-65 age groups were 76.4% and 97.2%, respectively. Mortality rates for those in the 18-to-65 and older-than-65 age groups who did not receive mechanical ventilation were 1.98% and 26.6%, respectively.[1623]

Compare the 76.4% of those 18 to 65 years old COVID-19 patients who were put on mechanical ventilators and subsequently died with only 1.98% of COVID-19 hospital patients 18 to 65 years old who were not ventilated and who died. We find that the mechanical ventilators caused a 39-fold increase in deaths.

Mechanical ventilation is a death sentence. Doctors have known for almost 200 years that mechanical ventilation is a dangerous and damaging practice. The federal authorities knew it full well beforehand and the greedy hospitals designed their protocols accordingly. Among the 2,634 COVID-19 New York City hospital patients who were discharged or died on or before April 4, 2020, approximately 12.2% (320) of them received invasive mechanical ventilation. That represents a $12,480,000 payout to the New York City hospitals.

One nurse working in a hospital in New York described the use of ventilators on COVID-19 patients as "murder."[1624] The

Daily Mail reported that a "frontline nurse working in New York on coronavirus patients claims the city is killing sufferers by putting them on ventilators." The nurse explained that "[t]he ventilators have high pressure, which then causes barotrauma, it causes trauma to the lungs." The Daily Mail further reported that "New York emergency room doctor Cameron Kyle-Sidell stepped down this month because he didn't want to follow the hospital's ventilator protocol."

Please make no mistake about it; mechanical ventilation is a deadly treatment. It is perverse to incentivize hospitals to administer such a dangerous protocol to treat a disease, unless you want to kill people. Hospitals who have been incentivized by the prospect of a financial windfall have turned to mechanical ventilation to treat COVID-19 when it is not otherwise appropriate.

Deaths from the ventilator offer the perfect cover for murder. The symptoms of pneumonia reported in severe COVID-19 patients (i.e., damaged air sacs in the lungs) are identical to the damage caused by mechanical ventilators.

Lest you think that this is some kind of fantastic exaggeration, USA Today, which is a left-wing liberal publication, did a fact check of Senator Jensen's allegations and determined the following:

> Our ruling: True[1625]
>
> We rate the claim that hospitals get paid more if patients are listed as COVID-19 and on ventilators as TRUE[1626]
>
> Hospitals and doctors do get paid more for Medicare patients diagnosed with COVID-19 or if it's considered presumed they have COVID-19

> absent a laboratory-confirmed test, and three times more if the patients are placed on a ventilator to cover the cost of care and loss of business resulting from a shift in focus to treat COVID-19 cases.[1627]

The behind-the-scenes scheme of the cabal pulling the strings of the government technocrats is to cause as much death and injury as possible to push a malicious agenda of mandatory vaccinations that will further kill and injure. In a December 6, 2021 interview with Bret Weinstein, world-renowned cardiologist Dr. Peter Mcullough agreed with Bret Weinstein's opinion that the actions of the government regulators indicate they have a vaccine agenda and a malicious and deliberate intent to harm and kill people.[1628] Dr. McCullough said:

> What you're really getting to right you're getting very close to an adjective which is nefarious, meaning are people actually intentionally trying to do harm. And the book to point to there I wrote one of the introductions is "COVID-19 and the Global Predators: We Are the Prey" by Peter Breggin. And I have to tell you, I think it's number one in a lot of the medical book listings right now. It has a thousand citations of evidence. This is a factual book. It's basically non-fiction, and it's laying out what almost certainly is, according to Bregin, nefarious intent. There is intent to make things worse. And you know I gave my interpretation to Tucker Carlson earlier this year. I was on [his show]. I said, "Tucker listen I'm just a doctor seeing this. But I think there is intentional suppression of early treatment. I think there is intentional promotion of masking, lockdowns, isolation, fear, suffering, hospitalization, and death in order to mass promote the vaccine." That was my interpretation now many months ago. And I

> gave Americans that interpretation on TV. So I am aligned with you, that it is more than just innocent incompetence. That there is an agenda. There is absolutely no doubt about it. There is a vaccine agenda that is being carried out.[1629]

Other than occasional fact-checking, the mainstream media rarely reports about dangerous ventilation and other unsafe and ineffective strategies of the CDC. Indeed, the tech companies act as gatekeepers making it challenging to find the truth on the internet. When searching for information about the dangerous practice of ventilation, you would find that Google is suppressing it. For example, this author watched an Instagram video[1630] in which the narrator referred to an article[1631] explaining that "nearly all COVID-19 patients who died in hospital during the early phase of the pandemic were killed as a direct result of being put on a ventilator."[1632]

This author wanted to read the article referenced in the Instagram post. On May 24, 2023, I did a Google search using the beginning quoted subtitle "nearly all covid-19 patients who died in hospitals" as the search term. But the Google search turned up zero (0) results. I then did a search using the same search term in a different search engine, Yandex, and the search result in Yandex showed the article in question as the first result. That is clear proof that Google is concealing the killing of COVID-19 patients by hospitals using ventilators.

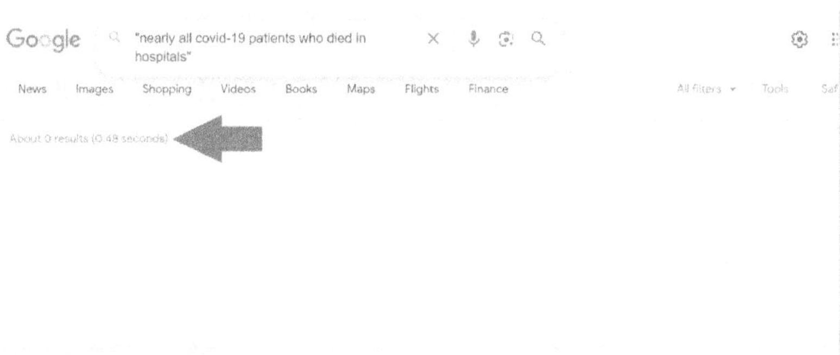

Above is a Google search showing zero results for search term: "nearly all covid-19 patients who died in hospitals". Below is a Yandex search of the same search term with the article about ventilator deaths being the first result. Clearly, Google is concealing the article that reveals that people were being killed in hospitals with ventilators.

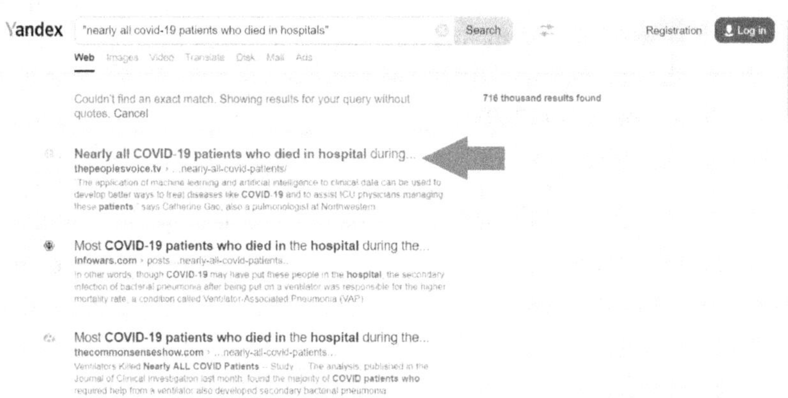

The article appearing in The People's Voice, cited a study in The Journal of Clinical Investigation.[1633] The Peoples Voice article revealed:

> So while COVID-19 may have put these patients in the hospital, it was actually a secondary infection brought on by the use of a mechanical ventilator that caused their deaths.[1634]

64 Euthanasia

It is not an overstatement to say that the medical establishment has introduced a program of euthanasia for those diagnosed with severe COVID-19. The official guidance on managing symptoms of COVID-19 from the National Institute for Health and Care Excellence (NICE) called for administering drugs to a COVID-19 patient, the only purpose of which would be to kill the patient.[1635] NICE claims it is an independent public body that provides national guidance and advice on medical and health care in England.[1636] However, NICE has a close interlocking relationship with the UK government. The Framework Agreement between NICE and the UK Department of Health & Social Care (DHSC) reveals that its "work is commissioned by Ministers or by NHS England."[1637] And DHSC funds NICE. He who pays the piper calls the tune. In any event, advice from NICE is generally considered authoritative medical guidance in England.

On page 12 of the NICE guidance for the treatment of COVID-19, it advises doctors to administer to the patient "an opioid and benzodiazepine." That combination is the worst possible combination of drugs to give someone with respiratory difficulty unless you aim to kill him.

The NICE document assumes that the patient is at the end of his life. But a doctor is not equipped to make that assessment for someone who is suffering from a recoverable illness like COVID-19. A doctor is in no position to determine that the patient is at the end of his life and thus should be hurried along in a comfortable death when the patient suffers from a condition with a reasonable likelihood of recovery. COVID-19 is not like terminal cancer. A meta-analysis involving 61 studies found that the median infection fatality rate (IFR) for COVID-19 was 0.27%.[1638] That means the COVID-19 survival rate for persons alleged to be ill, including undiagnosed, asymptomatic, and mild infections of COVID-19, is approximately 99.73%. According to the WHO June 2023 Coronavirus Dashboard, the worldwide case fatality rate (CFR) for COVID-19 is 0.9%. That means, according to the WHO, that 99.1% of all persons confirmed to have COVID-19 survive.[1639] The NICE document advises care as though a patient with difficulty breathing may be dying when he may simply be fighting through a difficult stage of the illness. The NICE document states, in pertinent part:

> Consider an opioid [e.g., morphine] and benzodiazepine [e.g., midazolam] combination for patients who:
>
> • are at the end of life and
> • have moderate to severe breathlessness and
> • are distressed.[1640]

The intent of that medical advice seems to be to kill the patient because page 13 of the NICE document states that **"[s]edation and opioid use should not be withheld because of a fear of causing respiratory depression."** That is an alarming statement. Respiratory depression will kill someone struggling to breathe from an illness that causes difficulty breathing. If you depress the patient, so he no longer struggles to breathe, he will suffer hypoxia, and death soon follows.

Midazolam is a dangerous drug that requires close monitoring of the patient. Midazolam slows a person's breathing. It is the last drug you would give to a patient struggling to get enough air unless you aim to kill the patient. The NIH National Library of Medicine provides the following red-box warning on its website about the danger of midazolam suppressing one's breathing after an injection.

> IMPORTANT WARNING:
> Midazolam injection may cause serious or life-threatening breathing problems such as shallow, slowed, or temporarily stopped breathing that may lead to permanent brain injury or death. You should only receive this medication in a hospital or doctor's office that has the equipment that is needed to monitor your heart and lungs and to provide life-saving medical treatment quickly if your breathing slows or stops. Your doctor or nurse will watch you closely after you receive this medication to make sure that you are breathing properly.[1641]

Dr. John Campbell, Ph.D., is a retired Nurse Teacher and accident and emergency (A&E) nurse based in England. He was shocked when he read the NICE instructions. He opined that they were instructions on how to administer euthanasia and not treat COVID-19. Dr. Campbell explains that COVID-19 is a recoverable condition and a person should never be given an opioid–benzodiazepine combination. Doing so will likely kill the patient. Dr. Campbell explains:

> If you give these two together [an opioid and benzodiazepine] that stops people breathing. Opioids and benzodiazepines will depress respiration. And given that a lot of these people that were breathless anyway, had acute respiratory

> distress syndrome, and you suppress their breathing ... you get respiratory depression. I don't think you need me to spell out the consequences of that: not enough oxygen tissue hypoxia and death would be the result.[1642]

The doctors who put that advice in the NICE publication are experts. It was not a mistake. They knew full well that administering a combination of an opioid and benzodiazepine to a patient who is struggling to breathe would likely kill him. And that is exactly what began happening when doctors followed that advice. Unsurprisingly, there was a spike in COVID-19 deaths in England as soon as the NICE advice was published, and the doctors blindly followed the NICE guidelines. Of course, the deaths were attributed to COVID-19, with the public unaware that the hospitals were killing the patients by suppressing their breathing using a combination of morphine and benzodiazepine. If that were not bad enough, the good doctors at NICE revised their recommendations. NICE maintained the deadly cocktail of an opioid and benzodiazepine in their revision, but they have added a recommendation for administering the poisonous "therapeutic" remdesivir.[1643]

It turns out that the plan was implemented apace as soon as COVID-19 was publicized. *The Expose* reported that "[a]s soon as the lockdown was declared in the United Kingdom on March 23rd 2020 deaths occurring in care homes in the weeks that followed skyrocketed." The media announced the deaths as COVID-19 deaths when in reality they were caused by euthanasia via the administration of midazolam. The Expose explained:

> Matt Hancock (the Health Secretary at the time) and Chris Whitty (the Chief Medical Officer) instructed hospitals to discharge as many patients as possible into care homes, the very place the patients loved ones were now banned from visiting,

> the very place a doctor was not required to visit to certify a death, the very place carers could not be held liable for a death as long as it was just suspected to be Covid-19.[1644]

Foreseeing the need for midazolam, the UK NHS scoured Europe for supplies of midazolam to administer under the new protocol. On or before March 2020, the NHS issued a regulatory waiver to allow French-labeled midazolam to be supplied to UK wholesalers.[1645] But that was not sufficient because by October 2020 the NHS had already burned through two years worth of midazolam, and the wholesalers in the UK were out of midazolam supplies.[1646]

The Expose reported new government rules prevented families of the elderly from visiting them at nursing care homes. With the coast clear of family interference, the NHS got busy following its newly framed protocols of administering midazolam to the elderly in nursing homes and vulnerable hospital patients who were now separated from family support or advocacy. The elderly and vulnerable decedents were then listed as COVID-19 deaths.[1647] *The Expose* explains that "whilst you stayed at home to protect the NHS, they were giving midazolam to the elderly and vulnerable, and telling you they were Covid-19 deaths."[1648]

The reported deaths fanned the flames of hysteria over the COVID-19 "pandemic." *The Expose* reported a direct correlation between midazolam prescriptions and deaths from January 2020 until March 2021. *The Expose* reported:

> The confidential NHS documents clearly show that the elderly and vulnerable were to be denied treatment and put on the end-of-life pathway in response to a pandemic, and the evidence clearly shows this was put into practice.[1649]

65 Vaccine Passports

There is a little-known plan by the U.S. Government to require vaccine passports. That plan is part of an international conspiracy to enslave all people. The world leaders at the G20 Summit, representing the 20 largest economic powers in the world, including the U.S., met on November 20, 2022, and signed a declaration that they would introduce vaccine passports for their respective countries. Vaccine Passports would be required for international travel and domestic business access. On March 28, 2021, Tom Pappert for National File reported:

> After months of speculation, today [March 28, 2021] The Washington Post[1650] confirmed that the Biden regime is developing a "vaccine passport" that Americans may need to present to prove they have received their COVID-19 vaccine before they will be allowed to engage in commerce in a "return to normalcy" that looks nothing like the past.
>
> According to The Washington Post, the Biden regime "and private companies are working to develop a standard way of handling credentials — often referred to as "vaccine passports" — that

> would allow Americans to prove they have been vaccinated against the novel coronavirus as businesses try to reopen."[1651]

The U.S. Government vaccine passport plan would include all manner of domestic commerce, from restaurants to schools and hospitals, etc., in addition to domestic travel. The apparent problem with the U.S. alone imposing vaccine passports for travel is that it would only work for travel within the U.S. For a vaccine passport system to apply to international travel, other countries must impose them on their citizens. It must become a universal requirement for international travel, as with ordinary passports, or it will not work. Undoubtedly, the G20 vaccine passports will also facilitate domestic restrictions on access to businesses for the unvaccinated.

At the G20 Summit in Indonesia on November 20, 2022, the twenty participating world leaders signed a declaration to introduce vaccine passports for their respective jurisdictions, with the intention of creating a global verification system to facilitate safe international travel. They agreed to a globalized 'vaccination passport.' This will be done under the framework of the International Health Regulations to "facilitate seamless international travel, interoperability, and recognizing digital solutions and non-digital solutions, including proof of vaccinations."[1652]

Sonia Hickey, writing for the Sydney Criminal Lawyers, reports that the leaders of the G20 countries "affirmed their respective countries' support of the World Health Organization mRNA Vaccine Technology Transfer hub, which aims to build capacity in low- and middle-income countries to produce mRNA vaccines."[1653] But the G20 then went full Orwellian. Stating that the countries want to have joint research and production of vaccines coupled with "a globalised 'vaccination passport.'"[1654] Sonia Hickey explains:

> Indonesia's Health Minister Budi Gunadi Sadikin said that a Digital Health Certificate using World Health Organization standards would be introduced during the next World Health Assembly in Geneva, in May next year.
>
> "If you have been vaccinated or tested properly, you can move around. So for the next pandemic, instead of stopping the movement of people 100%, you can still provide some movement of the people," Mr Sadikin said.
>
> Surprisingly, this news has not really grabbed the attention of mainstream media, despite its very serious implications for freedom of personal choice and freedom of movement.[1655]

Please understand that the planned vaccine passport will be required for all manner of commerce within your state. You will need it to travel, board a plane, board a train, board a bus, board a cruise ship, enter a hospital, enter a school, enter government buildings, enter a store, enter a bank, enter a hotel, enter a theatre, etc.

Of course, the major media outlets will not report on this. They are in on the conspiracy to enslave the world. The groundwork for medical passports was begun long before the November 20, 2022, G20 meeting. Undoubtedly, the world's governments have been working with technology companies to set the technical parameters needed for the coming vaccine passport.

The plans for a digital COVD-19 passport were reported in a press release published by a company in the Associated Press on May 8, 2020.[1656] At that time, the digital health passport was announced as simply a means to track and trace testing for COVID-19, as the EUA for vaccines had not yet been issued. But the digital health passport was designed with the eventuality of vaccine verification in mind. The press release stated, in pertinent part:

> The COVI-PASS™ Digital Health Passport works on an intelligent colour mapping system (green, amber, red) to authenticate and validate a COVID-19 test providing test history and relevant health information. This allows for accurate data metrics to assess those who have tested positive and negative and the location only of their testing. The COVI-PASS™ Digital Health Passport can be used as an authenticated gateway for Public Services, Businesses and Employees to manage a safe return to work, life, and safe travel.[1657]

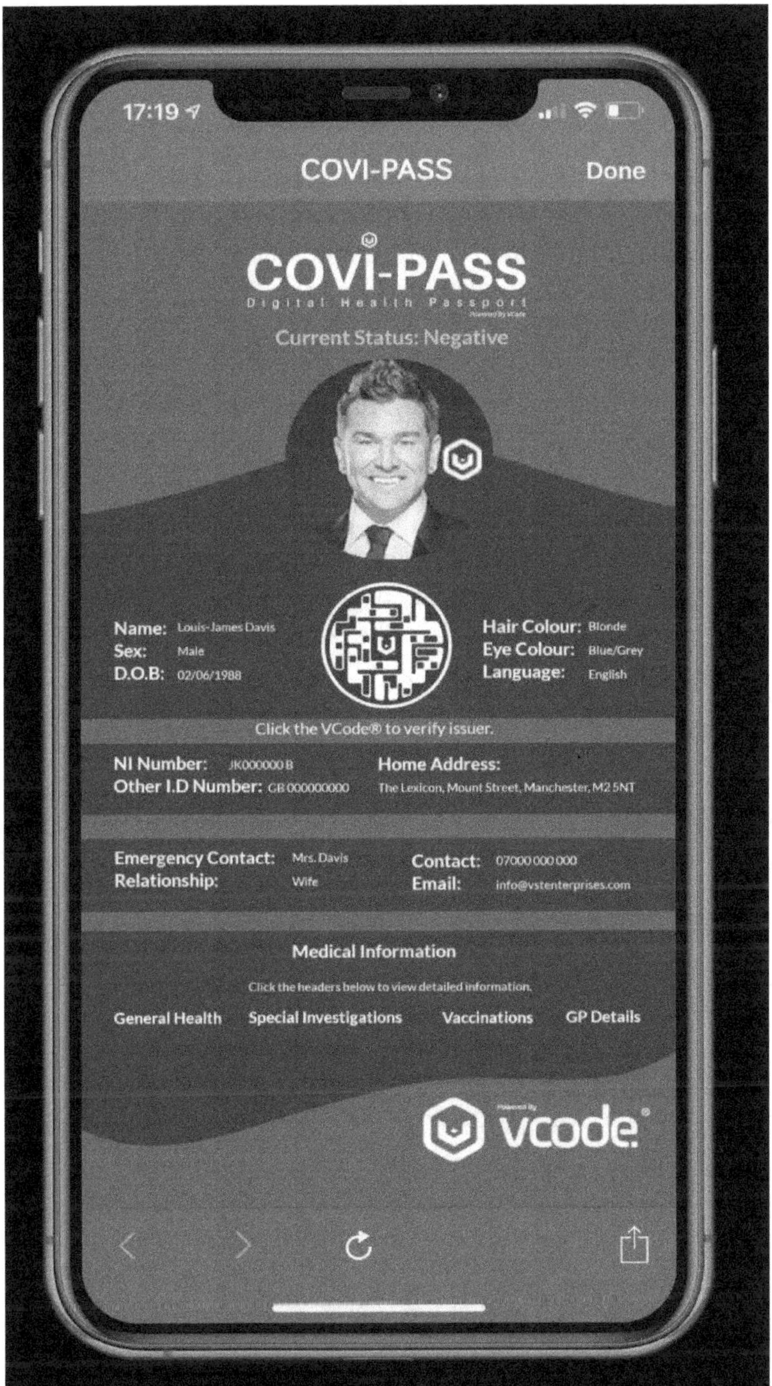
17:19
COVI-PASS
Done
COVI-PASS
Digital Health Passport
Current Status: Negative
Name: Louis-James Davis
Sex: Male
D.O.B: 02/06/1988
Hair Colour: Blonde
Eye Colour: Blue/Grey
Language: English
Click the VCode® to verify issuer.
NI Number: JK000000B
Other I.D Number: GB000000000
Home Address:
The Lexicon, Mount Street, Manchester, M2 5NT
Emergency Contact: Mrs. Davis
Relationship: Wife
Contact: 07000000000
Email: info@vstenterprises.com
Medical Information
Click the headers below to view detailed information.
General Health
Special Investigations
Vaccinations
GP Details
vcode

Initially, the COVI-PASS was planned to record COVID-19 test results. But the ultimate plan was that when a COVID-19 vaccine was developed, COVI-PASS would be used to verify that the person has been vaccinated with a COVID-19 vaccination. That vaccination information will then be a prerequisite to commerce and employment. The COVI-PASS website explained in July 2020, before the COVID-19 vaccine was tested or authorized:

> We are all waiting for the day that a **vaccine** can be found for this disease. Until then, COVI-PASS™ can be used to carry the COVID-19 test result. As this is a digital health pass it could also be used to show other tests and **vaccinations**. Some people have a booklet that has **a record of their vaccinations**. This is the same, but in digital format.[1658]

In response to the question about someone who decides not to obtain COVI-PASS, the COVI-PASS website states that you likely will not have a choice. The COVI-PASS may be required. Indeed, that is their business plan, which is why all of their efforts have been focused on marketing their product to governments. The consumer will be required to use COVI-PASS by the governments. COVI-PASS states:

> Having a COVID-19 test might be required if you are in a certain profession such as social care or retail for example. It might also be required at certain touch points in life, such as going on holiday. If you do require a test, you'll need a way to show the result. COVI-PASS™ is one way to do this. The result can also be shown on paper, although it's probably safer to store it digitally[1659]

The whole idea, as explained by COVI-PASS, is to "return to normal life and travel with peace of mind, knowing that your medical credentials are on hand, accessed only by the wallet holder's permission." Our overlords made our lives a living hell by shutting down businesses, requiring masks, issuing stay at home orders, and requiring social distancing. That was all part of the plan to coerce us into taking a COVID-19 vaccine. Although it is marketed as a digital health passport, it will not be limited to international travel. It will be a passport for every commercial transaction imaginable.

Raul Diego for Mint Press News explains that "COVI-PASS will determine whether you can go to a restaurant, if you need a medical test, or are due for a talking-to by authorities in a post-COVID world. Consent is voluntary, but enforcement will be compulsory."[1660]

Once a person takes the vaccine, he can "return to normal" and have his freedom back. At least, that is the promise. But it is a lie. The vaccine is just the first of a myriad of hoops that the sheep will need to jump through. Those who agree to take the vaccine will be circus animals running around the ring and obediently jumping through the hoops held by their trainers. Sadly, they will get sicker and weaker with each poisonous lap. As their liberties are forfeited and their health is ruined, they may find it too late to recover either before the poisonous needle claims their lives.

Tento Health is the company that developed COVI-PASS. The COVI-PASS was later rebranded as the Tento Health Wallet.[1661] Tento Health has now changed its name to Q-Servi. Q-Servi describes its service as one that "automates data management processes, distributes verified digital health documents and provides automated data reporting solutions."[1662] The company states some of the benefits of its digital services:

> Reduce delays at check-in with advanced visibility of **passengers [sic] health status prior to check-in**.
>
> Enable staff and customers to **share verified COVID vaccination information** digitally.
>
> **Receive vaccination details information** that is matched to a verified identity.[1663]

When Tento Health was renamed Q-Servi, its Tento Health Wallet was, in turn, rebranded as the Q-Wallet.[1664] Q-Servi describes its Q-Wallet as a digital wallet that will allow verification of health status, including but not limited to vaccine status. The Q-Wallet includes a digital vaccine passport, now available as a cell phone app on iPhones and Android devices. Q-Servi describes its Q-Wallet:

> The secure wallet enables individuals to control their personal data and share their **health pass** for entry such as concerts, casinos, theatre, sports or other large scale venues.
>
> Q-Wallet is a secure and contactless way to access amenities such as public transport, office buildings, construction or production sites, airlines, or events.
>
> The app only shows your photo, **your vaccination certificate expiry date**, and your test results. There is no personally identifiable information shared unless you decide that you want to share it.

The vaccine passport is not some wild conspiracy theory. It will be a dystopian reality unless the people resist it. Imagine what an oppressive regime would do with Q-Wallet (formerly COVI-PASS). Indeed, it seems that the government of communist

China has already instituted steps to incorporate COVID-19 track and tracing into their social credit scoring system. Paul Joseph Watson reported on Summit News:

> The local government of China's Jiangsu province has launched a new social control system that **combines the CCP's health code program** with the regime's **social credit system** to create what they're calling a civilization code. ...
>
> The new system ranks each citizen via a "civilization score" and then places them in a category which determines whether they get priority access to services or are punished and restricted.
>
> The new system represents an expansion of the social credit score and is being initially rolled out in the city of Suzhou and will apply to everyone over the age of 18.[1665]

Vaccine Passports will undoubtedly be useful to colleges and all other venues requiring vaccination for entrance. For example, beginning on or before April 2021 and continuing to the date of this writing (February 23, 2023), Brown University "requires all students who will be on campus or engage in any level of in-person instruction, whether in the U.S. or abroad, and all Brown students who are engaged in on-campus activities (education, jobs, research, or engaging in any in-person education or work with other Brown employees, students or visitors) to be up to date with COVID-19 vaccines."[1666]

Once you submit to the vaccine regimen, you cannot get off it. Brown students must get boosters. "Brown requires that students, faculty and staff receive the COVID-19 vaccine and (once eligible) a booster."[1667]

If you want to visit Brown University, you must be vaccinated. "Visitors to Brown, whether researchers, faculty, students or others, who are engaged in any sustained and consistent in-person contact with other Brown employees, students or visitors are required to be up to date with COVID-19 Vaccines."[1668]

Brown will not recognize any religious or medical exemption from vaccination for a visitor. "Exemptions for medical or religious grounds do not apply to visitors to the University."[1669]

The vaccine passport will be an invaluable convenience for visitors, students, and staff at places like Brown because those places will require proof of vaccination. All Brown students, staff, and visitors must "[p]rovide proof they have received a full course of a U.S. Food and Drug Administration or World Health Organization authorized COVID-19 vaccine; and provide proof they received a COVID-19 booster dose within 30 days of becoming eligible."[1670]

Dr. Robert Malone, the inventor of the mRNA technology used in several COVID-19 vaccines, has warned that the world's governments are laying the groundwork for their vaccine passports by using your vaccination records reported according to the International Classification of Diseases, known as ICD codes.[1671] Dr. Malone warns:

> The administrative state is busy building a vaccine passport system that will be active before most Americans are aware of what is being done to them.
>
> No one is going to knock on your door asking for your vaccine status because they already know. Do you remember on that form at the dentist or doctor's office asking for your vaccine status, as well as your social security number and date of

> birth when you checked in for your appointment? All the CDC needs to do is modify slightly the definition of what is a reportable event to include [ICD-10] Z28.310 and Z28.311 and they can use this information at will (if they aren't already under the COVID-19 Public Health Emergency executive order that has again been re-approved by Biden).[1672]

Dr. Malone explains that the "ICD system is used extensively in the USA and the world. With the passage by Congress of the Affordable Care Act (Obamacare) in 2012, the ICD coding system became fully integrated with the digitization of healthcare records in the USA." The ICD system is a classification system run by the WHO, not the U.S. Government. The WHO has given the U.S. Government permission to modify the ICD system to meet its needs. Dr. Malone reveals that in "April 2022, the federal Centers for Medicare and Medicaid (CMS) announced a new set of codes relating to vaccination status that are cause for concern. These ICD codes are not based on a disease or illness, but are based on COVID-19 vaccination status."

The codes are now being implemented and used by medical professionals. The National Association of Healthcare Revenue Integrity (NAHRI) posted troubling information about the new ICD codes. The information has since been removed from the website. This author retrieved the following information using the Wayback Machine - Internet Archive.[1673] The following is what this author found on the archived NAHRI website:

> Code Z28.310, Unvaccinated for COVID-19, may be assigned when the patient has not received at least one dose of any COVID-19 vaccine. Code Z28.311, Partially vaccinated for COVID-19, may be assigned when the patient has received at least one dose of a multi-dose COVID-19 vaccine regimen, but has not received the full set of doses

necessary to meet the CDC definition of "fully vaccinated" in place at the time of the encounter. For information, visit the CDC's website https://www.cdc.gov/coronavirus/2019-ncov/vaccines/.

The updated ICD-10-CM tabular instructions now includes the following information:

- Z28.3, underimmunization status
    - Use Additional code, if applicable, to identify:
        - immunization not carried out because of contraindication (Z28.0-)
        - immunization not carried out because of patient decision for other and unspecified reason (Z28.2-)
        - immunization not carried out because of patient decision for reasons of belief or group pressure (Z28.1)
        - immunization not carried out for other reason (Z28.8-)
- Z28.31, underimmunization for COVID-19 status
    - Note: These codes should not be used for individuals who are not eligible for the COVID-19 vaccines, as determined by the healthcare provider.
    - **Z28.310, unvaccinated for COVID-19**
    - **Z28.311, partially vaccinated for COVID-19**
- Z28.39, other underimmunization status

○ Delinquent immunization status
○ Lapsed immunization schedule status[1674] (bold emphasis added)

Dr. Malone explains that "[c]ode Number Z28.310 listed above is not a code for an illness or diagnosis, but rather for non-compliance of a medical procedure. This is an invasion of our right to privacy. There must be choice and that choice must be private."[1675] Those codes can now be entered into your medical record and be easily integrated into a vaccine passport that will prevent you from engaging in travel or commerce. The ICD codes even provide for counseling vaccine resisters. The American Academy of Pediatrics advises its members to "[u]se this code [ICD-10-CM-Z71.85] when reporting counseling provided to patients and caregivers who are vaccine hesitant."[1676] If you refuse a vaccine, the doctor can now bill you for trying to convince you to get vaccinated. Dr. Malone explains:

> There are not only ICD for those that are "under-immunized," but the World Health Organization and the Federal Centers for Medicare and Medicaid (CMS) have a solution to take care of that. They now have ICD codes to ensure immunization safety counseling. ... "Z71.85 is a billable ICD-10 code used to specify a medical diagnosis of encounter for immunization safety counseling." Yes, you too can undergo a "re-education" program, or maybe it will be a "re-education" camp targeting children. Yes, a camp has a must softer and gentler meaning, don't you think? and kids just love going to camp! (Brought to you by Pfizer)."[1677]

The World Health Organization (WHO) has announced a Global Digital Health Certification Network (GDHCN). That network will use a digital vaccination verification certificate. It will go beyond vaccine certification to include all health issues, including prescription verification and certifying who is a trusted physician. The WHO explains:

> The GDHCN can be used as an infrastructural building block to support additional use cases, which may include, for example, the digitisation of the International Certificate of Vaccination or Prophylaxis, verification of prescriptions across borders, the International Patient Summary, verification of vaccination certificates within and across borders, and certification of public health professionals (through WHO Academy).[1678]

The groundwork for the GDHCN was laid by the establishment of the digital European Union Digital COVID Certificate (EU DCC) system, which had been adopted across all Member States of the EU as well as 51 non-EU countries and territories during the COVID-19 alleged pandemic.[1679]

The GDHCN is a step closer to the mark of the beast. This author explains in the book *Antichrist: The Beast Revealed* that the prophecy regarding the mark of the beast points to the Pope of Rome being the Antichrist.

Notably, the Vatican has been granted permanent observer status at the UN and the WHO.[1680] The pope exercises significant influence over the WHO.[1681] Pope Francis has stated that getting a COVID-19 vaccination is a moral obligation.[1682] The pope denounces those who argue against getting vaccinated. The pope further said that "it is 'morally acceptable' for Catholics to receive COVID-19 vaccines based on research that used cells derived from aborted fetuses."[1683]

Indeed, the Vatican is on board with the digital health pass as evidenced by requiring a "Green Pass" for those seeking entry into its museums. Beginning on September 1, 2021, the "Vatican Museums requires all visitors to present the 'Green Pass' covid certification, or equivalent certificate, until further notice. The Green Pass, which comes in digital or paper versions, shows that people have been vaccinated, tested negative or recovered from Covid-19."[1684]

The Roman (Latin) letters are also Roman numerals. Latin, which was the official language of Rome and is also the official language of the Roman Catholic Church, is the logical first place to look for this number of the beast. The Vatican is concerned that people will learn the mystery that the number of the beast points directly to the pope of Rome. In order to throw people off the trail of the pope they have proposed an alternative reading of the number of the beast as "616" in Revelation 13:18. The Roman Catholic Jerusalem Bible contains a footnote to Revelation 13:18 that states:

> Var. '616'. In both Greek and Hebr., letters are used as numbers, the values corresponding to the place in the alphabet; by adding up the values of component letters the total 'number of a person's name' is obtained. Some commentators point out that in Hebr., the letters of Caesar Nero add up to 666, and in Greek, the letters of Caesar-God add up to 616 (an alternative reading).[1685]

The Catholic editors of the Jerusalem Bible do not explain the source of the alternative reading of "616." They simply announce in a footnote that there is one. The alternative should be seen as what it is. It is an obvious deception formulated to mislead readers and cause them to doubt that the pope is the beast of Revelation.

People should not be looking for simply three 6's in a row; the number of the beast is the number "**six hundred threescore**

and six." That means the beast's name must add up to six hundred sixty six.

According to the April 18, 1915, edition of *Our Sunday Visitor,* the largest circulated official Catholic publication in the United States, "[t]he letters inscribed in the pope's mitre are these: *Vicarius Filii Dei,* which is the Latin for the Vicar of the Son of God."[1686] When a new pope is crowned, some allege it is with the words *"Vicarius Filii Dei,"* others claim it with the words *"Vicarius Christi."*

Vicarius Filii Dei was used to refer to Peter and the popes in the medieval document that the Roman Catholic Church composed to claim that the Emperor Constantine transferred authority over Rome and the western part of the Roman Empire to the Pope. The document is known as the Donation of Constantine. The Donation of Constantine has been proven to be forged by agencies of the Roman Catholic Church in the 8th century A.D.

The official title of the Pope written in classical Latin is ***VICARIVS FILII DEI***. Notice that in classical Latin there is a V just before the S in *vicarius,* rather than a U. That is because there are only 23 letters in the classical Latin alphabet, it does not have the letters U, J, or W as in the English alphabet.[1687] The V is used in classical Latin when making the U sound.[1688] The values of Roman numerals are: D = 500, C = 100, L = 50, V = 5, I = 1. The values of the Roman numerals found in the Latin title for the Pope added together equals 666. V (used twice, 5 x 2 = 10) + C (100) + I (used 6 times, 1 x 6 = 6) + L (50) + D (500) = **666**.

The ubiquitous Universal Product Code (UPC) symbol contains the number 666 hidden within the lines of the symbol. The UPC depicted on this page is typical of the most common UPC seen on goods in the marketplace of today. The UPC has two sets of numbers. Each set has distinct computer codes that are represented by two parallel lines per number. In the second set of codes, the number 6 is represented by two equally thin parallel lines (**II**).

Notice that there are three double lines in the UPC symbol that do not have an Arabic number to identify them. One set of lines are in the middle and there are two other sets of lines, one on each end. Those three sets of lines together represent the number 666. Look at any product in your home and you will see the same hidden code for the number 666.

The numbers that appear on either end of the UPC symbol on this page (6 and 3) correspond to the double line codes that are inside the double line codes for the end 6's. Note that there are two sets of line codes for the numbers 0-9. The first set is to the left of the middle double lines (**II**), and the second set is to the right of the middle double lines. The 3 sets of double lines without numbers are always the line codes for the number 6 from the second set of codes. As you will notice, the 6 from the first set of codes is represented by a thin line on the left with a thick line on the right, whereas the line code for 6 from the second set of codes is represented by two thin lines (**II**).

Why is it that the only lines that do not have an Arabic number identifying are the lines that together read 666? Because the UPC symbol is part of the groundwork being laid to control the world's commerce. The world's goods are being marked with the number of the beast. It is a hidden code so as not to alarm the slumbering masses. The Bible states that one day people will be marked with a similar code in their right hand or forehead and that refusal to receive the mark will preclude them from being able to buy or sell anything. "And that no man might buy or sell, save he that had the mark, or the name of the beast, or the number of his name." (Revelation 13:17)

The Bible does not state that the mark will be *on* peoples foreheads or *on* their right hands but ***in*** their right hands or ***in*** their foreheads. Implantable biochips that are capable of storing several megabytes of data equal to thousands of pages of information have already been developed.[1689] These biochips allow the subject to be tracked and identified anywhere in the world. Could the present day UPC, with the hidden 666, be a key necessary to match a corresponding 666 code in an implantable biochip that would then allow a purchase of the item? Could it be that if there is no match, because the person has refused the 666 mark of the beast, then the person cannot purchase the item because "no man might buy or sell," unless he has the mark?

Once the governments of the world implement a mandatory identity card or digital tracking system like the WHO's proposed GDHCN, it would only be a matter of time before the convenience of an implantable chip is accepted. How close are we? The failed Health Security Card proposed by President Clinton was manufactured by Drexler Technology Corporation, Mountain View, California and was in fact a data storage card capable of storing 2,000 pages of information, including fingerprints, voice prints, and pictures.[1690]

The technology now exists to track persons and obtain massive amounts of information on them through an implantable chip. In 2004, the U.S. Food and Drug Administration approved the use of implantable radio frequency identification (RFID) chip in humans.[1691] The chip readers can scan the chip for information from great distances and they have the capability to read hundreds (eventually thousands) of chips at one time.

The manufacturer, VeriChip, is touting its chip as an easy and secure way to ensure that a person has their important medical data available in an emergency. VeriChip is an "implantable RFID microchip for patient identification."[1692] Thomas Green of *The Register* pointed out in 2004 the obvious Orwellian dangers. "Indeed, the medical care angle looks like a warm-and-fuzzy gimmick to speed adoption so that other, potentially more sinister, applications might follow."[1693]

It seems that the warm-and-fuzzy gimmick of using RFID chips in medical care is being pushed along by the U.S. Government. The digital health pass is a step toward an implantable chip, the groundwork for which was laid in 2004. With the characteristic timing of a tyranny, Jill Fisher revealed that shortly before the VeriChip RFID was approved by the FDA for implantation into Humans,"in April 2004, President Bush issued an executive order calling for the incorporation of health information technology into all medical practices nationwide and the creation of a National Health Information Technology Coordinator to oversee the process."[1694]

Fisher further reveals that VeriChip wasted no time in getting its implantable chip into hospitals. As of December 2005, the company had "agreements from 65 other medical facilities to begin implanting chips in patients in the near future.[1695] The idea behind an RFID implant is that patients can carry their medical records (or, more accurately, an identifier to access their records) with them wherever they go."[1696]

There had been much fear that the Obamacare law would require the implantation of RFID chips. The initial versions of the U.S. House of Representative health care bills (HR3200, HR3590, and HR4872) that eventually became Obamacare, did contain provisions for the discussed RFID chips. The language in those bills did not mandate the use of RFID chips, and only created a registry which would allow the Department of Health and Human

Services to collect data about and from RFID chips. That RFID provisions did not make it into the final Obamacare Law. Do not rest so easy. Each new contrived or real national security issue can be used as an excuse for new legislation for such a mandate.

And that seems to be what we see now with the World Health Organization's Global Digital Health Certification Network (GDHCN). If the proposed WHO global treaty on pandemic prevention, preparedness and response is ratified in the U.S., the GDNCN will be forced on U.S. citizens.[1697] Once the GDNCN is in place, the RFID implantation technology could be taughted and rolled out as a way to address what seem to be built-in provenance and authentication vulnerabilities with the GDNCN.

The WHO has instituted an arguably inadequate solution to the apparent authentication vulnerability with the GDNCN. Their solution is to use "software infrastructure that enables Member States to bilaterally verify the authenticity of digital records and health certificates through an interoperable trust architecture."[1698] Once the GDNCN is broadly adopted, the WHO could arrange a highly publicized exploitation of the authenticity vulnerability. When the propagandized authentication vulnerability is generally accepted, the WHO could push for the adoption of implantable RFID chips to remedy it. And the world's governments will be bound by treaty to force the implantable chip on their people.

In a March 25, 2014, Fox Business article, Peter Andrews revealed the new ultra-secure microchip technology that is being introduced into credit cards. After discussing the benefits of the microchips and other "mobile wallet" technologies, Andrews concludes the article with the following ominous prognostication:

> And, of course, ultimately you may not need to wear or carry a device at all. Although nobody's proposing such a thing at the moment, the

technology already exists that could allow you to have a radio frequency identification (RFID) chip implanted under your skin (maybe in that loose section between your thumb and your index finger), and one of those could, in the future, provide payment and ID services.

Many Americans would be appalled at such a prospect. And the likelihood of it being offered anytime soon receded with the wave of outrage that occurred when some mistakenly believed that "Obamacare" would make these subcutaneous RFID chips mandatory. That turned out to be a myth, but the violent reaction to it means it would now take a brave innovator to even tentatively suggest their introduction. One day, however…[1699]

In the Bible, God explains the consequences of worshiping the beast and receiving his mark:

And the third angel followed them, saying with a loud voice, If any man worship the beast and his image, and receive his mark in his forehead, or in his hand, The same shall drink of the wine of the wrath of God, which is poured out without mixture into the cup of his indignation; and he shall be tormented with fire and brimstone in the presence of the holy angels, and in the presence of the Lamb: And the smoke of their torment ascendeth up for ever and ever: and they have no rest day nor night, who worship the beast and his image, and whosoever receiveth the mark of his name. (Revelation 14:9-11)

66 Your Legal Rights Under Vaccine Mandates

President Joe Biden has issued unconstitutional executive orders and executive agency rules requiring federal workers, federal contractors, and the private sector to receive the COVID-19 vaccine.[1700] The problem is that under federal law, no person can be compelled to participate in a medical experiment without informed consent. Indeed, every COVID-19 vaccine manufacturer includes a notice that the recipient of the vaccine should be told that they have the option of accepting or refusing the experimental vaccines. For example, the Moderna fact sheet states: "It is your choice to receive or not receive the Moderna COVID-19 Vaccine. Should you decide not to receive it, it will not change your standard medical care."[1701] They do that because it is a legal requirement.

A person receiving the COVID-19 vaccine must be informed of its dangers and consent to being vaccinated. A person cannot be compelled to take the COVID-19 vaccine. 21 U.S. Code § 360bbb–3, which is the law governing the emergency use authorizations (EUA) of experimental vaccines, requires informed consent that is more limited than in the federal regulations on informed consent for medical experiments. But the statute nonetheless requires certain information be provided to the patient before vaccination, and the patient can withdraw consent and refuse to be vaccinated. The statute, 21 U.S.C. § 360bbb–3(e)(1)(A)(i), requires informed consent for vaccines authorized under an EUA. That code section provides:

> Appropriate conditions designed to ensure that individuals to whom the product is administered are **informed**—
> (I) that the Secretary has authorized the emergency use of the product;
> (II) of **the significant known and potential benefits and risks of such use**, and of the extent to which such benefits and risks are unknown; and
> (III) **of the option to accept or refuse administration of the product,** of the consequences, if any, of refusing administration of the product, and of the alternatives to the product that are available and of their benefits and risks.[1702]

Why is informed consent required for a vaccine under an EUA? Because those vaccines are investigational vaccines (a.k.a., experimental vaccines) whereby the manufacturers of the COVID-19 vaccines authorized under the EUA are under a continuing obligation to report all serious adverse events, including death and hospitalizations that result from the EUA administration of the COVID-19 vaccines. The vaccines are still being studied for safety and effectiveness. A person cannot be compelled to take the vaccine under the threat of any consequences for refusal.

The FDA's guidance on emergency use authorization of medical products requires the FDA to "ensure that recipients are informed to the extent practicable given the applicable circumstances … That **they have the option to accept or refuse the EUA product** …"[1703] In the same vein, when Dr. Amanda Cohn, the Executive Secretary of the CDC's Advisory Committee on Immunization Practices, was asked if Covid-19 vaccination can be required, she responded that under an EUA, **"vaccines are not allowed to be mandatory. So, early in this vaccination phase, individuals will have to be consented and they won't be able to be mandatory."**[1704] Cohn later affirmed that this prohibition on requiring the vaccines applies to organizations, including hospitals.[1705] The EUAs for COVID-19 vaccines require fact sheets to be given to vaccination providers and recipients. These fact sheets make clear that getting the vaccine is optional. For example, the fact sheet for recipients states that, "[i]t is your choice to receive or not receive the Covid-19 Vaccine," and if "you decide to not receive it, it will not change your standard of medical care." Attorney Aaron Siri points out that the FDA's position that the COVID-19 vaccines authorized under an EUA cannot be mandated is because informed consent is required by federal statute. Siri explains that "the same section of the Federal Food, Drug, and Cosmetic Act that authorizes the FDA to grant emergency use authorization also requires the secretary of Health and Human Services to **"ensure that individuals to whom the product is administered are informed ... of the option to accept or refuse administration of the product."**[1706]

FDA Interpretation of EUA Medical Experimentation Rules

Other regulatory provisions require informed consent for those participating in medical experiments. The FDA has taken the unofficial position that compliance with the other statutory provisions requiring informed consent are not required for an EUA vaccine. The FDA alleges:

> **Although informed consent as generally required under FDA regulations is not required for administration or use of an EUA product**, section 564 [21 U.S. Code § 360bbb–3] does provide EUA conditions to ensure that recipients are informed about the MCM [Medical

Countermeasure] they receive under an EUA.[1707]

The FDA further states:

> FDA must ensure that recipients of the vaccine under an EUA are informed, to the extent practicable given the applicable circumstances, that FDA has authorized the emergency use of the vaccine, of the known and potential benefits and risks, the extent to which such benefits and risks are unknown, that they have the option to accept or refuse the vaccine, and of any available alternatives to the product. Typically, this information is communicated in a patient "fact sheet." The FDA posts these fact sheets on our website.[1708]

The FDA thinks that providing a fact sheet to the recipients of the COVID-19 vaccines is sufficient. "Therefore, FDA recommends that a request for an EUA include a 'Fact Sheet' for recipients that includes essential information about the product."[1709]

The FDA is reading the statutory requirements under Section 564 [21 U.S. Code § 360bbb–3] for administering an unapproved MCM under an EUA as a waiver of the otherwise required informed consent. The FDA's position is presumably based on the following language in subsection (k) of 21 U.S. Code § 360bbb–3:

> If a product is the subject of an authorization under this section, the use of such product within the scope of the authorization shall not be considered to constitute a clinical investigation for purposes of section 355(i), 360b(j), or 360j(g) of this title or any other provision of this chapter or section 351 of the Public Health Service Act [42 U.S.C. 262].

DOJ OLC Opinion

Dawn Johnsen, Acting Assistant Attorney General Office of Legal Counsel, issued an opinion addressed to the Deputy Counsel to the President that public and private entities can legally mandate that employees get injected with the COVID-19 experimental vaccines as a condition of employment.[1710] That opinion seems to be the legal justification for the President's September 9, 2021 decision to mandate COVID-19 vaccinations for the federal workforce.

In the legal opinion, Ms. Johnsen focused on the language found under 21 U.S. C. § 360bbb–3(e)(1)(A)(i) that requires a recipient to be "informed … of the option to accept or refuse administration of the product, of the consequences, if any, of refusing administration of the product." Ms. Johnsen opines that a person can either "accept or reject" the vaccine, and a company can coerce the employee to make that decision as long as the company informs the employee "of the consequences, if any, of refusing administration of the product."

Ms. Johnsen reads the "option to accept or refuse" condition as merely informational and not conditional. That means the employer only needs to tell the employee the consequences of not taking the vaccine. Then, with that information known, the employee can decide whether to suffer the consequences of accepting or refusing the vaccine.

Ms. Johnsen opines: "These provisions all appear to require only that certain factual information be conveyed to those who might use the product."

DOJ Opines Employment Is Only a "Desirable Activity"

Ms. Johnsen says it is okay that the recipient of the information is faced with a choice at *Morton's Fork.* The worker is between the proverbial rock and a hard place. He is put there by the employer. Ms. Johnsen is okay with that. When someone is at Morton's Fork with two unpleasant choices, his choice cannot be characterized as a free choice. That is because the options are placed before him by the employer who wants him to choose vaccination. So the employer loads up the unpleasantness of not getting a vaccine to coerce him to get one. The employer controls the options. And so the choice is being coerced by the entity presenting the unpleasant options of accepting or refusing the vaccine. The employer wants the employee to take the vaccine and thus sets dire consequences for not doing so. He will be fired if he chooses not to be vaccinated. Thus, according to Ms. Johnsen, the option to accept or refuse the COVID-19 vaccine need not be voluntary.

Ms. Johnsen argues that getting fired or expelled from school is only a secondary consequence of refusal. DOJ characterizes getting fired from your job as simply exclusion from a "desirable activity." Ms. Johnsen thinks that your ability to feed your family is not a necessity, it is only a "desirable activity." Suppose you get fired for refusing to get vaccinated. In that case, DOJ considers you to have exercised your option, and to have chosen, of your own free will, to be excluded from a "desirable activity" of employment over getting vaccinated because you were told ahead of time you would be fired.

On the other hand, if you get vaccinated because you have been threatened with being fired, DOJ considers that exercising your free choice to get vaccinated. The coercive threat of losing your job is perfectly fine to DOJ. Your choice does not have to be voluntary, according to DOJ.

The very language of section 564 of the FDCA (21 U.S. Code § 360bbb-3) assumes that one has the right to refuse. Because it requires the recipient to be informed "of the option to accept or refuse administration of the product." The Congressional

Conference report on the legislation that created both section 564 of the FDCA (21 U.S. Code § 360bbb-3) and section 10 U.S.C. § 1107a interpreted the language in § 360bbb-3 requiring that patients be informed of the option to accept or refuse administration of the product as meaning they had the right to refuse the administration of the EUA product. Section 1107a allows a service member to refuse an EUA unless the President issues an overriding waiver of that right. In the context of explaining the meaning of the presidential waiver under § 1107a the Congressional Conference report states that:

> The amendment would authorize the President to waive **the right of service members to refuse administration of a product** if the President determines, in writing, that affording service members **the right to refuse the product** is not feasible, is contrary to the best interests of the members affected, or is not in the interests of national security.[1711]

Certainly, if the right to refuse found in § 360bbb-3, which applies to all service members and citizens, means that all citizens also have the right to refuse the administration of an EUA vaccine or other product. There is no Presidential waiver provisions for citizens.

The Department of Defense followed the guidance in the Congressional Conference Report. DOD stated in written legal guidance that DOD may not require service members to take an EUA product because they have a right to refuse the product unless the President exercises the waiver authority contained in 10 U.S.C. § 1107a.[1712]

DOJ agrees with the DOD position because of the consequences that a soldier would suffer if the notice of the option to refuse administration of an EUA vaccine was not interpreted to mean that the soldier had an absolute right to refuse administration. DOJ stated that DOD "understandably does not want to convey inaccurate or confusing information to service members—that is, telling them that they have the 'option' to refuse the COVID-19 vaccine if they effectively lack such an option."[1713] Indeed, that same logic would apply to civilians. What good is it to tell a civilian that he has the option to take a vaccine when exercising that option comes with the consequence of being fired? The civilian, like the soldier, in reality, lacks an option if there are detrimental consequences to exercising that option.

The only distinction between applying the option to refuse the EUA product between a soldier and a civilian is the difference in the consequences to a soldier and the consequences to a civilian. DOJ states that because of the concern that service members, unlike civilian employees, could face imprisonment for refusing an order of a superior officer, it would make no sense for a soldier to be told he has an option to refuse to get vaccinated if he did not have that option. An order that included a proviso that the soldier had the choice of getting a vaccine would be deceptive and confusing if the soldier exercised his right not to get the vaccine and was then punished for exercising the option. DOD and DOJ understand that informing a soldier he has the option to accept or refuse vaccination only to tell him he will be subjected to court-martial, dishonorable discharge, and possibly imprisonment is not a free choice. It is, by its nature, compulsion.

The only difference between a soldier and a civilian is the degree and kind of punishment he will suffer. A soldier could be subject to court martial and a dishonorable discharge from the service. In comparison, a civilian employee could be fired. They are functionally the same. The additional specter of imprisonment that a soldier would face does not change the nature of the right to refuse vaccination. In both civilian and military cases, the option to accept or refuse the administration of the product is meaningless if the person suffers severe consequences for exercising that option. It is nonsense for DOJ to characterize being fired and thus unable to support one's family as simply being excluded from a desirable activity. Only a tyrant thinks like that.

Indeed, even the FDA once understood that being informed of the option to accept or refuse administration of an EUA product in § 360bbb-3 assumes the patient has the right to refuse without compulsion or suffering any consequences. The FDA issued the following regulation in 2005 regarding the EUA Anthrax Vaccine Immunization Program for the Department of Defense:

> With respect to condition (3) [of § 360bbb-3], above, relating to the option to accept or refuse administration of AVA [Anthrax Vaccine Adsorbed], the AVIP [Anthrax Vaccine Immunization Program] will be revised to give personnel the option to refuse vaccination. Individuals who refuse anthrax vaccination will not be punished. Refusal may not be grounds for any disciplinary action under the Uniform Code of Military Justice. **Refusal may not be grounds for any adverse personnel action. Nor would either military or civilian personnel be considered non-deployable or processed for separation based on refusal of anthrax vaccination. There may be no penalty or loss of entitlement for refusing anthrax vaccination.**
>
> This information shall read in the trifold brochure provided to potential vaccine recipients as follows:
>
> You may refuse anthrax vaccination under the EUA, and you will not be punished. No disciplinary action or adverse personnel action will be taken. You will not be processed for separation, and you will still be deployable. There will be no

penalty or loss of entitlement for refusing anthrax vaccination.[1714]

Notice that the FDA interpretation of Section 564 [21 U.S. Code § 360bbb-3] that "[r]efusal may not be grounds for any adverse personnel action" applied to both civilian and military personnel. The FDA reaffirmed that interpretation in its extension of the Anthrax vaccine EUA for DOD personnel on August 3, 2005.[1715]

In its 2007 guidance on EUA products, the FDA made it clear that under 21 U.S. C. § 360bbb–3(e)(1)(A)(i) being informed of the option to accept or refuse administration of the product means that **"[r]ecipients must have an opportunity to accept or refuse the EUA product** and must be informed of any consequences of refusing administration of the product."[1716] Notice that the FDA viewed being informed of the option to accept or refuse the product means that the recipient must have the actual "opportunity to accept or refuse." An opportunity is defined as a convenient means of doing something.[1717] If you suffer for doing something, it is, by definition, inconvenient. If you are punished for doing something, that is the opposite of having an opportunity to do it. The opportunity to refuse is not genuine if the exercise of that opportunity is subjected to a penalty, like being fired or expelled from school.

But when it came to the COVID-19 vaccine, the same statute that the FDA said in 2015 precluded any penalty to service members for exercising the option to refuse vaccination and in 2007 said required an opportunity to accept or refuse a vaccine was suddenly interpreted by the FDA in 2020 to mean that citizens can be fired if they exercise the option to refuse vaccination.

DOJ vs. DOJ

The DOJ under the previous administration opined 14

months earlier, on May 30, 2020, that:

> There is no pandemic exception to the Constitution and its Bill of Rights. Indeed, "individual rights secured by the Constitution do not disappear during a public health crisis." *In re Abbott*, 954 F.3d at 784.[1718]

The above sentiment would preclude any opinion from the DOJ authorizing the coercion of federal workers to be vaccinated with an experimental vaccine under the threat of being subjected to masking, testing, social distancing, and travel prohibitions if they refused. DOJ taking the view that there is no pandemic exception to the Constitution, certainly would not issue an opinion that working to feed your family is simply a "desirable activity" and therefore it would be no great loss if you were fired because you decide not to be injected with an experimental vaccine.

Aaron Siri's Rebuttal

Aaron Siri, attorney for the Informed Consent Action Network, wrote a rebuttal to the DOJ OLC opinion. Mr. Siri wrote a letter of opinion to Dawn Johnsen, Acting Assistant Attorney General Office of Legal Counsel.[1719] Mr. Siri pointed out that the DOJ argument that expulsion from a job, school, and civil society are only "secondary consequences," which does not remove the "option to accept or refuse" defies common sense. He points out that the statutory framework and implementation of 21 U.S. Code § 360bbb-3 "all reflect that 'the option to accept or refuse' was intended to continue the longstanding principle that it is not permissible to coerce anyone to receive an unlicensed medical product."

Mr. Siri points out that the principle of informed consent "was carried forward when Congress included the words 'the right to accept or refuse' in Section 564 [21 U.S. Code § 360bbb-3] is reinforced by the legislative discussions surrounding the passing of Section 564 [21 U.S. Code § 360bbb-3]." He explained:

> On July 16, 2003, in deliberating Section 564, Representative Hays said, without any objection, that:
>
> > [A]ny authority to actually use experimental drugs or medical devices in emergency situations has to be defined and wielded with nothing less than surgical precision. Prior informed consent in connection with the administration of experimental therapy is a basic human right, a right no one should be asked to surrender.
>
> Similarly, on May 19, 2004, Senator Kennedy said while deliberating regarding Section 564 that "[t]he authorization for the emergency use of unapproved products also includes strong provisions on informed consent for patients."[1720]

The statements of Representative Hays and Senator Kennedy indicate that Congress thought that the requirement in Section 564 that the patient be informed of the "significant known and potential benefits and risks of such use" and "of the option to accept or refuse administration of the product" established a requirement of "informed consent." Indeed, Senator Kennedy and Representative Hays were adamant that informed consent be required before anyone was subjected to the administration of an unapproved medical product of any kind when it is authorized for use in an emergency. Senator Kennedy described the language in Section 564 as constituting "strong provisions" requiring informed consent. Informed consent is a higher degree of consent, and all consent must be voluntary to genuinely be consent.

The American Medical Association (AMA) states that "informed consent to medical treatment is fundamental in both ethics and law." The AMA states that when a physician is obtaining a patient's informed consent, he should: "Assess the patient's ability to understand relevant medical information and the implications of treatment alternatives and to make an independent, voluntary decision."

The concept of informed consent for medical experiment subjects is found in every state. For example, in Virginia, the state provides that an agency must obtain the informed consent of anyone taking part in a medical experiment. The Virginia statutes state that the consent must be unconstrained by any coercion: "Informed consent" means the knowing and voluntary agreement, without undue inducement or any element of force, fraud, deceit, duress, or other form of constraint or coercion, of a person who is capable of exercising free power of choice."[1721]

Informed consent in the context of experimental vaccines requires that the patient be fully informed. But regardless of the information provided, his decision to obtain the vaccine must be the product of an unencumbered will that is free of coercion. The litigation regarding the admissibility of confessions offers guidance as to what it means for consent to be voluntary. In *Culombe v. Connecticut*[1722], the U.S. Supreme Court stated that "[t]he ultimate test remains that which has been the only clearly established test in Anglo-American courts for two hundred years: the test of voluntariness. Is the confession the product of an essentially free and unconstrained choice by its maker?"[1723] The *Colombe* Court explained that "The line of distinction is that at which governing self-direction is lost and compulsion, of whatever nature or however infused, propels or helps to propel the confession."[1724] The critical distinction between a voluntary and an involuntary confession is whether the confessor was compelled to confess. For example, threatening to inform the prosecutor of a suspect's refusal to cooperate is viewed by courts to be coercive and render the resulting confession involuntary and inadmissible.[1725] That same concept is found in family law statutes. In Kentucky, voluntary, informed consent is defined by statute, in pertinent part, as:

> "Voluntary and informed consent" means that at the time of the execution of the consent, the consenting person was fully informed of the legal effect of the consent, that the consenting person was not given or promised anything of value except those expenses allowable under KRS 199.590(6), that the consenting person was not coerced in any way to execute the consent, and that the consent was voluntarily and knowingly given.[1726]

Coerced Vaccinations

Under no circumstances can the decision by a federal worker or anyone else to be vaccinated with a COVID-19 vaccine be considered voluntary when it is given under the threat that refusal to do so will result in them being "required to mask no matter where they work; test one or two times a week to see if they have ... acquired COVID; socially distance; and generally will not be allowed to travel for work,"[1727] as stated by President Biden.

Aaron Siri further explains:

> The FDA likewise viewed Section 564 as providing a substantive right to refuse when it explained the military exception:
>
> > [A]s a general rule, persons must be made aware of their right to refuse the product (or to refuse it for their

> children or others without the capacity to consent) and of the potential consequences, if any, of this choice. An exception to this rule is that the president, as commander in chief, can waive military personnel's right to refuse this product. If the right is not specifically waived by the president for a particular product given under EUA, military personnel have the same right to refuse as civilians.[1728]

The FDA thus makes clear that Section 564 provides a substantive right to refuse, and this right does not exist in the presence of a requirement that imposes negative consequences for refusing.

Similarly, the CDC's Advisory Committee on Immunization Practices ("ACIP") has interpreted Section 564 as a consent provision and not merely a requirement to inform. When responding to an inquiry regarding whether the COVID-19 vaccines can be required, the Executive Secretary of ACIP publicly stated that "under an EUA, vaccines are not allowed to be mandatory. Therefore, early in the vaccination phase individuals will have to be consented and cannot be mandated to be vaccinated."

ACIP's Executive Secretary then reaffirmed to the FDA's Vaccine and Related Biological Products Advisory Committee that no organization, public or private – including hospitals – can mandate the EUA COVID-19 Vaccines:

> Organizations, such as hospitals, with licensed products do have [the] capability of asking their workers to get the vaccine. But in the setting of an EUA, patients and individuals will have the right to refuse the vaccine.

> Consistent with the foregoing, the U.S. General Services Administration's ("GSA") Safer Federal Workforce website, applicable to all federal employees and contractors, expressly provided that the EUA COVID-19 vaccines cannot be mandatory.[1729]

The GSA's official position was that "COVID-19 vaccination should generally not be a pre-condition for employees or contractors at executive departments and agencies … to work in-person in Federal buildings, on Federal lands, and in other settings as required by their job duties."[1730]

Siri reveals that the GSA changed its interpretation of the statute after DOJ released its slip opinion. Now, GSA states that an unvaccinated person can be required to wear a mask, physical distance, be tested, restricted from travel, and even be quarantined.

The DOJ interpretation of Section 564 (21 U.S. Code § 360bbb-3) gives short shrift to the concept of freedom of choice. Section 564 (21 U.S. Code § 360bbb-3) allows "the **option** to accept or refuse administration of the product." "**Option**" is defined in the dictionary as "an act of choosing; the power or right to choose: freedom of choice."[1731] The DOJ opinion eliminates the "freedom of choice" by allowing the choice to be coerced by a threat of being fired, having to wear a mask, being tested, physical distance, etc.

Aaron Siri makes the common-sense observation that "[i]t is illogical that Congress would require that individuals be informed of a freedom of choice if that choice is illusory at the whim of any public or private entity."

National Research Act

Subsection (k) of 21 U.S. Code § 360bbb–3 indicates that an EUA is not to be considered a clinical investigation for purposes of section 355(i), 360b(j), or 360j(g) of this title or any other provision of this chapter or section 351 of the Public Health Service Act [42 U.S.C. 262]. But that language does affect other regulations that remain operative regarding an investigative vaccine under an EUA.

Aside from the misinterpretation of Section 564 (21 U.S. Code § 360bbb-3), coercing employees to get an experimental COVID-19 vaccine by the threat of masking, social distancing, medical testing, and travel prohibitions is a violation of the federal regulations and rulings passed under the authority of the National Research Act.[1732]

In the wake of the infamous Tuskegee Syphilis Study, which was terminated on November 14, 1972, Congress enacted The National Research Act.[1733] That law established a National Commission for the Protection of Human Subjects of Biomedical and Behavioral Research.

The commission was tasked with, among other things, conducting "a comprehensive investigation and study to identify the basic ethical principles which should underlie the conduct of biomedical and behavioral research involving human subjects."[1734] In carrying out that task the commission was ordered to "consider at least ... the nature and definition of informed consent in various research Settings."[1735]

The Belmont Report

The National Commission for the Protection of Human Subjects of Biomedical and Behavioral Research issued an authoritative report known as the Belmont Report.[1736] That report summarized the basic ethical principles identified by the Commission that were to be followed by researchers using human subjects in biomedical research.

The pertinent section of the Belmont Report is the section that addresses informed consent. The Belmont Report expressly states that any research subject must be informed of the risks and alternative treatments prior to entering a research study involving an experimental medical treatment. Notably, that informed consent is defined in the Belmont Report as voluntary consent that is free from coercion and undue influence. The report notes explicitly that consent from unjustifiable pressure is not valid consent. "Unjustifiable pressures usually occur when persons in positions of authority or commanding influence -- especially where possible sanctions are involved -- urge a course of action for a subject." The Pertinent language in the Belmont Report explaining informed consent is as follows:

> **Informed Consent.** -- Respect for persons requires that subjects, to the degree that they are capable, be given the **opportunity to choose** what shall or shall not happen to them. This opportunity is provided when adequate standards for **informed consent** are satisfied.
>
> While the importance of informed consent is unquestioned, controversy prevails over the nature and possibility of an informed consent. Nonetheless, there is widespread agreement that the consent process can be analyzed as containing three elements: information, comprehension and

> **voluntariness.**
>
> ***
>
> **Voluntariness.** An agreement to participate in research constitutes a **valid consent only if voluntarily given.** This element of informed consent requires conditions **free of coercion and undue influence.** Coercion occurs when an overt threat of harm is intentionally presented by one person to another in order to obtain compliance. Undue influence, by contrast, occurs through an offer of an excessive, unwarranted, inappropriate or improper reward or other overture in order to obtain compliance. Also, inducements that would ordinarily be acceptable may become undue influences if the subject is especially vulnerable.
>
> **Unjustifiable pressures usually occur when persons in positions of authority or commanding influence -- especially where possible sanctions are involved** -- urge a course of action for a subject. A continuum of such influencing factors exists, however, and it is impossible to state precisely where justifiable persuasion ends and undue influence begins. But undue influence would include actions such as manipulating a person's choice through the controlling influence of a close relative and threatening to withdraw health services to which an individual would otherwise be entitled.[1737] (emphasis added)

The U.S. Department of Health and Human Services has created a video wherein is explained the meaning and application of the Belmont Report. The video clarifies that "to deny someone autonomy is to deny them respect as an individual. ... Subjects must understand the extent of the risk they are taking. They must know that participation is **voluntary**, that they can withdraw from the research at any point if they choose. ... **Consent must be free of coercion or undue pressure.**"[1738]

The very actions that the President proposed and are being advocated by DOJ and the FDA constitute coercion and undue influence as defined by the Belmont Report. Federal employees are being coerced into being vaccinated under the penalty of being fired. The threat is being made by the employer who controls their job. The employee is under pressure to please his employer who is exercising undue influence over the employees as he decides whether to take part in the experimental COVID-19 vaccine program. Nothing in Section 564 (21 U.S. Code § 360bbb-3) excuses compliance for an EUA with the standards of informed consent in the Belmont Report.

Padma Nambisan explains that the "[t]he Belmont Report has served as an ethical framework for protecting human subjects and its recommendations incorporated into other guidelines. It is an essential reference document for Institutional Review Boards (IRBs) that review and ensure that research proposals involving human subjects conducted or supported by the Human & Health Services (HHS) meet the ethical standards of the regulations."[1739]

The ethical standards memorialized in the Belmont Report have been incorporated into Federal Regulations. The basic HHS Policy for Protecting Human Research Subjects "applies to all research involving human subjects conducted, supported, or otherwise subject to regulation by any Federal department or agency that takes appropriate administrative action to make the policy applicable to such research. This includes research conducted by Federal civilian employees or military personnel." 45 C.F.R. § 46.101(a). The regulations at 45 C.F.R. § 46.101, et seq., were enacted under the legislative authority of 5 U.S. Code

§ 301, 42 U.S.C. 300v-1(b), and 42 U.S. Code § 289.

45 C.F.R. § 46.101(i) provided that "[u]nless otherwise required by law, department or agency heads may waive the applicability of some or all of the provisions of this policy to specific research activities or classes of research activities otherwise covered by this policy, provided the alternative procedures to be followed are consistent with the principles of the **Belmont Report.**"[1740] That means that no agency of the federal government may drop their ethical protections of research subjects below that which is provided in the Belmont Report. Essentially, the Belmont Report sets the minimum standards beneath which no executive branch department may fall. Indeed, § 46.101(c) provides that "[d]epartment or agency heads retain final judgment as to whether a particular activity is covered by this policy and this judgment shall be exercised **consistent with the ethical principles of the Belmont Report.**" Thus no matter what an executive agency does, it must comply with the ethical standard of the Belmont Report, which includes the informed consent provisions. There is no wiggle room. The ethical standards of informed consent apply to all medical research involving human subjects.

45 C.F.R. §46.116 codifies, in part, the informed consent standards of the Belmont Report. That section provides in pertinent part:

> (1) Before involving a human subject in research covered by this policy, an investigator shall obtain the legally effective informed consent of the subject or the subject's legally authorized representative.
>
> (8) A statement that participation is voluntary, refusal to participate will involve no penalty or loss of benefits to which the subject is otherwise entitled, and the subject may discontinue

> participation at any time without penalty or loss of benefits to which the subject is otherwise entitled;[1741]

45 C.F.R. § 46.111(a)(5) requires that the informed consent must be documented in writing. The written documentation requirement can be waived but there is no allowance for a waiver of the informed consent requirement.

> Informed consent will be appropriately documented or appropriately waived in accordance with §46.117.

Please note that informed consent must be voluntary. If there is a penalty or loss of benefits of any kind, the consent is not voluntary.

Nuremberg Code

It is a well-established principle that non-consensual human medical experimentation violates the Nuremberg Code and customary international law. That principle was considered authoritative and applicable when determining the application of the Alien Tort Statute.[1742] The gravamen of the Nuremberg Code has been adopted in the United States in the *Belmont Report* and under 45 C.F.R. § 46.101, et seq.

The President may try to argue that he is informing the recipients of "the consequences, if any, of refusing the administration of the product." That is a misinterpretation of the statute. It would open the statute up to an interpretation that virtually any penalty is authorized as a punishment for refusing the vaccine as long as the patient is informed. It would turn restrictive statutory language on its head and make it permissive. It is basic that consent must be voluntary. The one obtaining the consent cannot threaten, cajole, or use undue influence. Otherwise, the consent is not voluntary.

21 U.S. Code § 360bbb–3(e)(1)(A)(I) requires informed consent. Such consent must be voluntary to be consent at all. All understand that fact. Indeed, as mentioned earlier, Dr. Amanda Cohn, the Executive Secretary of the CDC's Advisory Committee on Immunization Practices, stated that vaccines authorized under an EUA, "are not allowed to be mandatory. So, early in this vaccination phase, individuals will have to be consented and they won't be able to be mandatory." Informed consent is not informed consent if it is given under compulsion. The President can no more say that all who refuse the vaccine will be jailed until they agree to be vaccinated as he can require all who refuse to be vaccinated to be fired, wear a mask, be tested for COVID, social distance from others, and be prevented from traveling. That all assumes that the codification of the Nuremberg code in the Belmont Report and federal regulations is inapplicable to the EUA vaccines. Since they are applicable, it is clear that President Biden's edict is unlawful. 45 C.F.R. § 46.116(a)(1) explicitly states that "refusal to participate will involve no penalty or loss of benefits to which the subject is otherwise entitled."

No Emergency Exception to Constitutional Rights

The President's order stems from a declared state of emergency. There is no emergency exception to the Constitution. The U.S. Supreme Court has stated the legal maxim that "[t]he Constitution was adopted in a period of grave emergency. Its grants of power to the federal government and its limitations of the power of the States were determined in the light of emergency, and they are not altered by emergency." *Home Building & Loan Ass'n. v. Blaisdell.*[1743]

In the context of unconstitutional COVID-19 restrictions under executive orders issued by the Pennsylvania Governor, the Honorable William S. Stickman explained in *City of Butler v.*

Wolf[1744]:

> [G]ood intentions toward a laudable end are not alone enough to uphold governmental action against a constitutional challenge. Indeed, the greatest threats to our system of constitutional liberties may arise when the ends are laudable, and the intent is good—especially in a time of emergency. In an emergency, even a vigilant public may let down its guard over its constitutional liberties only to find that liberties, once relinquished, are hard to recoup and that restrictions—while expedient in the face of an emergency situation—may persist long after immediate danger has passed.[1745]

Judge Stickman concluded:

> [I]n an emergency, the authority of government is not unfettered. The liberties protected by the Constitution are not fair-weather freedoms—in place when times are good but able to be cast aside in times of trouble. There is no question that this Country has faced, and will face, emergencies of every sort. But the solution to a national crisis can never be permitted to supersede the commitment to individual liberty that stands as the foundation of the American experiment. The Constitution cannot accept the concept of a "new normal" where the basic liberties of the people can be subordinated to open-ended emergency mitigation measures. Rather, the Constitution sets certain lines that may not be crossed, even in an emergency. Actions taken by Defendants crossed those lines. It is the duty of the Court to declare those actions unconstitutional.[1746]

The President lacks any authority to mandate vaccinations of any kind.

Jacobson v. Massachusetts

This is a good point to address the alleged precedent of *Jacobson v. Massachusetts*.[1747] In *Jacobson*, the U.S. Supreme Court upheld a Massachusetts statute empowering municipal boards of health to require that smallpox vaccinations be given to all residents. Failure to obtain the vaccine subjected the violator to a civil fine.

The Honorable Judge Stickman in *City of Butler v. Wolf* explains the rather tenuous precedent of *Jacobson*:

> *Jacobson* was decided over a century ago. Since that time, there has been substantial development of federal constitutional law in the area of civil liberties. As a general matter, this development has seen a jurisprudential shift whereby federal courts have given greater deference to considerations of individual liberties, as weighed against the exercise of state police powers. That century of development has seen the creation of tiered levels of scrutiny for constitutional claims. They did not exist when *Jacobson* was decided. While Jacobson has been cited by some modern courts as ongoing support for a broad, hands-off deference to state authorities in matters of health and safety, other courts and commentators have questioned whether it remains instructive in light of the intervening jurisprudential developments.[1748]

In *Bayley's Campground, Inc. v. Mills*,[1749] where the court denied injunctive relief from COVID-19 restrictions, the court nonetheless stated:

> [T]he permissive *Jacobson* rule floats about in the air as a rubber stamp for all but the most absurd and egregious restrictions on constitutional liberties, free from the inconvenience of meaningful judicial review. This may help explain why the Supreme Court established the traditional tiers of scrutiny in the course of the 100 years since *Jacobson* was decided.[1750]

Justice Alito's dissent (joined by Justices Thomas and Kavanaugh) to the U.S. Supreme Court's denial of emergency injunctive relief in *Calvary Chapel Dayton Valley v. Sisolak*,[1751] calls into question whether *Jacobson* remains valid precedent. *Jacobson* is a phantom from a bygone era. Justice Alito argued that the Supreme Court should have granted the requested injunction: "We have a duty to defend the Constitution, and even a public health emergency does not absolve us of that responsibility."[1752] Justice Alito argued that "a public health emergency does not give Governors and other public officials *carte blanche* to disregard the Constitution for as long as the medical problem persists."[1753] Justice Alito warned that "it is a mistake to take language in *Jacobson* as the last word on what the Constitution allows public officials to do during the COVID–19 pandemic."[1754] Indeed, he viewed it "a considerable stretch to read the [Jacobson] decision as establishing the test to be applied when statewide measures of indefinite duration are challenged under the First Amendment or other provisions not at issue in that case."[1755]

Justice Gorsuch's concurrence in *Roman Cath. Diocese of Brooklyn v. Cuomo*[1756], questions *Jacobson's* continued viability as the sweeping precedent many ascribe to it. Justice Gorsuch stated that "Jacobson hardly supports cutting the Constitution loose during a pandemic."[1757] He had more to say:

> Why have some mistaken this Court's modest decision in *Jacobson* for a towering authority that

> overshadows the Constitution during a pandemic? In the end, I can only surmise that much of the answer lies in a particular judicial impulse to stay out of the way in times of crisis. But if that impulse may be understandable or even admirable in other circumstances, we may not shelter in place when the Constitution is under attack. Things never go well when we do.[1758]

As noted by the U.S. Court of Appeals for the Second Circuit in *Agudath Israel of Am. v. Cuomo*[1759]: "the *Jacobson* Court itself specifically noted that 'even if based on the acknowledged police powers of a state,' a public-health measure 'must always yield in case of conflict with ... any right which [the Constitution] gives or secures.'"[1760] (brackets in original).

Freedom of Religion

Requiring vaccination may also violate one's sincerely held religious beliefs. It is a violation of a person's sincerely held religious beliefs to require that he get a vaccine under penalty of masking, social distancing, testing, travel prohibition, or termination from employment.

Title VII of the Civil Rights Act of 1964[1761] prohibits employers with at least 15 employees from discriminating against applicants and employees based on religion, race, color, sex, and national origin. Title VII also applies to most federal executive employers, and through the Congressional Accountability Act, applies to most federal legislative employers.

The U.S. Equal Employment Opportunity Commission (EEOC) states that "Title VII of the Civil Rights Act of 1964 requires employers to make a reasonable accommodation for an employee's sincerely held religious beliefs as long as doing so does not pose an undue hardship on the employer."[1762] The courts in past cases had taken the view that an accommodation creates an undue hardship on an employer when it imposes "more than a *de minimis* [small or trifling] cost." But in June 2023, the U.S. Supreme Court, in *Groff v. DeJoy*[1763], ruled that to deny a religious accommodation because the accommodation would constitute an "undue hardship," an employer must show that the burden of accommodating the religious beliefs of the employee will **substantially** increase the costs to its business.

In a case involving a $300,000 judgment against a hospital for refusing to grant a religious exemption for an influenza vaccine, the EEOC has stated that "when considering requests for religious accommodation, the Health Center must adhere to the definition of 'religion' established by Title VII and controlling federal court decisions, a definition that **forbids employers from rejecting accommodation requests based on their disagreement with an employee's belief**; their opinion that the belief is unfounded, illogical, or inconsistent in some way; or their conclusion that an employee's belief is not an official tenet or endorsed teaching of any particular religion or denomination."[1764]

If a person asserts a sincere religious belief, it is not the function of courts to further explore that belief. The U.S. Supreme Court, in *Thomas v. Rev. Bd. of Indiana*[1765], explained that "the resolution of that question is not to turn upon a judicial perception of the particular belief or practice in question; religious beliefs need not be acceptable, logical, consistent, or comprehensible to others in order to merit First Amendment protection."[1766] The *Thomas* Court further stated that "it is not within the judicial function and judicial competence to inquire whether the petitioner or his fellow worker more correctly perceived the commands of their common faith. Courts are not arbiters of scriptural interpretation."[1767] The *Thomas* Court required that for the government to intrude on a person's religious liberty requires the government to show that "it is the least restrictive means of achieving some compelling state interest."[1768] That is a very high hurdle indeed.

Furthermore, for the government to allow a medical exemption for the vaccine, which it necessarily must since there are immunocompromised persons who cannot be vaccinated under any circumstances, it must also necessarily allow a religious exemption. The U.S. Supreme Court in Church of the *Lukumi Babalu Aye, Inc. v. City of Hialeah*[1769] explained:

> Neutrality and general applicability are interrelated, and, as becomes apparent in this case, failure to satisfy one requirement is a likely indication that the other has not been satisfied. A law failing to satisfy these requirements must be justified by a compelling governmental interest and must be narrowly tailored to advance that interest.[1770]

That strict scrutiny hurdle is virtually insurmountable, and the *Lukami* Court said so.

> A law that targets religious conduct for distinctive treatment or advances legitimate governmental interests only against conduct with a religious motivation will survive strict scrutiny only in rare cases.[1771]

The two factors, neutrality and generality, are closely related concepts. The vaccine rules of President Biden appear to be neutral on their face, but they are arguably not neutral in application. As the court stated in *Ward v. Polite,*[1772] "[a] double standard is not a neutral standard."[1773] The *Ward* court called for strict scrutiny when a secular exemption to a rule is allowed, but a religious exemption is disallowed. Even if facial neutrality is conceded, that is not enough. As the *Lukumi* Court held, the rule must also be of general application to avoid strict scrutiny. Here, there are medical exemptions allowed. If a medical exemption is allowed, then the rule is, by definition, not of general application. The *Lukumi* Court explained:

> Where government restricts only conduct protected by the First Amendment and fails to enact feasible measures to restrict other conduct producing substantial harm or alleged harm of the same sort, the interest given in justification of the restriction is not compelling. It is established in our strict scrutiny jurisprudence that "a law cannot be regarded as protecting an interest 'of the highest order' ... when it leaves appreciable damage to that supposedly vital interest unprohibited."[1774] (citation omitted)

Judge (now U.S. Supreme Court Justice) Alito applied that standard in a case where police officers were given medical exemptions from a department beard prohibition rule but not religious exemptions. In *Fraternal Ord. of Police Newark Lodge No. 12 v. City of Newark*,[1775] the court ruled that providing medical exemptions while refusing religious exemptions indicates discriminatory intent, which cannot survive even intermediate, let alone strict scrutiny. Allowing a medical exemption while denying a religious exemption puts the vaccine requirement outside the category of general applicability. It would be necessarily discriminatory against religious beliefs, which requires heightened scrutiny. If the government is going to allow an exemption for a secular medical reason, it must also allow an exemption for a religious reason as well, unless there is a compelling government reason to discriminate against a person's freedom of religion in the least intrusive means possible. No such showing has been, nor can be, made here.

The typically proposed accommodation is testing, masking and social distancing. The government cannot offer an option that violates federal workers' constitutional rights and then claim that option is a reasonable accommodation. The option of wearing a mask and being medically tested is not a reasonable accommodation because those procedures infringe on the constitutional rights of the workers. The U.S. Supreme Court in *Cruzan by Cruzan v. Missouri Dep't of Health*,[1776] has advised that "the patient generally possesses the right ... to refuse treatment." The FDA has determined that face masks are medical devices, including cloth face coverings and surgical masks worn for COVID-19 medical purposes.[1777] The *Cruzan* Court's ruling establishes a constitutional right to refuse to wear a medical device.[1778] The same reasoning applies to medical tests that require the insertion of a swab deep into the nostrils of a government employee once every three days.[1779] The federal worker has committed no crime, is not under arrest, is not even suspected of being ill. Such tests are a violation of a worker's bodily autonomy.

A little known fact is that the antigen tests that many employers require are also only allowed because they are have been authorized under an EUA.[1780] Because they are authorized under an EUA they come with the same informed consent restrictions as do the EUA vaccines, and the EUA masks. Thus, neither the government nor any other employer can require experimental masking or experimental testing when an employee refuses to take an experimental vaccine.

The masks recommended by the CDC are not approved. They are authorized by an EUA.[1781] The FDA explains: "On August 5, 2020, the FDA issued an umbrella EUA for certain disposable, single-use surgical masks."[1782] The CDC guidance for wearing FDA EUA masks is in accordance with the FDA power to authorize masks under its emergency powers. Such EUA masks are not FDA-approved medical devices. As such, masks cannot be mandated. EUA masks are unapproved experimental medical devices. The CDC references the definition from OSHA for what a facemask is. According to the pertinent part of the OSHA definition, a facemask means a "mask that is FDA-cleared, authorized by an FDA EUA, or offered or distributed as described in an FDA enforcement policy."[1783] The CDC recommendation of FDA EUA masks, come with the right to informed consent. Masks cannot be mandated.

Masks are medical devices.[1784] Any mask mandate is based on the FDA's emergency use authorization (EUA). The mask requirement is to prevent the spread of COVID-19 during the declared emergency. The mask requirement is for the purpose of following the FDA EUA mask guidance. While the FDA authorized masks under its emergency powers, such EUA masks are not FDA-approved medical devices.[1785] Mandating the use of an EUA medical device violates federal law. All EUA medical devices, including masks, come with the inherent legal right to refuse (21 U.S.C. 360bbb-3(e)(1)(A)(ii)(I-III)).

The FDA's blanket EUA mask letter clearly states that manufacturers cannot advertise masks as being safe or effective at diagnosing or preventing COVID-19.[1786] Indeed, the EUA authorizing letter from the FDA states that such mask manufacturers' "advertising and promotional materials, relating to the use of the product shall clearly and conspicuously state that [t]he product has not been FDA cleared or approved."[1787]

21 U.S.C. § 360bbb-3(e)(1)(A) provides that an EUA product can be used only when "[a]ppropriate conditions designed to ensure that individuals to whom the product is administered are informed ... of the significant known and potential benefits and risks of such use, and of the extent to which such benefits and risks are unknown; and ... of **the option to accept or refuse administration of the product**, of the consequences, if any, of refusing administration of the product, and of the alternatives to the product that are available and of their benefits and risks."

The federal government has violated federal law by:

1) not informing persons of the known and potential benefits and risks of wearing a mask,

2) not informing persons that they have **the option to accept or refuse to wear a mask**,

3) not informing persons of the consequences, in any, of not wearing a mask,

4) not informing persons of available alternatives to wearing a mask, and

5) not informing persons of the benefits and risks of the alternatives.

Feds for Medical Freedom v. Biden

Recall that on September 9, 2021, President Biden issued Executive Order # 14043.[1788] President Biden mandated that all federal employees get vaccinated against COVID-19 or lose their jobs. A non-profit organization, *Feds for Medical Freedom*, representing more than 6,000 federal workers and contractors, filed for a preliminary injunction. The United States District Court for the Southern District of Texas granted the request and issued a preliminary injunction.[1789] The injunction was based, in pertinent part, on the district court's finding that President Biden did not have the authority to require federal workers to be vaccinated. The *Feds for Medical Freedom* district court found that the President can regulate executive-branch employees' workplace conduct but not their general conduct. The court ruled that since getting vaccinated is not workplace conduct, the President has no authority to require vaccinations.

The *Feds for Medical Freedom* district court ruling was based partly on U.S. Supreme Court precedent in *NFIB v. OSHA*.[1790] In that case, the U.S. Supreme Court ruled that

COVID-19 is not a workplace risk. Rather, it is a "universal risk" that is "no different from the day-to-day dangers that all face from crime, air pollution, or any number of communicable diseases."[1791] Accordingly, the U.S. Supreme Court held that OSHA did not have the authority to require employees to vaccinate against COVID-19.

The *Feds for Medical Freedom* district court noted the curious fact that "even full-time remote federal workers are not exempt from the mandate." If the purpose of the mandate is to stop the spread of COVID-19 in the federal workplace, as alleged by the government, there seems no rational basis to mandate vaccinations for those who stay home.

More importantly, the Texas federal district court had little difficulty in finding that Article II of the Constitution does not grant any power to the President to impose medical procedures on civilian federal employees. The Government appealed the district court injunctive order and the district court ruling was reversed by a Fifth Circuit panel. That panel ruling was subsequently overturned by an *en banc* Fifth Circuit on March 23, 2023. A federal appeals court panel ruling involves three judges. An *en banc* federal appeals court decision involves all the judges for that particular circuit. In this case, nine judges. The *en banc* court affirmed the district court's ruling issuing the preliminary injunction.[1792] Thus, the nationwide injunction stopping the federal vaccine mandate remains as of this writing.

Mississippi Religious Exemption Ruling

On April 17, 2023, the Informed Consent Action Network (ICAN) secured a historic ruling from a federal court.[1793] The court ruled a Mississippi law unconstitutional. The law disallowed religious exemptions for childhood vaccinations. Children in Mississippi must obtain childhood vaccines before school enrollment. Violation of the vaccine requirement carried criminal penalties. The state statute allowed for medical exemptions but disallowed religious exemptions for the vaccine requirement. The federal district court issued an injunction preventing the enforcement of the law. The State of Mississippi must now afford its residents a religious exemption against having to vaccinate their children as a requirement to attend school.

The State of Mississippi statute made an unconstitutional value judgment that secular (i.e., medical) motivations for opting out of compulsory immunization are permitted but that religious grounds are not.[1794] That distinction unconstitutionally discriminates against a citizen's sincerely held religious beliefs. The U.S. Supreme Court has ruled that discriminating against a person's religious beliefs in that fashion is subject to strict scrutiny. The state must have a compelling reason to discriminate against someone based on his religious beliefs. The State of Mississippi could not make that showing. The U.S. Supreme Court has ruled that the government is prohibited from treating "any comparable secular activity more favorably than religious exercise."[1795]

The U.S. Supreme Court has issued similar rulings in recent COVID-19 cases. In *Tandon v. Newsom*,[1796] the U.S. Supreme Court ruled that it was unconstitutional for the State of California to issue regulations, ostensibly intended to slow the spread of COVID-19, that placed limits on religious gatherings but treated comparable non-religious activities – such as getting haircuts and retail shopping – more favorably. Similarly, the U.S. Supreme Court, in *Roman Catholic Diocese of Brooklyn v. Cuomo*,[1797] ruled that New York regulation that prohibited religious gatherings but permitted similar secular gatherings violated the First Amendment where the secular and religious activities in question presented comparable alleged contagion risks.

Please note that the restrictions in the *Newsom* and *Cuomo* cases were based on the unproven, mythical germ theory. The germ theory is a Satanic superstitious belief conjured to enslave the population. Governments will use that folklore to mask, lockdown, separate, and vaccinate its citizens, allegedly to protect the community from each new contrived boogeyman virus.

The State of Mississippi argued that it had an interest in stopping the spread of infectious disease, but it cannot discriminate against one's religious beliefs to accomplish that goal. The state argues that it wants to prevent the exposure of its vaccinated children to unvaccinated children. But the law does not do that because unvaccinated children with medical exemptions are not excluded from school. Those unvaccinated children would be mingling with the vaccinated children. Furthermore, teachers, administrators, and other adults in the schools are not required to be vaccinated; they have regular contact with the vaccinated children. Only those unvaccinated children with religious objections to vaccination are prohibited from entering the schools. That is unconstitutional religious discrimination.

Finally, the argument that unvaccinated children threaten vaccinated children with infection implicitly acknowledges that the vaccines do not work. If the vaccines worked to protect the vaccinated person, he should not care whether another is vaccinated.

67 The Right of the People to Peaceably Assemble

President Biden has become the bull in our china shop of rights. How so? One of the fragile rights violated by the laws he has passed in his vaccine coercion plan is the people's right to peaceably assemble. In his July 29, 2021 order, he mandated social distancing for the unvaccinated.

> [E]very federal government employee will be asked to attest to their vaccination status. Anyone who does not attest or is not vaccinated will be required to mask no matter where they work; test one or two times a week to see if they have a — they have acquired COVID; socially distance; and generally will not be allowed to travel for work.[1798]

The President's authority is limited. He does not have the constitutional authority to issue restrictions on the right of the people, wherever they are situated, to peaceably assemble.

The limitation on abridgment of the right of the people to peaceably assemble is found in the First Amendment to the U.S. Constitution. The United States Supreme Court has ruled that the First Amendment to the U.S. Constitution limits the authority of the government to infringe on the right of the people to assemble peaceably.[1799] The First Amendment to the U.S. Constitution prohibits "any law respecting an establishment of religion, or prohibiting the free exercise thereof; or abridging the freedom of speech, or of the press; or the right of the people peaceably to assemble, and to petition the Government for a redress of grievances."[1800]

The U.S. Supreme Court has found that freedom of assembly "cannot be denied without violating those fundamental principles of liberty and justice which lie at the base of all civil and political institutions."[1801] Indeed, the U.S. Supreme Court recognized, as should this court, that "[t]he very idea of a government, republican in form, implies a right on the part of its citizens to meet peaceably."[1802]

The Ninth Amendment to the U.S. Constitution provides that "[t]he enumeration in the Constitution, of certain rights, shall not be construed to deny or disparage others retained by the people."[1803]

William Pitt the Younger made a statement during a speech in the British House of Commons on November 18, 1783. "Necessity is the plea for every infringement of human freedom. It is the argument of tyrants; it is the creed of slaves." Indeed, that is true. Benjamin Franklin in reply to the Governor in the Pennsylvania Assembly on Nov. 11, 1755, put it this way: "Those who would give up essential Liberty, to purchase a little temporary safety, deserve neither Liberty nor Safety." Christopher Fox Graham puts it in plain terms: "[G]overnment tyranny invariably begins with popular support first to resisting a 'crisis' and then the tacit or explicit surrender of our liberties and freedoms in the name of safety and security."

But the announcement of "safety, safety, safety," rings from the White House to convince the people to surrender their freedom behind that shield of "safety." The gentle government is only looking out for the citizens' safety and just to make sure the citizens get that message, the sword is not far behind the shield. If a citizen does not want or need the safety offered by the gentle and caring government then he will be made to accept the offer of safety with force. The President is beginning with his employees. It matters not that the claim of peril is real or imagined, it all comes down to force. As George Orwell explained: "All tyrannies rule through fraud and force, but once the fraud is exposed they must rely exclusively on force."

The U.S. Supreme Court has foreclosed the "sky is falling" emergency excuse to infringe constitutional rights. "The Constitution was adopted in a period of grave emergency. Its grants of power to the federal government and its limitations of the power of the States were determined in the light of emergency, and they are not altered by emergency."[1804]

The Supreme Court of Wisconsin struck down the stay-at-home orders of the Secretary of the State Department of Health Services as being unlawful and unenforceable. In *dicta,* the court noted that "[a]s the United States Department of Justice has recently written in a COVID-19-related case raising constitutional issues, 'There is no pandemic exception ... to the fundamental liberties the Constitution safeguards. Indeed, 'individual rights secured by the Constitution do not disappear during a public health crisis.' These individual rights, including the protections in the Bill of Rights made applicable to the states through the Fourteenth Amendment, are always in force and restrain government action.'''[1805]

Justice Alito's dissent (joined by Justices Thomas and Kavanaugh) to the U.S. Supremen Court's denial of emergency injunctive relief to a church from the California Governor's COVID-19 restrictions, in *Calvary Chapel Dayton Valley v. Sisolak,*[1806] made the point that "[w]e have a duty to defend the

Constitution, and even a public health emergency does not absolve us of that responsibility."

But how could Justices Alito, Thomas, and Kavanaugh make such an argument in light of the precedent in *Jacobson v. Massachusetts*, 197 U.S. 11 (1905), that seemingly establishes a deferential approach to government action in a medical emergency? *Jacobson* seems to be the proverbial elephant in the room. But in reality, *Jacobson* is more a phantom than an elephant. And that phantom has been *de facto* abrogated by the U.S. Supreme Court over the past 100 years, although it has not been *de jure* overruled yet.

Indeed, in *City of Butler v. Wolf*, the Honorable William S. Stickman IV, explained the tenuousness of the precedent in *Jacobson* that still remains in light of more than 100 years of Supreme Court rulings that have eviscerated the guts from that opinion.[1807] The Honorable Judge Stickman explained that the "extraordinarily deferential standard based on *Jacobson* is not appropriate" when reviewing emergency executive orders. The *Butler* court ruled that intermediate constitutional scrutiny is the appropriate standard to apply to infringement of the right to assemble by medical emergency edicts. The *Butler* court stated: "Two considerations inform this decision—the ongoing and open-ended nature of the restrictions and the need for an independent judiciary to serve as a check on the exercise of emergency government power."[1808]

The factors that the *Butler* court considered for eschewing the deferential standard of *Jacobson* are factors that impeach the legitimacy of the President's order.

> First, the ongoing and indefinite nature of Defendants' [Governor's] actions weigh strongly against application of a more deferential level of review. The extraordinary emergency measures

> taken by Defendants in this case were promulgated beginning in March—six months ago. What were initially billed as temporary measures necessary to "flatten the curve" and protect hospital capacity have become open-ended and ongoing restrictions aimed at a very different end—stopping the spread of an infectious disease and preventing new cases from arising—which requires ongoing and open-ended efforts. Further, while the harshest measures have been "suspended," Defendants admit that they remain in-place and can be reinstated *sua sponte* as and when Defendants see fit. In other words, while not currently being enforced, Pennsylvania citizens remain subject to the re-imposition of the most severe provisions at any time. Further, testimony and evidence presented by Defendants does not establish any specified exit gate or end date to the emergency interventions. Rather, the record shows that Defendants view the presence of disease mitigation restrictions upon the citizens of Pennsylvania as a "new normal" and they have no actual plan to return to a state where all restrictions are lifted. It bears repeating; after six months, there is no plan to return to a situation where there are no restrictions imposed upon the people of the Commonwealth.[1809]

The *Butler* court was troubled by the virtually unlimited discretion given to the Governor of Pennsylvania. The deferential approach of *Jacobson* offered no check on that power.

> Absent a robust system of checks and balances, the guarantees of liberty set forth in the Constitution are just ink on parchment. There is no question that a global pandemic poses serious challenges for governments and for all Americans. But the

> response to a pandemic (or any emergency) cannot be permitted to undermine our system of constitutional liberties or the system of checks and balances protecting those liberties. Here, Defendants are statutorily permitted to act with little, if any, meaningful input from the legislature. For the judiciary to apply an overly deferential standard would remove the only meaningful check on the exercise of power.[1810]

The right to peaceably assemble has traditionally been given the same protection by the courts as the right to freedom of speech.[1811] In *De Jonge v. State of Oregon*,[1812] the U.S. Supreme Court stated that "[t]he right of peaceable assembly is a right cognate to those of free speech and free press and is equally fundamental."[1813] The *De Jonge* Court emphasized the importance of the right to peaceably assemble by noting that "the right is one that cannot be denied without violating those fundamental principles of liberty and justice which lie at the base of all civil and political institutions."[1814] Where the restrictions on speech only go to time, place, and manner, they are afforded intermediate scrutiny by courts. In *Butler*, the court viewed intermediate scrutiny, rather than strict scrutiny, as the appropriate standard to review restrictions on the right to assemble by the Pennsylvania Governor's COVID-19 orders because the orders were content neutral.

In order pass the intermediate scrutiny test, the orders of the President must be narrowly tailored to accomplish a substantial government interest.[1815] If the restriction by the government are not narrowly tailored to accomplish the "substantial" government interest then the restrictions are unconstitutional. In *Butler*, the court found that because the Pennsylvania Governor's orders permitted commercial gatherings at a percentage of occupancy, while other gatherings were limited based upon total number indicated that the orders were not narrowly tailored. The Butler court stated that "hundreds of people may congregate in stores, malls, large restaurants and other businesses based only on the occupancy limit of the building." The court found that incongruent with the hard numeric limitations on other activities. The *Butler* court ruled that "[t]he imposition of a cap on the number of people that may gather for political, social, cultural, educational and other expressive gatherings, while permitting a larger number for commercial gatherings limited only by a percentage of the occupancy capacity of the facility is not narrowly tailored and does not pass constitutional muster."[1816]

That very incongruency is found in the President's order. The President is treating those who do not get the vaccine as more likely to spread COVID-19. In fact, unimpeachable evidence proves that the COVID-19 vaccines are ineffective in preventing the spread of COVID-19. Thus, those who do not get the vaccine must be fired or offered some accommodation for their religious objections such as wearing masks, being tested, social distancing, and not traveling, when they are no more likely to spread COVID-19 than those who are vaccinated. A requirement to social distance does not accomplish the goal of preventing the spread of COVID-19. Indeed, the whole concept of social distancing is the threat of the asymptomatic spread of SARS-CoV-2. But the most authoritative study on that issue proves that there is no asymptomatic spread of SARS-CoV-2.[1817]

Actor Woody Harrelson used satire to illustrate the Orwellian reality in which we live. He appeared on the TV show Saturday Night Live. During his monologue, he lampooned an imaginary movie script as a metaphor that chillingly resembled the events surrounding the COVID-19 vaccine rollout. Harrelson explained the script:

> I started to read the craziest script. ... So the movie goes like this: The biggest drug cartels in the world get together and buy up all the media and all the

> politicians and force all the people in the world to stay locked in their homes, and people can only come out if they take the cartel's drugs and keep taking them over and over. I threw the script away. I mean, who was going to believe that crazy idea? Being forced to do drugs?[1818]

The bought and paid-for mockingbird media immediately criticized Harrelson. For example, *Rolling Stone* Magazine called Harrelson's monologue a reflection of his "strange" and "gonzo" views about COVID-19 and vaccines.[1819]

68 Social Distancing Is from the Mind of a Child

Social distancing is not based on rigorous science. The commonly accepted theory of illness spread by human contact is a theory. It has never been proven. Dr. Milton J. Rosenau's research in his landmark study in 1919 proved that the "Spanish Flu" was not transmissible.[1820] If that is the case, where did the government come up with the unconstitutional scheme of business and school shutdowns, self-isolation, and social distancing? That scheme was born from a 15-year-old child's high school science project, not from rigorous scientific studies.[1821]

You read that correctly; the basis for the social distancing to arrest the spread of COVID-19 came from the mind of a 15-year-old. Laura Glass was an Albuquerque High sophomore student in 2006 when she came up with the idea of social distancing and shut-downs for stopping the spread of pandemics. She laid out her plan in a science project. She received the third place prize in the Intel International Science and Engineering Fair.

At the time, Laura's father, Robert J. Glass, was working at the National Infrastructure Simulation and Analysis Center (NISAC) at Sandia. When the NISAC received a request to brief

Secretary Michael Chertoff of the U.S. Department of Homeland Security on how best to respond to bioterrorism, Glass ran his daughter's science project through the NISAC computers and presto-chango out came the theory of shut-downs and social distancing as the response to bioterrorism. After a review by the Centers for Disease Control (CDC), social distancing and business and school shutdowns became federal policy.

Michael Spenger disputes the science project story. He states that the CDC adopted social distancing as a policy in 2004. The CDC modeled that approach after the Chinese Communist Government's 2003 lockdown response to SARS.[1822] Spenger states that social distancing is simply the word used in Western countries to implement what is essentially the lockdown tyranny of the Chinese Communist Government. A lockdown is distinct from quarantine, which only affects the sick. A lockdown is imposed on the entire society. Once a lockdown becomes the policy of a government, each contrived "pandemic" offers the perfect excuse for a government to strip its citizens of their liberty.

In a study published in the Journal of Infectious Diseases on November 15, 2008, researchers determined that social distancing did not reduce febrile respiratory illness rates.[1823]

The researchers gathered data from "13,114 male military recruits (mean age, 19 years) at the Marine Corps Recruit Depot in San Diego, California"[1824] The data were collected between February 2004 and March 2005. The study involved military recruits that were distributed among a total of 196 housing units. The researchers explained that "[i]n the present study, we investigate the usefulness of social distancing in an environment in which high rates of febrile respiratory illness (FRI) are endemic."[1825] The researchers stated that "[b]ecause the primary means of transmission was presumed to be person-to-person transmission, we expected that groups that were socially distanced from potentially infectious individuals who were new to the group would incur rates of illness lower than those noted for groups that were not socially distanced."[1826] But the researchers found that not to be the case.

> The original hypothesis was rejected. There was not a statistically significant difference between the FRI [febrile respiratory illness] rates in the open and closed units as a whole, although the tendency was for the closed units to exhibit higher rates. The rejection of the hypothesis suggests that the primary route of transmission of FRI is not via the MCU/PCU recycling protocol (i.e., not via person-to-person contact between unit members and members newly introduced to the unit [i.e., potentially infectious convalescents]). The social distancing instituted in this setting was not successful in decreasing FRI rates.[1827]

Below is the opinion of an expert in the medical field on the approach of masking, testing, and social distancing. Dr. Roger Hodkinson, MA, MB, FRCPC, FCAP, is the CEO and medical director of Western Medical Assessments. Dr. Hodkinson explains:

> I'm a medical specialist in pathology which includes virology. I trained at Cambridge University in the U.K. I'm the ex-president of the pathology section of the Medical Association. I was previously an assistant professor in the Faculty of Medicine doing a lot of teaching. I was the chairman of the Royal College of Physicians of Canada Examination Committee and Pathology in Ottawa, but more to the point I'm currently the chairman of a biotechnology company in North Carolina selling the COVID-19 test.
>
> ***

There is no action of any kind needed other than what happened last year when we felt unwell. We stayed home, we took chicken noodle soup, we didn't visit granny, and we decided when we would return to work. We didn't need anyone to tell us.

Masks are utterly useless. There is no evidence base for their effectiveness whatsoever. Paper masks and fabric masks are simply virtue-signaling. They're not even worn effectively most of the time. It's utterly ridiculous. Seeing these unfortunate, uneducated people — I'm not saying that in a pejorative sense — seeing these people walking around like lemmings, obeying without any knowledge base, to put the mask on their face.

Social distancing is also useless because COVID is spread by aerosols which travel 30 meters or so before landing. Enclosures have had such terrible unintended consequences. Everywhere should be opened tomorrow as was stated in the Great Barrington Declaration that I circulated prior to this meeting.

And a word on testing: I do want to emphasize that I'm in the business of testing for COVID. I do want to emphasize that positive test results do not – underlined in neon – mean a clinical infection. It's simply driving public hysteria and **all testing should stop.** Unless you're presenting to the hospital with some respiratory problem.[1828]

Dr. Hodkins' opinion on this is not an isolated one. More than 14,879 medical and public health scientists and 43,804 public health practitioners have signed the Great Barrington Declaration against the prevailing COVID-19 masking, social distancing, and testing policies.[1829]

Dr. Paul E. Alexander is an expert in clinical epidemiology; he is a former COVID Pandemic Advisor to the WHO and the Pan American Health Organization; he was a former senior advisor on the COVID Pandemic in the Department of Health and Human Services during the Trump administration. Dr. Alexander states that there is no COVID pandemic, and the masking, social distancing, and vaccines recommended by the state and federal governments are unnecessary. He considers the alleged SARS-CoV-2 virus thought to cause COVID-19 no more virulent than the common flu.[1830]

69 Requiring Unsafe and Ineffective Masks

Requiring the unvaccinated to wear a mask to protect others makes no sense. If the vaccines were effective, the vaccinated would not need protection against the unvaccinated because they would be immune from the disease. Now that the vaccines have been proven ineffective, when required, masking rules are being applied across the board regardless of vaccine status. Mask requirements have been arbitrarily required and periodically relaxed, but the specter of mask requirements is an ever-present cloud over the liberty of the population. Masking is irrational, and mandating a mask is unconstitutional and otherwise illegal. Adding insult to injury, wearing a mask does not work to prevent illness. And masks are unsafe.

Masking is not based on science. The science is decidedly against masks. But politicians in government were lobbied with false propaganda to institute mask mandates. The concept of masking is a dystopian control mechanism. It is not surprising, therefore, to find that George Gao, the Director-General of the Communist Chinese Center for Disease Control and Prevention (China CDC) and participant in Event 201, taking the lead by using fraudulent and deception to advocate wearing the ineffective and unsafe masks to purportedly prevent the spread of COVID-19.[1831]

On September 16, 2020, the Director of the CDC, Robert Redfield, held up a disposable medical mask (a.k.a., surgical mask) while testifying before the U.S. Congress about the COVID-19 response and stated that "these face masks are the most important and powerful public health tool we have. And I will continue to appeal for all Americans, all individuals in our country, to embrace these face coverings. I said it; if we did it for 6, 8, 10, 12 weeks, we would bring this pandemic under control. We have clear scientific evidence that they work, and they are our best defense."[1832] Dr. Redfield's statement that there was "clear scientific evidence" that masks work was a bald-faced lie. In actuality, the CDC (of which he was the director) published an authoritative study on its website that concluded just the opposite; the study concluded that face masks do not work to prevent the spread of disease. That study had already been posted on the CDC website for many months when Dr. Redfield falsely testified before Congress that there was "clear scientific evidence" that masks work to prevent the spread of disease.

In May 2020, the CDC published a report in its *Emerging Infectious Diseases Journal* involving a systematic review of 10 randomized controlled studies that "reported estimates of the effectiveness of face masks in reducing laboratory-confirmed influenza virus infections."[1833] The researchers found "no significant reduction in influenza transmission with the use of face masks." The report reviewed studies involving disposable medical masks (the very same type of surgical mask held up by Dr. Redfield during his Congressional testimony) and found that "[t]here is limited evidence for their effectiveness in preventing influenza virus transmission either when worn by the infected person for source control or when worn by uninfected persons to reduce exposure." The researchers concluded that their "systematic review found no significant effect of face masks on transmission of laboratory-confirmed influenza."[1834]

A mask requirement is based on the premise that wearing a face mask is safe and effective. Upon examination of the science, we find that supporting data for wearing masks is not only lacking, but the weight of the scientific evidence is that wearing a mask is unsafe and ineffective.

Not only are masks ineffective in protecting the wearer they are also ineffective in protecting others. Indeed, there is no standard to even measure the effectiveness of a mask as source control to safeguard others from expired human-generated aerosols. The American Society for Testing Materials Standard Specification For Barrier Face Coverings (ASTM F3502-23a) states that there are no currently established methods for testing or measuring the outward leakage of masks as source control. Thus, no one can claim a mask will protect others from human-generated aerosols coming from the mask's wearer. ASTM states:

> There are currently no established methods for measuring outward leakage from a barrier face covering, medical mask, or respirator. Nothing in this specification addresses or implies a quantitative assessment of outward leakage and no claims can be made about the degree to which a barrier face covering reduces expired human-generated aerosols.[1835]

In a February 2023 Cochrane study, researchers at institutions in the U.K., Canada, Australia, Italy, and Saudi Arabia analyzed a total of 78 studies. The most recent studies included six that were conducted during the COVID-19 pandemic. The researchers concluded from their analysis of the studies that "[w]earing masks in the community probably makes little or no difference to the outcome of influenza-like illness (ILI)/COVID-19 like illness compared to not wearing masks." The researchers further found that "[t]here were no clear differences between the use of medical/surgical masks compared with N95/P2 respirators in healthcare workers when used in routine care to reduce respiratory viral infection."

In an April 5, 2023, meta-analytic study, researchers found that "blood oxygen is significantly lowered in mask use."[1836] They further concluded that "blood carbon dioxide (PtCO2, ETCO2, and PaCO2) is significantly elevated in mask use."[1837] The "meta-analysis clearly depicts that masks, and especially the N95 masks, significantly restrict O2 uptake and hinder CO_2 release."[1838]

The increase in CO_2 and decrease in O2 causes oxidative stress, which inhibits cell-mediated immune responses to fight viral infections. That causes immune suppression. That sets the stage for contracting diseases, "including SARS-CoV-2 and making the consequences of that infection much more severe. In essence, masks may put wearers at an increased risk of infection and severity."[1839]

The study further determined that "[o]phthalmological studies indicated risk of retinal damage from long-term use of masks."[1840] The researchers noted that "[n]eurologists observed changes in MRI brain signal baseline level due to face mask use. ... The MRI imaging revealed a significant drop in brain oxygenation."[1841] They likened the morphological change as being similar to that caused by holding one's breath.

Headway, a brain injury association, explains that "[t]he brain needs a continuous supply of oxygen to survive. If the oxygen supply is interrupted, the functioning of the brain is disturbed immediately and irreversible damage can quickly follow."[1842] Headache is the most commonly reported symptom of wearing a mask.[1843] Such headaches are indicative of a low-oxygen environment known as hypoxia. A low-oxygen environment (hypoxia) induced by wearing a mask over the mouth and nose causes brain cells to die. The brain cannot regenerate cells. Thus, hypoxia from wearing a mask will cause irreversible brain damage.

Interestingly, the researchers found that "[n]early 40% of main long-COVID-19 symptoms overlap with mask related complaints and symptoms."[1844] Thus, what has been called long-COVID may, in fact, be induced by the immune impairment caused by wearing masks that increase the CO_2 and lower the oxygen in the blood. The researchers opined, "[i]t is possible that some symptoms attributed to long-COVID-19 are predominantly mask-related."[1845]

Another study in a large U.K. hospital involved a group of hospital staff who did not wear masks for 40 weeks in 2022. The COVID-19 infection incidence in the study group was compared to the control group of hospital staff who continued to wear masks. The study concluded that "removal of the [hospital] mask policy was not associated with a statistically significant change in the rate of nosocomial [i.e., originating from the hospital] SARSCoV-2 infection in the study group."[1846] A notable detail is that during the 40-week study, the omicron COVID-19 variant was the dominant COVID-19 virus. That alleged variant was reputed to be the most infectious of the COVID-19 variants. Thus, if masks were to show efficacy, they would have done so during that study.

A landmark randomized study conducted in Denmark included a control group found that face masks are ineffective in preventing the spread of COVID-19. Carl Heneghan and Tom Jefferson, writng for *The Spectator*, summarized the study: "In the end, there was no statistically significant difference between those who wore masks and those who did not wear masks when it came to being infected by COVID-19. 1.8 percent of those wearing masks caught COVID, compared to 2.1 percent of the control Group."

The randomized and controlled Denmark study that Heneghan and Jefferson summarized contradicts the less scientific observational studies done in the Far East that alleged some benefit to wearing masks to prevent COVID-19. Observational studies have inherent deficiencies that often cause the observers to reach faulty conclusions. Heneghan and Jefferson point out that "observational studies are prone to recall bias: in the heat of a pandemic, not very many people will recall if and when they used masks and at what distance they kept from others. The lack of random allocation of masks can also 'confound' the results and might not account for seasonal effects."[1847] A randomized controlled study, like the Denmark mask study, removes the inherent unreliability that attends observational studies.

William Kaplan, was appointed as an arbitrator to decide a dispute between the Ontario Hospital Association (OHA) and the Ontario Nurse's Association (ONA). The collective bargaining agreement allowed the nurses working in the association hospitals to refuse influenza (flu) vaccination. The HOA imposed a new policy whereby if a nurse refused the influenza vaccine she would have to wear a mask while in the hospital. It was called a vaccine or mask policy (VOM). The ONA brought a complaint that the policy was coercive and, thus, in violation of the collective bargaining agreement.[1848]

The arbitrator in *St. Michael's Hospital* conducted 21 hearings spanning three years. He presided over testimony from many expert witnesses, reviewed many volumes of scientific studies, meta-analyses, commentaries, and expert commentaries. The arbitrator found that the VOM was not coercive, but he nonetheless struck it down because he determined that it was unreasonable.

In 2018 Kaplan rendered his opinion and determined that the scientific studies and expert testimony established that masks are ineffective in preventing nurses from spreading the flu to others. He further determined that masks are ineffective in protecting nurses from getting the flu. The arbitrator ruled that "[t]here is no persuasive evidence establishing a conclusive relationship between the use of surgical and procedural masks and protection against influenza transmission." The arbitrator cited one particular scientific study, which concluded that "there is a lack of substantial evidence to support claims that face-masks protect either patient or surgeon from infectious contamination." The arbitrator cited the U.S. Centers for Disease Control (CDC), which stated categorically: "No studies have definitively shown that mask use by either infectious patients or health-care personnel prevents influenza transmission."

Regarding the asymptomatic or pre-symptomatic transmission of the flu, the arbitrator stated that "[a]t best, the evidence indicates that asymptomatic transmission is not a significant factor in nosocomial [hospital-originating] influenza." The arbitrator cited to a credible expert witness who testified that "[t]he evidence that pre-symptomatic or asymptomatic infections contribute substantially to influenza transmission remains scant."

On April 1, 2020, the New England Journal of Medicine published an article that concluded that "wearing a mask outside health care facilities offers little, if any, protection from infection." The article went on to state that "[t]he chance of catching Covid-19 from a passing interaction in a public space is therefore minimal."[1849] The article was authored by:

> Michael Klompas, M.D., M.P.H.,
> Charles A. Morris, M.D., M.P.H.,
> Julia Sinclair, M.B.A.,
> Madelyn Pearson, D.N.P., R.N.,
> and Erica S. Shenoy, M.D., Ph.D.
>
> Author Affiliations: From the Department of Population Medicine, Harvard Medical School and Harvard Pilgrim Health Care Institute (M.K.), Brigham and Women's Hospital (M.K., C.A.M., J.S., M.P.), Harvard Medical School (M.K., C.A.M., E.S.S.), and the Infection Control Unit and

> Division of Infectious Diseases, Massachusetts General Hospital (E.S.S.) — all in Boston.

In a bizarre twist, the New England Journal of Medicine posted the following notice in a ribbon above the study:

> Editor's Note: This article was published on April 1, 2020, at NEJM.org. In a letter to the editor on June 3, 2020, the authors of this article state "We strongly support the calls of public health agencies for all people to wear masks when circumstances compel them to be within 6 ft of others for sustained periods."

That strange statement contradicts the conclusion drawn from their study that "[t]he chance of catching Covid-19 from a passing interaction in a public space is therefore minimal. In many cases, the desire for widespread masking is a reflexive reaction to anxiety over the pandemic." Their study with attributed authority says wearing a mask is ineffective, but later without citing any reason or authority, they make what seems to be a political statement saying to wear those ineffective masks anyway. That nonsense statement that contradicted the results of the study was obviously the result of institutional pressure.

Denis G. Rancourt, Ph.D., researched the effectiveness of wearing a mask and concluded that masks and respirators do not work in preventing influenza-like illnesses. Dr. Rancourt concluded:

> There have been extensive randomized controlled trial (RCT) studies, and meta-analysis reviews of RCT studies, which all show that masks and respirators do not work to prevent respiratory influenza-like illnesses, or respiratory illnesses believed to be transmitted by droplets and aerosol

particles.

***

> Furthermore, individuals should know that there is no known benefit arising from wearing a mask in a viral respiratory illness epidemic, and that scientific studies have shown that any benefit must be residually small, compared to other and determinative factors.[1850]

On September 20, 2022, the U.S. Centers for Disease Control (CDC) published a study showing that of the patients who tested positive for COVID-19, 85% (70.6% + 14.4% = 85%) of them either always wore a mask or often wore a mask. Thus, the study indicates that masks are largely ineffective in preventing the contraction of COVID-19.[1851] Another interesting outcome of the study is that 88.7% of non-COVID-19 participants either always wore a mask or often wore a mask. They, nonetheless, were symptomatic with flu-like illnesses. There seems to be a high correlation between wearing a mask and becoming ill from disease.[1852]

To assess community and close contact exposures associated with COVID-19, exposures reported by case-patients (154) were compared with exposures reported by control-participants (160). Case-patients were symptomatic adults (persons aged =18 years) with SARS-CoV-2 infection confirmed by reverse transcription–polymerase chain reaction (RT-PCR) testing. Control-participants were symptomatic outpatient adults from the same health care facilities who had negative SARS-CoV-2 test results.

Reported use of cloth face covering or mask 14 days before illness onset (missing = 2)

Characteristics	**Case Patients Symptomatic and Testing Positive for COVID-19** (n=154)	Control Participants Symptomatic But Testing Negative for COVID-19 (n=160)	P-Value
Never Wore Mask	6 (3.9%)	5 (3.1%)	0.86
Rarely Wore Mask	6 (3.9%)	6 (3.8%)	
Sometimes Wore Mask	11 (7.2%)	7 (14.5%)	
Often Wore Mask	22 **(14.4%)**	23 (14.5%)	
Always Wore Mask	109 **(70.6%)**	118 (74.2%)	

Above is the pertinent mask portion of the study published by the CDC on September 11, 2020, regarding COVID-19 contact exposures with the notable statistics highlighted, bold emphasis added, and the description from the study moved and appended above the chart. Notice that those who either often wore a mask or always wore a mask ended up being symptomatic with flu-like illnesses at a high rate. 85% tested positive for COVID-19 and 88.7% tested negative for COVID-19. But both groups who often or always wore masks got sick. As you can see from the above statistics, the longer a person wears a mask, the more likely he is to become ill.

With evidence in its own September 11, 2020, study showing that masks are ineffective (indeed detrimental), the CDC knew they had a problem. So, on February 4, 2022, the CDC conducted a new study it manipulated to falsely show that masks are effective. The chicanery in that study was so clear that Rafael King writing for Frontline News, concluded that "[t]he CDC's new study further erodes an already weak level of public trust in public health officials"[1853] A close reading of the actual data in the new study does not support the CDC's conclusion that masks are safe and effective that was falsely portrayed by the loud graphics published by the CDC. Vinay Prasad, M.D., MPH, hematologist-oncologist and Associate Professor in the Department of Epidemiology and Biostatistics at the University of California San Francisco, summed up the improprieties and data manipulations in the CDC study. "What happened to science? When the pandemic ends, and people have no faith in public health, it would be wrong to blame Joe Rogan. It's institutions like the CDC and our leaders who push bad info masquerading as science."[1854]

Dr. Russell Blaylock is a nationally recognized board-certified neurosurgeon, health practitioner, author, and lecturer. Dr. Blaylock stated on May 11, 2021 that "a recent careful examination of the literature, in which 17 of the best studies were analyzed, concluded that, 'None of the studies established a conclusive relationship between mask/respirator use and protection against influenza infection.' Keep in mind, no studies have been done to demonstrate that either a cloth mask or the N95 mask has any effect on transmission of the COVID-19 virus. Any recommendations, therefore, have to be based on studies of influenza virus transmission. And, as you have seen, there is no conclusive evidence of their efficiency in controlling flu virus transmission."[1855]

Dr. Brosseau is a national expert on respiratory protection and infectious diseases and professor (retired), University of Illinois at Chicago. Dr. Sietsema is also an expert on respiratory protection and an assistant professor at the University of Illinois at Chicago. The April 1, 2020, recommendation of the two doctors is based on a review of available literature and informed by professional expertise and consultation. These two eminent experts concluded: "Our review of relevant studies indicates that cloth masks will be ineffective at preventing SARS-CoV-2 transmission, whether worn as source control or as PPE [Personal Protective Equipment]."[1856]

The researchers further determined that "[t]here is no evidence that surgical masks worn by healthcare workers are effective at limiting the emission of small particles or in preventing contamination of wounds during surgery."[1857]

That in and of itself is an astounding finding since we are so accustomed to doctors wearing masks during surgery to prevent them from contaminating their patients. The two researchers determined that "[c]linical trials in the surgery theater have found no difference in wound infection rates with and without surgical masks. Despite these findings, it has been difficult for surgeons to give up a long-standing practice."[1858]

Checking the studies themselves bears out their conclusion. One research study conducted by Th. Goran Tunivall, M.D., spanned 115 weeks and involved 3,088 patients. There were 1,537 operations performed with face masks, resulting in 73 (4.7%) wound infections. But among the 1,551 operations performed without face masks, there were only 55 (3.5%) infections. Dr. Tunivall deemed the difference not to be statistically significant and confirmed the data from all other studies that face masks do not decrease postoperative infections. Indeed, Dr. Tunivall stated that "[i]t has never been shown that wearing surgical face masks decreases postoperative wound infections."[1859]

"The AAPS [American Association of Physicians and Surgeons], a national association of doctors founded in 1943, accurately delineates the physics and dynamics of face masks. Any government official that mandates the wearing of masks to prevent the spread of COVID-19 is acting in complete defiance of proven scientific facts."[1860]

The reason for requiring face masks is the alleged threat of asymptomatic transmission of SARS-CoV-2, the alleged virus purported to cause COVID-19. Asymptomatic transmission of SARS-C0V-2 is a theory that has never been proven. Indeed, it is a theory that an authoritative scientific study has refuted. A research study conducted between May 14 and June 1, 2020, involving almost 10 million residents of Wuhan, China, found zero transmission of SARS-Cov-2 from asymptomatic carriers of the alleged virus. The report revealed that "[a]ll city residents aged six years or older were eligible and 9,899,828 (92.9%) participated." The researchers identified 300 asymptomatic positive cases. The researchers then closely contact traced the asymptomatic persons who tested positive for SARS-CoV-2. They found that "[t]here were no positive tests amongst 1,174 close contacts of asymptomatic cases."[1861]

The ineffectiveness of masks is known among infectious disease experts. For example, In March 2020, Dr. Anthony Fauci, Director of the National Institute of Allergy and Infectious Diseases (NIAID), told CBS News chief medical correspondent Dr. Jonathan LaPook that there's no reason people in the U.S. should wear a mask. Fauci stated that "right now in the United States people should not be walking around with masks ... there is no reason to be walking around in a mask."[1862] Indeed, his statement is as true now as when he said it in March 2020. Dr. Fauci's advice has been confirmed as accurate by Dr. Juday Mikovits and Dr. Rahid Buttar.[1863] The advice not to wear a mask is advice that is also verified by infectious disease experts Drs. Dan Erickson and Atin Massihi.[1864] The World Health Organization (WHO) has also stated that "[t]he only people who should be wearing masks are healthy people who are taking care of someone who is sick or sick people who are coughing or sneezing when they are in public."[1865]

Former HHS Secretary Sylvia Burwell asked Anthony Fauci in an email, "I am traveling to [redacted]. Folks are suggesting I take a mask for the airport. Is this something I should do?" On February 5, 2020, Anthony Fauci responded in pertinent part:

> Masks are really for infected people to prevent them from spreading infection to people who are not infected rather than protecting uninfected people from acquiring infection. **The typical mask you buy in the drug store is not really effective in keeping out virus, which is small enough to pass through material.** It might, however, provide some slight benefit in keep out gross droplets if someone coughs or sneezes on you. **I do not recommend that you wear a mask**, particularly since you are going to a very low risk location.
>
> Safe travels,
> Best regards,
> Tony[1866]

On February 29, 2020, the U.S. Surgeon General Jerome Adams firmly tweeted, "Seriously people- STOP BUYING MASKS!" The Surgeon General explained in the tweet that masks "are NOT effective in preventing the general public from catching coronavirus."[1867] (Emphasis in original)

The Washington Post reported that the U.S. Surgeon General Jerome Adams said on "Fox & Friends" on Monday morning. **"There are things people can do to stay safe. There are things they shouldn't be doing. One of the things they shouldn't be doing, the general public, is going out and buying masks. It actually does not help, and it has not been proven to be effective in preventing the spread of coronavirus amongst the general public."**[1868]

The U.S. Surgeon General explains that the surgical masks worn in hospitals serve one function only, and "that is mostly intended to protect the patient or outside world from the wearer's respiratory emissions. It is not considered to provide respiratory protection for the wearer."[1869]

There is another kind of mask that is intended to partially protect a worker. An N-95 mask falls in that category. The Washington Post further reported that Surgeon General Adams said that as a health-care worker, he has to get "fit tested" when wearing protective masks, and those who do not wear the masks properly tend to fidget with them or touch their faces — **which "actually can increase the spread of coronavirus.**"[1870]

That is correct. The U.S. Surgeon General said that the surgical masks that are commonly worn by the public can actually increase the spread of coronovirus.

On March 31, 2020, Fox News reported the Surgeon General saying:

> "What the World Health Organization [WHO] and the CDC [The Centers for Disease Control and Prevention] have reaffirmed in the last few days is that they do not recommend the general public wear masks."

He then explained the reasons why.

> "On an individual level, there was a study in 2015 looking at medical students and medical students wearing surgical masks touch their face on average 23 times," Adams explained. "We know a major way that you can get respiratory diseases like coronavirus is by touching a surface and then touching your face so wearing a mask improperly can actually increase your risk of getting disease."[1871]

Both Dr. Fauci and Surgeon General Adams later equivocated on their original no-mask opinions. But their reason for flip-flopping was based on a now discredited theory that asymptomatic people can infect other people with coronavirus. President Donald Trump recognized the strange flip-flop of Dr. Fauci and the U.S. Surgeon General about wearing face masks; the president also recognized the danger of wearing face masks. During a July 19, 2020, interview with Fox News' Chris Wallace, President Trump stated: "Hey, Dr. Fauci said 'don't wear a mask.' Our surgeon general, a terrific guy, said 'don't wear a mask.' Everybody was saying 'don't wear a mask.' All of a sudden everybody's got to wear a mask. And as you know masks cause problems too."[1872]

On April 3, 2020, the U.S. Surgeon General changed course and stated that masks are recommended to prevent the spread of COVID-19. But he explained that the mask is not a protective device. He did not back off on his reason for initially stating that masks are unnecessary and ineffective. He reiterated that a mask does not prevent a person from being infected, the mask only prevents a person who has COVID-19 from spreading it to another person. A mask does not protect a healthy person. A mask only prevents a person wearing the mask who is a carrier of COVID-19 from spreading the disease to another person.[1873] He changed course because the CDC theorized that a person who does not have symptoms COVID-19 could, nonetheless, spread the disease to another. The theory that asymptomatic carriers of COVID-19 could spread the disease has now been proven False.[1874]

Face Masks Are Unsafe

Nationally-renowned board-certified neurosurgeon Dr. Russell Blaylock states that "[w]hile most agree that the N95 mask can cause significant hypoxia [reduction in blood oxygenation] and hypercapnia [elevation of CO_2 in the blood], another study of surgical masks found significant reductions in blood oxygen as well. In this study, researchers examined the blood oxygen levels in 53 surgeons using an oximeter. They measured blood oxygenation before surgery as well as at the end of surgeries. The researchers found that the mask reduced the blood oxygen levels (paO2) significantly. The longer the duration of wearing the mask, the greater the fall in blood oxygen levels."[1875]

Dr. Blaylock points out that "the importance of these findings is that a drop in oxygen levels (hypoxia) is associated with an impairment in immunity. Studies have shown that hypoxia can inhibit the type of main immune cells used to fight viral infections called the CD4+ T-lymphocyte. This occurs because the hypoxia increases the level of a compound called hypoxia inducible factor-1 (HIF-1), which inhibits T-lymphocytes and stimulates a powerful immune inhibitor cell called the Tregs. This sets the stage for contracting any infection, including COVID-19 and making the consequences of that infection much graver. In essence, your mask may very well put you at an increased risk of infections and if so, having a much worse outcome."[1876]

Dr. Blaylock warns:

> There is another danger to wearing these masks on a daily basis, especially if worn for several hours. When a person is infected with a respiratory virus, they will expel some of the virus with each breath. If they are wearing a mask, especially an N95 mask or other tightly fitting mask, they will be constantly rebreathing the viruses, raising the concentration of the virus in the lungs and the nasal passages. We know that people who have the worst reactions to the coronavirus have the highest concentrations of the virus early on. And this leads to the deadly cytokine storm in a selected number. It gets even more frightening. Newer evidence suggests that in some cases the virus can enter the brain. In most instances it enters the brain by way of the olfactory nerves (smell nerves), which connect directly with the area of the brain dealing with recent memory

> and memory consolidation. By wearing a mask, the exhaled viruses will not be able to escape and will concentrate in the nasal passages, enter the olfactory nerves and travel into the brain.[1877]

Dr. Blaylock specifically cites cancer as a risk of wearing a mask. Indeed, this has been known since Nobel Laureate Otto Warburg's discovery in 1931, and subsequent studies have confirmed that a reduction in oxygen level in the body increases the risk of cancer.

In a research study by Dr. Blaylock that was published by the National Institute of Health (NIH), Dr. Blaylock states that "[i]t is now known that angiogenesis [in cancer cells] is an early process and is driven by hypoxia."[1878] Angiogenesis is the formation of new blood vessels. Angiogenesis is "a hallmark of cancer, being necessary for both the growth (progression) and spread (metastasis) of cancer."[1879] Dr. Blaylock further found that "[h]ypoxia is also known to increase expression of CXCR4, which stimulates tumor cell migration and is associated with highly aggressive tumors and a poor prognosis."[1880]

Dr. Blaylock states that "[p]eople with cancer, especially if the cancer has spread, will be at a further risk from prolonged hypoxia as the cancer grows best in a microenvironment that is low in oxygen. Low oxygen also promotes inflammation which can promote the growth, invasion and spread of cancers."[1881]

Dr. Blaylock has further found that "[r]epeated episodes of hypoxia has been proposed as a significant factor in atherosclerosis and hence increases all cardiovascular (heart attacks) and cerebrovascular (strokes) diseases."[1882]

Furthermore, according to the Occupational Safety and Health Administration (OSHA), "[o]xygen deficient atmosphere means an atmosphere with an oxygen content below 19.5%."[1883]

Richard E. Fairfax, Director of the Directorate of Enforcement Programs for OSHA explains in an official post that "[p]aragraph (d)(2)(iii) of the Respiratory Protection Standard considers any atmosphere with an oxygen level below 19.5 percent to be oxygen-deficient and immediately dangerous to life or health."[1884]

What would cause such an oxygen-deficient condition? According to OSHA, "[o]xygen-deficient atmospheres may be created when oxygen is displaced by inerting gases, such as carbon dioxide."[1885]

That displacement of air by exhaled carbon dioxide is precisely the condition a person finds himself in when wearing a mask over his mouth and nose. Such a practice lowers the oxygen level below the safe limit of 19.5%, which OSHA has deemed to be "immediately dangerous to life." That fact seems to be the cause of the deleterious health effects of wearing masks found in the studies cited by Dr. Blaylock.

The typical oxygen level is approximately 20.9%. But when a mask is put over the wearer's mouth and nose, the oxygen level being breathed back in by the wearer of a mask drops to a range between 17% and 18%.[1886]

That reduced level of oxygen, according to OSHA, is "immediately dangerous to life." And it does not matter whether it is a surgical mask, an N95 mask, or a thin cloth covering. In tests using all different types of masks, the oxygen level for the wearer dropped to a level below 19.5%, which OSHA has determined is an "oxygen-deficient atmosphere" that is "immediately dangerous to life." Indeed, one woman wearing a mask while driving her car passed out unconscious from oxygen deprivation and crashed into a wooden telephone pole.[1887]

But when pressed about wearing masks to prevent the

spread of COVID, OSHA cleverly dodged the issue by stating that the oxygen level standards in their regulations "do not apply to the wearing of medical masks or cloth face coverings."[1888] But the issue is not whether the regulations apply to wearing masks. Nobody argued that they do. The issue is whether the standard under their regulations for a safe oxygen level is true. On that matter, OSHA has not backed down. According to OSHA, an oxygen level below 19.5 percent to be oxygen-deficient and immediately dangerous to life or health."[1889] Thus, wearing a mask that reduces the oxygen behind the mask to 17-18% is immediately dangerous to life.

Wearing masks creates an environment of moist warm air conducive to the incubation of pathogens. The breathing of those pathogens introduces them into the mouth and lungs and on the skin causing infections of the skin, tooth decay, and other illnesses. Some of those pathogens have been found to be resistant to antibiotics. For example, laboratory analysis of six face masks worn by children at a Florida school found that "five masks were contaminated with bacteria, parasites, and fungi, including three with dangerous pathogenic and pneumonia-causing bacteria."[1890] One-third (33%) of the pathogens found in the masks were determined to be antibiotic-resistant pathogens.[1891]

Dr. Margarite Griesz-Brisson M.D., Ph.D.,[1892] is a Consultant Neurologist and Neurophysiologist. She has a Ph.D. in Pharmacology, specializing in neurotoxicology, environmental medicine, neuroregeneration and neuroplasticity. Dr. Grisz-Brisson is the founder and medical director of the London Neurology and Pain Clinic. Dr. Griesz-Brisson holds membership in the American Academy of Neurology, the European Federation of Neurological Societies (EFNS), the General Medical Council, United Kingdom, the German Medical Association, the Swiss Medical Society, the European Academy for Environmental Medicine, and the International Board for Clinical Metal Toxicology. Dr. Griesz-Brisson holds medical licenses in Germany, USA,

Switzerland, United Kingdom, Qatar, and Norway. She is one of the foremost experts in the world on the effects of oxygen deprivation on the brain. Dr. Griesz-Brisson states that wearing a mask over one's mouth and nose creates an oxygen deficiency and an increased intake of carbon dioxide. It causes an oxygen deficiency for the brain cells.[1893] In essence, the brain is being suffocated, which causes irreversible degeneration of the brain. Depriving the developing brain of needed oxygen causes brain damage that "cannot be reversed." Dr. Griesz-Brisson unequivocally warned that prolonged mask-wearing for hours on end will cause irreversible brain damage. She explains that the effects of oxygen deprivation are irreversible. Dr. Griesz-Brisson stated:

> The rebreathing of our exhaled air will without a doubt create oxygen deficiency and flooding of carbon dioxide. We know that the human brain is very sensitive to oxygen deprivation. There are nerve cells for example in the hippocampus that can't be longer than 3 minutes without oxygen – they cannot survive. The acute warning symptoms are headaches, drowsiness, dizziness, issues in concentration, slowing down of the reaction time – reactions of the cognitive system.
>
> However, when you have chronic oxygen deprivation, all of those symptoms disappear because you get used to it. But your efficiency will remain impaired, and the undersupply of oxygen in your brain continues to progress.
>
> We know that neurodegenerative diseases take years to decades to develop. If today you forget your phone number, the breakdown in your brain would have already started 20 or 30 years ago.

> While you're thinking that you have gotten used to wearing your mask and rebreathing your own exhaled air, the degenerative processes in your brain are getting amplified as your oxygen deprivation continues.
>
> The second problem is that the nerve cells in your brain are unable to divide themselves normally. So in case our governments will generously allow us to get rid of the masks and go back to breathing oxygen freely again in a few months, the lost nerve cells will no longer be regenerated. What is gone is gone.
>
> ***
>
> When in ten years, dementia is going to increase exponentially, and the younger generations couldn't reach their God-given potential, it won't help to say "we didn't need the masks."

Sayer Ji, writing for *Green Med Info*, reports that a Meta-Analysis of 65 scientific studies reveals that wearing a face mask induces a serious medical condition that has been labeled: Mask-Induced Exhaustion Syndrome (MIES).[1894] The research report, published in the *International Journal of Environmental Research and Public Health*, was written by eight doctors and researchers with broad scientific expertise in cellular anatomy, neuroscience, pathology, pathophysiology, psychology, and medicine.[1895]

The research paper reveals that "mask-related changes in respiratory physiology can have an adverse effect on the wearer's blood gases sub-clinically and in some cases also clinically manifest and, therefore, have a negative effect on the basis of all aerobic life, external and internal respiration, with an influence on a wide variety of organ systems and metabolic processes with physical, psychological and social consequences for the individual human being."[1896]

Masks Make Breathing Difficult: The study proves that due to airway resistance of the mask, "the mask acts as a disturbance factor in breathing and makes the observed compensatory reactions with an increase in breathing frequency and simultaneous feeling of breathlessness plausible (increased work of the respiratory muscles). This extra strain due to the amplified work of breathing against bigger resistance caused by the masks also leads to intensified exhaustion with a rise in heart rate and increased CO_2 production."[1897]

Neurological Disorders from Wearing Masks: The restricted airflow causes a significant drop in oxygen intake and a concomitant increase in carbon dioxide intake. This causes the mask wearer to be confused, disoriented, and drowsy. The researchers found that these neurological impairments were a direct result of mask-wearing. "In view of the scientific data, this connection also appears to be indisputable."[1898] The study shows that "masks also restrict the cognitive abilities of the individual (measured using a Likert scale survey) accompanied by a decline in psycho-motoric abilities and consequently a reduced responsiveness (measured using a linear position transducer) as well as an overall reduced performance capability (measured with the Roberge Subjective Symptoms-during-Work Scale)."[1899]

Susceptibility to Accidents While Wearing Masks: The researchers determined that masks caused the wearer to suffer "confusion, impaired thinking, disorientation ... and in some cases a decrease in maximum speed and reaction time .... This can become clinically relevant especially with regard to the further reduced ability to react and the additional increased susceptibility to accidents of such patients when wearing masks."[1900]

Bacterial Infections from Masks: It was found that "germs (bacteria, fungi and viruses) accumulate on the outside and inside of the masks due to the warm and moist environment. They can cause clinically relevant fungal, bacterial or viral infections." The researchers cited a New York study that evaluated a random sample of 343 participants. The study found that frequent wearing of surgical mask type and N95 masks among healthcare workers during the COVID-19 pandemic "caused headache in 71.4% of participants, in addition to drowsiness in 23.6%, detectable skin damage in 51% and acne in 53% of mask users."

Mask Mouth: The researchers further also noted what has been come to be known as "mask mouth." "There are reports from dental communities about negative effects of masks and are accordingly titled 'mask mouth.' Provocation of gingivitis (inflammation of the gums), halitosis (bad breath), candidiasis (fungal infestation of the mucous membranes with Candida albicans) and cheilitis (inflammation of the lips), especially of the corners of the mouth, and even plaque and caries are attributed to the excessive and improper use of masks."[1901] The researchers found that "the main trigger of the oral diseases mentioned is an increased dry mouth due to a reduced saliva flow and increased breathing through the open mouth under the mask. Mouth breathing causes surface dehydration and reduced salivary flow rate. Dry mouth is scientifically proven due to mask wear. The bad habit of breathing through the open mouth while wearing a mask seems plausible because such breathing pattern compensates for the increased breathing resistance, especially when inhaling through the masks. In turn, the outer skin moisture with altered skin flora, which has already been described under dermatological side effects, is held responsible as an explanation for the inflammation of the lips and corners of the mouth (cheilitis). This clearly shows the disease-promoting reversal of the natural conditions caused by masks. The physiological internal moisture with external dryness in the oral cavity converts into internal dryness with external moisture."[1902]

Voice Disorders: The report noted that "masks act like an acoustic filter and provoke excessively loud speech. This causes a voice disorder. The increased volume of speech also contributes to increased aerosol production by the mask wearer."[1903]

Masks Increase the Spread of Germs: The researchers found that masks increase germs because "the masks act like nebulizers and contribute to the production of very fine aerosols. Smaller particles, however, spread faster and further than large ones for physical reasons. Of particular interest in this experimental reference study was the finding that a test subject wearing a single-layer fabric mask was also able to release a total of 384% more particles (of various sizes) when breathing than a person without."[1904]

Masks Cause Depression in Wearers: There were also found severe psychological effects of mask-wearing. "[M]asks also frequently cause anxiety and psycho-vegetative stress reactions in children—as well as in adults—with an increase in psychosomatic and stress-related illnesses and depressive self-experience, reduced participation, social withdrawal and lowered health-related self-care. Over 50% of the mask wearers studied had at least mild depressive feelings."[1905]

There is reasonable medical certainty that wearing a face mask will cause hypoxia, hypercapnia, and other conditions that would be dangerous to my health.

Dr. Zacharias Fögen, MD, conducted a study where he compared counties in Kansas that instituted mask mandates with counties in Kansas that did not institute mask mandates.[1906] The comparative study showed that there was a significantly increased fatality rate from COVID-19 in those counties that required the wearing of masks. The report states: "Results from this study strongly suggest that mask mandates actually caused about 1.5 times the number of deaths or ~50% more deaths compared to no mask mandates."[1907] Dr. Fogen concluded that "[t]hese findings suggest that mask use might pose a yet unknown threat to the user instead of protecting them, making mask mandates a debatable epidemiologic intervention."[1908]

Dr. Fogen theorized the increased death rate was from the spread of virions deeper into the respiratory tract due to "deep inhalation of hypercondensed droplets or pure virions caught in facemasks."[1909] The report states:

> A rationale for the increased RR [risk ratio] by mandating masks is probably that virions that enter or those coughed out in droplets are retained in the facemask tissue, and after quick evaporation of the droplets, hypercondensed droplets or pure virions (virions not inside a droplet) are re-inhaled from a very short distance during inspiration.[1910] (endnote citation deleted)

Basically, the mask wearers are re-inhaling a hypercondensed aerosol of germs trapped by the mask. The mask acts as a petri-dish over the mouth and nose of the wearer, who then inhales the contaminants that have coagulated inside the mask.

Masks Contain Toxic Substances

Chris Schaefer is a respirator specialist and recognized authority on respirators and masks. He has taught fit testing for respirators for more than 20 years. His company, SafeCom Training Services Inc., has clients that include the Canadian government and military. Schaefer opines that the masks that have been mandated are not truly masks but rather breathing barriers that block the wearer's air. Schaefer states that the mask "captures carbon dioxide that you exhale, forces you to re-inhale it, causing a reduction in your inhaled oxygen levels and causes excessive carbon dioxide. So they're not safe to wear."[1911]

But Schaefer mentions another risk of wearing masks that is often overlooked. Melt-blown fabric is the core material used in the production of surgical masks, and its major component is polypropylene (PP). As surgical masks are worn, those microscopic PP particles are inhaled by the wearer. Shaefer states:

> As far as whether it could cause somebody to inhale the polypropylene fibres that are used to make this and synthetic polymers that are used to make the filtration of these devices — absolutely. Take a pair of scissors and cut one open. You can see that in between the two main covers that are encapsulating, these loose fibres are breaking away. They're becoming dislodged from the cover itself, just through normal wear and tear and the agitation of putting it on and taking it off.
>
> The heat and moisture that it captures will cause the degradation of those fibres to break down smaller. Absolutely, people are inhaling [microplastic particles]. I've written very extensively on the hazards of these breathing barriers the last two years, I've spoken to scientists [and other] people for the last two years about people inhaling the fibres. If you get the sensation that you've gotten a little bit of cat hair, or any type of irritation in the back of your throat after wearing them. That means you're inhaling the fibres.[1912]

Amanda Brown, reporting for Western Standard, revealed that a recent study from Great Britain seems to confirm the opinion of Schaefer.

> Microplastic fibres were found deep in the lower

lungs of living human beings in almost every person sampled in a recent UK study.

The study from Great Britain discovered microplastic particles — present in many COVID-19 masks — in the lung tissue of 11 out of 13 patients undergoing surgery.

Polypropylene (PP) and polyethylene terephthalate (PET) were the most prevalent substances present in the lungs.

The microscopic plastic fragments and fibres were discovered by scientists at Hull York Medical School in the UK. Some of the filaments were two millimetres long in patients undergoing surgery whose lung tissue they sampled.

The plastic dust and microscopic debris comprises the same plastics used to manufacture the ubiquitous surgical masks worn by hundreds of millions of people around the world as mandated by governments in an attempt to halt the spread of COVID-19.

The material most commonly used to make these masks is PP — PP fabric is made from a "thermoplastic" polymer, meaning that it's easy to work with and shape at high temperatures.

Blue surgical masks can also be made of polystyrene, polycarbonate, polyethylene, or polyester, all of which are types of fabrics derived from thermoplastic polymers.

Disposable blue masks are to be found littering

> almost every city street in the developed world after two years of COVID-19 mandates ruled that masks should be worn in most indoor environments much of the time. Healthy adults, children, the immunocompromised, and the elderly have all been subject to mask mandates.[1913]

The authors of another study that was designed to measure the effectiveness of masks did not make a finding of masks being the source of inhaled plastic micro fibers, but warned:

> Surgical masks have three layers. The front and back covers are made of PP, with a fiber diameter of approximately 20 μm. The middle layer of surgical masks is melt-blown fabric, which is the core material for virus rejection. Microplastics or nanoplastics can be generated during the use and reuse of masks made from the aforementioned materials. This condition can lead to the risk of microplastic inhalation via breathing.[1914] (citations omitted)

Dr. Colleen Huber warns:

> If widespread masking continues, then the potential for inhaling mask fibers and environmental and biological debris continues on a daily basis for hundreds of millions of people. This should be alarming for physicians and epidemiologists knowledgeable in occupational hazards.[1915]

Dr. Carla Peters, who earned a Ph.D. in Immunology, reveals that "[m]any scientific studies and analysis all arrive at the same conclusion: the wearing of masks by healthy people cannot stop the spread of a virus."[1916] But ineffectiveness is not the end of the story. Research has shown that wearing masks drives and increases what has been characterized as COVID-19.

As we have seen, the masks create a hypoxic and hypercapnic environment that makes people ill. It is, therefore, no surprise that they would be diagnosed with COVID-19. But there is another danger posed by masks that is also driving illnesses. Dr. Peters reveals that masks produced throughout the world used by medical personnel and the general public contain "a diversity of plastics, toxic and cancerous compounds like perfluorocarbon, aniline, phthalate, formaldehyde, bisfenol A as well as heavy metals, biocides (zinc oxide, graphene oxide) and nanoparticles."[1917]

Fifteen scientists did a study of batches of disposable masks from twelve different manufacturers sourced from around the world. The scientists found that 70% of the disposable masks contain titanium dioxide (TiO_2), a suspected human carcinogen, that, when inhaled, poses a danger to the health of the mask wearers.[1918] The scientists explained that TiO_2 is commonly applied in face masks to improve stability to ultraviolet light, as a white colorant, or as a matting agent.[1919] The scientists revealed that "[i]n animal experiments, toxic effects were reported when TiO_2 particles were inhaled."[1920]

Dr. Carla Peters revealed that "the Belgian Sciensano found titanium dioxide in 24 different single and reusable types of facemasks meant for the general public systemically exceeded the acceptable exposure level by inhalation when masks are worn intensively."[1921] Dr. Peters further explained:

> In Germany, The Netherlands and Canada millions of masks have been retracted from the market due to the presence of graphene-oxide known in ECHA as a substance causing eye irritation, skin irritation and may cause respiratory irritation. In a review on graphene nanoparticles the underlying toxicity has

> been revealed, for instance physical destruction, oxidative stress, DNA damage, inflammatory response, apoptosis, autophagy and necrosis.[1922]

Dr. Peters states that "''[t]he large part of available current literature indicates that graphene-based nanomaterials are cytotoxic.''[1923] A study cited by Dr. Peters explains the damage that can be done through inhaled graphene oxide:

> The lungs are a potential entrance for graphene nanoparticles into the human body through [the] airway. The inhaled GO [graphene oxide] nanosheets can destroy the ultrastructure and biophysical properties of pulmonary surfactant (PS) film, which is the first line of host defense, and emerge their potential toxicity. ... GO can result in acute inflammation response and chronic injury by interfering with the normal physiological functions of important organs.[1924]

Dr. Peters reveals the many illnesses caused by titanium dioxide exposure.

> A recent publication in Gut[1925] showed that exposure to titanium dioxide could exacerbate inflammation of the colon (Colitis Ulcerosa) weakening the innate immune system. Furthermore, titanium dioxide can enter directly into the brain and cause oxidative stress in glial cells (or mast cells), cells with an important role in the proper functioning of the innate immune system and nervous system. Maternal exposure to titanium dioxide during pregnancy may result in impaired memory in the infant. Long-term exposure and high concentrations could even cause DNA damage. Unfortunately, masks with titanium dioxide are still

available on the market.[1926]

Inflating the COVID-19 Statistics

In December 2020, Tyler Durden reported that researcher Justin Hart had determined that "states with mask mandates had a greater number of COVID cases per 100,000 people than states without mandates." Hart "looked at cases on days where mask mandates were in place vs when they were not. We calculated the cases per day adjusted for population." Hart found that "[w]ith mandates in place states say 10 more cases per 100K population." That amounts to a 38% increase in COVID-19 cases when masks are mandated over when masks are not mandated.[1927]

Why is there an increase in COVID-19 cases when masks are mandated? It is because the masks cause the same symptoms indicative of COVID-19.

It is interesting to note that many of the listed clinical criteria for a COVID-19 probable case, as defined by the CDC, are symptoms that are common for persons who wear masks. For example, one of the listed clinical symptoms of COVID-19 is a headache. Cove, a professional medical blog devoted to migraine and headache relief, reveals:

> A 2006 study[1928] of 212 healthcare workers required to wear the medical-grade N95 face mask found that 37% said the mask gave them headaches, and 32% of those people had headaches more than six times a month. In a newer study[1929] at the National University Hospital in Singapore, 81% of medical personnel who wore the N95 mask for 6 hours a day developed headaches. 23% of participants said their headaches included migraine symptoms[1930] like nausea and photophobia.[1931]

The headaches caused by wearing a mask are a direct result of the lowered oxygen in the blood (hypoxia) and the raised carbon dioxide in the blood (hypercapnia). As long as people continue to wear masks and display the flu-like symptoms that result from the hypoxia and hypercapnia caused by the masks, those people will be classified as probable COVID-19 cases. Dr. Russell Blaylock explains that hypoxia can inhibit the immune cells that fight viral infections.[1932] The hypoxic environment in the body sets the stage for symptoms that would be diagnosed as COVID-19.

That means that the same masks people wear to prevent COVID-19 may cause many diseases, including what is thought to be influenza or what is thought to be COVID-19. People who wear masks may show up at their doctor's office with the flu because they wore a mask.

Under the new probable case[1933] definition, the same symptoms typical of the flu and caused by the masks would be deemed COVID-19. Indeed, it seems that the alleged COVID-19 cases are actually influenza cases being misdiagnosed as COVID-19 cases. That explains why influenza disappeared during the 2020-2021 influenza season. People who wear masks may show up at their doctor's office with the flu because they wore a mask.

Under the new "probable case"[1934] definition for COVID-19 from the CDC, a person would be listed as a COVID-19 case if he has a headache (which is a typical side effect of wearing a mask) and also has a fever or muscle aches or a sore throat or difficulty smelling things or difficulty tasting things and was within the last 14 days in close contact with another person who was deemed to be a "probable case" for COVID-19.[1935]

A person with the above symptoms does not even need to have been in contact with a person who was deemed a probable COVID-19 case. Under the new CDC criteria for diagnosing

COVID-19, a person who manifests the above symptoms could be considered a probable COVID-19 case if he traveled to or had a residence "in an area with sustained, ongoing community transmission" of COVID-19.[1936]

The government is pulling a slick trick. It mandates people to wear masks. The masks cause symptoms that the government lists as indicative of a probable case of COVID-19. The doctors follow the CDC guidance on what is a probable case of COVID-19 and diagnose the person with COVID-19. Thus, the government can inflate its COVID-19 statistics to keep the phony pandemic going.[1937]

On May 26, 2020, Collin County, Texas, Judge Chris Hill remarked how easy it was to classify someone with COVID-19 under the new CDC rules for a probable case. He said: "It is remarkable how low the standard is now."[1938] The concern of county officials was that "[t]he increase in false positives will result in more residents quarantined for insignificant reasons and will raise public distrust of the state's reporting."[1939] The county officials do not understand that increasing false positives is not a bureaucratic snafu. It is the plan. Below are slides from Collin County, Texas, that graphically reveals the scam being run by the CDC, with its new scheme of counting "probable"[1940] cases. The liars at the CDC were successful in getting officials nationwide to inflate their COVID-19 cases through a definitional trick.

Current Case Definition

- Confirmed case of COVID-19
  - Positive PCR lab result for COVID-19

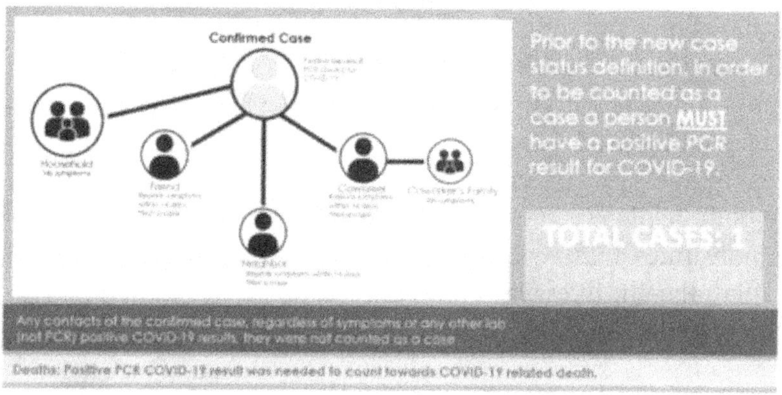

NEW Probable Case Definition

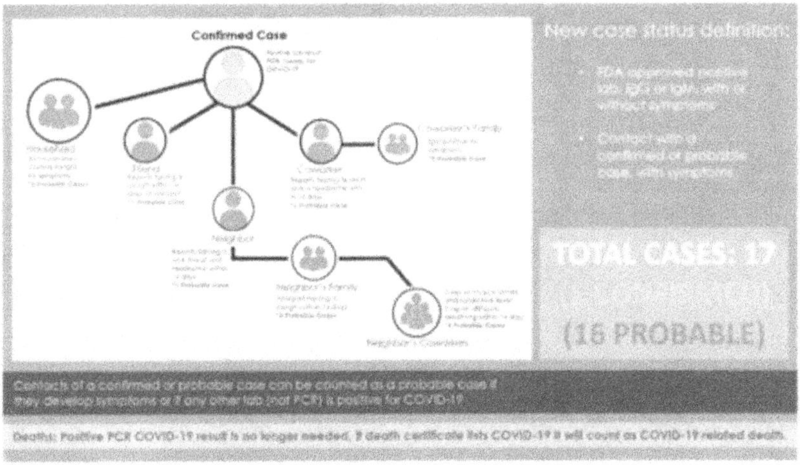

Above are slides from Collin County, Texas, Showing how the new CDC definition of a COVID-19 case includes "probable" cases. By changing how the cases are reported, the CDC can create hysteria over a pandemic that does not truly exist. In the hypothetical case on the slide, one confirmed case can turn into 17 cases (1 confirmed case + 16 probable cases = 17 total cases).

We have entered Alice's Wonderland, where Humpty Dumpty scornfully said, "When I use a word, it means just what I choose it to mean — neither more nor less." If the CDC uses the word COVID-19, it means what the CDC chooses it to mean—neither more nor less.

The Virginia Department of Health graph provided by Ian Miller shows the sudden drop in COVID-19 cases among school children once the mask mandate in Virginia schools was ended.[1941] The graph shows an explosion in reported COVID-19 cases among school children after the school mask mandate was instituted. That was followed by a precipitous drop of 93% in reported COVID-19 cases immediately after the school mask mandate was lifted. This demonstrates that when people wear masks, they develop and display the flu-like symptoms that result from the hypoxia and hypercapnia caused by the masks. These Virginia schoolchildren were being classified as probable COVID-19 cases. Once the mask mandate for school children ended, the reported COVID-19 cases among school children dropped precipitously.

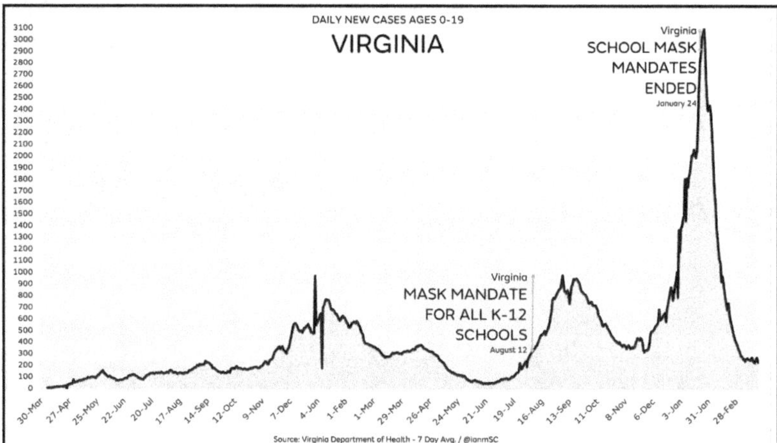

Graph from the Virginia Department of Health shows a sharp increase in reported COVID-19 cases among school children after the school mask mandate was instituted on August 12, 2021. And when the mask mandate was ended on January 24, 2022, the reported COVID-19 cases dropped precipitously by 93%.

States can classify someone with COVID-19 even though they have not tested positive for COVID-19. The longer a person wears a mask, the more likely they will display flu-like symptoms caused by hypoxia and hypercapnia. The mask-wearers who show flu-like symptoms are then added to the probable COVID-19 numbers, even though they do not have COVID-19. This has the effect of artificially inflating COVID-19 statistics. It is a vicious never-ending cycle of deception. Thankfully, the newly elected Governor of Virginia ended the cycle of deception, and in doing so, he exposed the scam.

On March 29, 2022, Frankie Stockes reported for National File about the stunning reversal in reported COVID-19 cases among the Virginia School children once the school mask mandate was lifted.[1942]

> Newly reported cases of COVID-19 in Virginia's children have dropped by a whopping 93% since Governor Glenn Youngkin ordered an end to school mask mandates upon taking office this January.
>
> A graph from the Virginia Department of Health charting newly reported COVID-19 cases in Virginians aged 0-19 was recently released showing the wild success of Republican Governor Glenn Youngkin's executive order bringing an end to Virginia's school mask mandates, which were enforced on children against the will of their parents.
>
> Despite hysterical warnings from those who claimed countless teachers and children would die were face freedom restored to Virginia's youth, newly reported COVID cases in the state's 0-19 age

> bracket have dropped by a whopping 93% since Governor Youngkin's executive order restoring parental rights went into effect. Though a number of left-wing school districts resisted Youngkin's order, claiming that state law allowed them the right to forcibly cover kids' faces, Youngkin later signed a bill passed by the state's legislature that made face freedom in schools the law of the land.
>
> ***
>
> According to a Virginia Department of Health graph shared on Twitter by [Ian] Miller, cases of COVID among Virginians aged 0-19 peaked under ex-Governor Ralph Northam and the Democrats' school mask mandates. Some days, thousands of new childhood COVID cases were reported as kids were forced to sit in school for hours with a germ-collecting mask pressed to their face – and no right to remove it!
>
> Immediately following the January 24th executive order to end school mask mandates in Virginia, the number of newly reported childhood COVID cases, which had reached as many as over 3,000 in one day, began a steady decline. By the end of February, cases had leveled out towards the bottom of the graph.[1943]

Despite the clear evidence that masks cause and exacerbate illnesses, some hysterical superstitious zealots treat the CDC masking advice[1944] as an *ex-cathedra* infallible pronouncement that must be believed and obeyed at all costs. Outrageously, a Virginia judge believed the nonsense that masks are efficacious and ordered that healthy school children be masked to protect the children of ignorant zealots. Stockes reports:

Despite the good news that Virginia's school kids are both safe and free to show their faces, some districts and pro-maskers within them have fought tooth and nail to keep masks on the faces of other people's children. Just recently, US District Court Judge Norman Moon ruled that 12 medically unwell children in Virginia can force their classes to make "reasonable modifications" to their setting, including the forced masking of other children against their own will and that of their parents.

That case was brought to the court by pro-mask parents and the far-left ACLU, who celebrated the ruling, boasting that it will serve as a "blueprint" for the continued forced masking of kids in school.[1945]

70 Compelling Symbolic Speech

Masks do not prevent the spread of COVID-19, because asymptomatic carriers cannot spread COVID-19, and thus, it is pointless for healthy people to wear masks. In addition, the masks do not prevent the wearer from being infected. Why then is the CDC now recommending that the public wear masks?

There is a reason for wearing masks that has been revealed by government officials. They explain that masks are symbolic. In essence, the mask is virtue signaling. USA Today reported that "[t]op infectious disease specialist Dr. Anthony Fauci said Wednesday that he wears a mask as a **'symbol'** of what 'you should be doing' during the coronavirus pandemic."[1946] You read that correctly. The mask is largely symbolic. Dr. Fauci elaborated:

> "I want to protect myself and protect others, and also because **I want to make it be a symbol for people to see that that's the kind of thing you should be doing,"** Fauci told CNN.[1947]

Dr. Fauci knows that the masks are not effective. He is on record saying so. Dr. Fauci views mask wearing a way to show respect for others.

> When asked by host Jim Sciutto if his wearing of a mask encouraged their use, Fauci acknowledged masks aren't "100% effective" but are a "valuable safeguard" and part of **"respect for another person."**[1948]

CNN explained that "[a]mid coronavirus surge, health officials urge people to wear masks as a symbol of respect."[1949] CNN argued that government health officials think that "[a] face mask is more than a piece of cloth. It's a sign of respect."[1950] CNN quotes Dr. Fauci saying **"It signifies one common good and that is care for the public health."**[1951] The article continues:

> "This is not about politics," said Dr. Leana Wen, Baltimore's former health commissioner, an emergency physician and public health professor at George Washington University. "This is about each of us **showing that we care about one another, that we respect one another."**
>
> Noting that behavior change takes time, Dr. Joshua Barocas, an infectious diseases physician at Boston Medical Center, says wearing a mask can help reduce transmission, help form a good habit and serve as a **sign of respect**. "I think beyond simply the viral transmission, **wearing a mask can just be a symbol**," said Barocas. **"It can show people that you are committed to the cause,** that you're committed to fighting Covid-19 as a community... committed to protecting other people's lives and their children's lives and their families' lives... committed to having a strong economy open when we're fully ready."
>
> Dr. Jessica Justman, an infectious diseases specialist and epidemiologist at Columbia

> University and attending physician at the Columbia University Irving Medical Center, says that **messaging plays an important role in the implementation of public health strategies**, like this one. She says that **it can make a difference when a leader dons a face mask as an example to others.**[1952]

Jeremy Howard, part of the Word Economic Forum Young Global Leaders program advocated for following the lead of the communist Chinese government in the U.S. response to COVID-19. Howard joined with Zeynep Tufekci, who thinks that when a social media company cancels an account "it's not an infringement of free speech."[1953] Howard and Tufekci were the two most instrumental influencers prodding governments to mandate masks. They also advocated that citizens follow the example of communist China and shut down businesses and institutions to stop the spread of COVID-19. The problem is that science did not support masking. But that did not stop Howard and Tufekci from falsely claiming that science had established that masking was effective.

It seems that the real reason for masking was symbolic. Howard and Tofekci argued that masking of citizens was primarily to convey a message. Howard and Tufekci considered masking to be important as "symbols of altruism and solidarity" and that "[r]itual and solidarity are important in human societies and can combine with visible signals to shape new societal behaviors."[1954] They advocated for mask mandates because they would "be highly effective in shaping new societal norms."[1955] The masks acted more as "a visible signal and reminder of the pandemic" than an effective way to stop the spread of COVID-19.

Masks are essentially symbolic. Symbols are inherently communicative. A symbol is defined in the Merriam-Webster Dictionary as "an authoritative summary of faith or doctrine:

creed."[1956] The definition continues: "a visible sign of something invisible. ... an object or act representing something in the unconscious mind that has been repressed ... an act, sound, or object having cultural significance and the capacity to excite or objectify a response"[1957] Thus, wearing a mask is symbolic of some invisible idea, and most significantly, religious doctrines or faith.

Everyone wearing a mask communicates an invisible idea or doctrine to others. When the government forces a person to wear a mask, it forces that person to communicate an idea. The government medical professionals acknowledge that fact. They have stated that wearing a mask is the communication part of the public health strategy The mask communicates that the wearer is "committed to the cause," that you "care for the public health" and as a "sign of respect." But what if a person disagrees with the public health strategy? Should a dissenting person be forced to wear a mask that falsely communicates to the world that they are "committed to the cause?" Certainly not! Just as a Democrat should not be forced to campaign on behalf of a Republican, a person should not be forced to wear a mask that communicates that he is committed to a cause to which he is certainly not committed. Government mask mandates are essentially government compelled speech. To compel speech is to violate a citizen's Constitutional First Amendment Right to free speech.

The U.S. Supreme Court has ruled that "[j]ust as the First Amendment may prevent the government from prohibiting speech, the Amendment may prevent the government from compelling individuals to express certain views."[1958] The U.S. Supreme Court has been strident on that point. "The right to speak and the right to refrain from speaking are complementary components of the broader concept of 'individual freedom of mind.'"[1959] The state cannot require a person to carry an ideological message on his private property[1960], in like manner, the state cannot require a person to wear a symbolic mask on his face that conveys an ideological message.

Mask Mandate Violates Freedom of Religion

Professor William Schaffner, a preventive medicine professor at the Vanderbilt University School of Medicine, revealed one of the impulses to wear masks. Dr. Shaffner explained that it comes down to psychology. He said that "[b]y getting masks and wearing them, we move the locus of control somewhat to ourselves."[1961] The masks don't do any good. They just make the wearer feel better. And that is just what Dr. Fauci said. Masks evoke an emotional response from the wearer.

Indeed, the Encyclopedia Britannica explains that mask-wearing is essentially a religious practice. Earlier in the Merriam-Webster Dictionary definition of symbol, we saw that symbols primarily convey "an authoritative summary of faith or doctrine: creed."[1962] The government medical authorities mandating masks admit that the masks are primarily symbolic. The Encyclopedia Britannica explains that the concept of masks having medical efficacy is closely associated with social convention and religious superstition. "Many masks are primarily associated with ceremonies that have religious and social significance or are concerned with funerary customs, fertility rites, or the **curing of sickness**."[1963] Masks are often worn by those taking part in occult and satanic rituals. According to Gayland Hurst, Ph.D., one of the characteristics of occult-related homicide is that the body is found wearing a mask.[1964] The symbolic wearing of a mask causes the person to take on an alter-ego, whereby a spirit being (i.e., a devil) acts through him. The Encyclopedia Britannica explains the religious meaning behind the wearing of masks:

> The person who wears the mask is also considered to be in direct association with the mask's spirit force and is consequently exposed to like personal danger of being affected by it. ... Upon donning the mask, the wearer sometimes undergoes a psychic change and as in a trance assumes the spirit

> character depicted by the mask. Usually, however, the wearer skillfully becomes a "partner" of the character he is impersonating, giving to the mask not only an important spark of vitality by the light flashing from his own eyes but also bringing it alive by his movements and poses. But often the wearer seems to become psychologically one with the character he is helping to create. He seems to become an automaton, without his own will, which has become subservient to that of the personage of the mask. At all times there remains some important, even if sub rosa, association between the mask and its wearer.[1965]

The practice of Satanists evidences that mask-wearing is an occult superstition. Those who practice Satanism are noted for non-conformity and rebellion against social and moral norms. But when it comes to wearing masks and being vaccinated, they suddenly become sticklers for conformity. That is because vaccination and masking are heathen religious practices. Satanic beliefs are the source of the vaccine and masking requirement, so it should not be surprising to find that Satanists strictly adhere to those practices. For example, the Satanic Temple sponsors a Satan Conference (Satancon). The Satanic Temple requires all attendees at their April 28-30, 2023 Satan Conference to be vaccinated and masked. The Satan Conference promotional website posts the warning:

> Satancon attendees must be 18 or over and have proof of COVID vaccination. Attendees must wear an N-95, KN-95, or disposable surgical mask. Gaiters, bandanas, and cloth masks will not be allowed.[1966]

As we have seen, the wearing of a mask is not medically efficacious. The government medical professionals claim the masks are efficacious but acknowledge that wearing a mask is primarily symbolic. Thus mask-wearing is, in essence, communicative. But the mask also has a spiritual effect on its wearer. To mandate the wearing of a mask is to impose a religious effect on the wearer in contravention of the wearer's Constitutional First Amendment right to freedom of religion and violates the establishment clause.[1967]

A Christian could have a sincerely held religious belief that the mask mandate is part of Satan's plan to subjugate the world under the rule of his Antichrist. Jesus describes Satan as the father of lies. "When he speaketh a lie, he speaketh of his own: for he is a liar, and the father of it." John 8:44. The mask mandate is based on a lie. Wearing a mask gives testimony to the world that the wearer is "committed to the cause."[1968] If a person is NOT "committed to the cause" because he understands that the cause is a deception, he should not be required to wear a mask.

To signify to the world that one is committed to the cause when one is not is a lie. To force someone to wear an ineffective and unsafe mask that only symbolizes his agreement with the COVID-19 deception that is contrary to his sincerely held religious beliefs violates the wearer's First Amendment rights to freedom of religion and freedom of speech. Forcing the objector to wear a mask makes the objector engage in compelled speech that he sincerely believes is a lie. Such compelled speech is a sin and an affront to religious liberty and freedom of speech. A Christian is called on to walk uprightly and not in a twisted deceitful way. "He that walketh uprightly walketh surely: but he that perverteth his ways shall be known." Proverbs 10:9. To walk with a mask that testifies to a lie is to walk in darkness. "If we say that we have fellowship with him, and walk in darkness, we lie, and do not the truth." 1 John 1:6. The mask has all of the appearance of evil, of which a Christian is called on to eschew. "Abstain from all appearance of evil." 1 Thessalonians 5:22.

Philip Buckler explains in his book, *The Book on Masks* that the the emotional-blackmail used to push compulsory vaccination and masking is eerily reminiscent of Johann Tetzel's indulgence sales tactics.[1969] It was those corrupt methods that led Martin Luther into posting his 95 theses, one of the notable events of the Protestant Reformation. Indulgences were sold to allegedly ease the suffering of those supposedly residing in a mythical place called purgatory. The money was given to the Roman Catholic Church who would then used its spiritual grace to influence God to lessen the time in the torments of purgatory and speed the resident toward his release from torments into heaven. Buckler explains that Johann Tetzel was one of the most effective in the business of selling indulgences:

> Don't you hear the voices of your wailing dead parents and others who say, 'Have mercy upon me, have mercy upon me, because we are in severe punishment and pain. From this you could redeem us with a small alms and yet you do not want to do so.' Open your ears as the father says to the son and the mother to the daughter, 'We have created you, fed you, cared for you, and left you our temporal goods. Why then are you so cruel and harsh that you do not want to save us, though it only takes a little? You let us lie in flames so that we only slowly come to the promised glory.'[1970]

Buckler explains:

> This is, at its core, the same basic argument that was used to "sell" masks and vaccines to avoid COVID-19 parallels between Johann Tetzel's sales pitch for indulgences and the public health browbeating to get people to participate in masking and vaccination during COVID are obvious. In modern terms, Tetzel's slogan was: "We have a

> moral obligation to buy indulgences to protect our family members," and "We don't have the right to keep people in purgatory." Compare this to: "We don't have the right to infect others," with all its underlying fallacious reasoning relating to causality and ultimate responsibility.[1971]

Philip Buckler explains in his *The Book on Masks* why a Christian should not wear a mask.

> It is not loving to cater to an untrue belief by pretending that it is true. That is dysfunctional enabling. A psychiatrist who makes an elaborate show of searching his office for surveillance devices before beginning counseling does nothing to help a patient who is suffering from paranoia . such actions merely validate that paranoia. If you have a friend who is convinced that investing their life savings in a particular stock is a good idea, and you have knowledge or even reasonable grounds to suspect the investment is a bad idea, it is not loving to reinforce their belief by purchasing some of that stock yourself, even if they ask you to do so. In cases where you and your neighbor both vehemently disagree about the factual basis of certain beliefs, the most loving thing is to tolerate their beliefs and practices while vigorously challenging them by argument and example. In the case of COVID or any other disease, this may include wearing or not wearing a mask, and vaccinating or refusing vaccination.[1972]

The argument against masks is very much similar to the Christian argument against vaccination. Vaccination has much in common with the religion of Molech. It is the sacrifice of the few to protect the many. Doctors know that a certain percentage of children will die and be injured by vaccines. But as with the sacrifice of children to Molech, the medical community claims that "the benefits outweigh the risks." As with the worship of Molech, the few must be sacrificed for the benefit of society. Vaccination is the perverse ethic of doing evil that good may result. God calls such an ethic a damnable heresy. *See* Romans 3:8. God condemns it. The child sacrifices to Molech were ineffectual; they were based on mythology. In like manner, vaccination is ineffectual; it is also based on mythology. Just as Molech was no threat, so also viruses pose no threat. The sacrifice of the few to Molech did nothing to protect the many. In like manner, sacrificing the few to vaccination does nothing to protect the many. The same could be said for masking. It is a sin to do evil, wearing a mask that could cause illness, in order to gain some future benefit of allegedly preventing an illness.

Many hospitals (e.g., Inova) require staff who are relgiously exempt from vaccination to wear a mask. Wearing a mask in lieu of vaccination announces to the world that the wearer agrees with the heathen religious superstition that a mask is safe, effective, and necessary because the mask wearer is unvaccinated and the mask is needed to protect from viruses. It is an implicit affirmation of the falsehood that vaccines are efficacious and safe. Christians are called on to "[a]bstain from all appearance of evil." 1 Thessalonians 5:22. Wearing a mask, without question, is the appearance of evil.

The government has acknowledged that the vaccines they are mandating do not prevent the infection or spread of COVID-19. They have given an exemption from wearing a mask to a vaccinated person who is just as likely to be infected and spread COVID-19 as the unvaccinated person. As explained in the FREEDOM OF RELIGION section, *supra*, since the government allows a secular medical exemption for the masks (vaccination), it must also necessarily allow a religious exemption. There is also the medical exemption allowed for those with medical conditions who cannot wear a mask. The U.S. Supreme Court in *Church of the Lukumi Babalu Aye, Inc. v. City of Hialeah*[1973] explained:

> Where government restricts only conduct protected by the First Amendment and fails to enact feasible measures to restrict other conduct producing substantial harm or alleged harm of the same sort, the interest given in justification of the restriction is not compelling. It is established in our strict scrutiny jurisprudence that "a law cannot be regarded as protecting an interest 'of the highest order' ... when it leaves appreciable damage to that supposedly vital interest unprohibited."[1974] (citation omitted)

Furthermore, If the person who must wear the mask is tested and shown not to have COVID-19, there is no threat of the spread of COVID-19 from the wearer, even if one were to believe the discredited theory of asymptomatic spread. That is because an asymptomatic carrier would necessarily test positive for COVID-19. Testing positive for COVID-19 but not having symptoms of the disease is what it means to be an asymptomatic carrier. It is not a reasonable accommodation to force someone who tests negative for COVID-19 to nonetheless wear a mask. Since the person has tested negative for COVID-19, the mask serves no useful purpose. An uninfected person cannot spread COVID-19. It is irrational to require him to wear a mask. That suggests that the mask is a punishment for refusing to be vaccinated and not a reasonable accommodation.

The evidence is against the efficacy and safety of wearing masks to prevent COVID-19 and the only other reason for the mask is symbolic. Consequently, all who object on religious grounds should be granted religious exemptions from wearing a mask. Furthermore, the mask requirement acts as a punishment for exercising one's constitutional right not to be vaccinated.

71 Abridging the Freedom of Speech

The First Amendment to the U.S. Constitution provides:

> Congress shall make no law respecting an establishment of religion, or prohibiting the free exercise thereof; or abridging the freedom of speech, or of the press; or the right of the people peaceably to assemble, and to petition the Government for a redress of grievances.[1975]

In *Gitlow v. New York*,[1976] the U.S. Supreme Court ruled that "freedom of speech and of the press—which are protected by the First Amendment from abridgment by Congress—are among the fundamental personal rights and 'liberties' protected by the due process clause of the Fourteenth Amendment from impairment by the States." Id. at 666.

An expected mask requirement as an accommodation in lieu of a vaccine restrains verbal and non-verbal speech, both of which are critical for the ability of the citizens to communicate effectively. Both of which are protected by the U.S. Constitution.

Facial coverings severely limit the volume and reach of speech. It unconstitutionally impairs speech and discourages people from speaking or communicating with others because the mask makes it difficult to hear the speaker's muffled voice. The speaker is restrained from conversion because the difficulty in breathing when wearing the suffocating mask requires the wearer to cut the conversation shorter than otherwise would be the case. Such mask requirements "abridge" the free speech rights of the people in violation of the Virginia and U.S. Constitutions.

Furthermore, non-verbal communication is protected by the right to free speech because facial expressions carry communicative information. While that truth is common sense, it is supported by studies that have shown that facial expressions carry communication. For example, a study by the Wellcome Trust Centre for Neuroimaging at UCL, Centre of Functionally Integrative Neuroscience, University of Aarhus concluded that "[t]he emotional expressions presented by faces are not simply reflexive, but also have a communicative component."[1977] "For example, empathic expressions of pain are not simply a reflexive response to the sight of pain in another, since they are exaggerated when the empathizer knows he or she is being observed. It seems that we want people to know that we are empathic. Of especial importance among facial expressions are ostensive gestures such as the eyebrow flash, which indicate the intention to communicate. These gestures indicate, first, that the sender is to be trusted and, second, that any following signals are of importance to the receiver."[1978]

The U.S. Supreme Court has recognized that the right to free speech includes the right to express oneself in ways that do not involve talking. For example, in *Tinker v. Des Moines Indep. Cmty. Sch. Dist.*,[1979] the U.S. Supreme Court struck down a school regulation that prohibited the wearing of black armbands to protest the Vietnam war. The Court stated that the armbands, although they did not involve the use of words, were nonetheless protected by the Constitution as free speech because they were expressions of ideas and thoughts.

In *Texas v. Johnson,*[1980] the U.S. Supreme Court stated that the First Amendment protects any conduct if "that conduct may be sufficiently imbued with elements of communication to fall within the scope of the First and Fourteenth Amendments."[1981] The *Johnson* Court further stated that "the State's argument cannot depend here on the distinction between written or spoken words and nonverbal conduct. That distinction, we have shown, is of no moment where the nonverbal conduct is expressive."[1982]

The mask regulation does limit free communication. But the mask mandate is not specifically designed to regulate speech. And thus it should be reviewed under the intermediate scrutiny standard, rather than the strict scrutiny standard required when the content of speech is being regulated.

To pass the intermediate scrutiny test, the President's orders must be narrowly tailored to accomplish a substantial government interest.[1983] If the restrictions by the President are not narrowly tailored to accomplish the "substantial" government interest, then the restrictions are unconstitutional.

The President's order requires all federal employees to be vaccinated.

A masking requirement in lieu of a vaccine, as will likely be proposed for those who claim a religious exemption from vaccination, is not narrowly tailored to address the federal government's alleged interest in stopping the spread of COVID-19, since masks are ineffective. Thus, a requirement to wear a mask is irrational. That truth is confirmed when one looks at the research reports establishing that masks are neither safe nor effective in preventing the spread of infectious diseases.

In a given context, a facial expression of a smile is as much communication of approval as would be spoken words. In a given context, a facial expression of a frown would be just as much a communication of disapproval as spoken words. To order that federal employees' faces be covered so they cannot communicate with others through their facial expressions is an infringement of freedom of expression in violation of the U.S. Constitution. Covering the face also isolates hearing-impaired people who must read lips to communicate.

Under Article VI of the U.S. Constitution, all state and federal officials are bound by an oath or affirmation to support the U.S. Constitution. The Bill of Rights is part of that Constitution. Thus, all state and federal officials are solemnly obligated to protect your rights. They should be reminded often of that fact.

The Bill of Rights enumerate your God-given rights to life, liberty, and property. You must assert those rights, or they will be lost. We should follow the ensample of Paul, who asserted his rights as a Roman citizen and appealed to Caesar. *See* Acts 25:10-12. We should likewise assert our God-given rights, which are a limit on government action.

Jesus said: "Behold, I send you forth as sheep in the midst of wolves: be ye therefore wise as serpents, and harmless as doves." Matthew 10:16.

Christians are sheep among wolves. That does not mean that we are to act like sheep. Jesus told us how to act. Jesus said we are to be harmless as doves and wise as serpents. Okay, so be harmless, and be wise. The gospel is the entire Bible. Matthew 10:16 is not all God said about how we should act. He also told us to be bold as lions. "The wicked flee when no man pursueth: but the righteous are bold as a lion." Proverbs 28:1-3.

Thus we are to be wise as serpents, harmless as doves, and

bold as lions. Remember what God said about going along with the evil of this world. "Whosoever therefore will be a friend of the world is the enemy of God." James 4:4. Only three verses later, God tells us to "submit yourselves therefore to God. Resist the devil, and he will flee from you." James 4:7. Submit to God, resist the devil.

How can we be any of those things without knowledge? We can't. We must be informed.

> My people are destroyed for lack of knowledge: because thou hast rejected knowledge, I will also reject thee. Hosea 4:6.

> Wisdom is the principal thing; therefore get wisdom: and with all thy getting get understanding. Proverbs 4:7.

There is a time for everything under the sun. there is "a time to keep silence, and a time to speak." Ecclesiastes 3:7. Now is the time to speak. Get knowledge; be harmless as doves; be wise and serpents; be bold as lions; speak out against this tyranny that is about to befall us.

> Humble yourselves in the sight of the Lord, and he shall lift you up. James 4:10.

> Pray without ceasing. 1 Thessalonians 5:17.

Appendix

The following article was written by Dr. Russell L. Blaylock and published on April 22, 2022, in the Journal of Surgical Neurology International.[1984] Dr. Russell Blaylock is the author of The Blaylock Wellness Report newsletter. He is a nationally recognized board-certified neurosurgeon, health practitioner, author, and lecturer. For 26 years, Dr. Blaylock practiced neurosurgery and had a nutritional practice. He recently retired from his neurosurgical duties to devote full attention to nutritional research. Dr. Blaylock has authored four books, Excitotoxins: The Taste That Kills, Health and Nutrition Secrets That Can Save Your Life, Natural Strategies for Cancer Patients, and his most recent work, Cellular and Molecular Biology of Autism Spectrum Disorders.

Dr. Blaylock's article is a treasure of information from a medical doctor with years of experience who has the expertise to identify and explain medical malfeasance that reared its ugly head during the COVID-19 "pandemic."

COVID UPDATE: What is the truth?[1985]

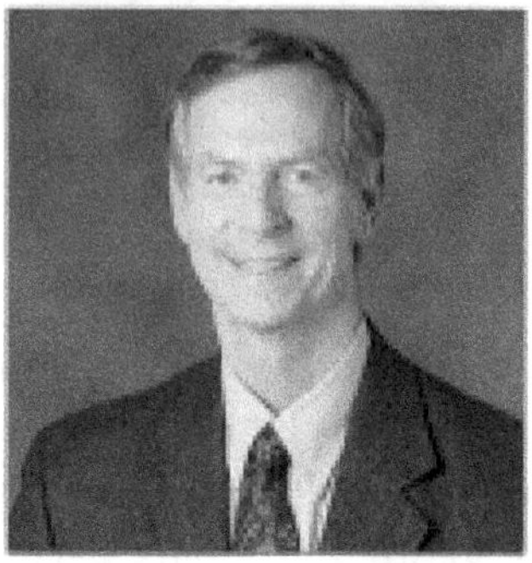

Dr. Russell L. Blaylock

The COVID-19 pandemic is one of the most manipulated infectious disease events in history, characterized by official lies in an unending stream led by government bureaucracies, medical associations, medical boards, the media, and international agencies.[1986] We have witnessed a long list of unprecedented intrusions into medical practice, including attacks on medical experts, destruction of medical careers among doctors refusing to participate in killing their patients and a massive regimentation of health care, led by non-qualified individuals with enormous wealth, power and influence.

For the first time in American history a president, governors, mayors, hospital administrators and federal bureaucrats are determining medical treatments based not on accurate scientifically based or even experience based information, but rather to force the acceptance of special forms of care and "prevention"—including remdesivir, use of respirators and ultimately a series of essentially untested messenger RNA vaccines. For the first time in history, medical treatment protocols are not being formulated based on the experience of the physicians treating the largest number of patients successfully, but rather individuals and bureaucracies that have never treated a single patient—including Anthony Fauci, Bill Gates, EcoHealth Alliance, the CDC, WHO, state public health officers and hospital administrators.[1987]

The media (TV, newspapers, magazines, etc), medical societies, state medical boards and the owners of social media have appointed themselves to be the sole source of information concerning this so-called "pandemic". Websites have been removed, highly credentialed and experienced clinical doctors and scientific experts in the field of infectious diseases have been demonized, careers have been destroyed and all dissenting information has been labeled "misinformation" and "dangerous lies", even when sourced from top experts in the fields of virology, infectious diseases, pulmonary critical care, and epidemiology. These blackouts of truth occur even when this information is backed by extensive scientific citations from some of the most qualified medical specialists in the world.[1988] Incredibly, even individuals, such as Dr. Michael Yeadon, a retired ex-Chief Scientist, and vice-president for the science division of Pfizer Pharmaceutical company in the UK, who charged the company with making an extremely dangerous vaccine, is ignored and demonized. Further, he, along with other highly qualified scientists have stated that no one should take this vaccine.

Dr. Peter McCullough, one of the most cited experts in his field, who has successfully treated over 2000 COVID patients by using a protocol of early treatment (which the so-called experts completely ignored), has been the victim of a particularly vicious assault by those benefiting financially from the vaccines. He has published his results in peer reviewed journals, reporting an 80% reduction in hospitalizations and a 75% reduction in deaths by using early treatment.[1989] Despite this, he is under an unrelenting series of attacks by the information controllers, none of which have treated a single patient.

Neither Anthony Fauci, the CDC, WHO nor any medical governmental establishment has ever offered any early treatment other than Tylenol, hydration and call an ambulance once you have difficulty breathing. This is unprecedented in the entire history of medical care as early treatment of infections is critical to saving lives and preventing severe complications. Not only have these medical organizations and federal lapdogs not even suggested early treatment, they attacked anyone who attempted to initiate such treatment with all the weapons at their disposal—loss of license, removal of hospital privileges, shaming, destruction of reputations and even arrest.[1990]

A good example of this outrage against freedom of speech and providing informed consent information is the recent suspension by the medical board in Maine of Dr. Meryl Nass' medical license and the ordering of her to undergo a psychiatric evaluation for prescribing Ivermectin and sharing her expertise in this field.[1991] I know Dr. Nass personally and can vouch for her integrity, brilliance and dedication to truth. Her scientific credentials are impeccable. This behavior by a medical licensing board is reminiscent of the methodology of the Soviet KGB during the period when dissidents were incarcerated in psychiatric gulags to silence their dissent.

OTHER UNPRECEDENTED ATTACKS

Another unprecedented tactic is to remove dissenting doctors from their positions as journal editors, reviewers and retracting of their scientific papers from journals, even after these papers have been in print. Until this pandemic event, I have never seen so many journal papers being retracted— the vast majority promoting alternatives to official dogma, especially if the papers question vaccine safety. Normally a submitted paper or study is reviewed by experts in the field, called peer review. These reviews can be quite intense and nit picking in detail, insisting that all errors within the paper be corrected before publication. So, unless fraud or some other major hidden problem is discovered after the paper is in print, the paper remains in the scientific literature.

We are now witnessing a growing number of excellent scientific papers, written by top experts in the field, being retracted from major medical and scientific journals weeks, months and even years after publication. A careful review indicates that in far too many instances the authors dared question accepted dogma by the controllers of scientific publications—especially concerning the safety, alternative treatments or efficacy of vaccines.[1992] These journals rely on extensive adverting by pharmaceutical companies for their revenue. Several instances have occurred where powerful pharmaceutical companies exerted their influence on owners of these journals to remove articles that in any way question these companies' products.[1993]

Worse still is the actual designing of medical articles for promoting drugs and pharmaceutical products that involve fake studies, so-called ghostwritten articles.[1994] Richard Horton is quoted by the Guardian as saying "journals have devolved into information laundering operations for the pharmaceutical industry."[1995] Proven fraudulent "ghostwritten" articles sponsored by pharmaceutical giants have appeared regularly in top clinical journals, such as JAMA, and New England Journal of Medicine—never to be removed despite proven scientific abuse and manipulation of data.[1996]

Ghostwritten articles involve using planning companies whose job it is to design articles containing manipulated data to support a pharmaceutical product and then have these articles accepted by high-impact clinical journals, that is, the journals most likely to affect clinical decision making of doctors. Further, they supply doctors in clinical practice with free reprints of these manipulated articles. The Guardian found 250 companies engaged in this ghostwriting business. The final step in designing these articles for publication in the most prestigious journals is to recruit well recognized medical experts from prestigious institutions, to add their name to these articles. These recruited medical authors are either paid upon agreeing to add their name to these pre- written articles or they do so for the prestige of having their name on an article in a prestigious medical journal.[1997]

Of vital importance is the observation by experts in the field of medical publishing that nothing has been done to stop this abuse. Medical ethicists have lamented that because of this widespread practice "you can't trust anything." While some journals insist on disclosure information, most doctors reading these articles ignore this information or excuse it and several journals make disclosure more difficult by requiring the reader to find the disclosure statements at another location. Many journals do not police such statements and omissions by authors are common and without punishment.

As concerns the information made available to the public, virtually all the media is under the control of these pharmaceutical giants or others who are benefitting from this "pandemic". Their stories are all the same, both in content and even wording. Orchestrated coverups occur daily and massive data exposing the lies being generated by these information controllers are hidden from the public. All data coming over the national media (TV, newspaper and magazines), as well as the local news you watch every day, comes only from "official" sources—most of which are lies, distortions or completely manufactured out of whole cloth—all aimed to deceive the public.

Television media receives the majority of its advertising budget from the international pharmaceutical companies—this creates an irresistible influence to report all concocted studies supporting their vaccines and other so-called treatments.[1998] In 2020 alone the pharmaceutical industries spent 6.56 billion dollars on such advertising.[1999] Pharma TV advertising amounted to 4.58 billion, an incredible 75% of their budget. That buys a lot of influence and control over the media. World famous experts within all fields of infectious diseases are excluded from media exposure and from social media should they in any way deviate against the concocted lies and distortions by the makers of these vaccines. In addition, these pharmaceutical companies spend tens of millions on social media advertising, with Pfizer leading the pack with $55 million in 2020.[2000]

While these attacks on free speech are terrifying enough, even worse is the virtually universal control hospital administrators have exercised over the details of medical care in hospitals. These hirelings are now instructing doctors which treatment protocols they will adhere to and which treatments they will not use, no matter how harmful the "approved" treatments are or how beneficial the "unapproved" treatments are.[2001]

Never in the history of American medicine have hospital administrators dictated to its physicians how they will practice medicine and what medications they can use. The CDC has no authority to dictate to hospitals or doctors concerning medical treatments. Yet, most physicians complied without the slightest resistance.

The federal Care Act encouraged this human disaster by offering all US hospitals up to 39,000 dollars for each ICU patient they put on respirators, despite the fact that early on it was obvious that the respirators were a major cause of death among these unsuspecting, trusting patients. In addition, the hospitals received 12,000 dollars for each patient that was admitted to the ICU—explaining, in my opinion and others, why all federal medical bureaucracies (CDC, FDA, NIAID, NIH, etc) did all in their power to prevent life-saving early treatments.[2002] Letting patients deteriorate to the point they needed hospitalization, meant big money for all hospitals. A growing number of hospitals are in danger of bankruptcy, and many have closed their doors, even before this "pandemic".[2003] Most of these hospitals are now owned by national or international corporations, including teaching hospitals.[2004]

It is also interesting to note that with the arrival of this "pandemic" we have witnessed a surge in hospital corporate chains buying up a number of these financially at-risk hospitals.[2005] It has been noted that billions in Federal Covid aid is being used by these hospital giants to acquire these financially endangered hospitals, further increasing the power of corporate medicine over physician independence. Physicians expelled from their hospitals are finding it difficult to find other hospitals staffs to join since they too may be owned by the same corporate giant. As a result, vaccine mandate policies include far larger numbers of hospital employees. For example, Mayo Clinic fired 700 employees for exercising their right to refuse a dangerous, essentially untested experimental vaccine.[2006] Mayo Clinic did this despite the fact that many of these employees worked during the worst of the epidemic and are being fired when the Omicron variant is the dominant strain of the virus, has the pathogenicity of a common cold for most and the vaccines are ineffective in preventing the infection.

In addition, it has been proven that the vaccinated asymptomatic person has a nasopharyngeal titer of the virus as high as an infected unvaccinated person. If the purpose of the vaccine mandate is to prevent viral spread among the hospital staff and patients, then it is the vaccinated who present the greatest risk of transmission, not the unvaccinated. The difference is that a sick unvaccinated person would not go to work, the asymptomatic vaccinated spreader will.

What we do know is that major medical centers, such as Mayo Clinic, receive tens of millions of dollars in NIH grants each year as well as monies from the pharmaceutical makers of these experimental "vaccines." In my view, that is the real consideration driving these policies. If this could be proven in a court of law the administrators making these mandates should be prosecuted to the fullest extent of the law and sued by all injured parties.

The hospital bankruptcy problem has grown increasingly acute due to hospitals vaccine mandates and resulting large number of hospitals staff, especially nurses, refusing to be forcibly vaccinated.[2007] This is all unprecedented in the history of medical care. Doctors within hospitals are responsible for the treatment of their individual patients and work directly with these patients and their families to initiate these treatments. Outside organizations, such as the CDC, have no authority to intervene in these treatments and to do so exposes the patients to grave errors by an organization that has never treated a single COVID-19 patient.

When this pandemic started, hospitals were ordered by the CDC to follow a treatment protocol that resulted in the deaths of hundreds of thousands of patients, most of whom would have recovered had proper treatments been allowed.[2008] The majority of these deaths could have been prevented had doctors been allowed to use early treatment with such products as Ivermectin, hydroxy-chloroquine and a number of other safe drugs and natural compounds. It has been estimated, based on results by physicians treating the most covid patients successfully, that of the 800,000 people that we are told died from Covid, 640,000 could have not only been saved, but could have, in many cases, returned to their pre-infection health status had mandated early treatment with these proven methods been used. This neglect of early treatment constitutes mass murder. That means 160,000 would have actually died, far less than the number dying at the hands of bureaucracies, medical associations and medical boards that refused to stand up for their patients. According to studies of early treatment of thousands of patients by brave, caring doctors, seventy-five to eighty percent of the deaths could have been prevented.[2009]

Incredibly, these knowledgeable doctors were prevented from saving these Covid-19 infected people. It should be an embarrassment to the medical profession that so many doctors mindlessly followed the deadly protocols established by the controllers of medicine.

One must also keep in mind that this event never satisfied the criteria for a pandemic. The World Health Organization changed the criteria to make this a pandemic. To qualify for a pandemic status the virus must have a high mortality rate for the vast majority of people, which it didn't (with a 99.98% survival rate), and it must have no known existing treatments—which this virus had—in fact, a growing number of very successful treatments.

The draconian measures established to contain this contrived "pandemic" have never been shown to be successful, such as masking the public, lockdowns, and social distancing. A number of carefully done studies during previous flu seasons demonstrated that masks, of any kind, had never prevented the spread of the virus among the public.[2010]

In fact, some very good studies suggested that the masks actually spread the virus by giving people a false sense of security and other factors, such as the observation that people were constantly breaking sterile technique by touching their mask, improper removal and by leakage of infectious aerosols around the edges of the mask. In addition masks were being disposed of in parking lots, walking trails, laid on tabletops in restaurants and placed in pockets and purses.

Within a few minutes of putting on the mask, a number of pathogenic bacteria can be cultured from the masks, putting the immune suppressed person at a high risk of bacterial pneumonia and children at a higher risk of meningitis.[2011] A study by researchers at the University of Florida cultured over 11 pathogenic bacteria from the inside of the mask worn by children in schools.[2012]

It was also known that children were at essentially no risk of either getting sick from the virus or transmitting it.

In addition, it was also known that wearing a mask for over 4 hours (as occurs in all schools) results in significant hypoxia (low blood oxygen levels) and hypercapnia (high CO_2 levels), which have a number of deleterious effects on health, including impairing the development of the child's brain.[2013]

We have known that brain development continues long after the grade school years. A recent study found that children born during the "pandemic" have significantly lower IQs—yet school boards, school principals and other educational bureaucrats are obviously unconcerned.[2014]

TOOLS OF THE INDOCTRINATION TRADE

The designers of this pandemic anticipated a pushback by the public and that major embarrassing questions would be asked. To prevent this, the controllers fed the media a number of tactics, one of the most commonly used was and is the "fact check" scam. With each confrontation with carefully documented evidence, the media "fact checkers" countered with the charge of "misinformation", and an unfounded "conspiracy theory" charge that was, in their lexicon, "debunked". Never were we told who the fact checkers were or the source of their "debunking" information—we were just to believe the "fact checkers". A recent court case established under oath that facebook "fact checkers" used their own staff opinion and not real experts to check "facts".[2015] When sources are in fact revealed they are invariably the corrupt CDC, WHO or Anthony Fauci or just their opinion. Here is a list of things that were labeled as "myths" and "misinformation" that were later proven to be true.

- The asymptomatic vaccinated are spreading the virus equally as with unvaccinated symptomatic infected.
- The vaccines cannot protect adequately against new variants, such as Delta and Omicron.
- Natural immunity is far superior to vaccine immunity and is most likely lifelong.
- Vaccine immunity not only wanes after several

months, but all immune cells are impaired for prolonged periods, putting the vaccinated at a high risk of all infections and cancer.

- COVID vaccines can cause a significant incidence of blood clots and other serious side effects.
- The vaccine proponents will demand numerous boosters as each variant appears on the scene.
- Fauci will insist on the covid vaccine for small children and even babies.
- Vaccine passports will be required to enter a business, fly in a plane, and use public transportation.
- There will be internment camps for the unvaccinated (as in Australia, Austria and Canada).
- The unvaccinated will be denied employment.
- There are secret agreements between the government, elitist institutions, and vaccine makers.
- Many hospitals were either empty or had low occupancy during the pandemic.
- The spike protein from the vaccine enters the nucleus of the cell, altering cell DNA repair function.
- Hundreds of thousands have been killed by the vaccines and many times more have been permanently damaged.
- Early treatment could have saved the lives of most of the 700,000 who died.
- Vaccine-induced myocarditis (which was denied initially) is a significant problem [...].
- Special deadly lots (batches) of these vaccines are mixed with the mass of other Covid-19 vaccines.

Several of these claims by those opposing these vaccines now appear on the CDC website—most still identified as "myths". Today, extensive evidence has confirmed that each of these so-called "myths" were in fact true. Many are even admitted by the "saint of vaccines", Anthony Fauci. For example, we were told, even by our cognitively impaired President, that once the vaccine was released all the vaccinated people could take off their masks. Oops! We were told shortly afterward— the vaccinated have high concentrations (titers) of the virus in their noses and mouths (nasopharynx) and can transmit the virus to others in which they come into contact—especially their own family members. On go the masks once again— in fact double masking is recommended. The vaccinated are now known to be the main superspreaders of the virus and hospitals are filled with the sick vaccinated and people suffering from serious vaccine complications.[2016]

Another tactic by the vaccine proponents is to demonize those who reject being vaccinated for a variety of reasons. The media refers to these critically thinking individuals as "anti-vaxxers", "vaccine deniers", "Vaccine resisters", "murder[er]s", "enemies of the greater good" and as being the ones prolonging the pandemic. I have been appalled by the vicious, often heartless attacks by some of the people on social media when a parent or loved one relates a story of the terrible suffering and eventual death, they or their loved one suffered as a result of the vaccines. Some psychopaths tweet that they are glad that the loved one died or that the dead vaccinated person was an enemy of good for telling of the event and should be banned. This is hard to conceptualize. This level of cruelty is terrifying, and signifies the collapse of a moral, decent, and compassionate society.

It is bad enough for the public to sink this low, but the media, political leaders, hospital administrators, medical associations and medical licensing boards are acting in a similar morally dysfunctional and cruel way.

LOGIC, REASONING, AND SCIENTIFIC EVIDENCE HAS

DISAPPEARED IN THIS EVENT

Has scientific evidence, carefully done studies, clinical experience and medical logic had any effect on stopping these ineffective and dangerous vaccines? Absolutely not! The draconian efforts to vaccinate everyone on the planet continues (except the elite, postal workers, members of Congress and other insiders).[2017]

In the case of all other drugs and previous conventional vaccines under review by the FDA, the otherwise unexplained deaths of 50 or less individuals would result in a halt in further distribution of the product, as happened on 1976 with the swine flu vaccine. With over 18,000 deaths being reported by the VAERS system for the period December 14, 2020 and December 31st, 2021 as well as 139,126 serious injuries (including deaths) for the same period there is still no interest in stopping this deadly vaccine program.[2018] Worse, there is no serious investigation by any government agency to determine why these people are dying and being seriously and permanently injured by these vaccines.[2019] What we do see is a continuous series of coverups and evasions by the vaccine makers and their promoters.

The war against effective cheap and very safe repurposed drugs and natural compounds, that have proven beyond all doubt to have saved millions of lives all over the world, has not only continued but has stepped up in intensity.[2020]

Doctors are told they cannot provide these life-saving compounds for their patients and if they do, they will be removed from the hospital, have their medical license removed or be punished in many other ways. A great many pharmacies have refused to fill prescriptions for lvermectin or hydroxychloroquine, despite the fact that millions of people have taken these drugs safely for over 60 years in the case of hydroxy chloroquine and decades for Ivermectin.[2021] This refusal to fill prescriptions is unprecedented and has been engineered by those wanting to prevent alternative methods of treatment, all based on protecting vaccine expansion to all. Several companies that make hydroxychloroquine agreed to empty their stocks of the drug by donating them to the Strategic National Stockpile, making this drug far more difficult to get.[2022] Why would the government do that when over 30 well-done studies have shown that this drug reduced deaths anywhere from 66% to 92% in other countries, such as India, Egypt, Argentina, France, Nigeria, Spain, Peru, Mexico, and others?[2023]

The critics of these two life-saving drugs are most often funded by Bill Gates and Anthony Fauci, both of which are making millions from these vaccines.[2024]

To further stop the use of these drugs, the pharmaceutical industry and Bill Gates/Anthony Fauci funded fake research to make the case that hydroxy chloroquine was a dangerous drug and could damage the heart.[2025] To make this fraudulent case the researchers administered the sickest of covid patients a near lethal dose of the drug, in a dose far higher than used on any covid patient by Dr. Kory, McCullough and other "real", and compassionate doctors, physicians who were actually treating covid patients.[2026]

The controlled, lap-dog media, of course, hammered the public with stories of the deadly effect of hydroxy- chloroquine, all with a terrified look of fake panic. All these stories of ivermectin dangers were shown to be untrue and some of the stories were incredibly preposterous.[2027]

The attack on Ivermectin was even more vicious than against hydroxychloroquine. All of this, and a great deal more is meticulously chronicled in Robert Kennedy, Jr's excellent new book—*The Real Anthony Fauci: Bill Gates, Big Pharma, and the Global War on Democracy and Public Health.*[2028] If you are truly concerned with the truth and with all that has occurred since this atrocity started, you must not only read, but study this book carefully. It is fully referenced and covers all topics in great detail.

This is a designed human tragedy of Biblical proportions by some of the most vile, heartless, psychopaths in history.

Millions have been deliberately killed and crippled, not only by this engineered virus, but by the vaccine itself and by the draconian measures used by these governments to "control the pandemic spread". We must not ignore the "deaths by despair" caused by these draconian measures, which can exceed hundreds of thousands. Millions have starved in third world countries as a result. In the United States alone, of the 800,000 who died, claimed by the medical bureaucracies, well over 600,000 of these deaths were the result of the purposeful neglect of early treatment, blocking the use of highly effective and safe repurposed drugs, such as hydroxy-chloroquine and Ivermectin, and the forced use of deadly treatments such as remdesivir and use of ventilators. This does not count the deaths of despair and neglected medical care caused by the lockdown and hospital measures forced on healthcare systems.

To compound all this, because of vaccine mandates among all hospital personnel, thousands of nurses and other hospital workers have resigned or been fired.[2029] This has resulted in critical shortages of these vital healthcare workers and dangerous reductions of ICU beds in many hospitals. In addition, as occurred in the Lewis County Healthcare System, a specialty-hospital system in Lowville, N.Y., closed its maternity unit following the resignation of 30 hospital staff over the state's disastrous vaccine mandate orders. The irony in all these cases of resignations is that the administrators unhesitatingly accepted these mass staffing losses despite rantings about suffering from short staffing during a "crisis". This is especially puzzling when we learned that the vaccines did not prevent viral transmission and the present predominant variant is of extremely low pathogenicity.

DANGERS OF THE VACCINES ARE INCREASINGLY REVEALED BY SCIENCE

While most researchers, virologists, infectious disease researchers and epidemiologists have been intimidated into silence, a growing number of high integrity individuals with tremendous expertise have come forward to tell the truth—that is, that these vaccines are deadly.

Most new vaccines must go through extensive safety testing for years before they are approved. New technologies, such as the mRNA and DNA vaccines, require a minimum of 10 years of careful testing and extensive follow-up. These new so-called vaccines were "tested" for only 2 months and then the results of these safety tests were and continue to be kept secret. Testimony before Senator Ron Johnson by several who participated in the 2 months study indicates that virtually no follow-up of the participants of the pre-release study was ever done.[2030] Complaints of complications were ignored and despite promises by Pfizer that all medical expenses caused by the "vaccines" would be paid by Pfizer, these individuals stated that none were paid.[2031] Some medical expenses exceed 100,000 dollars.

As an example of the deception by Pfizer, and the other makers of mRNA vaccines, is the case of 12-year-old Maddie de Garay, who participated in the Pfizer vaccine pre-release safety study. At Sen. Johnson's presentation with the families of the vaccine injured, her mother told of her child's recurrent seizures, that she is now confined to a wheelchair, must be tube fed and suffers permanent brain damage. On the Pfizer safety evaluation submitted to the FDA her only side effect is listed as having a "stomachache". Each person submitted similar horrifying stories.

The Japanese resorted to a FOIA (Freedom of Information Act) lawsuit to force Pfizer to release its secret biodistribution study. The reason Pfizer wanted it kept secret is that it demonstrated that Pfizer lied to the public and the regulatory agencies about the fate of the injected vaccine contents (the mRNA enclosed nano-lipid carrier). They claimed that it remained at the site of the injection (the shoulder), when in fact their own study found that it rapidly spread throughout the entire body by the bloodstream within 48 hours.

The study also found that these deadly nano-lipid carriers collected in very high concentrations in several organs, including the reproductive organs of males and females, the heart, the liver, the bone marrow, and the spleen (a major immune organ). The highest concentration was in the ovaries and the bone marrow. These nano-lipid carriers also were deposited in the brain.

Dr. Ryan Cole, a pathologist from Idaho reported a dramatic spike in highly aggressive cancers among vaccinated individuals, (not reported in the Media). He found a frighteningly high incidence of highly aggressive cancers in vaccinated individuals, especially highly invasive melanomas in young people and uterine cancers in women.[2032] Other reports of activation of previously controlled cancers are also appearing among vaccinated cancer patients.[2033] Thus far, no studies have been done to confirm these reports, but it is unlikely such studies will be done, at least studies funded by grants from the NIH.

The high concentration of spike proteins found in the ovaries in the biodistribution study could very well impair fertility in young women, alter menstruation, and could put them at an increased risk of ovarian cancer. The high concentration in the bone marrow, could also put the vaccinated at a high risk of leukemia and lymphoma. The leukemia risk is very worrisome now that they have started vaccinating children as young as 5 years of age. No long-term studies have been conducted by any of these makers of Covid-19 vaccines, especially as regards the risk of cancer induction. Chronic inflammation is intimately linked to cancer induction, growth and invasion and vaccines stimulate inflammation.

Cancer patients are being told they should get vaccinated with these deadly vaccines. This, in my opinion, is insane. Newer studies have shown that this type of vaccine inserts the spike protein within the nucleus of the immune cells (and most likely many cell types) and once there, inhibits two very important DNA repair enzymes, BRCA1 and 53BP1, whose duty it is to repair damage to the cell's DNA.[2034] Unrepaired DNA damage plays a major role in cancer.

There is a hereditary disease called xeroderma pigmentosum in which the DNA repair enzymes are defective. These ill-fated individuals develop multiple skin cancers and a very high incidence of organ cancer as a result. Here we have a vaccine that does the same thing, but to a less extensive degree.

One of the defective repair enzymes caused by these vaccines is called BRCA1, which is associated with a significantly higher incidence of breast cancer in women and prostate cancer in men.

It should be noted that no studies were ever done on several critical aspects of this type of vaccine.

- They have never been tested for long term effects
- They have never been tested for induction of autoimmunity
- They have never been properly tested for safety during any stage of pregnancy
- No follow-up studies have been done on the babies of vaccinated women
- There are no long-term studies on the children of vaccinated pregnant women after their birth (Especially as neurodevelopmental milestone occur).
- It has never been tested for effects on a long list of medical conditions:
    - Diabetes
    - Heart disease

•Atherosclerosis
•Neurodegenerative diseases
•Neuropsychiatric effects
•Induction of autism spectrum disorders and schizophrenia
•Long term immune function
•Vertical transmission of defects and disorders
•Cancer
•Autoimmune disorders

Previous experience with the flu vaccines clearly demonstrates that the safety studies done by researchers and clinical doctors with ties to pharmaceutical companies were essentially all either poorly done or purposefully designed to falsely show safety and coverup side effects and complications. This was dramatically demonstrated with the previously mentioned phony studies designed to indicate that hydroxy Chloroquine and Ivermectin were ineffective and too dangerous to use.[2035] These fake studies resulted in millions of deaths and severe health disasters worldwide. As stated, 80% of all deaths were unnecessary and could have been prevented with inexpensive, safe repurposed medications with a very long safety history among millions who have taken them for decades or even a lifetime.[2036]

It is beyond ironic that those claiming that they are responsible for protecting our health approved a poorly tested set of vaccines that has resulted in more deaths in less than a year of use than all the other vaccines combined given over the past 30 years. Their excuse when confronted was—"we had to overlook some safety measures because this was a deadly pandemic".[2037]

In 1986 President Reagan signed the National Childhood Vaccine Injury Act, which gave blanket protection to pharmaceutical makers of vaccines against injury litigation by families of vaccine injured individuals. The Supreme Court, in a 57-page opinion, ruled in favor of the vaccine companies, effectively allowing vaccine makers to manufacture and distribute dangerous, often ineffective vaccines to the population without fear of legal consequences. The court did insist on a vaccine injury compensation system which has paid out only a very small number of rewards to a large number of severely injured individuals. It is known that it is very difficult to receive these awards. According to the Health Resources and Services Administration, since 1988 the Vaccine Injury Compensation Program (VICP) has agreed to pay 3,597 awards among 19,098 vaccine injured individuals applying amounting to a total sum of $3.8 billion. This was prior to the introduction of the Covid-19 vaccines, in which the deaths alone exceed all deaths related to all the vaccines combined over a thirty-year period.

In 2018 President Trump signed into law the "right-to-try" law which allowed the use of experimental drugs and all unconventional treatments to be used in cases of extreme medical conditions. As we have seen with the refusal of many hospitals and even blanket refusal by states to allow Ivermectin, hydroxy-chloroquine or any other unapproved "official" methods to treat even terminal Covid-19 cases, these nefarious individuals have ignored this law.

Strangely, they did not use this same logic or the law when it came to Ivermectin and Hydroxy Chloroquine, both of which had undergone extensive safety testing by over 30 clinical studies of a high quality and given glowing reports on both efficacy and safety in numerous countries. In addition, we had a record of use for up to 60 years by millions of people, using these drugs worldwide, with an excellent safety record. It was obvious that a group of very powerful people in conjunction with pharmaceutical conglomerates didn't want the pandemic to end and wanted vaccines as the only treatment option. Kennedy's book makes this case using extensive evidence and citations.[2038]

Dr. James Thorpe, an expert in maternal-fetal medicine, demonstrates that these COVID-19 vaccines given during pregnancy have resulted in a 50-fold higher incidence of miscarriage than reported with all other vaccines combined.[2039] When we examine his graph on fetal malformations there was a 144-fold higher incidence of fetal malformation with the Covid-19 vaccines given during pregnancy as compared to all other vaccines combined. Yet, the American Academy of Obstetrics and Gynecology and the American College of Obstetrics and Gynecology endorse the safety of these vaccines for all stages of pregnancy and among women breast feeding their babies.

It is noteworthy that these medical specialty groups have received significant funding from Pfizer pharmaceutical company. The American College of Obstetrics and Gynecology, just in the 4th quarter of 2010, received a total of $11,000 from Pfizer Pharmaceutical company alone.[2040] Funding from NIH grants are much higher.[2041] The best way to lose these grants is to criticize the source of the funds, their products or pet programs. Peter Duesberg, because of his daring to question Fauci's pet theory of AIDS caused by HIV virus, was no longer awarded any of the 30 grant applications he submitted after going public. Prior to this episode, as the leading authority on retroviruses in the world, he had never been turned down for an NIH grant.[2042] This is how the "corrupted" system works, even though much of the grant money comes from our taxes.

HOT LOTS—DEADLY BATCHES OF THE VACCINES

A new study has now surfaced, the results of which are terrifying.[2043] A researcher at Kingston University in London, has completed an extensive analysis of the VAERs data (a subdepartment of the CDC which collects voluntary vaccine complication data), in which he grouped reported deaths following the vaccines according to the manufacturer's lot numbers of the vaccines. Vaccines are manufactured in large batches called lots.

What he discovered was that the vaccines are divided into over 20,000 lots and that one out of every 200 of these batches (lots) is demonstrably deadly to anyone who receives a vaccine from that lot, which includes thousands of vaccine doses.

He examined all manufactured vaccines—Pfizer, Moderna, Johnson and Johnson (Janssen), etc. He found that among every 200 batches of the vaccine from Pfizer and other makers, one batch of the 200 was found to be over 50x more deadly than vaccines batches from other lots. The other vaccine lots (batches) were also causing deaths and disabilities, but nowhere near to this extent. These deadly batches should have appeared randomly among all "vaccines" if it was an unintentional event. However, he found that 5% of the vaccines were responsible for 90% of the serious adverse events, including deaths. The incidence of deaths and serious complications among these "hot lots" varied from over 1000% to several thousand percent higher than comparable safer lots. If you think this was by accident—think again. This is not the first time "hot lots" were, in my opinion, purposefully manufactured and sent across the nation—usually vaccines designed for children. In one such scandal, "hot lots" of a vaccine ended up all in one state and the damage immediately became evident. What was the manufacture's response? It wasn't to remove the deadly batches of the vaccine. He ordered his company to scatter the hot lots across the nation so that authorities would not see the obvious deadly effect.

All lots of a vaccine are numbered—for example Modera labels them with such codes as 013M20A. It was noted that the batch numbers ended in either 20A or 21A. Batches ending in 20A were much more toxic than the ones ending in 21A. The batches ending in 20A had about 1700 adverse events, versus a few hundred to twenty or thirty events for the 21A batches. This example explains why some people had few or no adverse events after taking the vaccine while others are either killed or severely and permanently harmed. To see the researcher's explanation, go to https://www.bitchute.com/video/6xIYPZBkydsu/ In my opinion these examples strongly suggest an intentional alteration of the production of the "vaccine" to include deadly batches.

I have met and worked with a number of people concerned with vaccine safety and I can tell you they are not the evil anti-vaxxers you are told they are. They are highly principled, moral, compassionate people, many of which are top researchers and people who have studied the issue extensively. Robert Kennedy, Jr, Barbara Lou Fisher, Dr. Meryl Nass, Professor Christopher Shaw, Megan Redshaw, Dr. Sherri Tenpenny, Dr. Joseph Mercola, Neil Z. Miller, Dr. Lucija Tomjinovic, Dr. Stephanie Seneff, Dr. Steve Kirsch and Dr. Peter McCullough just to name a few. These people have nothing to gain and a lot to lose. They are attacked viciously by the media, government agencies, and elite billionaires who think they should control the world and everyone in it.

WHY DID FAUCI WANT NO AUTOPSIES OF THOSE WHO DIED AFTER VACCINATION?

There are many things about this "pandemic" that are unprecedented in medical history. One of the most startling is that at the height of the pandemic so few autopsies, especially total autopsies, were being done. A mysterious virus was rapidly spreading around the world, a selected group of people with weakened immune systems were getting seriously ill and many were dying and the one way we could rapidly gain the most knowledge about this virus—an autopsy, was being discouraged.

Guerriero noted that by the end of April, 2020 approximately 150,000 people had died, yet there were only 16 autopsies performed and reported in the medical literature.[2044] Among these, only seven were complete autopsies, the remaining 9 being partial or by needle biopsy or incisional biopsy. Only after 170,000 deaths by Covid-19 and four months into the pandemic were the first series of autopsies actually done, that is, more than ten. And only after 280,000 deaths and another month, were the first large series of autopsies performed, some 80 in number.[2045] Sperhake, in a call for autopsies to be done without question, noted that the first full autopsy reported in the literature along with photomicrographs appeared in a medico-legal journal from China in February 2020.[2046] Sperhake expressed confusion as to why there was a reluctance to perform autopsies during the crisis, but he knew it was not coming from the pathologists. The medical literature was littered with appeals by pathologist for more autopsies to be performed.[2047] Sperhake further noted that the Robert Koch Institute (The German health monitoring system) at least initially advised against doing autopsies. He also knew that at the time 200 participating autopsy institutions in the United States had done at least 225 autopsies among 14 states.

Some have claimed that this dearth of autopsies was based on the government's fear of infection among the pathologists, but a study of 225 autopsies on Covid-19 cases demonstrated only one case of infection among the pathologist and this was concluded to have been an infection contracted elsewhere.[2048] Guerriero ends his article calling for more autopsies with this observation: "Shoulder to shoulder, clinical and forensic pathologists overcame the obstructions of autopsy studies in Covid-19 victims and hereby generated valuable knowledge on the pathophysiology of the interaction between the SARS-CoV-2 and the human body, thus contributing to our understanding of the disease."[2049]

Suspicion concerning the worldwide reluctance of nations to allow full post mortem studies of Covid-19 victims may be based on the idea that it was more than by chance. There are at least two possibilities that stand out. First, those leading the progression of this "non-pandemic" event into a perceived worldwide "deadly pandemic", were hiding an important secret that autopsies could document. Namely, just how many of the deaths were actually caused by the virus? To implement draconian measures, such as mandated mask wearing, lockdowns, destruction of businesses, and eventually mandated forced vaccination, they needed very large numbers of covid-19 infected dead. Fear would be the driving force for all these destructive pandemic control programs.

Elder et al in his study classified the autopsy findings into four groups.[2050]

1. Certain Covid-19 death
2. Probably Covid-19 death
3. Possible Covid-19 death
4. Not associated with Covid-19, despite the positive test.

What possibly concerned or even terrified the engineers of this pandemic was that autopsies just might, and did, show that a number of these so-called Covid-19 deaths in truth died of their comorbid diseases. In the vast majority of autopsy studies reported, pathologists noted multiple comorbid conditions, most of which at the extremes of life could alone be fatal. Previously it was known that common cold viruses had an 8% mortality in nursing homes.

In addition, valuable evidence could be obtained from the autopsies that would improve clinical treatments and could possibly demonstrate the deadly effect of the CDC mandated protocols all hospitals were required to follow, such as the use of respirators and the deadly, kidney-destroying drug remdesivir. The autopsies also demonstrated accumulating medical errors and poor-quality care, as the shielding of doctors in intensive care units from the eyes of family members inevitably leads to poorer quality care as reported by several nurses working in these areas.[2051]

As bad as all this was, the very same thing is being done in the case of Covid vaccine deaths—very few complete autopsies have been done to understand why these people died, that is, until recently. Two highly qualified researchers, Dr. Sucharit Bhakdi a microbiologist and highly qualified expert in infectious disease and

Dr. Arne Burkhardt, a pathologist who is a widely published authority having been a professor of pathology at several prestigious institutions, recently performed autopsies on 15 people having died after vaccination. What they found explains why so many are dying and experiencing organ damage and deadly blood clots.[2052]

They determined that 14 of the fifteen people died as a result of the vaccines and not of other causes. Dr. Burkhardt, the pathologist, observed widespread evidence of an immune attack on the autopsied individuals' organs and tissues— especially their heart. This evidence included extensive invasion of small blood vessels with massive numbers of lymphocytes, which cause extensive cell destruction when unleashed. Other organs, such as the lungs and liver, were observed to have extensive damage as well. These findings indicate the vaccines were causing the body to attack itself with deadly consequences. One can easily see why Anthony Fauci, as well as public health officers and all who are heavily promoting these vaccines, publicly discouraged autopsies on the vaccinated who subsequently died. One can also see that in the case of vaccines, that were essentially untested prior to being approved for the general public, at least the regulatory agencies should have been required to carefully monitor and analyze all serious complications, and certainly deaths, linked to these vaccines. The best way to do that is with complete autopsies.

While we learned important information from these autopsies what is really needed are special studies of the tissues of those who have died after vaccination for the presence of spike protein infiltration throughout the organs and tissues. This would be critical information, as such infiltration would result in severe damage to all tissues and organs involved—especially the heart, the brain, and the immune system. Animal studies have demonstrated this. In these vaccinated individuals the source of these spike proteins would be the injected nanolipid carriers of the spike protein producing mRNA. It is obvious that the government health authorities and pharmaceutical manufacturers of these "vaccines" do not want these critical studies done as the public would be outraged and demand an end to the vaccination program and prosecution of the involved individuals who covered this up.

CONCLUSIONS

We are all living through one of the most drastic changes in our culture, economic system, as well as political system in our nation's history as well as the rest of the world. We have been told that we will never return to "normal" and that a great reset has been designed to create a "new world order". This has all been outlined by Klaus Schwab, head of the World Economic Forum, in his book on the "Great Reset".[2053] This book gives a great deal of insight as to the thinking of the utopians who are proud to claim this pandemic "crisis" as their way to usher in a new world. This new world order has been on the drawing boards of the elite manipulators for over a century.[2054] In this paper I have concentrated on the devastating effects this has had on the medical care system in the United States, but also includes much of the Western world. In past papers I have discussed the slow erosion of traditional medical care in the United States and how this system has become increasingly bureaucratized and regimented.[2055] This process was rapidly accelerating, but the appearance of this, in my opinion, manufactured "pandemic" has transformed our health care system over night.

As you have seen, an unprecedented series of events have taken place within this system. Hospital administrators, for example, assumed the position of medical dictators, ordering doctors to follow protocols derived not from those having extensive experience in treating this virus, but rather from a medical bureaucracy that has never treated a single COVID-19 patient. The mandated use of respirators on ICU Covid-19 patients, for example, was imposed in all medical systems and dissenting physicians were rapidly removed from their positions as caregivers, despite their demonstration of markedly improved treatment methods. Further, doctors were told to use the drug remdesivir despite its proven toxicity, lack of effectiveness and high complication rate. They were told to use drugs that impaired respiration and mask every patient, despite the patient's impaired breathing. In each case, those who refused to abuse their patients were removed from the hospital and even faced a loss of license—or worse.

For the first time in modern medical history, early medical treatment of these infected patients was ignored nationwide. Studies have shown that early medical treatment was saving 80% of higher number of these infected people when initiated by independent doctors.[2056] Early treatment could have saved over 640,000 lives over the course of this "pandemic". Despite the demonstration of the power of these early treatments, the forces controlling medical care continued this destructive policy.

Families were not allowed to see their loved ones, forcing these very sick individuals in the hospitals to face their deaths alone. To add insult to injury, funerals were limited to a few grieving family members, who were not allowed to even sit together. All the while large stores, such as Walmart and Cosco were allowed to operate with minimal restrictions. Nursing home patients were also not allowed to have family visitations, again being forced to die a lonely death. All the while, in a number of states, the most transparent being in New York state, infected elderly were purposefully transferred from hospitals into nursing homes, resulting in a very high death rates of these nursing home residents. At the beginning of this "pandemic" over 50% of all death were occurring in nursing homes.

Throughout this "pandemic" we have been fed an unending series of lies, distortions and disinformation by the media, the public health officials, medical bureaucracies (CDC, FDA and WHO) and medical associations. Physicians, scientists, and experts in infectious treatments who formed associations designed to develop more effective and safer treatments, were regularly demonized, harassed, shamed, humiliated, and experience a loss of licensure, loss of hospital privileges and, in at least one case, ordered to have a psychiatric examination.[2057]

Anthony Fauci was given essentially absolute control of all forms of medical care during this event, including insisting that drugs he profited from be used by all treating physicians. He ordered the use of masks, despite at first laughing at the use of masks to filter a virus. Governors, mayors, and many businesses followed his orders without question.

The draconian measures being used, masking, lockdowns, testing of the uninfected, use of the inaccurate PCR test, social distancing, and contact tracing had been shown previously to be of little or no use during previous pandemics, yet all attempts to reject these methods were to no avail. Some states ignored these draconian orders and had either the same or fewer cases, as well as deaths, as the states with the most strictly enforced measures. Again, no amount of evidence or obvious demonstration along these lines had any effect on ending these socially destructive measures. Even when entire countries, such as Sweden, which avoided all these measures, demonstrated equal rates of infections and hospitalization as nations with the strictest, very draconian measures, no policy change by the controlling institutions occurred. No amount of evidence changed anything.

Experts in the psychology of destructive events, such as economic collapses, major disasters and previous pandemics demonstrated that draconian measures come with an enormous cost in the form of "deaths of despair" and in a dramatic increase in serious psychological disorders. The effects of these pandemic measures on children's neurodevelopment is catastrophic and to a large extent irreversible.

Over time tens of thousands could die as a result of this damage. Even when these predictions began to appear, the controllers of this "pandemic" continued full steam ahead. Drastic increases in suicides, a rise in obesity, a rise in drug and alcohol use, a worsening of many health measures and a terrifying rise in psychiatric disorders, especially depression and anxiety, were ignored by the officials controlling this event.

We eventually learned that many of the deaths were a result of medical neglect. Individuals with chronic medical conditions, diabetes, cancer, cardiovascular disease, and neurological diseases were no longer being followed properly in their clinics and doctor's offices. Non-emergency surgeries were put on hold. Many of these patients chose to die at home rather than risk going to the hospitals and many considered hospitals "death houses".

Records of deaths have shown that there was a rise in deaths among those aged 75 and older, mostly explained by Covid-19 infections, but for those between the ages of 65 to 74, deaths had been increasing well before the pandemic onset.[69] Between ages of 18 and aged 65 years, records demonstrate a shocking hike in non-Covid-19 deaths. Some of these deaths were explained by a dramatic increase in drug-related deaths, some 20,000 more than 2019. Alcohol related deaths also increased substantially, and homicides increased almost 30% in the 18 to 65-year group.

The head of the insurance company OneAmerica stated that their data indicated that the death rate for individuals aged 18 to 64 had increased 40% over the pre-pandemic period.[2058] Scott Davidson, the company's CEO, stated that this represented the highest death rate in the history of insurance records, which does extensive data collections on death rates each year. Davidson also noted that this high of a death rate increase has never been seen in the history of death data collection. Previous catastrophes of monumental extent increased death rates no more than 10 percent, 40% is unprecedented.

Dr. Lindsay Weaver, Indiana's chief medical officer, stated that hospitalizations in Indiana are higher than at any point in the past five years. This is of critical importance since the vaccines were supposed to significantly reduce deaths, but the opposite has happened. Hospitals are being flooded with vaccine complications and people in critical condition from medical neglect caused by the lockdowns and other pandemic measures.[2059]

A dramatic number of these people are now dying, with the spike occurring after the vaccines were introduced. The lies flowing from those who have appointed themselves as medical dictators are endless. First, we were told that the lockdown would last only two weeks, they lasted over a year. Then we were told that masks were ineffective and did not need to be worn. Quickly that was reversed. Then we were told the cloth mask was very effective, now it's not and everyone should be wearing an N95 mask and before that that they should double mask. We were told there was a severe shortage of respirators, then we discover they are sitting unused in warehouses and in city dumps, still in their packing crates. We were informed that the hospitals were filled mostly with the unvaccinated and later found the exact opposite was true the world over. We were told that the vaccine was 95% effective, only to learn that in fact the vaccines cause a progressive erosion of innate immunity.

Upon release of the vaccines, women were told the vaccines were safe during all states of pregnancy, only to find out no studies had been done on safety during pregnancy during the "safety tests" prior to release of the vaccine. We were told that careful testing on volunteers before the EUA approval for public use demonstrated extreme safety of the vaccines, only to learn that these unfortunate subjects were not followed, medical complications caused by the vaccines were not paid for and the media covered this all up.[2060] We also learned that the pharmaceutical makers of the vaccines were told by the FDA that further animal testing was unnecessary (the general public would be the Guinea pigs.) Incredibly, we were told that the Pfizer's new mRNA vaccines had been approved by the FDA, which was a clever deception, in that another vaccine had approval (comirnaty) and not the one being used, the BioNTech vaccine. The approved comirnaty vaccine was not available in the United States. The national media told the public that the Pfizer vaccine had been approved and was no longer classed as experimental, a blatant lie. These deadly lies continue. It is time to stop this insanity and bring these people to justice.

Endnotes

1.Dr. Archie Kalokerinos, Interview---- International Vaccine Newsletter June 1995, http://www.whale.to/v/kalokerinos.html.

2.Medicine man Edward Jenner was the father of modern vaccination!, https://www.reformation.org/vaccine.html (last visited on January 6, 2023). See also Charles Ceeithton, M.D., Jenner and Vaccination, 1889, http://www.whale.to/vaccines/creighton_b.html.

3.Eleanor McBean, The Poisoned Needle (1957), http://www.whale.to/a/mcbean.html.

4.Medicine man Edward Jenner, supra.

5.Charles Creighton, M.A., M.D., Encyclopedia Britannica, Ninth Edition, 1875-1889, http://www.whale.to/a/creighton4.html.

6.Id.

7.Id.

8.Eleanor McBean, The Poisoned Needle (1957), http://www.whale.to/a/mcbean.html, quoting Thomas Morgan, Medical Delusions (p. 48-49).

9.Eleanor McBean, supra.

10.Eleanor McBean, supra.

11.Eleanor McBean, supra, quoting Thomas Morgan, Medical Delusions (p. 48-49).

12.Smallpox Vaccination, CDC, https://www.cdc.gov/vaccines/vpd/smallpox/index.html (last visited on January 9, 2013).

13.Smallpox, Mayo Clinic, https://www.mayoclinic.org/diseases-conditions/smallpox/symptoms-causes/syc-20353027 (last visited on January 9, 2023).

14.Smallpox, Mayo Clinic, https://www.mayoclinic.org/diseases-conditions/smallpox/symptoms-causes/syc-20353027 (last visited on January 9, 2023).

15.Kerry Evans, From variolation to vaccination, Labroots, January 1, 2017, https://www.labroots.com/trending/microbiology/4928/variolation-vaccination.

16.R.B. Pearson, The Dream & Lie of Louis Pasteur (1942) (origninally titled: Pasteur, Plagiarist, Imposter), http://www.whale.to/a/b/pearson.html.

17.Burrough Wellcome & Co., Lecture Memoranda, 17th International Congress of Medicine, London, The History of Inoculation and Vaccination for the Prevention of Disease (1913).

18.Burrough Wellcome & Co., supra at 17-18.

19.Ralph W. Nicholas, The Goddess Sitala and Epidemic Smallpox in Bengal, Journal of Asian Studies (1981) 41 (1): 21–44. https://doi.org/10.2307/2055600.

20.Burrough Wellcome & Co., supra at 16.

21.Steve Halbrook, Vaccine Pandemic: Part 1: The Inoculation Controversy of the 1700s, Vaccines and Christianity, January 25, 2019, https://www.vaccinesandchristianity.org/2019/01/25/vaccine-pandemic-part-1-the-inoculation-controversy-of-the-1700s/, quoting James Martin Peebles, Vaccination a Curse and a Menace to Personal Liberty: With Statistics Showing Its Dangers and Criminality (Los Angeles, CA: Peebles Publishing Company, 1913), 14.

22.Steve Halbrook, Vaccine Pandemic: Part 1: The Inoculation Controversy of the 1700s, Vaccines and Christianity, January 25, 2019, https://www.vaccinesandchristianity.org/2019/01/25/vaccine-pandemic-part-1-the-inoculation-controversy-of-the-1700s/, citing William H. York, Health and Wellness in Antiquity Through the Middle Ages (Santa Barbara, CA: ABC-CLIO, 2012), 105, 106.

23.Steve Halbrook, Vaccine Pandemic: Part 1: The Inoculation Controversy of the 1700s, Vaccines and Christianity, January 25, 2019, https://www.vaccinesandchristianity.org/2019/01/25/vaccine-pandemic-part-1-the-inoculation-controversy-of-the-1700s/, quoting James Martin Peebles, Vaccination a Curse and a Menace to Personal Liberty: With Statistics Showing Its Dangers and Criminality (Los Angeles, CA: Peebles Publishing Company, 1913), 14-15.

24.Vaccinia (Smallpox) Vaccines, CDC, https://www.cdc.gov/vaccines/vpd/smallpox/hcp/vaccines.html (last visited on July 30, 2023).

25.Burrough Wellcome & Co., supra at 13-14.

26.Dominik Wujastyk, 'A Pious Fraud': The Indian claims for pre-Jennerian smallpox vaccination, https://www.academia.edu/451964/_A_Pious_Fraud_The_Indian_Claims_for_pre_Jennerian_Smallpox_Vaccination (last visited on July 30, 2023).

27.Dominik Wujastyk, supra.

28.Raymond Obomsawin, Ph.D., Immunity, Infectious Disease, and Vaccination. Video Re-Posted by Edward Hendrie Under Article Heading: The History of Vaccines Proving They Are Ineffective and Dangerous, May 26, 2021, https://greatmountainpublishing.com/2021/05/26/the-history-of-vaccines-proving-they-are-ineffective-and-dangerous/. See also, Ida Honorof and Eleanor McBean, Vaccination, The Silent Killer: A Clear and Present Danger (1977), https://archive.org/details/vaccinationsilen00hono, and Eleanor McBean, The Poisoned Needle (1957), http://www.whale.to/a/mcbean.html.

29.Eleanor McBean, supra.

30.Herbert Shelton, Vaccines and Serum Evils (c1940's), http://www.whale.to/vaccines/shelton3.html (last visited on August 3, 2023).

31.Id.

32.Steve C. Halbrook, Vaccine Pandemic: Part 2: Opposition to Vaccines by Doctors and Others in History, January 25, 2019, https://www.vaccinesandchristianity.org/2019/01/25/vaccine-pandemic-part-2-opposition-to-vaccines-by-doct ors-and-others-in-history/, citing George Starr White, A Lecture Course to Physicians on Natural Methods in Diagnosis and Treatment: Aids to Human Helpers (Los Angeles, CA: George Star White, M.D., 1918), 1032.

33.Steve C. Halbrook, Part 2, supra, quoting Charles Creighton, Jenner and Vaccination: A Strange Chapter of Medical History (London: Swan Sonnenschein & Co., 1889), 353.

34.Charles Creighton, M.A., M.D., Encyclopedia Britannica, Ninth Edition, 1875-1889, http://www.whale.to/a/creighton4.html.

35.Steve C. Halbrook, Part 2, supra, quoting George Starr White, A Lecture Course to Physicians on Natural Methods in Diagnosis and Treatment: Aids to Human Helpers (Los Angeles, CA: George Star White, M.D., 1918), 1032, 1033.

36.Steve C. Halbrook, Part 2, supra.

37.Steve C. Halbrook, Part 2, supra, quoting John W. Hodge, The Vaccination Superstition: Prophylaxis to be Realized Through the Attainment of Health, Not by the Propagation of Disease; Can Vaccination Produce Syphilis? (Niagara Falls, NY: 1902) (Read before the Western New York Homeopathic Medical Society In Buffalo April 11, 1902), 44.

38.Steve C. Halbrook, Part 2, supra, quoting James Martin Peebles, Vaccination a Curse and a Menace to Personal Liberty: With Statistics Showing Its Dangers and Criminality (Los Angeles, CA: Peebles Publishing Company, 1913), 303.

39.Dr. William Howard Hay, Address to The Medical Freedom Society (June 25, 1937), http://www.whale.to/v/hay1.html.

40.Brett Wilcox, Jabbed, How the Vaccine Industry, Medical Establishment and Government Stick It to You and Your Family, at 224 (2018).

41.Brett Wilcox, supra, chapter 1.

42.Brett Wilcox, Jabbed, supra at chapter 23.

43.Brett Wilcox, Jabbed, supra at chapter 23.

44.Brett Wilcox, Jabbed, supra at chapter 23.

45.Edward Hendrie, Antichrist: The Beast Revealed (2015).

46.Physician Group Practice Demonstration, Influenza Vaccination Strategies, CMS, at 6, https://innovation.cms.gov/files/x/pgp-flu-vaccination.pdf (last visited on April 10, 2023).

47.Readers sound off on coed classrooms, vaccines and 'Sesame Street', New York Daily News, November 7, 2015, https://www.nydailynews.com/opinion/nov-7-coed-classrooms-vaccines-sesame-street-article-1.2426184.

48.AMA Supports Tighter Limitations on Immunization Opt Outs, AMA, June 8, 2015, https://web.archive.org/web/20150614042738/https://www.ama-assn.org/ama/pub/news/news/2015/2015-06-08-tighter-limitations-immunization-opt-outs.page.

49.Rong-Gong Lin II, Rosanna Xia, Vaccines required for daycare workers under new California law. Los

Angeles Times, October 13, 2015, https://www.latimes.com/local/lanow/la-me-ln-vaccines-required-for-daycare-workers-under-new-california-law-20151012-story.html.

50.Smallpox, CDC, https://www.cdc.gov/smallpox/index.html#:~:text=Thousands%20of%20years%20ago%2C%20variola,United%20States%20occurred%20in%201949. (last visited on February 11, 2023).

51.Dr. A.R. Campbell, M.D. -- Discoverer of the Cause of Smallpox, https://www.reformation.org/campbell.html (last visited on February 11, 2023).

52.Dr. A.R. Campbell, M.D., supra.

53.Smallpox, CDC, https://www.cdc.gov/smallpox/index.html#:~:text=Thousands%20of%20years%20ago%2C%20variola,United%20States%20occurred%20in%201949. (last visited on February 11, 2023).

54.Tomas S. Cowan and Sally Morell, The Contaigion Myth, at 30 (2020).

55.Toby Rogers, Pfizer COVID Vaccine Fails Risk-Benefit Analysis in Children 5 to 11, The Defender, November 5, 2021, https://childrenshealthdefense.org/defender/fda-pfizer-covid-vaccine-risk-benefit-analysis-nntv-children/.

56.Coronavirus disease (COVID-19): Herd immunity, lockdowns and COVID-19, World Health Organization, 31 December 2020, https://www.who.int/news-room/questions-and-answer

s/item/herd-immunity-lockdowns-and-covid-19.

57.Remarks by President Biden on the COVID-19 Response and the State of Vaccinations, The White House, April 21, 2021, https://www.whitehouse.gov/briefing-room/speeches-remarks/2021/04/21/remarks-by-president-biden-on-the-covid-19-response-and-the-state-of-vaccinations-2/.

58.Koplan JP. Benefits, risks and costs of immunization programmes. Ciba Found Symp. 1985;110:55-68. doi: 10.1002/9780470720912.ch5. PMID: 3921321.

59.Miller NZ, Goldman GS. Infant mortality rates regressed against number of vaccine doses routinely given: is there a biochemical or synergistic toxicity? Hum Exp Toxicol. 2011 Sep;30(9):1420-8. doi: 10.1177/0960327111407644. Epub 2011 May 4. Erratum in: Hum Exp Toxicol. 2011 Sep;30(9):1429. PMID: 21543527; PMCID: PMC3170075, https://www.ncbi.nlm.nih.gov/pmc/articles/PMC3170075/.

60.Dan Olmstead, The Age of Polio. Explosion., https://www.ageofautism.com/the-age-of-polio-explosion.html (last visited on February 11, 2023).

61.Dan Olmstead, supra.

62.Tomas S. Cowan and Sally Morell, The Contaigion Myth, at 30 (2020).

63.Jason Bergerhouse, The Germ Theory Is Bogus!, March 27, 2021, https://thrivespinecenter.com/the-germ-theory-is-bogus/, citing Jim West, Thomas S. Cowan, M.D., and Sally

Fallon Morell.

64.Suzanne Humphries, M.D., Roman Bystrianyk, Dissolving Illusions, at 242 (2015).

65.Suzanne Humphries, M.D., supra.

66.Jim West, Pesticides and Polio: A Critique of Scientific Literature, August 2, 2003, https://somosbacteriasyvirus.com/pdf/polioyddt.pdf.

67.Jim West, supra.

68.Jim West, supra.

69.Jim West, supra .

70.Suzanne Humphries, M.D., Roman Bystrianyk, Dissolving Illusions, at 222-92 (2015).

71.Suzanne Humphries, M.D., supra.

72.Suzanne Humphries, M.D., supra.

73.Jim West, Pesticides and Polio: A Critique of Scientific Literature, August 2, 2003, https://somosbacteriasyvirus.com/pdf/polioyddt.pdf.

74.Dhiman R, Prakash SC, Sreenivas V, Puliyel J. Correlation between Non-Polio Acute Flaccid Paralysis Rates with Pulse Polio Frequency in India. Int J Environ Res Public Health. 2018 Aug 15;15(8):1755. doi: 10.3390/ijerph15081755. PMID: 30111741; PMCID: PMC6121585. https://pubmed.ncbi.nlm.nih.gov/30111741/.

75.Eleanor McBean, The Poisoned Needle (1957).

76.Jefferey Jaxen, 491,000 Children Paralyzed Over 17 Years, Indian Polio Vaccine Program Study Suggests, GreenMedinfo, September 13th 2018, https://greenmedinfo.com/blog/491000-children-paralyzed-over-17-years-indian-polio-vaccine-program-study-sugges.

77.Helen Branswell, 'The switch' was supposed to be a major step toward eradicating polio. Now it's a quandary, STAT, September 13, 2019, https://www.statnews.com/2019/09/13/the-switch-polio-eradication-quandary/.

78.Brian Shilhavy, Big Pharma and Corporate Media Finally Admit the Oral Polio Vaccine is a Failure – Causes Polio Instead of Preventing It, Health Impact News, Novermber 20, 2019, https://healthimpactnews.com/2019/big-pharma-and-corporate-media-finally-admit-the-oral-polio-vaccine-is-a-failure-causes-polio-instead-of-preventing-it/.

79.More polio cases now caused by vaccine than by wild virus, AP, November 25, 2019, https://apnews.com/article/health-united-nations-ap-top-news-pakistan-international-news-7d8b0e32efd0480fbd12acf27729f6a5.

80.Brian Shilhavy, Big Pharma and Corporate Media Finally Admit the Oral Polio Vaccine is a Failure – Causes Polio Instead of Preventing It, Health Impact News, Novermber 20, 2019, https://healthimpactnews.com/2019/big-pharma-and-corporate-media-finally-admit-the-oral-polio-vaccine-is-a-failure-causes-polio-instead-of-preventing-it/.

81.Polio Vaccination—Still Causing Polio After All These Years, Children's Health Defense, September

24, 2019, https://childrenshealthdefense.org/news/childrens-health/polio-vaccination-still-causing-polio-after-all-these-years/.

82.Measles, Mumps, and Rubella (MMR) Vaccination: What Everyone Should Know, CDC, https://www.cdc.gov/vaccines/vpd/mmr/public/index.html (last visited on February 12, 2023).

83.Measles, Mumps, and Rubella (MMR), supra.

84.Dave Mihalovic, Biologist wins Supreme Court case proving that the measles virus does not exist, SOTT, 27 January 2017, https://www.sott.net/article/340948-Biologist-wins-Supreme-Court-case-proving-that-the-measles-virus-does-not-exist.

85.Dave Mihalovic, SOTT, supra.

86.Dave Mihalovic, SOTT, supra.

87.Germany court orders measles sceptic to pay 100,000 euros, BBC, 12 March 2015, https://www.bbc.com/news/world-europe-31864218.

88.Dave Mihalovic, SOTT, supra.

89.Dave Mihalovic, SOTT, supra.

90.Dave Mihalovic, SOTT, supra.

91.Mike Adams, MMR measles vaccine clinical trial results FAKED by Big Pharma - shocking U.S. court documents reveal all, Janaury 25, 2015, https://graviolateam.blogspot.com/2017/02/mmr-measles-vaccine-clinical-trial.html. Complaint For Violation

of the Federal False Claims Act, United States, ex rel., Stephen Kahling and Joan A. Wlochowski v. Merck, U.S. District Court for the District of Eastern Districe of Pennsylvania, Civil Action No. 10 4374, August 27, 2010,
https://www.naturalnews.com/gallery/documents/Merck-False-Claims-Act.pdf.

92.Chatom Primary Care v. Merck, Civil Action No. 12 3555, Class Action Complaint, June 12, 2012, https://www.naturalnews.com/gallery/documents/Chatom-Lawsuit-Merck-Mumps.pdf.

93.Mike Adams, January 25, 2015, supra.

94.Joseph Mercola, Two Lawsuits Accuse Merck of Lying about Vaccine Effectiveness, Vaccine Impact, July 10, 2012,
https://vaccineimpact.com/2012/two-lawsuits-accuse-merck-of-lying-about-vaccine-effectiveness/.

95.Immunization: The Basics, CDC,
https://www.cdc.gov/vaccines/vac-gen/imz-basics.htm (last visited on Janaury 5, 2023).

96.Vaccine Knowledge Project, University of Oxford, https://vk.ovg.ox.ac.uk/vk/vaccine-ingredients#Active%20ingredients (last visited on January 5, 2023).

97.Antigen, Oxford Learner's Dictionaries, https://www.oxfordlearnersdictionaries.com/us/definition/english/antigen (last visited on January 5, 2023).

98.Immunization: The Basics, CDC, https://web.archive.org/web/20210826113846/https://www.cdc.gov/vaccines/vac-gen/imz-basics.htm (August 26, 2021 archive).

99.Vaccine Knowledge Project, University of Oxford, https://vk.ovg.ox.ac.uk/vk/vaccine-ingredients#Active%20ingredients (last visited on January 5, 2023).

100.Claire Gillespie, Fetal Cell Lines Were Used to Make the Johnson & Johnson COVID Vaccine—Here's What That Means, Health, March 4, 2021, https://www.health.com/condition/vaccines/johnson-and-johnson-fetal-cells-vaccine.

101.Vaccines, Merck, https://www.merck.com/research/vaccines/ (last visited on February 23, 2023).

102.Vaccines, Merck, https://www.merck.com/research/vaccines/ (last visited on February 23, 2023).

103.About our company, Merck, https://www.merck.com/company-overview/ (last viewed on February 23, 2023).

104.Hope Changes Lives, Pfizer, https://www.pfizer.com/ (last visited on February 23, 2023).

105.Pharmaceutical Products, The Janssen Pharmaceutical Companies of Johnson & Johnson, Infectious Diseases & Vaccines, https://www.jnj.com/healthcare-products/prescription. (last visited on February 23, 2023).

106.Moderna Reports Fourth Quarter and Fiscal Year 2022 Financial Results and Provides Business Updates, Moderna, February 23, 2023, https://investors.modernatx.com/news/news-details/20

23/Moderna-Reports-Fourth-Quarter-and-Fiscal-Year-2022-Financial-Results-and-Provides-Business-Updates/default.aspx.

107.Medicine, American Dictionary of the English Language, https://webstersdictionary1828.com/Dictionary/medicine (last visited on February 23, 2023).

108.Medicine, supra.

109.Pharmaceutical, American Dictionary of the English Language, https://webstersdictionary1828.com/Dictionary/Pharmaceutic (last visited on February 23, 2023).

110.Pharmaceutical, Online Etymology Dictionary, https://www.etymonline.com/search?q=pharmaceutical (last visited on February 23, 2023).

111.Pharmacy, Online Etymology Dictionary, https://www.etymonline.com/word/pharmaceutical#etymonline_v_14832 (last visited on February 23, 2023).

112.Vioxx: Revisiting Merck's History of Manipulating Science for Profit, Regardless of Public Health Risk, The New Atlantean, Substack, October 11, 2021, https://newatlantean.substack.com/p/vioxx-revisiting-mercks-history-of.

113.Snigdha Prakash, Timeline: The Rise and Fall of Vioxx, NPR, November 10, 2007, https://www.npr.org/2007/11/10/5470430/timeline-the-rise-and-fall-of-vioxx. Vioxx: Revisiting Merck's History of Manipulating Science for Profit, Regardless of Public Health Risk, The New Atlantean, Substack,

October 11, 2021, https://newatlantean.substack.com/p/vioxx-revisiting-mercks-history-of.

114.Gregory D. Curfman, M.D., Stephen Morrissey, Ph.D., and Jeffrey M. Drazen, M.D., Expression of Concern: Bombardier et al., "Comparison of Upper Gastrointestinal Toxicity of Rofecoxib and Naproxen in Patients with Rheumatoid Arthritis," N Engl J Med 2000;343:1520-8., N Engl J Med 2005; 353:2813-2814, DOI: 10.1056/NEJMe058314, December 29, 2005, https://www.nejm.org/doi/full/10.1056/NEJMe058314.

115.Snigdha Prakash, Timeline: The Rise and Fall of Vioxx, NPR, November 10, 2007, https://www.npr.org/2007/11/10/5470430/timeline-the-rise-and-fall-of-vioxx.

116.U.S. Pharmaceutical Company Merck Sharp & Dohme to Pay Nearly One Billion Dollars Over Promotion of Vioxx®, Merck to Pay $950 Million for Illegal Marketing, Department of Justice Office of Public Affairs, November 22, 2011, https://www.justice.gov/opa/pr/us-pharmaceutical-company-merck-sharp-dohme-pay-nearly-one-billion-dollars-over-promotion.

117.Pfizer's $2.3 Billion Settlement Leaves Victims in the lurch, Alliance for Human Research Protection, https://ahrp.org/pfizers-2-3-billion-settlement-leaves-victims-in-the-lurch/ (last visited on February 24, 2023).

118.Pfizer's $2.3 Billion Settlement, supra.

119.Justice Department Announces Largest Health Care Fraud Settlement in Its History, Pfizer to Pay $2.3

Billion for Fraudulent Marketing, September 2, 2009, https://www.justice.gov/opa/pr/justice-department-announces-largest-health-care-fraud-settlement-its-history.

120.Sammy Almashat, et. al., Twenty-Seven Years of Pharmaceutical Industry Criminal and Civil Penalties: 1991 Through 2017, Public Citizen, March 14, 2018, https://www.citizen.org/wp-content/uploads/2408.pdf.

121.Curis Wayant, Risperdal Lawsuit, Consumer Safety, https://www.consumersafety.org/drug-lawsuits/risperdal/ (last visited on February 24, 2023).

122.Johnson & Johnson to Pay More Than $2.2 Billion to Resolve Criminal and Civil Investigations, U.S. Department of Justice, November 4, 2013, https://www.justice.gov/opa/pr/johnson-johnson-pay-more-22-billion-resolve-criminal-and-civil-investigations.

123.Jack Fortier and Brian Mann, Johnson & Johnson Ordered To Pay Oklahoma $572 Million In Opioid Trial, NPR, August 26, 2019, https://www.npr.org/sections/health-shots/2019/08/26/754481268/judge-in-opioid-trial-rules-johnson-johnson-must-pay-oklahoma-572-million.

124.Jack Fortier and Brian Mann, Johnson & Johnson Ordered To Pay Oklahoma $572 Million In Opioid Trial, NPR, August 26, 2019, https://www.npr.org/sections/health-shots/2019/08/26/754481268/judge-in-opioid-trial-rules-johnson-johnson-must-pay-oklahoma-572-million.

125.Justice Department Announces Global Resolution of Criminal and Civil Investigations with Opioid

Manufacturer Purdue Pharma and Civil Settlement with Members of the Sackler Family, Press Release, Ocober 21, 2020, https://www.justice.gov/opa/pr/justice-department-announces-global-resolution-criminal-and-civil-investigations-opioid.

126.Dina Kraft, Sackler Name Is Everywhere at Tel Aviv U., but Not the Opioid Controversy Plaguing the Family, Haaretz, March 4, 2019, https://www.haaretz.com/israel-news/2019-03-04/ty-article/.premium/at-tel-aviv-u-sackler-name-is-everywhere-not-the-opioid-controversy/0000017f-ea91-d0f7-a9ff-eed536350000.

127.Ronny Linder, Tel Aviv University Resists Pressure to Remove Sackler Name Over Opioid Crisis, Haaretz, November 18, 2021, https://www.haaretz.com/israel-news/2021-11-18/ty-article/.premium/tel-aviv-university-resists-pressure-to-remove-sackler-name-over-opioid-crisis/0000017f-e0e2-d7b2-a77f-e3e7fc580000.

128.Harriet Ryan, Lisa Girion and Scott Glover, OxyContin goes global — "We're only just getting started", Los Angeles Times, December 18, 2016, https://www.latimes.com/projects/la-me-oxycontin-part3/.

129.Harriet Ryan, December 18, 2016, supra.

130.Brett Wilcox, Jabbed, How the Vaccine Industry, Medical Establishment and Government Stick It to You and Your Family, at 43-44 (2018).

131.Memo From Alan Bernstein to Larry Hewlett, Regading DTP Vaccine, Wyeth, August 27, 1979, https://www.ageofautism.com/files/wyeth79.pdf.

132.Brett Wilcox, Jabbed, How the Vaccine Industry, Medical Establishment and Government
Stick It to You and Your Family, at 43-44 (2018).

133.Brett Wilcox, Jabbed, How the Vaccine Industry, Medical Establishment and Government
Stick It to You and Your Family, at 30 (2018), quoting Executive Reorganization and Government Research of the Committee on Government Operations United States Senate, Ninety-Second Congress, Second Session, pages 499-505, April 20-21 and May 3-4, 1972.

134.Brett Wilcox, Jabbed, How the Vaccine Industry, Medical Establishment and Government
Stick It to You and Your Family, at 29 (2018), quoting Richard Carter, Breakthrough: The Saga of Jonas Salk, Trident Press, New York, 1965, pp. 318-319.

135.Brett Wilcox, Jabbed, at 28, supra.

136.The Satanic Temple Presents Satancon, https://archive.is/zf48L#selection-1389.0-1389.195 (last visited on February 22, 2023).

137.Brett Wilcox, Jabbed, supra at p. 233.

138.American Medical Association, Source Watch, Center for Media and Democracy, https://www.sourcewatch.org/index.php/American_Medical_Association#cite_note-5 (last visited on April 7, 2023).

139.AMA, Source Watch, supra.

140.Richard Shulze, Forbidden words, and diagnosis, http://whale.to/a/cure_word.html (last visited on April 7, 2023).

141.Pakcage Insert, Gardasil [Quadrivalent Human Papillomavirus (Types 6, 11, 16, 18) Recombinant Vaccine], Merck, http://web.archive.org/web/20060614111131/http://www.merck.com/product/usa/pi_circulars/g/gardasil/gardasil_pi.pdf (last visited on March 15, 2023).

142.Placebo, Merriam-Webster, https://www.merriam-webster.com/dictionary/placebo (last visited on March 16, 2023).

143.Beecher Hk. The Powerful Placebo. JAMA. 1955;159(17):1602–1606. doi:10.1001/jama.1955.02960340022006, https://jamanetwork.com/journals/jama/article-abstract/303530.

144.Doshi P, Bourgeois F, Hong K, et alAdjuvant-containing control arms in pivotal quadrivalent human papillomavirus vaccine trials: restoration of previously unpublished methodologyBMJ Evidence-Based Medicine 2020;25:213-219, https://ebm.bmj.com/content/25/6/213.

145.Package Insert, Gardasil [Human Papillomavirus Quadrivalent (Types 6, 11, 16, and 18) Vaccine, Recombinant], Merck, http://web.archive.org/web/20080916044911/http://www.merck.com/product/usa/pi_circulars/g/gardasil/gardasil_pi.pdf (las visited on March 15, 2023).

146.Doshi P, Bourgeois F, Hong K, et alAdjuvant-containing control arms in pivotal quadrivalent human papillomavirus vaccine trials: restoration of previously unpublished methodologyBMJ Evidence-Based Medicine 2020;25:213-219, https://ebm.bmj.com/content/25/6/213.

147.Doshi, supra.

148.Doshi, supra.

149.Doshi, supra.

150.Doshi, supra.

151.Anonymous, Turtles All the Way Down, at 52 (2022).

152.Vaccine (Shot) for Hepatitis A, CDC, https://www.cdc.gov/vaccines/parents/diseases/hepa.html (last visited on March 15, 2023).

153.VAQTA® (Hepatitis A Vaccine, Inactivated), Suspension for Intramuscular Injection, Package Insert, Merck & Co.

154.Diphtheria, Tetanus, and Pertussis Vaccines, Vaccine Safety, CDC, https://www.cdc.gov/vaccinesafety/vaccines/dtap-tdap-vaccine.html (last visited on March 15, 2023).

155.Dr. William H. Gaunt, M.D., How to cheat and lie with Vaccine Science, https://nexusnewsfeed.com/article/health-healing/how-to-cheat-and-lie-with-vaccine-science/ (last visited on March 14, 2023).

156.Antonia Geber, M.D., Clinical Review of Biological License Application DAPTACEL (CPDT), Division of Vaccines and Related Products Applications, Office of Vaccines Research and Review, Center for Biologics Evaluation and Research, Food and Drug Administration, at 54 and 61, 9 April 2002.

157.Antonia Geber, M.D., supra at p. 55.

158.Investigational Drug, NIH, National Cancer Institute, https://www.cancer.gov/publications/dictionaries/cancer-terms/def/investigational-drug (last visited on March 14, 2023).

159.Package Insert, Pneumococcal 7-valent Conjugate Vaccine (Diphtheria CRM197 Protein) Prevnar®, For Pediatric Use Only, For Intramuscular Injection Only.

160.Anonymous, Turtles All the Way Down, at 61 (2022), citing Black S, Shinefield H, Fireman B, Lewis E, Ray P, Hansen JR, Elvin L, Ensor KM, Hackell J, Siber G, Malinoski F, Madore D, Chang I, Kohberger R, Watson W, Austrian R, Edwards K. Efficacy, safety and immunogenicity of heptavalent pneumococcal conjugate vaccine in children. Northern California Kaiser Permanente Vaccine Study Center Group. Pediatr Infect Dis J. 2000 Mar;19(3):187-95. doi: 10.1097/00006454-200003000-00003. PMID: 10749457.

161.Package Insert, Prevnar.

162.PREVNAR-13 Package Insert, PREVNAR 13 (Pneumococcal 13-valent Conjugate Vaccine [Diphtheria CRM197 Protein]) Suspension for intramuscular injection Initial US Approval: 2010.

163.PREVNAR-13 Package Insert, supra.

164.Ransdell Pierson, U.S. advisory panel recommends Prevnar 13 vaccine for elderly, Reuters, August 13, 2014, https://www.reuters.com/article/us-pfizer-prevnar-idUSKBN0GD23I20140813.

165.Jeremy Howick, Coronavirus vaccine: why it's important to know what's in the placebo, The Conversation, September 21, 2020, https://theconversation.com/coronavirus-vaccine-why-its-important-to-know-whats-in-the-placebo-146365.

166.Study # NCT04368728 (v1), Sponsor BioNTech, Study to Describe the Safety, Tolerability, Immunogenicity, and Potential Efficacy of RNA Vaccine Candidates Against COVID-19 in Healthy Adults, April 29, 2020, https://clinicaltrials.gov/ct2/history/NCT04368728?V_1=View#StudyPageTop.

167.Study # NCT04368728 (v1), supra.

168.Letter from Sarah Kotler, Director Division of Freedom of Information, FDA to ICAN, Request Number: 2020-3738, Subject of Request: ingredients of the ‘placebo’ in the clinical trial NCTR04368728, June 3, 2020, https://icandecide.org/wp-content/uploads/2021/06/Denial-of-Information-Regarding-Placebo-in-Pfizer-COVID-19-Vaccine-Trial.pdf.

169.Vinu Arumugham, Evidence that Food Proteins in Vaccines Cause the Development of Food

Allergies and Its Implications for Vaccine Policy (2015) https://www.longdom.org/open-access/evidence-that-food-proteins-in-vaccines-cause-the-development-of-foodallergies-and-its-implications-for-vaccine-policy-2329-6631-1000137.pdf.

170.Id.

171.Id.

172.American College of Allergy, Asthma, and Immunology, Milk Allergy Affects Half of US Food-Allergic Kids under Age 1: Most children with a milk allergy don't carry epinephrine, ScienceDaily, 16 November 2018, www.sciencedaily.com/releases/2018/11/181116083208.htm.

173.Brett Wilcox, Jabbed, How the Vaccine Industry, Medical Establishment and Government Stick It to You and Your Family, at 41-42 (2018), citing Heather Fraser, The Peanut Allergy Epidemic: What's Causing It and How to Stop It (2011).

174.Robyn Charron, How to Cause a Peanut Allergy Epidemic in 4 Easy Steps, The Thinking Moms' Revolution, August 18, 2015, https://thinkingmomsrevolution.com/whats-really-behind-peanut-allergy-epidemic/.

175.Robyn Charron, August 18, 2015, supra.

176.Steve Zauderer, 69+ Autism Statistics: How Many People Have Autism?, Key Autism Statistics: Rates Of Autism In 2021 and 2022, December 28, 2022, https://www.crossrivertherapy.com/autism-statistics.

177.Child and Adolescent Immunization Schedule by Age, CDC, https://www.cdc.gov/vaccines/schedules/hcp/imz/child-adolescent.html#note-mening (last visited on February 14, 2023).

178.Child and Adolescent Immunization Schedule by Age, CDC, https://www.cdc.gov/vaccines/schedules/hcp/imz/child-adolescent.html#note-mening (last visited on February 14, 2023).

179.Autism & Aluminum Adjuvants in Vaccines, How Aluminum Adjuvants in Vaccines Can Cause, August 18, 2017, Autismhttp://vaccinepapers.org/wp-content/uploads/Autism-and-aluminum-adjuvants-in-vaccines-1.pdf.

180.Vaccine Aluminum Travels Into The Brain, February 10, 2015, http://vaccinepapers.org/vaccine-aluminum-travels-to-the-brain/.

181.Vaccine Aluminum Travels Into The Brain, supra.

182.Matthew Mold, et al., Aluminium in brain tissue in autism, Journal of Trace Elements in Medicine and Biology, 46 (2018) 76-82, http://vaccinepapers.org/wp-content/uploads/Mold-2018-Aluminium-aluminum-in-brain-tissue-in-autism.pdf.

183.Vaccine Aluminum Travels Into The Brain, February 10, 2015, http://vaccinepapers.org/vaccine-aluminum-travels-to-the-brain/.

184.Gallagher CM, Goodman MS. Hepatitis B vaccination of male neonates and autism diagnosis, NHIS 1997-2002. J Toxicol Environ Health A. 2010;73(24):1665-77. doi: 10.1080/15287394.2010.519317. PMID: 21058170. https://pubmed.ncbi.nlm.nih.gov/21058170/.

185.Mawson AR, Ray BD, Bhuiyan AR, Jacob B (2017) Pilot comparative study on the health of vaccinated and unvaccinated 6- to 12-year-old U.S. children. J Transl Sci 3: DOI: 10.15761/JTS.1000186, April 24, 2017, https://www.oatext.com/Pilot-comparative-study-on-the-health-of-vaccinated-and-unvaccinated-6-to-12-year-old-U-S-children.php#gsc.tab=0.

186.Edward Hendrie, Vaccines Cause Autism and Allergies, August 5, 2020, https://greatmountainpublishing.com/2020/08/05/vaccines-cause-autism-and-allergies/.

187.Edward Hendrie, August 5, 2020, supra.

188.Andrew Wakefield, et al., Ileal-lymphoid-nodular hyperplasia, non-specific colitis, and pervasive developmental disorder in children, The Lancet, Volume 351, ISSUE 9103, P637-641, February 28, 1998, https://www.thelancet.com/journals/lancet/article/PIIS0140673697110960/fulltext. DOI:https://doi.org/10.1016/S0140-6736(97)11096-0.

189.Anders Hvid, et al., Measles, Mumps, Rubella Vaccination and Autism, 16 April 2019, https://www.acpjournals.org/doi/full/10.7326/M18-2101.

190.Anders Hvid, et al., supra.

191.Anders Hvid, et al., supra.

192.Novo Nordsk Foundation, Who Are We?, https://novonordiskfonden.dk/en/who-we-are/ (last visited on February 13, 2023).

193.Novo Holdings A/S, Annual Report, 2021, https://www.novoholdings.dk/wp-content/uploads/Novo-Holdings-Annual-Report-2021.pdf.

194.Novo Nordisk Foundation, Open Philanthropy, and Bill & Melinda Gates Foundation Launch Initiative to Support New Antiviral Medicines for Future Pandemics, Bill & Melinda Gates Foundation, https://www.gatesfoundation.org/ideas/media-center/press-releases/2022/03/funding-new-antiviral-medicines-and-preventing-future-pandemics (last visited on February 13, 2023).

195.Quats Application, Novo Nordisk A/S/, https://novonordiskpharmatech.com/products/vaccine-production/ (last visited on February 14, 2023). See also What is Cetrimonium bromide (CTAB)?, Novo Nordisk Pharmaceuticals A/S/, https://novonordiskpharmatech.com/products/ctab/ (last visited on February 14, 2023).

196.Quats Application, Novo Nordisk A/S/, https://novonordiskpharmatech.com/products/vaccine-production/ (last visited on February 14, 2023). See also What is Cetrimonium bromide (CTAB)?, Novo Nordisk Pharmaceuticals A/S/, https://novonordiskpharmatech.com/products/ctab/ (last visited on February 14, 2023).

197.Quats Application, supra.

198.Anders Hvid, et al., Measles, Mumps, Rubella Vaccination and Autism, 16 April 2019, https://www.acpjournals.org/doi/full/10.7326/M18-2101.

199.New in Denmark, Health Guidelines for Parents with small Children, Danish Health Authority, 2016, https://www.sst.dk/-/media/Udgivelser/2016/Ny-i-et-fremmed-land/Engelsk_Ny-i-et-fremmed-land.ashx.

200.Rob Stein, A Large Study Provides More Evidence That MMR Vaccines Don't Cause Autism, NPR, March 4, 2019, https://www.npr.org/sections/health-shots/2019/03/04/699997613/a-large-study-provides-more-evidence-that-mmr-vaccines-dont-cause-autism.

201.Rob Stein, March 4, 2019, supra.

202.New in Denmark, Health Guidelines for Parents with small Children, Danish Health Authority, 2016, https://www.sst.dk/-/media/Udgivelser/2016/Ny-i-et-fremmed-land/Engelsk_Ny-i-et-fremmed-land.ashx.

203.Danish Health Authority Guidelines, 2016, supra.

204.Anders Hvid, et al., Measles, Mumps, Rubella Vaccination and Autism, 16 April 2019, https://www.acpjournals.org/doi/full/10.7326/M18-2101.

205.Rob Stein, A Large Study Provides More Evidence That MMR Vaccines Don't Cause Autism, NPR, March 4, 2019, https://www.npr.org/sections/health-shots/2019/03/04/699997613/a-large-study-provides-more-evidence-that-mmr-vaccines-dont-cause-autism.

206.Rob Stein, March 4, 2019 supra.

207.Comment of Pedro Alcantara, Asociacion Espanola de Pediatria, 9 May 2019. Anders Hvid, et al., Measles, Mumps, Rubella Vaccination and Autism, 16 April 2019, https://www.acpjournals.org/doi/full/10.7326/M18-2101.

208.Comment of Anthony R. Mawson, Department of Epidemiology and Biostatistics, School of Public Health, Jackson State University, 28 March 2019. Anders Hvid, et al., Measles, Mumps, Rubella Vaccination and Autism, 16 April 2019, https://www.acpjournals.org/doi/full/10.7326/M18-2101.

209.Brett Wilcox, Jabbed, How the Vaccine Industry, Medical Establishment and Government Stick It to You and Your Family, at 32-33 (2018).

210.Wilcox, Jabbed, supra.

211.Wilcox, Jabbed, supra.

212.Vaccination Recommendations by the AAP, https://www.aap.org/en/patient-care/immunizations/vaccination-recommendations-by-the-aap/ (last visited on June 17, 2023).

213.COVID-19 Vaccines in Infants, Children, and Adolescents, AAP, August 29, 2022, https://doi.org/10.1542/peds.2022-058700.

214.VAERS COVID Vaccine Adverse Event Reports, June 2, 2023, https://openvaers.com/covid-data.

215.Brian Peckford, American Academy of Pediatrics tries hiding Pfizer funding, August 27, 2021, https://peckford42.wordpress.com/2021/08/27/american-academy-of-pediatrics-tries-hiding-pfizer-funding/.

216.Brian Peckford, August 27, 2021, supra.

217.Vaccination Recommendations by the AAP, https://www.aap.org/en/patient-care/immunizations/vaccination-recommendations-by-the-aap/ (last visited on June 17, 2023).

218.Vaccines—Autism Toolkit, AAP, 2021, https://publications.aap.org/patiented/article-abstract/doi/10.1542/peo_document599/82016/Vaccines-Autism-Toolkit?redirectedFrom=fulltext.

219.Robert E. Weibel, et al., Acute Encephalopathy Followed by Permanent Brain Injury or Death Associated With Further Attenuated Measles Vaccines: A Review of Claims Submitted to the National Vaccine Injury Compensation Program, AAP, March 1998, https://doi.org/10.1542/peds.101.3.383.

220.How Do Vaccines Cause Autism?, https://howdovaccinescauseautism.org/ (last visited on June 17, 2023). See also Ginger Taylor, 214 Research Papers Supporting The Vaccine/Autism Link, April 28, 2014, https://www.scribd.com/doc/220807175/214-Research-Papers-Supporting-the-Vaccine-Autism-Link?utm_source=substack&utm_medium=email#.

221.Steve Kirsch, If vaccines don't cause autism, then how do you explain all this evidence?, June 17, 2023, https://stevekirsch.substack.com/p/if-vaccines-dont-cause-autism-then?utm_source=post-email-title&publicati

on_id=548354&post_id=128881554&isFreemail=true &utm_medium=email.

222.Steve Kirsch, June 17, 2023, supra.

223.Steve Kirsch, June 17, 2023, supra.

224.Steve Kirsch, June 17, 2023, supra.

225.Steve Kirsch, June 17, 2023, supra.

226.Steve Kirsch, June 17, 2023, supra.

227.Thimerosal FAQs, CDC, https://www.cdc.gov/vaccinesafety/concerns/thimerosal/faqs.html#:~:text=make%20us%20sick.-,Is%20thimerosal%20safe%3F,in%20vaccines%20for%20many%20years. (last visited on April 6, 2023).

228.Autism and Vaccines, CDC, https://www.cdc.gov/vaccinesafety/concerns/autism.html (last visited on April 6, 2023).

229.Thomas M. Verstraeten, R. Davies, D. Gu, F DeStefano, Increased risk of developmental neurologic impairment after high exposure to thimerosalcontaining vaccine in first month of life, 1999, https://yale62.org/wp-content/uploads/2021/06/Verstraeten-Thomas-M.D.-et-al-CDC-1999.pdf.

230.Hooker B, Kern J, Geier D, Haley B, Sykes L, King P, Geier M. Methodological issues and evidence of malfeasance in research purporting to show thimerosal in vaccines is safe. Biomed Res Int. 2014;2014:247218. doi: 10.1155/2014/247218. Epub 2014 Jun 4. PMID: 24995277; PMCID: PMC4065774, https://www.ncbi.nlm.nih.gov/pmc/articles/PMC40657

74/#B20.

231.Thimerosal and Vaccines, CDC, https://www.cdc.gov/vaccinesafety/concerns/thimerosal/index.html (last visited on April 5, 2023).

232.Mary Holland, Louis Conte, Robert Krakow, and Lisa Colin, Unanswered Questions from the Vaccine Injury Compensation Program: A Review of Compensated Cases of Vaccine-Induced Brain Injury, 28, Pace Envtl. L. Rev. 480 (2011), Available at: http://digitalcommons.pace.edu/pelr/vol28/iss2/6.

233.Mary Holland, supra.

234.42 U.S.C. § 300aa-11.

235.42 U.S.C. § 300aa-11.

236.42 U.S.C. §§ 300aa-11 and 300aa-21.

237.42 U.S.C. § 300aa-22(c).

238.Mary Holland, Vaccine-Induced Brain Injury, 2011, supra.

239.Ginger Taylor, Adventures in Autism, September 17, 2010, http://adventuresinautism.blogspot.com/2010/09/vaccines-don't-cause-autism-and-guns.html.

240.Ginger Taylor, Adventures in Autism, September 17, 2010, http://adventuresinautism.blogspot.com/2010/09/vaccines-don't-cause-autism-and-guns.html.

241.Court says vaccine not to blame for autism, NBC News, AP, February 12, 2009, https://www.nbcnews.com/health/health-news/court-says-vaccine-not-blame-autism-flna1c9454805.

242.Brett Wilcox, Jabbed, How the Vaccine Industry, Medical Establishment and Government Stick It to You and Your Family, at 175 (2018).

243.Brett Wilcox, Jabbed, supra.

244.Don Olmstead, Weekly Wrap: Standing Up for Yates, Age of Autism, https://www.ageofautism.com/2013/11/standing-up-for-yates.html (last visited on April 6, 2023).

245.Don Olmstead, supra.

246.Mary Holland, Vaccine-Induced Brain Injury, 2011, supra.

247.Vaccine Excipient Summary, Appendix B, CDC, https://www.cdc.gov/vaccines/pubs/pinkbook/downloads/appendices/b/excipient-table-2.pdf (last visited on January 28, 2023).

248.Vaccine Excipient Summary, supra.

249.Vaccine Excipient Summary, supra.

250.Medical Management Guidelines for Formaldehyde, CDC, https://wwwn.cdc.gov/TSP/MMG/MMGDetails.aspx?mmgid=216&toxid=39#:~:text=The%20exact%20mechanism%20of%20action,which%20results%20in%20cell%20death (last visited on January 28, 2023).

251.Center for Disease Control, Vaccine Excipient Summary, February 2020, https://www.cdc.gov/vaccines/pubs/pinkbook/downloa

ds/appendices/b/excipient-table-2.pdf?fbclid=IwAR2cxiqnMzWzyV_YCGjFoQ0Qv4kF0V13aO8qe-IH3D8IwHx0dpp6-KTKL_o.

252.Id.

253.Calvin C. Willhite, Nataliya A. Karyakina, Robert A. Yokel, Nagarajkumar Yenugadhati, Thomas M. Wisniewski, Ian M. F. Arnold, Franco Momoli, and Daniel Krewski1, Systematic Review of Potential Health Risks Posed by Pharmaceutical, Occupational and Consumer Exposures to Metallic and Nanoscale Aluminum, Aluminum Oxides, Aluminum Hydroxide and its Soluble Salts, US National Library of Medicine, National Institutes of Health, August 25, 2016, https://www.ncbi.nlm.nih.gov/pmc/articles/PMC4997813/#R40.

254.Howard Frumkin M.D., Dr.P.H., Director, National Center for Environmental Health/Agency for Toxic Substances and Disease Registry, Julie Louise Gerberding, M.D., M.P.H., Administrator, Agency for Toxic Substances and Disease Registry, TOXICOLOGICAL PROFILE FOR ALUMINUM, September 2008, https://www.atsdr.cdc.gov/toxprofiles/tp22.pdf.

255.Id.

256.Id.

257.Anne Dachel, Dachel Interview: Dr. Paul Thomas, Age of Autism, https://www.ageofautism.com/2017/02/dachel-interview-dr-paul-thomas.html (last visited on April 8, 2023).

258.Thimerosal and Vaccines, CDC, https://www.cdc.gov/vaccinesafety/concerns/thimerosal/index.html (last visited on April 5, 2023).

259.Center for Disease Control, Vaccine Excipient Summary, February 2020, https://www.cdc.gov/vaccines/pubs/pinkbook/downloads/appendices/b/excipient-table-2.pdf?fbclid=IwAR2cxiqnMzWzyV_YCGjFoQ0Qv4kF0V13aO8qe-IH3D8IwHx0dpp6-KTKL_o.

260.Thimerosal and Vaccines, FDA, content current as of February 1, 2018, https://www.fda.gov/vaccines-blood-biologics/safety-availability-biologics/thimerosal-and-vaccines.

261.Thimerosal in Vaccines, FDA, archived page from October 2, 2016, https://web.archive.org/web/20161002220751/http://www.fda.gov/BiologicsBloodVaccines/SafetyAvailability/VaccineSafety/UCM096228 (last visited on April 4, 2023).

262.Geier, David A., Sykes, Lisa K. and Geier, Mark R. (2007) 'A Review of Thimerosal (Merthiolate) and its Ethylmercury Breakdown Product: Specific Historical Considerations Regarding Safety and Effectiveness', Journal of Toxicology and Environmental Health, Part B, 10:8, 575 - 596, DOI: 10.1080/10937400701389875, https://web.archive.org/web/20170727232138/http://www.progressiveconvergence.com/Review%20of%20Thimerosal%20and%20its%20Ethylmercury%20Breakdown%20Product.pdf. See also M.M. Powell and W.A. Jamieson, Merthiolate as a Germicide, American Jounal of Hygiene, 1931 Vol. 13, pp. 296-310, ref. 3. ISSN: 0096-5294, Record Number: 19312701068, https://www.cabdirect.org/cabdirect/abstract/19312701068. Thmerosal and Autism Timeline, Slide Share, April 11, 2014, https://www.slideshare.net/ashotoftruth/a-shot-of-truth-thimerosal-timeline-33423446. Thimerosal and Autism Timeline, Before It's News, Tuesday, October 21, 2014, https://beforeitsnews.com/terrorism/2014/10/thimerosal-and-autism-timeline-2451042.html.

263.Brett Wilcox, Jabbed, How the Vaccine Industry, Medical Establishment and Government Stick It to You and Your Family, at 125 (2018).

264.Thimerosal and Autism Timeline, supra.

265.Brett Wilcox, Jabbed, supra at 125.

266.Thomas M. Verstraeten, R. Davies, D. Gu, F DeStefano, Increased risk of developmental neurologic impairment after high exposure to thimerosalcontaining vaccine in first month of life, 1999, https://yale62.org/wp-content/uploads/2021/06/Verstraeten-Thomas-M.D.-et-al-CDC-1999.pdf.

267.Hooker B, Kern J, Geier D, Haley B, Sykes L, King P, Geier M. Methodological issues and evidence of malfeasance in research purporting to show thimerosal in vaccines is safe. Biomed Res Int. 2014;2014:247218. doi: 10.1155/2014/247218. Epub 2014 Jun 4. PMID: 24995277; PMCID: PMC4065774, https://www.ncbi.nlm.nih.gov/pmc/articles/PMC4065774/#B20.

268.Fact Sheet for Recipients and Caregivers, Emergency Use Authorization (EUA) of the Moderna

COVID-19 Vaccine to Prevent Coronavirus Disease 2019 (COVID-19) in Individuals 18 Years of Age and Older, https://www.fda.gov/media/144638/download. Fact Sheet for Recipients and Caregivers, Emergency Use Authorization (EUA) of the Pfizer-BioNTech COVID-19 Vaccine to Prevent Coronavirus Disease 2019 (COVID-19) in Individuals 18 Years of Age and Older, https://www.fda.gov/media/144414/download.

269.Cosby A. Stone, M.D., M.P.H., et al., Immediate Hypersensitivity to Polyethylene Glycols and Polysorbates: More Common Than We Have Recognized, The Journal of Allergy and Clinical Immunology: In Practice, Volume 7, Issue 5, 2019 May-June, https://www.ncbi.nlm.nih.gov/pmc/articles/PMC6706272/ and https://www.sciencedirect.com/science/article/abs/pii/S2213219818308237?via%3Dihub.

270.These 'Inactive' Ingredients in COVID Vaccines Could Trigger Allergic Reactions, March 12, 2021, https://childrenshealthdefense.org/defender/inactive-ingredients-covid-vaccines-allergic-reactions/.

271.Angel A. Justiz Vaillant, et. al., Immediate Hypersensitivity Reactions, January 2021, https://pubmed.ncbi.nlm.nih.gov/30020687/.

272.These 'Inactive' Ingredients in COVID Vaccines Could Trigger Allergic Reactions, March 12, 2021, https://childrenshealthdefense.org/defender/inactive-ingredients-covid-vaccines-allergic-reactions/.

273.RFK, Jr. Warned FDA Three Months Ago About Ingredient in Pfizer COVID Vaccine That Likely Caused Life-Threatening Reaction in Two UK

Healthcare Workers, December 11, 2020, https://childrenshealthdefense.org/defender/pfizer-covid-vaccine-reaction-fda-peg/.

274.Fact Sheet for Recipients and Caregivers, Emergency Use Authorization (EUA) of the Janssen COVID-19 Vaccine to Prevent Coronavirus Disease 2019 (COVID-19) in Individuals 18 Years of Age and Older, https://www.fda.gov/media/146305/download.

275.Vaccine Excipient Summary, Excipients Included in U.S. Vaccines, by Vaccine, 2019-2020 Norther Hemisphere Formulations, CDC, https://www.cdc.gov/vaccines/pubs/pinkbook/downloads/appendices/b/excipient-table-2.pdf?fbclid=IwAR2cxiqnMzWzyV_YCGjFoQ0Qv4kF0V13aO8qe-IH3D8IwHx0dpp6-KTKL_o.

276.Cosby A. Stone, M.D., M.P.H., et al., Immediate Hypersensitivity to Polyethylene Glycols and Polysorbates: More Common Than We Have Recognized, The Journal of Allergy and Clinical Immunology: In Practice, Volume 7, Issue 5, 2019 May-June, https://www.ncbi.nlm.nih.gov/pmc/articles/PMC6706272/ and https://www.sciencedirect.com/science/article/abs/pii/S2213219818308237?via%3Dihub.

277.These 'Inactive' Ingredients in COVID Vaccines Could Trigger Allergic Reactions, March 12, 2021, https://childrenshealthdefense.org/defender/inactive-ingredients-covid-vaccines-allergic-reactions/.

278.Angel A. Justiz Vaillant, et. al., Immediate Hypersensitivity Reactions, January 2021, https://pubmed.ncbi.nlm.nih.gov/30020687/.

279.Berkely Lovelace, Jr., J&J Says Two Trial Participants Had Severe Allergic Reactions after Getting Covid Vaccine, CNBC, February 26, 2021, https://www.cnbc.com/2021/02/26/jj-says-two-people-had-severe-allergic-reactions-after-getting-covid-vaccine.html.

280.Brett Wilcox, Jabbed, How the Vaccine Industry, Medical Establishment and Government Stick It to You and Your Family, at 41-42 (2018).

281.Eleanor McBean, The Poisoned Needle (1957).

282.Eleanor McBean, The Poisoned Needle (1957).

283.Lioness of Judah Ministry, MIND-BLOWING REVELATION: Why It's IMPOSSIBLE to "Vaccinate" Against Anything and Why "Vaccines" Are the PERFECT POISONS, Ocober 2, 2024, https://lionessofjudah.substack.com/p/mind-blowing-revelation-why-its-impossible?publication_id=581065&utm_campaign=email-post-title&r=2q45gw&utm_medium=email.

284.Id.

285.Id.

286.Id.

287.Arumugham, Vinu, Evidence that Food Proteins in Vaccines Cause the Development of Food Allergies and Its Implications for Vaccine Policy (2015). Journal of Developing Drugs, 2015, DOI: 10.4172/2329-6631.1000137, Available at SSRN: https://ssrn.com/abstract=3571073.

288.Charles Richet Facts, The Nobel Prize in Physiology or Medicine 1913, https://www.nobelprize.org/prizes/medicine/1913/richet/facts/ (last visited on October 7, 2024).

289.Id.

290.Poison, Merriam Webster Dictionary, https://www.merriam-webster.com/dictionary/poison (last visited on December 13, 2024).

291.ICD-10-CM, CDC, June 7, 2024, https://www.cdc.gov/nchs/icd/icd-10-cm/index.html.

292.ICD-9-CM Dignosis Code 978, https://www.icd10data.com/search?s=978&codebook=icd9volume1 (last visited on December 13, 2024).

293.Convert ICD-9-CM Diagnosis 978.4 to ICD-10-CM, https://www.icd10data.com/Convert/978.4 (last visited on December 13, 2024).

294.ICD-9-CM Dignosis Code 978, https://www.icd10data.com/search?s=978&codebook=icd9volume1 (last visited on December 13, 2024).

295.Convert ICD-9-CM Diagnosis 978.5 to ICD-10-CM, https://www.icd10data.com/Convert/978.5 (last visited on December 13, 2024).

296.ICD-9-CM Diagnosis Code 979.4, https://www.icd10data.com/Search?s=979.4&codebook=icd9volume1 (last visited on December 13, 2024).

297.2025 ICD-10-CM Diagnosis Code T50.B91A, https://www.icd10data.com/ICD10CM/Codes/S00-T88

/T36-T50/T50-/T50.B91A (last visited on December 13, 2024).

298.Convert ICD-9-CM Diagnosis 979.5 to ICD-10-CM, https://www.icd10data.com/Convert/979.5 (last visited on December 13, 2024).

299.Vaccine Ingredients – Fetal Cells, Vaccine Education Center, CHOP, https://www.chop.edu/centers-programs/vaccine-education-center/vaccine-ingredients/fetal-tissues (last visited on January 28, 2023).

300.Overview of COVID-19 Vaccines, CDC, November 1, 2022, https://www.cdc.gov/coronavirus/2019-ncov/vaccines/different-vaccines/overview-COVID-19-vaccines.html?CDC_AA_refVal=https%3A%2F%2Fwww.cdc.gov%2Fcoronavirus%2F2019-ncov%2Fvaccines%2Fdifferent-vaccines%2FModerna.html.

301.ImmunizeBC, https://immunizebc.ca/ask-us/questions/are-there-any-animal-products-including-pork-covid-19-vaccines (last visited on January 29, 2023).

302.Claire Gillespie, Fetal Cell Lines Were Used to Make the Johnson & Johnson COVID Vaccine—Here's What That Means, Health, March 4, 2021, https://www.health.com/condition/vaccines/johnson-and-johnson-fetal-cells-vaccine.

303.Danielle Ong, Johnson & Johnson Vaccine Did Use Aborted Fetal Cell Lines: What Does This Mean?, International Business Times, March 4, 2021, https://www.ibtimes.com/johnson-johnson-vaccine-did-use-aborted-fetal-cell-lines-what-does-mean-3156846.

304.Claire Gillespie, March 4, 2021, supra.

305.Kyle Christopher McKenna, Ph.D, Use of Aborted Fetal Tissue in Vaccines and Medical Research Obscures the Value of All Human Life, US National Library of Medicine
National Institutes of Health, March 28, 2018, https://www.ncbi.nlm.nih.gov/pmc/articles/PMC6027112/.

306.Id.

307.Id.

308.Vaccines, Abortion, & Fetal Tissue, Right to Life of Michigan, https://rtl.org/educational-materials/vaccines-abortion/, July 9, 2020, quoting Transcript of the Vaccines and Related Biological Products Advisory Committee of the U.S. Food and Drug Administration, hearing date 16 May 2001, 91. See also, https://www.ohiolife.org/vaccines_abortion_fetal_tissue, October 27, 2017.

309.Jack Jenkins, New Novavax Shot Could Appeal to Pro-Life Christian Skeptics, Religious News Service, February 18, 2022, https://www.christianitytoday.com/news/2022/february/novavax-covid-vaccine-cell-lines-pro-life-abortion-christia.html.

310.McKenna KC. Use of Aborted Fetal Tissue in Vaccines and Medical Research Obscures the Value of All Human Life. Linacre Q. 2018 Feb;85(1):13-17. doi:

10.1177/0024363918761715. Epub 2018 Mar 28. PMID: 29970932; PMCID: PMC6027112. Also found at Lyle Christopher McKenna, Use of Aborted Fetal Tissue in Vaccines and Medical Research Obscures the Value of All Human Life, NIH, March 28, 2018, https://www.ncbi.nlm.nih.gov/pmc/articles/PMC6027112/.

311.Sandhya Bangaru, et al., Structural analysis of full-length SARS-CoV-2 spike protein from an advanced vaccine candidate, 20 October 2020, https://www.science.org/doi/10.1126/science.abe1502.

312.Sandhya Bangaru, et al., Structural analysis of full-length SARS-CoV-2 spike protein from an advanced vaccine candidate, 20 October 2020, https://www.science.org/doi/10.1126/science.abe1502.

313.Jack Jenkins, New Novavax Shot Could Appeal to Pro-Life Christian Skeptics, Religious News Service, February 18, 2022, https://www.christianitytoday.com/news/2022/february/novavax-covid-vaccine-cell-lines-pro-life-abortion-christia.html.

314.Sarah Quale, Yes, Novavax Used HEK293, an Aborted Fetal Cell Line, Personhood Alliance, February 2, 2022, https://personhood.org/yes-novavax-used-hek293-an-aborted-fetal-cell-line-2/.

315.Sara Quale, February 2, 2022, supra.

316.562 U.S. 223 (2011), https://www.supremecourt.gov/opinions/10pdf/09-152.pdf.

317.42 U.S.C. § 300aa–22, https://www.law.cornell.edu/uscode/text/42/300aa-22.

318.National Vaccine Injury Compensation Program, Children's Health Defense, https://childrenshealthdefense.org/national-vaccine-injury-compensation-program/ (last visited on January 6, 2021).

319.Mary S. Holland, Liability for Vaccine Injury: The United States, the European Union, and the Developing World, Emory Law Journal, Vol 67, 2018, https://scholarlycommons.law.emory.edu/elj/vol67/iss3/3/.

320.Mary S. Holland, supra.

321.National Vaccine Injury Compensation Program, Children's Health Defense, https://childrenshealthdefense.org/national-vaccine-injury-compensation-program/ (last visited on January 6, 2021).

322.Mary S. Holland, supra.

323.Mary S. Holland, supra. Quoting Gayle DeLong, Is "Delitigation" Associated with a Change in Product Safety? The Case of Vaccines, Rev. Ind. Org. (June 14, 2017).

324.42 U.S.C. § 300aa–22, https://www.law.cornell.edu/uscode/text/42/300aa-22.

325.42 U.S.C. § 300aa–27, https://www.law.cornell.edu/uscode/text/42/300aa-27.

326.42 U.S.C. § 300aa–27.

327.42 U.S.C. § 300aa–27.

328.42 U.S.C. § 300aa–27.

329.RFK, Jr. Proves HHS is in Violation of the "Mandate for Safer Childhood Vaccines" as Stipulated in the Vaccine Injury Compensation Act, Children's Health Defense, September 13, 2018, https://childrenshealthdefense.org/child-health-topics/federal-failures/rfk-jr-proves-hhs-is-in-violation-of-the-mandate-for-safer-childhood-vaccines-as-stipulated-in-the-vaccine-injury-compensation-act/. ICAN v. HHS, Complaint for Declaratory and Injunctive Relief, April 12, 2018, https://childrenshealthdefense.org/wp-content/uploads/rfk-complaint-against-united-states-department-of-health-and-human-services.pdf. See also ICAN & RFK, Jr. Call Out DHHS for Vaccine Safety Violations, Texans for Vaccine Choice, July 18, 2018, https://texansforvaccinechoice.com/ican-rfk-jr-call-out-dhhs-for-vaccine-safety-violations/.

330.ICAN v. HHS, Stipulation, July 9, 2018, https://childrenshealthdefense.org/wp-content/uploads/rfk-hhs-stipulated-order-july-2018.pdf.

331.RFK, Jr. Proves HHS is in Violation of the "Mandate for Safer Childhood Vaccines" as Stipulated in the Vaccine Injury Compensation Act, Children's Health Defense, September 13, 2018, https://childrenshealthdefense.org/child-health-topics/federal-failures/rfk-jr-proves-hhs-is-in-violation-of-the-mandate-for-safer-childhood-vaccines-as-stipulated-in-the-vaccine-injury-compensation-act/.

332.Edward Hendrie, Study Shows That Vaccinated Children Are Significantly Less Healthy Than

Unvaccinated Children, December 20, 2020, https://greatmountainpublishing.com/2020/12/20/study-shows-that-vaccinated-children-are-significantly-less-healthy-than-unvaccinated-children/. Edward Hendrie, Vaccines Increase Mortality of Infants, August 17, 2020, https://greatmountainpublishing.com/2020/08/17/vaccines-increase-mortality-of-children/. Edward Hendrie, Vaccines Cause Autism and Allergies, August 5, 2020, https://greatmountainpublishing.com/2020/08/05/vaccines-cause-autism-and-allergies/.

333.Pfizer to Acquire Arena Pharmaceuticals, December 13, 2021, https://www.pfizer.com/news/press-release/press-release-detail/pfizer-acquire-arena-pharmaceuticals.

334.Edward Hendrie, Follow the SILENCE: Paper Proving That COVID-19 Vaccines Cause Myocarditis Is Removed From Publication Without Explanation, October 31, 2021, https://greatmountainpublishing.com/2021/10/31/follow-the-silence-paper-proving-that-covid-19-vaccines-cause-myocarditis-is-removed-from-publication-without-explanation/. See also Edward Hendrie, The FDA and Pfizer Concealed Evidence That COVID-19 Vaccines Will Cause Myocarditis in Children, November 7, 2021, https://greatmountainpublishing.com/2021/11/07/the-fda-and-pfizer-concealed-evidence-that-covid-19-vaccines-will-cause-myocarditis-in-children/.

335.Pfizer buys immuno-inflammatory firm Arena Pharmaceuticals for $6.7b, December 13, 2021, Outsourcing-Pharma, https://www.outsourcing-pharma.com/Article/2021/12/13/Pfizer-buys-immuno-inflammatory-firm-Arena-for-

6.7b.

336.Edward Hendrie, Doctor Finds That His Patients Have Permanent Organ Damage from Blood Clots Caused by COVID-19 Vaccines, Great Mountain Publishing, October 23, 2021, https://greatmountainpublishing.com/2021/10/23/doctor-finds-that-his-patients-have-permanent-organ-damage-from-blood-clots-caused-by-covid-19-vaccines/, quoting CFT Team, Doctor Warns How COVID mRNA 'Vaccines' Will Cause Delayed Strokes & Heart Attacks — 'The Worst Is Yet To Come', July 14, 2021, https://christiansfortruth.com/doctor-warns-how-covid-mrna-vaccines-will-soon-cause-strokes-heart-attacks-the-worst-is-yet-to-come/.

337.Harvey Eisner, Firehouse Magazine, archived October 7, 1999 page, https://web.archive.org/web/19991007180848/https://www.firehouse.com/magazine/archives/1998/September/progress2.html.

338.Firefighter Arson, USFA-TR-141/January 2003, Special Report, U.S. Fire Administration, FEMA, archived page from November 9, 2004, ttps://web.archive.org/web/20041109074057/https://www.usfa.fema.gov/downloads/pdf/publications/tr-141.pdf.

339.Pfizer Completes Acquisition of Global Blood Therapeutics, Pfizer, October 05, 2022, https://www.pfizer.com/news/press-release/press-release-detail/pfizer-completes-acquisition-global-blood-therapeutics.

340.Top Pathologist confirms Cancer, Infertility & Strange Blood Clots are common side effects of Covid-19 Vaccination, The Expose, April 22, 2023, https://expose-news.com/2023/04/22/cancer-infertility-blood-clots-due-to-covid-vaccination/?cmid=b9c65fea-8808-4668-80f8-1e76ab03f676.

341.Official Government Reports prove the COVID Vaccines cause Cancer. The Expose, August 21, 2021, https://expose-news.com/2022/08/21/gov-reports-prove-covid-vaccines-cause-cancer/. See also Lynn Redwood, Researchers Show How COVID Damages Immune System, Increasing Cancer Risks — Science Says Vaccines May Do the Same, The Defender, December 20, 2021, https://childrenshealthdefense.org/defender/covid-vaccines-immune-system-cancer-risks/, citing Jiang H, Mei Y-F. SARS–CoV–2 Spike Impairs DNA Damage Repair and Inhibits V(D)J Recombination In Vitro. Viruses. 2021; 13(10):2056. https://doi.org/10.3390/v13102056 (Published: 13 October 2021 / Retracted: 10 May 2022).

342.Eustace Mullins, Murder by Injection, The Story of the Medical Conspiracy Against America, at 82 (1988).

343.Eustace Mullins, Murder by Injection, The Story of the Medical Conspiracy Against America, at 82 (1988).

344.Phil Taylor, The top 10 biopharma M&A deals in 2021, January 18, 2022, Fierce Pharma, https://www.fiercepharma.com/special-report/top-10-biopharma-m-a-deals-2021.

345.Pfizer Invests $43 Billion to Battle Cancer, Pfizer, March 13, 2023, https://www.pfizer.com/news/press-release/press-release-detail/pfizer-invests-43-billion-battle-cancer.

346.McKenzie Sigalos, You Can't Sue Pfizer or Moderna If You Have Severe Covid Vaccine Side Effects. The Government Likely Won't Compensate You for Damages Either, CNBC, December 17, 2020, https://www.cnbc.com/2020/12/16/covid-vaccine-side-effects-compensation-lawsuit.html.

347.Zachary Stieber, Few, If Any, Doses of Spikevax or Comirnaty Available in United States, Despite FDA Approvals, The Epoch Times, February 2, 2022, https://archive.ph/Ry0Xh. See also SpikeVax COVID-19 Vaccine (Moderna), Updated May 28, 2022, https://www.precisionvaccinations.com/vaccines/spikevax-covid-19-vaccine-moderna. "As of July 11, 2022, Moderna's SpikeVax was **available** in Poland, Czech Republic, Caribbean, Denmark, Romania, Hungary, Bulgaria, Slovenia, Slovakia, Croatia, Estonia, Latvia, Lithuania, Serbia, Ukraine, Moldova, Albania, Bosnia-Herzegovina, Kosovo, North Macedonia, Montenegro, Israel, France, the African Union, Australian, Spain, Switzerland, South Korea, the United Kingdom, Switzerland, and was **Approved in the U.S.**" Id.

348.MacKenzie Sigalos, You Can't Sue Pfizer or Moderna If You Have Severe Covid Vaccine Side Effects. The Government Likely Won't Compensate You for Damages Either, CNBC, December 17, 2020, https://www.cnbc.com/2020/12/16/covid-vaccine-side-effects-compensation-lawsuit.html.

349.Mary S. Holland, *Liability for Vaccine Injury: The United States, the European Union, and the Developing World*, 67 Emory L. J. 415 (2018). Available at: https://scholarlycommons.law.emory.edu/elj/vol67/iss3/3.

350.Countermeasures Injury Compensation Program, Request for Benefits Form Instructions, OMB Control No. 0915-0334, Expiration Date: 3/31/2023, https://www.hrsa.gov/sites/default/files/hrsa/cicp/cicp-request-form-instructions.pdf.

351.Id.

352.MacKenzie Sigalos, You Can't Sue Pfizer or Moderna If You Have Severe Covid Vaccine Side Effects. The Government Likely Won't Compensate You for Damages Either, CNBC, December 17, 2020, https://www.cnbc.com/2020/12/16/covid-vaccine-side-effects-compensation-lawsuit.html.

353.A Vaccine Progress Report, The Wall Street Jounal, July 22, 2020, https://www.wsj.com/articles/a-vaccine-progress-report-11595461075?mod=searchresults&page=1&pos=5.

354.Edmund Massey, A Sermon Against the Dangerous and Sinful Practice of Inoculation, at 6 (1722).

355.Edmund Massey, A Sermon Against the Dangerous and Sinful Practice of Inoculation, at 7 (1722).

356.Edmund Massey, A Sermon Against the Dangerous and Sinful Practice of Inoculation, at 13

(1722).

357.Edmund Massey, A Sermon Against the Dangerous and Sinful Practice of Inoculation, at 15 (1722).

358.Eustace Mullins, Murder by Injection, The Story of the Medical Conspiracy Against America, at 82 (1988).

359.WE, THE PEOPLE@HD283271, Twitter, January 13, 2023, https://mobile.twitter.com/HD283271/status/1614002688802308097.

360.Eleanor McBean, The Poisoned Needle (1957), http://www.whale.to/a/mcbean.html.

361.Eleanor McBean, supra.

362.Eleanor McBean, supra.

363.Eleanor McBean, supra.

364.Eleanor McBean, supra.

365.Eustace Mullins, Murder by Injection, The Story of the Medical Conspiracy Against America, at 81 (1988).

366.Eustace Mullins, Murder by Injection, supra.

367.Rhoda Wilson, Big Study Finds Non-Vaccinated are Healthier than Vaccinated, The Expose, April 11, 2022, https://expose-news.com/2022/04/11/study-finds-non-vaccinated-are-healthier-than-vaccinated/.

368.The Control Group, https://www.thecontrolgroup.org/.

369.The Control Group, https://www.thecontrolgroup.org/.

370.Eleanor McBean, supra.

371.Eleanor McBean, supra.

372.Eleanor McBean, supra.

373.Eleanor McBean, supra.

374.Eleanor McBean, supra.

375.Eleanor McBean, supra.

376.Eleanor McBean, supra.

377.Eleanor McBean, supra.

378.Sharon Rikin, et al., Assessment of temporally-related acute respiratory illness following influenza vaccination, Elsevier, Volume 36, Issue 15, April 2018, https://www.sciencedirect.com/science/article/pii/S0264410X18303153?via%3Dihub#t0010.

379.Sharon Rikin, et al., supra.

380.Surender Khurana, Vaccine-Induced Anti-HA2 Antibodies Promote Virus Fusion and Enhance Influenza Virus Respiratory Disease, Science Translational Medicine, Vol 5, Issue 200, 28 August 2013, https://www.science.org/doi/10.1126/scitranslmed.3006366.

381.Surender Khurana, supra.

382.Brett Wilcox, Jabbed, How the Vaccine Industry, Medical Establishment and Government Stick It to You and Your Family, at 178 (2018)

383.Influenza, CDC, https://www.cdc.gov/nchs/fastats/flu.htm (last visited on April 6, 2023). See also, https://web.archive.org/web/20230406133028/https://www.cdc.gov/nchs/fastats/flu.htm.

384.Glen Nowak, Planning for the 2004-05 Influenza Vaccination Season: A Communication Situation Analysis, archived September 5, 2004 page, https://web.archive.org/web/20040905095426/https://www.ama-assn.org/ama1/pub/upload/mm/36/2004_flu_nowak.pdf.

385.Laheij RJF, Sturkenboom MCJM, Hassing R, Dieleman J, Stricker BHC, Jansen JBMJ. Risk of Community-Acquired Pneumonia and Use of Gastric Acid–Suppressive Drugs. JAMA. 2004;292(16):1955–1960. doi:10.1001/jama.292.16.1955, https://jamanetwork.com/journals/jama/article-abstract/199672.

386.Jon Rappoport, Bombshell: 18 people died of the flu, not 36,000, September 8, 2012, https://www.naturalnews.com/037129_influenza_death_statistics_CDC.html.

387.Influenza: The Disease, CDC, archived September 27, 2008, page, https://web.archive.org/web/20080927045351/http://www.cdc.gov/flu/about/disease/.

388.Kenneth Stoller, CDC — Influenza Deaths: Request for Correction (RFC), https://aspe.hhs.gov/cdc-influenza-deaths-request-correction-rfc (last visited on April 6, 2023).

389.Seasonal Influenza: The Disease, CDC, archived April 7, 2010, page, https://web.archive.org/web/20100407203929/http://www.cdc.gov/flu/about/disease/.

390.Glen Nowak, Planning for the 2004-05 Influenza Vaccination Season: A Communication Situation Analysis, archived September 5, 2004 page, https://web.archive.org/web/20040905095426/https://www.ama-assn.org/ama1/pub/upload/mm/36/2004_flu_nowak.pdf.

391.Glen Nowak, supra.

392.Glen Nowak, supra.

393.Seasonal Flu Vaccines, CDC, https://www.cdc.gov/flu/prevent/flushot.htm#:~:text=Everyone%206%20months%20and%20older,the%202010%2D2011%20flu%20season. (last visited on April 7, 2023).

394.Brett Wilcox, Jabbed, supra at 180, citing Vittorio Demicheli, et al., Vaccines for preventing influenza in healthy adults, February 1, 2018, https://doi.org/10.1002/14651858.CD001269.pub6.

395.Brett Wilcox, Jabbed, supra at 181.

396.Brett Wilcox, Jabbed, supra at 181.

397.Congressional Record, 113th Congress, Vol. 159, No. 59, at E576, April 26, 2013, https://www.govinfo.gov/content/pkg/CREC-2013-04-26/pdf/CREC-2013-04-26.pdf.

398.Dan Burton, "Mercury in Medicine," Congressional Record (May 20, 2003): E1011, E1014, https://www.aapsonline.org/vaccines/mercinmed.pdf.

399.Influenza (Flu) Vaccine and Pregnancy, CDC, https://www.cdc.gov/vaccines/pregnancy/hcp-toolkit/flu-vaccine-pregnancy.html (last visited on April 7, 2023).

400.Brett Wilcox, Jabbed, supra.

401.Daniel Neides, Make 2017 the year to avoid toxins (good luck) and master your domain: Words on Wellness, Cleveland Clinic, January 6, 2017, https://www.cleveland.com/lyndhurst-south-euclid/2017/01/make_2017_the_year_to_avoid_to.html.

402.Statement from Cleveland Clinic, Affirming our support of vaccinations, Cleveland Clinic, January 8, 2017, https://newsroom.clevelandclinic.org/2017/01/08/statement-cleveland-clinic/.

403.Brett Wilcox, Jabbed, supra at 248.

404.Brett Wilcox, Jabbed, How the Vaccine Industry, Medical Establishment and Government Stick It to You and Your Family, at 249 (2018).

405.Brett Wilcox, Jabbed, supra at 247-48.

406.Brett Wilcox, Jabbed supra at 183.

407.FLUARIX QUADRIVALENT (Influenza Vaccine) injectable suspension, for intramuscular use

2022-2023 Formula Initial U.S. Approval: 2012, at 16, https://www.fda.gov/media/79278/download.

408.FLUARIX QUADRIVALENT (Influenza Vaccine) injectable suspension, for intramuscular use 2022-2023 Formula Initial U.S. Approval: 2012, https://gskpro.com/content/dam/global/hcpportal/en_US/Prescribing_Information/Fluarix_Quadrivalent/pdf/FLUARIX-QUADRIVALENT.PDF.

409.Edmund Massey, A Sermon Against the Dangerous and Sinful Practice of Inoculation, at 14 (1722).

410.Edmund Massey, supra at p. 15.

411.Paul Offit, Biography, https://www.paul-offit.com/about-paul-offit-md (last visited on January 29, 2023).

412.Are Fetal Cells Used to Make Vaccines?, https://www.chop.edu/centers-programs/vaccine-education-center/video/are-fetal-cells-used-make-vaccines (last visited on January 29, 2023).

413.Patrick Reilly, *Assessing the Catholic Campaign for Human Development, Human Events,* November 20, 1998.

414.*Id.*

415.*Id.*

416.*Id.*

417.*Id.*

418.Katheryn Jean Lopez, *Catholic Campaign for Human Development: Still Entranced by Leftist Activism, Despite Growing Unrest, Human Events,* November 10, 2000.

419.*Id.*

420.*Id.*

421.*Id.*

422.*Id.*

423.KERRI HOUSTON AND PATRICIA FAVA, ALL GORE, AMERICA IN THE BALANCE, p. 59 (2000).

424.Walt Murray, A medical Mort Sahl, Press-Telegram, January 21, 1983, https://thepeoplesdoctor.net/wp-content/uploads/2016/01/ASC17293.pdf.

425.Brett Wilcox, Jabbed, How the Vaccine Industry, Medical Establishment and Government Stick It to You and Your Family (2018), quoting Robert S. Mendelsohn, Confessions of a Medical Heretic (1979).

426.Brett Wilcox, supra, quoting Robert S. Mendelsohn, Confessions of a Medical Heretic (1979).

427.Richard Moskowitz, The Case Against Immunizations, https://sites.google.com/site/doctorrmosk/the-case-against-immunizations (last visited on March 26, 2023).

428.Brett Wilcox, supra, quoting Olivier Clerc, Modern Medicine: The New World Religion: How

Beliefs Secretly Influence Medical Dogmas and Practices (2004).

429.Brett Wilcox, quoting Oliver Clerc, supra.

430.Brett Wilcox, Jabbed, How the Vaccine Industry, Medical Establishment and Government Stick It to You and Your Family (2018).

431.Wilcox, supra.

432.Wilcox, supra.

433.Marco Cáceres, The Toxic Logic of Water and Applesauce, The Vaccine Reaction, December 8, 2015, https://thevaccinereaction.org/2015/12/the-toxic-logic-of-water-and-applesauce/.

434.Marco Cáceres, December 8, 2015, supra.

435.Claudia Kalb, Dr. Paul Offit: Debunking the Vaccine-Autism Link, Newsweek, October 24, 2008, https://www.newsweek.com/dr-paul-offit-debunking-vaccine-autism-link-91933.

436.Parents Pack Newsletter, Children's Hospital of Philadelphia, October 2005, archive of September 7, 2006 page, http://web.archive.org/web/20060907100428/http://www.chop.edu/consumer/jsp/division/generic.jsp?id=81553.

437.Andrew Zuckerman, How Panicked Parents Skipping Shots Endanger Us All, Wired, October 19, 2009, https://www.wired.com/2009/10/ff-waronscience/.

438.J.B. Handley, Dr. Paul Offit, The Autism Expert. Doesn't See Patients with Autism?, Age of Autism, October 26, 2009, https://www.ageofautism.com/2009/10/dr-paul-offit-the-autism-expert-doesnt-see-patients-with-autism.html.

439.Brett Wilcox, Jabbed, How the Vaccine Industry, Medical Establishment and Government Stick It to You and Your Family, at 20 (2018).

440.Medication Health Fraud, FDA, https://www.fda.gov/drugs/buying-using-medicine-safely/medication-health-fraud (last visited on February 9, 2023).

441.Medication Health Fraud, FDA, https://www.fda.gov/drugs/buying-using-medicine-safely/medication-health-fraud#:~:text=The%20FDA%20defines%20health%20fraud%20as%20the%20deceptive,scientifically%20proven%20safe%20and%20effective%20for%20such%20purposes (last visited on February 9, 2023).

442.21 U.S.C. § 360bbb–3.

443. Advisory Committee on Immunization Practices, CDC National Center for Immunization & Respiratory Diseases, October 20, 2022, https://www.cdc.gov/vaccines/acip/meetings/downloads/slides-2022-10-19-20/04-influenza-chung-olson-lewis-508.pdf.

444. Advisory Committee on Immunization Practices, CDC National Center for Immunization & Respiratory Diseases, October 20, 2022, https://www.cdc.gov/vaccines/acip/meetings/downloads/slides-2022-10-19-20/04-influenza-chung-olson-lewi

s-508.pdf.

445.Rochelle Walensky, MD, MPH, @CDCDirector, Twitter, November 11, 2022, https://twitter.com/CDCDirector/status/1591157419576467456.

446.Mary Kay Linge, CDC director Dr. Rochelle Walensky comes down with COVID a month after booster shot, New York Post, October 22, 2022, https://nypost.com/2022/10/22/cdc-director-dr-rochelle-walensky-comes-down-with-covid-a-month-after-booster/.

447.Medication Health Fraud, FDA, https://www.fda.gov/drugs/buying-using-medicine-safely/medication-health-fraud (last visited on February 9, 2023).

448.Igor Chudov, Influenza Vaccine is Perfect Example of MEDICAL QUACKERY at the FDA and the CDC, November 12, 2022, https://igorchudov.substack.com/p/influenza-vaccine-is-perfect-example?utm_source=substack&utm_campaign=post_embed&utm_medium=web.

449.Medicare Part B 2023, https://www.youtube.com/watch?v=5QFK24hMqP4&t=1s. (last visited on February 9, 2023).

450.FDA Grants Accelerated Approval for Alzheimer's Drug, FDA, June 7, 2021, https://www.fda.gov/news-events/press-announcements/fda-grants-accelerated-approval-alzheimers-drug.

451.Medication Health Fraud, FDA, https://www.fda.gov/drugs/buying-using-medicine-safe

ly/medication-health-fraud (last visited on February 9, 2023).

452.Pam Belluck and Rebecca Robbins, Three F.D.A. Advisers Resign Over Agency's Approval of Alzheimer's Drug, June 10, 2021, New York Times, updated September 2, 2021, https://www.nytimes.com/2021/06/10/health/aduhelm-fda-resign-alzheimers.html#:~:text=Three%20F.D.A.-,Advisers%20Resign%20Over%20Agency's%20Approval%20of%20Alzheimer's%20Drug,evidence%20that%20it%20helps%20patients.&text=As%20a%20subscriber%2C%20you%20have,articles%20to%20give%20each%20month.

453.Pam Belluck and Rebecca Robbins, supra.

454.Raymond Obomsawin, Ph.D., Immunity, Infectious Disease, and Vaccination. Video Re-Posted by Edward Hendrie Under Article Heading: The History of Vaccines Proving They Are Ineffective and Dangerous, May 26, 2021, https://greatmountainpublishing.com/2021/05/26/the-history-of-vaccines-proving-they-are-ineffective-and-dangerous/. See also, Ida Honorof and Eleanor McBean, Vaccination, The Silent Killer: A Clear and Present Danger (1977), https://archive.org/details/vaccinationsilen00hono, and Eleanor McBean, The Poisoned Needle (1957), http://www.whale.to/a/mcbean.html.

455.Brett Wilcox, Jabbed, How the Vaccine Industry, Medical Establishment and Government Stick It to You and Your Family (2018), quoting James Howenstine, M.D., A Physicians Guide to Natural Health Products (2002),

456.Edward Hendrie, Study Shows That Vaccinated Children Are Significantly Less Healthy Than Unvaccinated Children, December 20, 2020, https://greatmountainpublishing.com/2020/12/20/study-shows-that-vaccinated-children-are-significantly-less-healthy-than-unvaccinated-children/.

457.Id.

458.James Lyons-Weiler and Paul Thomas, Relative Incidence of Office Visits and Cumulative Rates of Billed Diagnoses Along the Axis of Vaccination, 22 November 2020, https://www.mdpi.com/1660-4601/17/22/8674/htm.

459.Retraction: Lyons-Weiler, J.; Thomas, P. Relative Incidence of Office Visits and Cumulative Rates of Billed Diagnoses along the Axis of Vaccination. Int. J. Environ. Res. Public Health 2020, 17, 8674, https://www.mdpi.com/1660-4601/18/15/7754/htm.

460.Lyons-Weiler, J., & Russell L, B. (2022). Revisiting Excess Diagnoses of Illnesses and Conditions in Children Whose Parents Provided Informed Permission to Vaccinate Them. International Journal of Vaccine Theory, Practice, and Research, 2(2), 603–618. https://doi.org/10.56098/ijvtpr.v2i2.59. See also https://ijvtpr.com/index.php/IJVTPR/article/view/59/118.

461.Steve Kirsch, The data is clear: the more vaccines you give your child, the more likely it is that they will develop chronic diseases including autism, May 30, 2023, https://stevekirsch.substack.com/p/the-data-is-clear-the-more-vaccines?utm_source=post-email-title&publicati

on_id=548354&post_id=124853131&isFreemail=true &utm_medium=email.

462.Oregon Medical Board, "In the Matter of Paul Norman Thomas, MD, License No. MD15689: Order of Emergency Suspension," State of Oregon, December 3, 2020, https://omb.oregon.gov/Clients/ORMB/OrderDocuments/e579dd35-7e1b-471f-a69a-3a800317ed4c.pdf.

463.James Lyons-Weiler and Paul Thomas, "Relative Incidence of Office Visits and Cumulative Rates of Billed Diagnoses Along the Axis of Vaccination", International Journal of Environmental Research and Public Health, November 22, 2020, https://doi.org/10.3390/ijerph17228674.

464.Retraction: Lyons-Weiler, J.; Thomas, P. Relative Incidence of Office Visits and Cumulative Rates of Billed Diagnoses along the Axis of Vaccination. Int. J. Environ. Res. Public Health 2020, 17, 8674, https://www.mdpi.com/1660-4601/18/15/7754/htm.

465.Jeremy Hammond, March 26, 2021, Oregon Medical Board Suspends Dr. Paul Thomas for Practicing Informed Consent, https://www.jeremyrhammond.com/2021/03/26/oregon-medical-board-suspends-dr-paul-thomas-for-practicing-informed-consent/.

466.Jeremy Hammond, March 26, 2021, supra.

467.IPAK, https://ipaknowledge.org/ (last visited on December 20, 2020).

468.Rhoda Wilson, Big Study Finds Non-Vaccinated are Healthier than Vaccinated, The Expose, April 11,

2022,
https://expose-news.com/2022/04/11/study-finds-non-vaccinated-are-healthier-than-vaccinated/.

469.The Control Group,
https://www.thecontrolgroup.org/.

470.Garner v. Trump, Verified Petition for Declaratory and Injunctive Relief, December 14, 2020,
https://informedconsentdefense.files.wordpress.com/2020/12/verified-petition-filed.pdf.

471.The Control Group Litigation, Update October 4, 2022, https://informedconsentdefense.org/.

472.Rhoda Wilson, Big Study Finds Non-Vaccinated are Healthier than Vaccinated, The Expose, April 11, 2022,
https://expose-news.com/2022/04/11/study-finds-non-vaccinated-are-healthier-than-vaccinated/.

473.Brian S. Hooker, Analysis of health outcomes in vaccinated and unvaccinated children: Developmental delays, asthma, ear infections and gastrointestinal disorders, May 27, 2020,
https://journals.sagepub.com/doi/10.1177/2050312120925344.

474.Anthony Mawson, Pilot comparative study on the health of vaccinated and unvaccinated 6- to 12-year-old U.S. children, Journal of Translational Science, 2017,
https://childrenshealthdefense.org/wp-content/uploads/Unvaccinated-vaccinated-ASD-ADHD-study-Mawson-2017.pdf.

475.State of health of unvaccinated children, https://www.vaccineinjury.info/survey/results-unvaccinated/results-illnesses.html (last visited on May 31, 2023).

476.Steve Kirsch, The data is clear: the more vaccines you give your child, the more likely it is that they will develop chronic diseases including autism, May 30, 2023, https://stevekirsch.substack.com/p/the-data-is-clear-the-more-vaccines?utm_source=post-email-title&publication_id=548354&post_id=124853131&isFreemail=true&utm_medium=email.

477.Cal-Oregon Unvaccinated Survey, Generation Rescue, June 26, 2007, https://www.lynneshealth.com/resources/Autism/Vacination%20Study.pdf.

478.Robert F. Kennedy Jr., Fully Vaccinated vs. Unvaccinated — Part 1, Children's Health Defense, June 25, 2019, https://childrenshealthdefense.org/child-health-topics/exposing-truth/fully-vaccinated-vs-unvaccinated/.

479.Secret CDC Verstraeten study shows neurological developmental disorders with mercury in vaccines, https://www.vaccineinjury.info/news/978-secret-cdc-verstraeten-study-shows-neurological-developmental-disorders-with-mercury-in-vaccines.html (last visited on September 23, 2024).

480.Id.

481.Robert F. Kennedy Jr., Fully Vaccinated vs. Unvaccinated — Part 1, supra.

482.Secret CDC Verstraeten study, supra.

483.Verstraeten T, Davis RL, DeStefano F, Lieu TA, Rhodes PH, Black SB, Shinefield H, Chen RT; Vaccine Safety Datalink Team. Safety of thimerosal-containing vaccines: a two-phased study of computerized health maintenance organization databases. Pediatrics. 2003 Nov;112(5):1039-48. Erratum in: Pediatrics. 2004 Jan;113(1):184. PMID: 14595043.

484.State of health of unvaccinated children, https://www.vaccineinjury.info/survey/results-unvaccinated/results-illnesses.html (last visited on May 31, 2023).

485.Kreesten Meldgaard Madsen and Anders Hviid, et al., A Population-Based Study of Measles, Mumps, and Rubella Vaccination and Autism, NEJM, November 7, 2002, N Engl J Med 2002; 347:1477-1482, DOI: 10.1056/NEJMoa021134, https://www.nejm.org/doi/full/10.1056/nejmoa021134

486.Steven Kirsch, Proof: author of #1 paper showing no link between vaccines and autism is corrupt, May 29, 2023, https://stevekirsch.substack.com/p/key-paper-showing-no-link-between?utm_source=post-email-title&publication_id=548354&post_id=124221729&isFreemail=true&utm_medium=email.

487.Something Is Rotten in Denmark. October 2003, https://childrenshealthdefense.org/wp-content/uploads/5.15-SOMETHING-IS-ROTTEN-IN-DENMARK.pdf.

488.Paul Thorsen, https://oig.hhs.gov/fraud/fugitives/poul-thorsen/ (last visited on May 31, 2023).

489.Aaby P, Mogensen SW, Rodrigues A, Benn CS. Evidence of Increase in Mortality After the Introduction of Diphtheria-Tetanus-Pertussis Vaccine to Children Aged 6-35 Months in Guinea-Bissau: A Time for Reflection? Front Public Health. 2018 Mar 19;6:79. doi: 10.3389/fpubh.2018.00079. PMID: 29616207; PMCID: PMC5868131, https://www.ncbi.nlm.nih.gov/pmc/articles/PMC5868131/.

490.Aaron Siri Letter Re: Death of Infants in Certain Developing Countries by Systematic Use of a Biologic to Special Rapporteur on Torture and Other Cruel, Inhuman or Degrading Treatment or Punishment, Janauary 28, 2021, https://icandecide.org/wp-content/uploads/2021/06/2021.01.28-Letter-to-Special-Rapporteur-on-Torture.pdf.

491.Aaby P, et al., 2018 March 19, supra.

492.Aaron Siri Letter, January 28, 2021, supra.

493.Koepke R, Eickhoff JC, Ayele RA, Petit AB, Schauer SL, Hopfensperger DJ, Conway JH, Davis JP. Estimating the effectiveness of tetanus-diphtheria-acellular pertussis vaccine (Tdap) for preventing pertussis: evidence of rapidly waning immunity and difference in effectiveness by Tdap brand. J Infect Dis. 2014 Sep 15;210(6):942-53. doi: 10.1093/infdis/jiu322. Epub 2014 Jun 5. PMID: 24903664, https://pubmed.ncbi.nlm.nih.gov/24903664/.

494.Igor Chudov, Are Childhood Vaccines Safe? DTP Vaccine Was Not - and Was Given for Decades!, May

26, 2023, https://igorchudov.substack.com/p/are-childhood-vaccines-safe-dtp-vaccine?utm_source=post-email-title&publication_id=441185&post_id=123856103&isFreemail=true&utm_medium=email.

495.Aaron Siri Letter, January 28, 2021, supra.

496.Aaron Siri Letter, January 28, 2021, supra.

497.What is SIDS?, NIH, https://safetosleep.nichd.nih.gov/about/sids-definition (last visited on June 23, 2023).

498.What is SIDS?, NIH, supra.

499.A Midwestern Doctor, Healthy Adults are Not the Only Ones Who Have Been Killed by Vaccines, June 16, 2023, https://amidwesterndoctor.substack.com/p/healthy-adults-are-not-the-only-ones?utm_source=profile&utm_medium=reader2.

500.A Midwestern Doctor, The Century of Evidence That Vaccines Cause Infant Deaths, August 24, 2022, https://amidwesterndoctor.substack.com/p/a-century-of-evidence-has-accumulated.

501.Igor Chudov, Florida "Vaccine Hesitancy" REDUCED Infant Mortality in 2021, March 14, 2022, https://igorchudov.substack.com/p/florida-vaccine-hesitancy-reduced.

502.Carina Blackmore, Director, Divisionof Disease Controland Health Protection, Assessment of County Health Department Immunization Coverage Levels in 2-Year-OldChildren (2021), Florida Health Department, June 4, 2021, https://www.floridahealth.gov/programs-and-services/immunization/resources/surveys/_documents/chd-assessment-2021.pdf.

503.Florida Death Statistics in 2021, https://deadorkicking.com/death-statistics/us/florida/2021/ (last visited on May 28, 2023).

504.Carina Blackmore, June 4, 2021, supra.

505.Igor Chudov, March 14, 2021, supra.

506.Edward Hendrie, Most Pediatricians Refuse to Treat Unvaccinated Children Because They Are Paid a Bounty for Every Fully Vaccinated Child in Their Practice above a Certain Threshold, October 16, 2022, https://hendrie.substack.com/p/most-pediatricians-refuse-to-treat.

507.EO 8.7 Routine Universal Immunization of Physicians, Code of Medical Ethics, Immunization, AMA, https://policysearch.ama-assn.org/policyfinder/detail/immunization?uri=%2FAMADoc%2FEthics.xml-E-8.7.xml.

508.Edward Hendrie, The AMA Is Working to Stop Religious Exemptions and Requires Doctors to Encourage Patients to Get Vaccinated, November 19, 2021, https://greatmountainpublishing.com/2021/11/19/the-ama-is-working-to-stop-religious-exemptions-and-requires-doctors-to-encourage-patients-to-get-vaccinated/.

509.AMA Code of Medical Ethics, https://code-medical-ethics.ama-assn.org/faq (last visited on May 28, 2023).

510.Lessons from the Lockdown—Why Are So Many Fewer Children Dying?, Children's Health Defense, June 18, 2020, https://childrenshealthdefense.org/news/lessons-from-the-lockdown-why-are-so-many-fewer-children-dying/.

511.Id.

512.Santoli, Jeanne M et al. Effects of the COVID-19 Pandemic on Routine Pediatric Vaccine Ordering and Administration — United States, 2020. cdc.gov. https://www.cdc.gov/mmwr/volumes/69/wr/mm6919e2.htm#F1_down.

513.Lessons from the Lockdown, supra.

514.Miller NZ, Goldman GS. Infant mortality rates regressed against number of vaccine doses routinely given: is there a biochemical or synergistic toxicity? Hum Exp Toxicol. 2011 Sep;30(9):1420-8. doi: 10.1177/0960327111407644. Epub 2011 May 4. Erratum in: Hum Exp Toxicol. 2011 Sep;30(9):1429. PMID: 21543527; PMCID: PMC3170075, https://www.ncbi.nlm.nih.gov/pmc/articles/PMC3170075/.

515.Brett Wilcox, Jabbed, How the Vaccine Industry, Medical Establishment and Government
Stick It to You and Your Family (2018), quoting James Howenstine, M.D., A Physicians Guide to Natural Health Products (2002),

516.Id.

517.EO 8.7 Routine Universal Immunization of Physicians, Code of Medical Ethics, Immunization, AMA, https://policysearch.ama-assn.org/policyfinder/detail/immunization?uri=%2FAMADoc%2FEthics.xml-E-8.7.xml.

518.Immunization: The Basics, CDC, September 1, 2021, https://www.cdc.gov/vaccines/vac-gen/imz-basics.htm.

519.AFLD et al., v. Xavier Becerra, et al., Complaint, United States District Court for the Northern District of Alabama, Case 2:21-cv-00702-CLM, http://www.opensourcetruth.com/wp-content/uploads/2021/06/Doc-10-Original-AFLDs-Complaint.pdf.

520.AFLD et al., v. Xavier Becerra, et al., supra.

521.AFLD et al., v. Xavier Becerra, et al., supra.

522.Monique A. Spillman, MD, Chair, Report of the Council on Ethical and Judicial Affairs, Reference Committee on Amendments to Constitution and Bylaws, CEJA Report 2, November 2020, https://www.ama-assn.org/system/files/2020-12/nov2020-ceja-report-2.pdf.

523.Monique A. Spillman, supra.

524.Monique A. Spillman, supra.

525.Nonmedical Exemptions from Immunizations H-440.970, Public Health, AMA, 2021, https://policysearch.ama-assn.org/policyfinder/detail/H-440.970?uri=%2FAMADoc%2FHOD.xml-0-3985.xml.

526.Virginia Pediatrics Group, https://www.vapg.com/service/vaccines-specialist (last visited on October 19, 2022).

527.Virginia Pediatric Group, https://web.archive.org/web/20200923183720/http://www.vapg.com/docs/VPG%20Vaccination%20Policy%209-2019.pdf (last visited on October 19, 2022).

528.The Real Agenda Behind American Academy of Pediatrics: Weaponizing Children's Mental Health and Vaccines for Profit, The Defender, December 8, 2022, https://childrenshealthdefense.org/defender/profit-american-academy-pediatrics-childrens-mental-health-vaccines/.

529.Ensuring Comprehensive Care and Support for Transgender and Gender-Diverse Children and Adolescents, AAP, October 1, 2008, https://doi.org/10.1542/peds.2018-2162.

530.Sample Vaccine Policy Statement, Immunization Action Coalition, https://www.immunize.org/catg.d/p2067.pdf (last visited on October 19, 2022).

531.Sample Vaccine Policy Statement, supra.

532.The Immunization Action Coalition, https://www.immunize.org/aboutus/ (last visited on Ocober 19, 2022).

533.CDC and WHO Corrupt Financial Entanglements with the Vaccine Industry, Children's Health Defense, https://childrenshealthdefense.org/cdc-who/ (last visited on October 19, 2022).

534.Alex Pietroski, Proof Surfaces Insurance Co Pays Massive Bonuses to Doctors for Vaccinating Babies, Waking Times, August 8, 2017, http://www.wakingtimes.com/proof-surfaces-insurance

-co-pays-massive-bonuses-doctors-vaccinating-babies/.

535.Doctors to Texas parents: No vaccination, no office visit, AP, March 13, 2019, https://abc13.com/measles-vaccination-texas-doctors-doctor-refuse-to-see-un-vaccinated-children/5189002/.

536.Vaccine Refusal: AAP Changes Stance on Patient Dismissal, Consulant 360, https://www.consultant360.com/exclusives/vaccine-refusal-aap-changes-stance-patient-dismissal (last visited on October 2, 2022).

537.David Weissman, No vaccination, no service: Some SC pediatricians turning away kids for parents' decisions, Greenville News, May 7, 2019, https://www.greenvilleonline.com/story/news/2019/05/07/some-sc-pediatricians-refuse-service-if-children-dont-get-vaccine-anti-vaxxer-parents/1128830001/.

538.David Weissman, May 7, 2019, supra.

539.Brian Argo, LinkedIn, https://www.linkedin.com/in/brian-argo-2ba882b (last visited on October 2, 2022).

540.2016 Performance Recognition Program, Provider Incentive Program, Blue Cross Blue Shield, at 15, http://www.whale.to/c/2016-BCN-BCBSM-Incentive-Program-Booklet.pdf (last visited on October 1, 2022).

541.Id.

542.Alison B. Bocian, et al., Size and Age-Sex Distribution of Pediatric Practice: A Study From Pediatric Research in Office Settings, JAMA, January 1999, https://jamanetwork.com/journals/jamapediatrics/fullar

ticle/344727.

543.WE, How Much Money Do Pediatricians Really Make From Vaccines?, Wellness and Equality, June 20, 2016, https://wellnessandequality.com/2016/06/20/how-much-money-do-pediatricians-really-make-from-vaccines/.

544.WE, How Much Money Do Pediatricians Really Make From Vaccines?, Wellness and Equality, June 20, 2016, https://wellnessandequality.com/2016/06/20/how-much-money-do-pediatricians-really-make-from-vaccines/. No Results Found, 2016 Blue Cross Blue Shield Performance Recognition Program removed from: https://thephysicianalliance.org/wp-content/uploads/2016/03/2016-BCN-BCBSM-Incentive-Program-Booklet.pdf (last visited on February 23, 2023). 2016 Blue Cross Blue Shield Performance Recognition Program available at: https://greatmountainpublishing.com/wp-content/uploads/2021/05/2016-BCN-BCBSM-Incentive-Program-Booklet.pdf (last visited on February 23, 2023). 2016 Blue Cross Blue Shield Performance Recognition Program also available at: http://www.whale.to/c/2016-BCN-BCBSM-Incentive-Program-Booklet.pdf (last visited on February 23, 2023).

545.J.B. Handley, Vaccines Don't Cause Autism, Pediatricians Do., Age of Autism, https://www.ageofautism.com/2010/01/vaccines-dont-cause-autism-pediatricians-do.html (last visited on April 8, 2023).

546.Brett Wilcox, Jabbed, How the Vaccine Industry, Medical Establishment and Government

Stick It to You and Your Family, at 250 (2018).

547.Thomas Massey, Your primary care provider was bribed to suggest you should take the COVID vaccine, Twitter, @RepThomasMassie, https://twitter.com/RepThomasMassie/status/1646696738013454336?utm_source=substack&utm_medium=email.

548.Michael Nevradakis, Exclusive: She Made 'The Real Anthony Fauci' Required Reading for Her Students. Here's What Happened Next., The Defender, April 25, 2023, https://childrenshealthdefense.org/defender/lynn-comerford-the-real-anthony-fauci-required-reading-students-csueb/?utm_source=luminate&utm_medium=email&utm_campaign=defender-wk&utm_id=20230430.

549.Michael Nevradakis, The Defender, April 26, 2023, supra.

550.COVID-19 Vaccination Policy, Yale University, February 7, 2023, https://covid19.yale.edu/covid-19-vaccination-policy#:~:text=The%20university%20requires%20all%20students,within%2014%20days%20of%20eligibility.

551.U.S. Department of Health and Human Services Launches Nationwide Network of Trusted Voices to Encourage Vaccination in Next Phase of COVID-19 Public Education Campaign, April 1, 2021, archive copy from April 1, 2021, https://web.archive.org/web/20210401225102/https:/www.hhs.gov/about/news/2021/04/01/hhs-launches-nationwide-network-trusted-voices-encourage-vaccination-next-phase-covid-19-public-education-campaign.html.

552.Maggie Thorp and Jim Thorp, FOIA Reveals Troubling Relationship between HHS/CDC & the American College of Obstetricians and Gynecologists, America Out Loud, May 7, 2023, https://www.americaoutloud.com/foia-reveals-troubling-relationship-between-hhs-cdc-the-american-college-of-obstetricians-and-gynecologists/?utm_source=substack&utm_medium=email.

553.Maggie Thorp and Jim Thorp, May 7, 2023, supra.

554.Maggie Thorp and Jim Thorp, May 7, 2023, supra.

555.Maggie Thorp and Jim Thorp, May 7, 2023, supra.

556.COVID-19 Vaccines and Pregnancy: Conversation Guide, ACOG, https://www.acog.org/covid-19/covid-19-vaccines-and-pregnancy-conversation-guide-for-clinicians (last visited on May 10, 2023).

557.COVID-19 Vaccines and Pregnancy, supra.

558.Maggie Thorp and Jim Thorp, May 7, 2023, supra.

559.David Bell, M.D., Brownstone Institute, COVID Vaccines Were Never Safe for Pregnant Women, Pfizer's Own Data Show, The Defender, April 28, 2023, https://childrenshealthdefense.org/defender/pfizer-covid-vaccine-pregnancy/.

560.David Bell, supra.

561.Amy Kelly, Report 69: BOMBSHELL – Pfizer and FDA Knew in Early 2021 That Pfizer mRNA COVID "Vaccine" Caused Dire Fetal and Infant Risks, Including Death. They Began an Aggressive Campaign to Vaccinate Pregnant Women Anyway., April 29, 2023, https://dailyclout.io/bombshell-pfizer-and-the-fda-knew-in-early-2021-that-the-pfizer-mrna-covid-vaccine-caused-dire-fetal-and-infant-risks-they-began-an-aggressive-campaign-to-vaccinate-pregnant-women-anyway/.

562.Amy Kelly, April 29, 2023, supra.

563.Amy Kelly, April 29, 2023, supra.

564.Amy Kelly, April 29, 2023, supra.

565.Supporting CDC and Public Health, CDC Foundation, https://www.cdcfoundation.org/supporting-cdc (last visited on May 11, 2023).

566.Corporations, Foundations & Organizations, CDC Foundation, https://www.cdcfoundation.org/FY2018/organizations (last visited on May 11, 2023).

567.Doctors Are No Experts on Vaccines. Get Over it., November 22, 2015, https://idsent.wordpress.com/2015/11/22/doctors-are-no-experts-on-vaccines-get-over-it/#_edn1.

568.Id.

569.Brett Wilcox, Jabbed, How the Vaccine Industry, Medical Establishment and Government
Stick It to You and Your Family, at 246 (2018).

570.Kathryn A. Hale , I saw VAXXED and I was shattered!, https://www.abundanthealthlife.com/blog/vaxxed (last visite on April 8, 2023).

571.Kathryn A. Hale , I saw VAXXED and I was shattered!, https://www.abundanthealthlife.com/blog/vaxxed (last visite on April 8, 2023).

572.*United States v. Heredia*, 483 F.3d 913, 918, n. 4 (9th Cir. 2007) (en banc) (citations omitted).

573.Global Tech. v. SEB S.A., 563 U.S, 754, 766 (2011).

574.Medical Doctor: Blood of Every Vaccine Injured or Killed Child on Hands of Murder-by-Vaccine Pediatricians, October 22, 2017, https://healthimpactnews.com/2017/medical-doctor-blood-of-every-vaccine-injured-or-killed-child-on-hands-of-murder-by-vaccine-pediatricians/.

575.J.B. Handley, Vaccines Don't Cause Autism, Pediatricians Do., Age of Autism, https://www.ageofautism.com/2010/01/vaccines-dont-cause-autism-pediatricians-do.html (last visited on April 8, 2023).

576.Barbara Loe Fisher, Baylor's Doc Hotez Bullies Parents of Vaccine Injured Children, March 10, 2018, https://www.nvic.org/newsletter/mar-2018/baylor%E2%80%99s-doc-hotez-bullies-parents-of-vaccine-injured-children#_edn8.

577.Barbara Loe Fisher, supra.

578.Peter J. Hotez, Will an American-Led Anti-Vaccine Movement Subvert Global Health?, Scientific American, March 3, 2017, https://blogs.scientificamerican.com/guest-blog/will-an-american-led-anti-vaccine-movement-subvert-global-h ealth/.

579.Sivan Gazit, et. al., Comparing SARS-CoV-2 Natural Immunity to Vaccine-Inducted Immunity: Reinfections Versus Breakthrough Infections, August 25, 2021, https://www.scribd.com/document/521947447/2021-08-24-21262415v1-full#from_embed. Also at: https://www.medrxiv.org/content/10.1101/2021.08.24.21262415v1.

580.Meredith Wadman, Having SARS-CoV-2 Once Confers Much Greater Immunity than a Vaccine—but No Infection Parties, Please, Science, Aug. 26, 2021. Original article at: https://web.archive.org/web/20210827005111/https://www.sciencemag.org/news/2021/08/having-sars-cov-2-once-confers-much-greater-immunity-vaccine-no-infection-parties. Updated article at: https://www.sciencemag.org/news/2021/08/having-sars-cov-2-once-confers-much-greater-immunity-vaccine-no-infection-parties.

581.Jackson S. Turner, et. al., Sars-cov-2 Infection Induces Long-lived Bone Marrow Plasma Cells in Humans, Nature, May 24, 2021, https://www.nature.com/articles/s41586-021-03647-4. Also available at Turner, J.S., Kim, W., Kalaidina, E. et al. SARS-CoV-2 Infection Induces Long-lived Bone Marrow Plasma Cells in Humans. Nature 595, 421–425 (2021). https://doi.org/10.1038/s41586-021-03647-4.

582.Lasting Immunity Found after Recovery from COVID-19, NIH, January 26, 2021, https://www.nih.gov/news-events/nih-research-matters/lasting-immunity-found-after-recovery-covid-19.

583.Andrea Radbruch, et. al., A Long-term Perspective on Immunity to COVID, Nature, June 14, 2021, https://www.nature.com/articles/d41586-021-01557-z?error=cookies_not_supported&code=1802a619-93cb-4e6d-81fe-fc1df8891542.

584.Paul Elias Alexander, 141 Research Studies Affirm Naturally Acquired Immunity to Covid-19: Documented, Linked, and Quoted, October 17, 2021, https://brownstone.org/articles/79-research-studies-affirm-naturally-acquired-immunity-to-covid-19-documented-linked-and-quoted/.

585.Nabin K. Shrestha, et al., Necessity of COVID-19 Vaccination in Previously Infected Individuals, June 5, 2021, MedRXiv, https://www.medrxiv.org/content/10.1101/2021.06.01.21258176v2.

586.E.g., Gabor David Kelen, M.D., Lisa Maragakis, M.D., M.P.H., COVID-19 Vaccine: What You Need to Know, Johns Hopkins, Updated on November 1, 2022, https://www.hopkinsmedicine.org/health/conditions-and-diseases/coronavirus/covid-19-vaccine-what-you-need-to-know#:~:text=Yes%2C%20evidence%20continues%20to%20indicate,had%20COVID%2D19%20or%20not.

587.E.g., Richard Gray, This is how new Covid-19 variants are changing the pandemic, BBC, 27 January 2021, https://www.bbc.com/future/article/20210127-covid-19-variants-how-mutations-are-changing-the-pandemic.

588.Raji Suri, COVID-19 Survivors May Possess Wide-ranging Resistance to the Disease, Emory University, Woodruff Health Sciences Center, July 22,

2021,
https://news.emory.edu/stories/2021/07/covid_survivors_resistance/index.html.

589.Mild COVID-19 Induces Lasting Antibody Protection, Study Finds, May 24, 2021, https://www.sciencedaily.com/releases/2021/05/210524110135.htm.

590.Jennifer M. Dann, et. al., Immunological Memory to SARS-CoV-2 Assessed for Up to 8 Months After Infection, Science, 5 February 2021, https://science.sciencemag.org/content/371/6529/eabf4063.

591.Paul Elias Alexander, 160 Plus Research Studies Affirm Naturally Acquired Immunity to Covid-19: Documented, Linked, and Quoted, Brownstone Institute, October 17, 2021, https://brownstone.org/author/paul-elias-alexander/.

592.Paul Elias Alexander, October 17, 2021, supra.

593.Nabin K Shrestha, Patrick C Burke, Amy S Nowacki, Paul Terpeluk, Steven M Gordon, Necessity of Coronavirus Disease 2019 (COVID-19) Vaccination in Persons Who Have Already Had COVID-19, Clinical Infectious Diseases, Volume 75, Issue 1, 1 July 2022, Pages e662–e671, https://doi.org/10.1093/cid/ciac022. Also found at https://www.medrxiv.org/content/10.1101/2021.06.01.21258176v2.

594.Sivan Gazit, Roei Shlezinger, Galit Perez, Roni Lotan, Asaf Peretz, Amir Ben-Tov, Esma Herzel, Hillel Alapi, Dani Cohen, Khitam Muhsen, Gabriel Chodick, Tal Patalon, Severe Acute Respiratory

Syndrome Coronavirus 2 (SARS-CoV-2) Naturally Acquired Immunity versus Vaccine-induced Immunity, Reinfections versus Breakthrough Infections: A Retrospective Cohort Study, Clinical Infectious Diseases, Volume 75, Issue 1, 1 July 2022, Pages e545–e551, https://doi.org/10.1093/cid/ciac262. Also found at https://www.medrxiv.org/content/10.1101/2021.08.24.21262415v1.full.

595.COVID-19 Vaccine Booster Shot, CDC, August 20, 2021, https://www.cdc.gov/coronavirus/2019-ncov/vaccines/booster-shot.html.

596.Frequently Asked Questions about COVID-19 Vaccination, CDC, August 19, 2021, https://www.cdc.gov/coronavirus/2019-ncov/vaccines/faq.html.

597.Alyson M. Cavanaugh, et. al., Reduced Risk of Reinfection with SARS-CoV-2 After COVID-19 Vaccination — Kentucky, May–June 2021, Morbidity and Mortality Weekly Report, August 13, 2021, https://www.cdc.gov/mmwr/volumes/70/wr/pdfs/mm7032e1-H.pdf. See also Suggested citation for this article: Cavanaugh AM, Spicer KB, Thoroughman D, Glick C, Winter K. Reduced Risk of Reinfection with SARS-CoV-2 After COVID-19 Vaccination — Kentucky, May–June 2021. MMWR Morb Mortal Wkly Rep 2021;70:1081-1083. DOI: http://dx.doi.org/10.15585/mmwr.mm7032e1.

598.Frequently Asked Questions about COVID-19 Vaccination, FDA, August 19, 2021, https://www.cdc.gov/coronavirus/2019-ncov/vaccines/faq.html#:~:text=Yes%2C%20you%20should%20be%2

0vaccinated,ve%20already%20had%20COVID%2D19
. See also

599.Alyson M. Cavanaugh, et. al., supra.

600.Alyson M. Cavanaugh, et. al., supra.

601.Megan Redshaw, Scientists Challenge Health Officials on Vaccinating People Who Already Had COVID, The Defender, April 5, 2021, https://childrenshealthdefense.org/defender/scientists-challenge-health-officials-on-vaccinating-covid/?utm_source=salsa&eType=EmailBlastContent&eId=f9f42235-fc83-4837-a2e2-c8362cc97140.

602.Megan Redshaw, April 5, 2021, supra.

603.Megan Redshaw, April 5, 2021, supra.

604.Megan Redshaw, April 5, 2021, supra.

605.Vaccines and Related Biological Products Advisory Committee Meeting December 17, 2020, FDA Briefing Document, Moderna COVID-19 Vaccine, at 15, https://www.fda.gov/media/144434/download.

606.Id. at 12.

607.Megan Redshaw, April 5, 2021, supra.

608.Sivan Gazit, et. al., Comparing SARS-CoV-2 Natural Immunity to Vaccine-Inducted Immunity: Reinfections Versus Breakthrough Infections, August 25, 2021, https://www.scribd.com/document/521947447/2021-08-24-21262415v1-full#from_embed. Also at: https://www.medrxiv.org/content/10.1101/2021.08.24.

21262415v1.

609.Anthony Fauci, Albany Medical College, https://www.amc.edu/PR/Current_News_Stories/fauci-story.cfm (last visited on September 13, 2021).

610.Anthony Fauci, Albany Medical College, https://www.amc.edu/PR/Current_News_Stories/fauci-story.cfm (last visited on September 13, 2021).

611.Anderson Cooper 360 Degrees, CNN, Aired September 09, 2021 - 20:00 ET, https://transcripts.cnn.com/show/acd/date/2021-09-09/segment/01.

612.Anthony Fauci, Albany Medical College, https://www.amc.edu/PR/Current_News_Stories/fauci-story.cfm (last visited on September 13, 2021).

613.Jack Phillips, Pfizer Board Member: 'Natural Immunity' Against COVID-19 Needs to Be Included in Policy Discussions, Epoch Times, August 30, 2021, https://www.theepochtimes.com/pfizer-board-member-natural-immunity-against-covid-needs-to-be-included-in-policy-discussions_3971383.html.

614.CDC Admits They Have No Records of Any Person with Recovered Immunity Every Trasnmitting The COVID-19 Virus, The Last Refuge, November 11, 2021, https://theconservativetreehouse.com/blog/2021/11/11/cdc-admits-they-have-no-records-of-any-person-with-recovered-immunity-ever-transmitting-the-covid-19-virus/, quoting November 5, 2021 Letter to Elizabeth Brenm from Roger Andoh, CDC/ATSDR FOIA Officer. See also Aaron Siri, CDC Admits Crushing Rights of Naturally Immune Without Proof They

Transmit the Virus, November 11, 2021, https://aaronsiri.substack.com/p/cdc-admits-crushing-rights-of-naturally.

615.Id.

616.Cahterine Brown, et al., Outbreak of SARS-CoV-2 Infections, Including COVID-19 Vaccine Breakthrough Infections, Associated with Large Public Gatherings - Barnstable County, Massachusetts, July 2021, August 6, 2021, https://pubmed.ncbi.nlm.nih.gov/34351882/.

617.Nguyen Van Vinh Chau, et al., Transmission of SARS-CoV-2 Delta Variant Among Vaccinated Healthcare Workers, Vietnam, Volume 41, November 2021, 11043, https://doi.org/10.1016/j.eclinm.2021.101143, and also at: https://papers.ssrn.com/sol3/papers.cfm?abstract_id=3897733.

618.Carla Saade, et al., Live virus neutralization testing in convalescent patients and subjects vaccinated against 19A, 20B, 20I/501Y.V1 and 20H/501Y.V2 isolates of SARS-CoV-2, December 2021, https://pubmed.ncbi.nlm.nih.gov/34176436/.

619.Kasen K. Riemersma, et al., Shedding of Infectious SARS-CoV-2 Despite Vaccination, August 24, 2021, https://www.medrxiv.org/content/10.1101/2021.07.31.21261387v4.full.pdf.

620.Immunization: The Basics, CDC, https://www.cdc.gov/vaccines/vac-gen/imz-basics.htm (last visited on December 7, 2022).

621.Immunization: The Basics, CDC, supra.

622.The World's Best Hospitals 2023, Newsweek, 2023, https://www.newsweek.com/rankings/worlds-best-hospitals-2023.

623.Nabin K. Shrestha, et al., Effectiveness of the Coronavirus Disease 2019 (COVID-19) Bivalent Vaccine, medRxiv preprint doi: https://doi.org/10.1101/2022.12.17.22283625; December 19, 2022, https://www.medrxiv.org/content/10.1101/2022.12.17.22283625v1.full.pdf.

624.Nabin K. Shrestha, supra.

625.Steve Kirsch, Very large Cleveland Clinic study shows more vaccines make you more likely to get COVID, January 19, 2023, https://stevekirsch.substack.com/p/very-large-cleveland-clinic-study#%C2%A7the-original-pfizer-study-showed-you-were-at-least-x-more-likely-to-get-covid-if-you-got-the-shots.

626.Steve Kirsch, January 19, 2023, supra.

627.Vaccines and Related Biological Products Advisory Committee Meeting, FDA Briefing Document, Application for licensure of a booster dose for COMIRNATY (COVID-19 Vaccine, mRNA), September 17, 2021, https://www.fda.gov/media/152176/download?utm_source=substack&utm_medium=email.

628.Steve Kirsch, January 19, 2023, supra.

629.CDC Endorses ACIP's Updated COVID-19 Vaccine Recommendations, CDC, Media Statement, December 16, 2021, https://www.cdc.gov/media/releases/2021/s1216-covid-19-vaccines.html.

630.Fiona P. Havers, et al., Laboratory-Confirmed COVID-19–Associated Hospitalizations Among Adults During SARS-CoV-2 Omicron BA.2 Variant Predominance — COVID-19–Associated Hospitalization Surveillance Network, 14 States, June 20, 2021–May 31, 2022, CDC, August 26, 2022, https://www.cdc.gov/mmwr/volumes/71/wr/mm7134a3.htm?s_cid=mm7134a3_x.

631.Fiona P. Havers, et al., supra.

632.Edward Hendrie, The CDC Falsely Counts Vaccinated COVID Deaths as Unvaccinated COVID Deaths, December 27, 2021, https://greatmountainpublishing.com/2021/12/27/the-cdc-falsely-counts-vaccinated-covid-deaths-as-unvaccinated-covid-deaths/.

633.Jennifer B. Griffin, Ph.D., et al., SARS-CoV-2 Infections and Hospitalizations Among Persons Aged =16 Years, by Vaccination Status — Los Angeles County, California, May 1–July 25, 2021, Morbidity and Mortality Weekly Report / August 27, 2021 / Vol. 70 / No. 34, https://www.cdc.gov/mmwr/volumes/70/wr/pdfs/mm7034e5-H.pdf.

634.Monitoring COVID-19 Vaccine Effectiveness, CDC, https://www.cdc.gov/coronavirus/2019-ncov/vaccines/effectiveness/how-they-work.html. The language that had been posted on the CDC website on or before September 3, 2021 at that URL, has been deleted from the CDC website. But See the Washoe County Health District COVID-19 Facts, which quotes from the language since deleted from the CDC website, https://experience.arcgis.com/experience/6b88f7dff38a44d8b174e89a7ce25352/page/page_4/. (last visited on February 3, 2023).

635.Joseph Mercola, Shockingly, CDC Now Lists Vaccinated Deaths as Unvaccinated, Flyby News, September 15, 2021, https://flybynews.wordpress.com/2021/09/15/shockingly-cdc-now-lists-vaccinated-deaths-as-unvaccinated/. Article also found at: https://greatmountainpublishing.com/2021/12/27/the-cdc-falsely-counts-vaccinated-covid-deaths-as-unvaccinated-covid-deaths/.

636.Joseph Mercola, September 15, 2021, supra.

637.Joseph Mercola, September 15, 2021, supra.

638.Edward Hendrie, "Breakthrough" Cases in the Vaccinated Population Are Actually Symptoms of Antibody-Dependent Enhancement Caused by the Covid-19 Vaccines, September 1, 2021, https://greatmountainpublishing.com/2021/09/01/breakthrough-cases-in-the-vaccinated-population-are-actually-symptoms-of-antibody-dependent-enhancement-caused-by-the-covid-19-vaccines/.

639.Nobel Prize Winner French Virologist Luc Montagnier Explains How COVID-19 Vaccines Are Creating Variants, May 21, 2021, https://greatgameindia.com/covid-19-vaccines-creating-variants/.

640.80% of the nuns in this Kentucky convent got COVID 2 days after vaccine, Lifesite News, February 25, 2021, https://www.lifesitenews.com/news/several-nuns-die-after-taking-first-shot-of-covid-vaccine/.

641.Washoe County COVID-19 Facts, https://experience.arcgis.com/experience/6b88f7dff38a44d8b174e89a7ce25352/page/page_4/. (last visited on February 3, 2023). See also Agenda Packet, Office of the District Health Officer District Health Officer Staff Report Board Meeting Date: July 22, 2021, Appendix, at page 421, https://www.washoecounty.gov/health/about-us/board-committees/district-board-of-health/2021/files/Agenda-Packet-07-22-2021.pdf.

642.COVID-19 Vaccine Breakthrough Case Investigation and Reporting, CDC, https://www.cdc.gov/vaccines/covid-19/health-departments/breakthrough-cases.html (last visited on August 28, 2021).

643.*CDC 2019-Novel Coronavirus (2019-nCoV) Real-Time RT-PCR Diagnostic Panel*, Catalog # 2019-nCoVEUA-01 1000 reactions, 7, 13, 2020, https://www.fda.gov/media/134922/download.

644.Vincent Racaniello, *TWiV 641: COVID-19 with Dr. Anthony Fauci*, July 16, 2020, https://www.youtube.com/watch?time_continue=260&v=a_Vy6fgaBPE&feature=emb_logo.

645.COVID-19 Vaccine Breakthrough Case Investigation and Reporting, CDC, https://www.cdc.gov/vaccines/covid-19/health-departments/breakthrough-cases.html (last visited on August

28, 2021).

646.Joseph Mercola, September 15, 2021, supra.

647.Kit Knightly, How the CDC Is Manipulating Data to Prop-up "Vaccine Effectiveness," Off Guardian, May 18, 2021, https://off-guardian.org/2021/05/18/how-the-cdc-is-manipulating-data-to-prop-up-vaccine-effectiveness/.

648.Deaths by Vaccination Status, England, Office for National Statistics, Dataset, https://www.ons.gov.uk/peoplepopulationandcommunity/birthsdeathsandmarriages/deaths/datasets/deathsbyvaccinationstatusengland (last visited on November 22, 2021).

649.Alex Berenson, Vaccinated English Adults under 60 Are Dying at Twice the Rate of Unvaccinated People the Same Age, Novemer 20, 2021, https://alexberenson.substack.com/p/vaccinated-english-adults-under-60.

650.Alex Berenson, November 20, 2021, supra.

651.Alex Berenson, November 20, 2021, supra.

652.Deaths by Vaccination Status, England, UK Office for National Statistics, https://www.ons.gov.uk/peoplepopulationandcommunity/birthsdeathsandmarriages/deaths/datasets/deathsbyvaccinationstatusengland (last visited on November 26, 2021).

653.James Lyons-Weiler, et al., Relative Incidence of Office Visits and Cumulative Rates of Billed Diagnoses Along the Axis of Vaccination, 14 November 2020, https://www.mdpi.com/1660-4601/17/22/8674. On 16 July 2021, the MDPI retracted the article with the following cryptic notice. "The journal retracts the article 'Relative Incidence of Office Visits and Cumulative Rates of Billed Diagnoses along the Axis of Vaccination' cited above. Following publication, concerns were brought to the attention of the editorial office regarding the validity of the conclusions of the published research. Adhering to our complaints procedure, an investigation was conducted that raised several methodological issues and confirmed that the conclusions were not supported by strong scientific data. The article is therefore retracted. This retraction is approved by the Editor in Chief of the journal. The authors did not agree to this retraction." https://www.mdpi.com/1660-4601/18/15/7754/htm. The MDPI did not indicate what were the "methodological issues" or specify how the conclusions "were not supported by strong scientific data." That lack of specificity for such an extraordinary action suggests the retraction of the article by the MDPI was not due to methodological issues or that it was not supported by strong scientific data but was rather due to financial and political pressure put on MDPI.

654.Gunter Kampf, The Epidemiological Relevance of the COVID-19-Vaccinated Population Is Increasing, Tha Lancet, November 19, 2021, https://www.thelancet.com/journals/lanepe/article/PIIS2666-7762(21)00258-1/fulltext.

655.Gunter Kampf, November 19, 2021, supra.

656.Robert Koch-Institut. Wochentlicher Lagebericht des RKI zur Coronavirus-Krank-heit-2019 (COVID-19). AKTUALISIERTER STAND FUR

DEUTSCHLAND 22. Juli 2021. https://www.rki.de/DE/Content/InfAZ/N/Neuartiges_Coronavirus/Situationsberichte/Wochenbericht/Wochenbericht_2021-07-22.pdf?__blob=publicationFile (accessed 28. September 2021).

657.The Robert Koch Institute, Tasks and Aims, https://www.rki.de/EN/Content/Institute/institute_node.html;jsessionid=A6B6D73428CC04A2F8D992C80F881F61.internet061 (last visited on December 31, 2021).

658.Stunning Omicron Data Emerges From Germany Showing Negative COVID-19 Vaccine Efficacy, January 1, 2022, https://lorphicweb.com/stunning-omicron-data-emerges-from-germany-showing-negative-covid-19-vaccine-efficacy/.

659.Id.

660.Ethan Huff, Lancet Science Paper Destroys False Narrative of COVID Vaccines, Reveals Vaccinated Are Perpetuating the Pandemic, NEWSTARGET, December 21, 2021, https://www.newstarget.com/2021-12-21-lancet-paper-destroys-false-narrative-covid-vaccines.html.

661.Coronavirus Disease 2019 (COVID-19) Outbreak, Maryland Department of Health, https://coronavirus.maryland.gov/#Vaccine (last visited on October 24, 2021).

662.Joe Hoft, EXCLUSIVE: Analysis Shows More COVID Deaths in 2021 than 2020 with Large Percent of 2021 Deaths Fully Vaccinated, October 22, 2021, https://www.thegatewaypundit.com/2021/10/exclusive-analysis-shows-covid-deaths-2021-2020-large-percent-

2021-deaths-fully-vaccinated/?utm_source=Email&utm_medium=the-gateway-pundit&utm_campaign=dailypm&utm_content=daily.

663.Joe Hoft, EXCLUSIVE: Analysis Shows More COVID Deaths in 2021 than 2020 with Large Percent of 2021 Deaths Fully Vaccinated, October 22, 2021, https://www.thegatewaypundit.com/2021/10/exclusive-analysis-shows-covid-deaths-2021-2020-large-percent-2021-deaths-fully-vaccinated/?utm_source=Email&utm_medium=the-gateway-pundit&utm_campaign=dailypm&utm_content=daily.

664.Jim Hoft, Former CDC Director Robert Redfield Claims More Than 40% COVID-19 Deaths in Maryland Were Fully Vaccinated, The Gateway Pundit, October 27, 2021, https://www.thegatewaypundit.com/2021/10/former-cdc-director-robert-redfield-claims-40-deaths-cases-maryland-fully-vaccinated/.

665.Jim Hoft, October 27, 2021, supra.

666.Coronavirus Disease 2019 (COVID-19) Outbreak, Maryland Department of Health, https://coronavirus.maryland.gov/#Vaccine (last visited on October 24, 2021).

667.Joe Hoft, EXCLUSIVE: Analysis Shows More COVID Deaths in 2021 than 2020 with Large Percent of 2021 Deaths Fully Vaccinated, October 22, 2021, https://www.thegatewaypundit.com/2021/10/exclusive-analysis-shows-covid-deaths-2021-2020-large-percent-2021-deaths-fully-vaccinated/?utm_source=Email&utm_medium=the-gateway-pundit&utm_campaign=dailypm&utm_content=daily.

668.Joe Hoft, October 22, 2021, supra.

669.The United Kingdom Health Security Agency COVID-19 Vaccine Surveillance Report, Publishing Reference: GOV-10158, at 4-6, October 14, 2021, https://assets.publishing.service.gov.uk/government/uploads/system/uploads/attachment_data/file/1025358/Vaccine-surveillance-report-week-41.pdf

670.Alex Berenson, Vaccinated English Adults under 60 Are Dying at Twice the Rate of Unvaccinated People the Same Age, Novemer 20, 2021, https://alexberenson.substack.com/p/vaccinated-english-adults-under-60.

671.Dr. Anthony Fauci: Fully Vaccinated People Carry As Much Virus As Unvaccinated For Delta Variant, MSNBC, July 27, 2021, https://rumble.com/vlt9b1-dr.-anthony-fauci-fully-vaccinated-people-carry-as-much-virus-as-unvaccinat.html.

672.Kyle Becker, Becker News, CDC Director Changes Her Story, Now Admits COVID Vaccines Don't Prevent Virus Transmission, August 7, 2021, https://beckernews.com/cdc-director-changes-her-story-now-admits-covid-vaccines-dont-prevent-virus-transmission-40754/.

673.Yasmeen Abutaleb, et.al., The War Has Changed': Internal CDC Document Urges New Messaging, Warns Delta Infections Likely More Severe, The Washington Post, July 29, 2021, https://www.washingtonpost.com/health/2021/07/29/cdc-mask-guidance/.

674.Boris Johnson Admits That Covid-1984 Jab DOES NOT Protect You From Anything - So What Is

The Point?, April 9, 2021,
https://www.bitchute.com/video/OQBS0IAIrXEa/.

675.Andrew White, UK's Boris Johnson Admits Vaccines Do Not Prevent Contracting, Spreading COVID-19, National File, October 23, 2021, https://nationalfile.com/uks-boris-johnson-admits-vaccines-do-not-prevent-contracting-spreading-covid-19/.

676.Remarks by President Biden Laying Out the Next Steps in Our Effort to Get More Americans Vaccinated and Combat the Spread of the Delta Variant, July 29, 2021, 4:23 p.m. EDT, https://www.whitehouse.gov/briefing-room/speeches-remarks/2021/07/29/remarks-by-president-biden-laying-out-the-next-steps-in-our-effort-to-get-more-americans-vaccinated-and-combat-the-spread-of-the-delta-variant/.

677.Natalie Rahhal, Pfizer CEO Admits He Is 'Not Certain' Their COVID-19 Shot Will Prevent Vaccinated People from Spreading the Virus - as the Firm Cuts the Number of Doses it Will Ship this Year, Daily Mail, December 4, 2020, https://www.dailymail.co.uk/health/article-9018547/Pfizer-CEO-not-certain-covid-shot-prevents-transmission.html.

678.AXIOS on HBO: Moderna Chief Medical Officer Tal Zaks (Clip) | HBO, November 23, 2020, https://www.youtube.com/watch?v=po7qt9BZz0s&t=65s.

679.60% of People Being Admitted to UK Hospitals Are Unvaccinated - Adviser, Reuters, July 19, 2021, https://www.reuters.com/business/healthcare-pharmaceuticals/60-people-being-admitted-uk-hospitals-had-two

-covid-jabs-adviser-2021-07-19/.

680.Canada: COVID-19 Outbreak at Retirement Home Where 82% of Residents Are "Vaccinated", March 12, 2021, https://thecovidblog.com/2021/03/12/canada-covid-19-outbreak-at-retirement-home-where-82-of-residents-are-vaccinated/.

681.CDC Issues First Set of Guidelines on How Fully Vaccinated People Can Visit Safely with Others, March 8, 2021, https://archive.is/PrcRy#selection-455.0-455.94.

682.Shannon Pettypiece, et al., CDC Recommends the Vaccinated Wear Masks in Areas with Low Vaccination Rates, NBC News, July 27, 2021, https://www.nbcnews.com/politics/white-house/biden-administration-recommend-vaccinated-wear-masks-areas-low-vaccination-rates-n1275012.

683.Emily Kopp, CDC report shows vaccinated people can spread COVID-19, Roll Call, July 30, 2021, https://www.rollcall.com/2021/07/30/cdc-report-shows-vaccinated-people-can-spread-covid-19/.

684.Outbreak of SARS-CoV-2 Infections, Including COVID-19 Vaccine Breakthrough Infections, Associated with Large Public Gatherings — Barnstable County, Massachusetts, July 2021, CDC, August 6, 2021, https://www.cdc.gov/mmwr/volumes/70/wr/mm7031e2.htm.

685.Nina Pierpont, Covid-19 Vaccine Mandates Are Now Pointless: Covid-19 Vaccines Do Not Keep People from Catching the Prevailing Delta Variant and

Passing it to Others, September 9, 2021, https://theexpose.uk/wp-content/uploads/2021/09/Pierpont-Why-mandated-vaccines-are-pointless-final-1.pdf.

686.https://www.instagram.com/tv/CYpnmfioB2K/?utm_medium=copy_link.

687.https://www.instagram.com/tv/CYpnmfioB2K/?utm_medium=copy_link.

688.Jeff Faraudo, Cal Football: Bears Expecting Everyone Back From COVID-19 for the Big Game, Sports Illustrated, November 13, 2021, https://www.si.com/college/cal/news/cal-covid-update-111321.

689.University of California 2021 Football Roster, https://calbears.com/sports/football/roster.

690.Carol Rosenberg and Aishvarya Kavi, a U.S. Navy Combat Ship Is Stranded in Guantánamo Bay with a Virus Outbreak, The New York Times, December 25, 2021, https://www.nytimes.com/2021/12/25/world/navy-ship-covid-guantanamo-bay.html.

691.Darling v. Sacred Heart Health System, 3:21-CV-1787/TKW, (N.D. Fl. 2021), ruling from the bench of U.S. District Court Judge T. Kent Wetherell, II denying motion for preliminary injunction.

692.COVID-19 Vaccine Breakthrough Infections Reported to CDC — United States, January 1–April 30, 2021, CDC, May 28, 2021, https://www.cdc.gov/mmwr/volumes/70/wr/mm7021e3.htm.

693.Letter from Seanator Edward J. Markey to Dr. Dr. Rochelle P. Walletnsky, Director, CDC, July 22, 2021, https://www.markey.senate.gov/imo/media/doc/cdc_breakthrough_cases_letter.pdf.

694.The Expose, Whilst you were distracted by Boris resigning, the UK Gov. quietly published a report confirming the Vaccinated account for 94% of all COVID-19 Deaths since April, 90% of which were Triple/Quadruple Jabbed, July 11, 2022, https://expose-news.com/2022/07/11/boris-distraction-uk-gov-revealed-triple-vaccinated-94percent-covid-deaths/.

695.The Expose, July 11, 2022, supra.

696.Deaths by vaccination status, England. Office for National Statistics, https://www.ons.gov.uk/peoplepopulationandcommunity/birthsdeathsandmarriages/deaths/datasets/deathsbyvaccinationstatusengland, Release date: 06 July 2022.

697.UK Government quietly confirms Triple+ Vaccinated accounted for 92% of COVID Deaths in 2022, The Expose, March 26, 2023, https://expose-news.com/2023/03/26/uk-gov-confirms-vaccinated-accounted-for-92-percent-of-covid-deaths-in-2022/.

698.Guy Page, 76% of September COVID-19 Deaths Are Vax Breakthroughs, Vermont Daily Chronicle, September 30, 2021, https://vermontdailychronicle.com/2021/09/30/76-of-september-covid-19-deaths-are-vaxxed-breakthroughs/.

699.Protect Yourself & Others, Vermont Department of Public Health, https://www.healthvermont.gov/covid-19/protect-yourself-others (last visited on October 14, 2021).

700.Hall Turner Radio Show, Newsdesk, November 9, 2021, https://halturnerradioshow.com/index.php/en/news-page/world/hospitals-in-antwerp-belgium-75-6-vaxxed-are-now-reporting-100-of-their-covid-cases-are-double-vaccinated.

701.Id.

702.Id.

703.EXCLUSIVE – 89% of COVID-19 Deaths in the past 4 Weeks Were among the Fully Vaccinated According to the Latest Public Health Data, The Expose, November 11, 2021, https://theexpose.uk/2021/11/11/89-percent-of-covid-19-deaths-were-among-the-fully-vaccinated-in-the-past-month/.

704.Public Health Scotland, COVID-19 & Winter Statistical Report, As at 17 January 2022, Publication Date: 19 January 2022, https://publichealthscotland.scot/media/11223/22-01-19-covid19-winter_publication_report.pdf.

705.Id.

706.Id.

707.Id.

708.Public Health Scotland, COVID-19 & Winter Statistical Report, As at 17 January 2022, Publication Date: 19 January 2022, archived from January 19, 2022, https://web.archive.org/web/20220119160752/https://publichealthscotland.scot/media/11223/22-01-19-covid19-winter_publication_report.pdf

709.Public Health Scotland COVID-19 & Winter Statistical Report As at 14 February 2022 Publication date: 16 February 2022, https://publichealthscotland.scot/media/11916/22-02-16-covid19-winter_publication_report.pdf.

710.Ana Da Silva, Health bosses to stop publishing Covid deaths by vaccine status after 'misrepresentation' of figures, The Press and Jounal, February 17, 2022, https://www.pressandjournal.co.uk/fp/politics/scottish-politics/3966759/health-bosses-to-stop-publishing-covid-deaths-by-vaccine-status/.

711.Steve Kirsch, Think vaccines work?, Substack, February 23, 2022, https://stevekirsch.substack.com/p/think-vaccines-work?utm_source=url.

712.Public Health Scotland COVID-19 & Winter Statistical Report As at 10 January 2022 Publication date: 12 January 2022, https://publichealthscotland.scot/media/11076/22-01-12-covid19-winter_publication_report.pdf.

713.Edward Hendrie, COVER-UP: Scotland Health Authorities Will Stop Reporting COVID Deaths by Vaccine Status, February 25, 2022, https://greatmountainpublishing.com/2022/02/25/coverup-scotland-health-authorities-will-stop-reporting-covid-deaths-by-vaccine-status/.

714.5.3.6 CUMULATIVE ANALYSIS OF POST-AUTHORIZATION ADVERSE EVENT REPORTS OF PF-07302048 (BNT162B2) RECEIVED THROUGH 28-FEB-2021, https://drtrozzi.org/wp-content/uploads/2022/01/Pfizer-Cumulative-Analysis-of-Post-authorization-Adverse-Event-Reports.pdf.

715.Compare COVID-19 epidemiology update, July 29, 2022, https://health-infobase.canada.ca/covid-19/, with COVID-19 epidemiology update, June 17, 2022, https://web.archive.org/web/20220622061056/https://health-infobase.canada.ca/covid-19/.

716.Trudeau's Government confirms the Quadruple/Triple Vaccinated have accounted for 90% of Covid-19 Deaths across Canada since the beginning of June, The Expose, July 29, 2022, https://expose-news.com/2022/07/29/trudeau-90percent-covid-deaths-vaccinated-canada/?cmid=60835409-a89a-4896-82cd-c51b2d11c704.

717.Id.

718.Id.

719.Cahterine Brown, et al., Outbreak of SARS-CoV-2 Infections, Including COVID-19 Vaccine Breakthrough Infections, Associated with Large Public Gatherings - Barnstable County, Massachusetts, July 2021, August 6, 2021, https://pubmed.ncbi.nlm.nih.gov/34351882/.

720.Nguyen Van Vinh Chau, et al., Transmission of SARS-CoV-2 Delta Variant Among Vaccinated Healthcare Workers, Vietnam, Volume 41, November 2021, 11043,

https://doi.org/10.1016/j.eclinm.2021.101143, and also at:
https://papers.ssrn.com/sol3/papers.cfm?abstract_id=3897733.

721.Carla Saade, et al., Live virus neutralization testing in convalescent patients and subjects vaccinated against 19A, 20B, 20I/501Y.V1 and 20H/501Y.V2 isolates of SARS-CoV-2, December 2021, https://pubmed.ncbi.nlm.nih.gov/34176436/.

722.Kasen K. Riemersma, et al., Shedding of Infectious SARS-CoV-2 Despite Vaccination, August 24, 2021, https://www.medrxiv.org/content/10.1101/2021.07.31.21261387v4.full.pdf.

723.The United Kingdom Health Security Agency COVID-19 Vaccine Surveillance Report, Publishing Reference: GOV-10227, at 12, October 21, 2021, https://assets.publishing.service.gov.uk/government/uploads/system/uploads/attachment_data/file/1027511/Vaccine-surveillance-report-week-42.pdf.

724.The United Health Kingdom Health Security Agency COVID-19 Vaccine Surveillance Report, Publishing Reference: GOV-10227, at 13, October 21, 2021, https://assets.publishing.service.gov.uk/government/uploads/system/uploads/attachment_data/file/1027511/Vaccine-surveillance-report-week-42.pdf.

725.Latest UK Health Security Agency report Shows the COVID-19 Vaccines Have NEGATIVE Effectiveness As Low As MINUS 124%, The Expose, October 22, 2021, https://theexpose.uk/2021/10/22/covid-19-vaccines-ha

ve-negative-effectiveness-as-low-as-minus-124-percent/.

726.Official Government Reports Suggest the Fully Vaccinated Will Develop Acquired Immunodeficiency Syndrome by Christmas, The Expose, Ocober 27, 2021, https://theexpose.uk/2021/10/27/official-government-reports-suggest-the-fully-vaccinated-will-develop-acquired-immunodeficiency-syndrome-by-christmas/.

727.COVID-19 Vaccine Surveillance Report, Week 42, UK Health Security Agency, Publishing reference: GOV-10227, 21 October 2021, https://assets.publishing.service.gov.uk/government/uploads/system/uploads/attachment_data/file/1027511/Vaccine-surveillance-report-week-42.pdf.

728.Official Government Reports Suggest the Fully Vaccinated Will Develop Acquired Immunodeficiency Syndrome by Christmas, The Expose, Ocober 27, 2021, https://theexpose.uk/2021/10/27/official-government-reports-suggest-the-fully-vaccinated-will-develop-acquired-immunodeficiency-syndrome-by-christmas/.

729.S. V. Subramanian and Akhil Kumar, Increases in COVID-19 Are Unrelated to Levels of Vaccination Across 68 Countries and 2947 Counties in the United States, September 30, 2021, https://www.ncbi.nlm.nih.gov/pmc/articles/PMC8481107/#CR1.

730.S. V. Subramanian and Akhil Kumar, supra.

731.S. V. Subramanian and Akhil Kumar, supra.

732.Barbara A. Cohn, et al., Breakthrough SARS-CoV-2 infections in 620,000 U.S. Veterans, February 1, 2021 to August 13, 2021, October 14, 2021, https://www.medrxiv.org/content/10.1101/2021.10.13.21264966v1.

733.Joseph A. Ladapo, M.D., Ph.D., State Surgeon General, Guidance for Pediatric COVID-19 Vaccines, March 8, 2022, http://ww11.doh.state.fl.us/comm/_partners/covid19_report_archive/press-release-assets/g2-jtr_QWBT4hJpqr_20220308-1923.pdf.

734.Joseph A. Ladapo, March 8, 2022, supra.

735.Joseph A. Ladapo, March 8, 2022, supra.

736.Joseph A. Ladapo, March 8, 2022, supra.

737.Stay Up to Date with COVID-19 Vaccines Including Boosters, CDC, October 4, 2022, https://www.cdc.gov/coronavirus/2019-ncov/vaccines/stay-up-to-date.html#children.

738.Interim Infection Prevention and Control Recommendations for Healthcare Personnel During the Coronavirus Disease 2019 (COVID-19) Pandemic, September 23, 2022, CDC, COVID-19, https://www.cdc.gov/coronavirus/2019-ncov/hcp/infection-control-recommendations.html#.

739.Catherine J Frompovich, An Interview With Research Immunologist Tetyana Obukhanych, PhD, Part 1 of 3, https://studylib.net/doc/7772112/an-interview-with-research-immunologist-tetyana-obukhanyc... (last visited on April 3, 2023).

740.Brett Wilcox, Jabbed, How the Vaccine Industry, Medical Establishment and Government Stick It to You and Your Family, at 97 (2018).

741.Brett Wilcox, Jabbed, supra, at 88.

742.America's Frontline Doctors et al., v. Xavier Becerra, Secretary of the U.S. Department of Health and Human Services, et al., Civil Action No. 2:21-cv-00702-CLM (N.D. Alabama 2021), https://www.courtlistener.com/docket/59929233/americas-frontline-doctors-etc-v-becerra/.

743.Immunization: The Basics, CDC, September 1, 2021, https://www.cdc.gov/vaccines/vac-gen/imz-basics.htm.

744.Immunization: The Basics, CDC, August 24, 2021 archive date, https://web.archive.org/web/20210824024512/https://www.cdc.gov/vaccines/vac-gen/imz-basics.htm.

745.Immunization: The Basics, CDC, September 1, 2021, https://www.cdc.gov/vaccines/vac-gen/imz-basics.htm.

746.Getting Your COVID-19 Vaccine, CDC, https://www.cdc.gov/coronavirus/2019-ncov/vaccines/expect.html?s_cid=11781:when%20to%20get%20vaccine%20after%20having%20covid:sem.ga:p:RG:GM:gen:PTN:FY22.

747.Nabin K. Shrestha, et al., Necessity of COVID-19 vaccination in previously infected individuals, June 5, 2020, https://www.medrxiv.org/content/10.1101/2021.06.01.

21258176v2.

748.Dr. Scot Youngblood at San Diego City Council Meeting, September 20, 2022, https://www.bitchute.com/video/H3onzCie2198/.

749.Id.

750.Megan Loe, Yes, the CDC changed its definition of vaccine to be 'more transparent', News West 9, February 4, 2022, https://www.newswest9.com/article/news/verify/coronavirus-verify/cdc-changed-vaccine-definition-more-transparent/536-03ce7891-2604-4090-b548-b1618d286834.

751.Vaccine, Merriam-Webster Dicitonary, January 18, 2021, https://web.archive.org/web/20210118193104/https://www.merriam-webster.com/dictionary/vaccine.

752.Vaccine, Merriam-Webster Dicitonary, https://www.merriam-webster.com/dictionary/vaccine (last visited on February 2, 2023).

753.Biological Weapon, Merriam-Webster Dictionary, https://www.merriam-webster.com/dictionary/biological%20weapon#medicalDictionary (last visited on February 2, 2023).

754.Peter Loftus, As Covid-19 Vaccine Development Pushes Ahead, Researchers Probe Safety, The Wall Street Journal, July 12, 2020, https://www.wsj.com/articles/as-covid-19-vaccine-development-pushes-ahead-researchers-probe-safety-11594546201

755.Peter Loftus, July 12, 2020, supra.

756.Daniel Payne, Moderna COVID-19 vaccine induced adverse reactions in 'more than half' of trial participants, Just the News, July 15, 2022, https://justthenews.com/nation/science/moderna-covid-19-vaccine-induced-adverse-reactions-more-half-trial-participants?utm_source=justthenews.com&utm_medium=feed&utm_campaign=external-news-aggregators

757.Lisa A. Jackson, et al., An mRNA Vaccine against SARS-CoV-2 — Preliminary Report, NEJM, N Engl J Med 2020; 383:1920-1931
DOI: 10.1056/NEJMoa2022483, November 12, 2020, https://www.nejm.org/doi/full/10.1056/NEJMoa2022483#figures_media. See also July 14, 2020 article posting at:
http://web.archive.org/web/20200714232719/https://www.nejm.org/doi/full/10.1056/NEJMoa2022483.

758.Lisa A. Jackson, et al., An mRNA Vaccine against SARS-CoV-2 — Preliminary Report, NEJM, N Engl J Med 2020; 383:1920-1931
DOI: 10.1056/NEJMoa2022483, November 12, 2020, https://www.nejm.org/doi/full/10.1056/NEJMoa2022483#figures_media.

759.Lazarus, Ross, et al., Grant ID: R18 HS 017045, Final Report, Electronic Support for Public Health–Vaccine Adverse Event Reporting System (ESP:VAERS), at 6, 2/01/07 - 09/30/10, Submitted to: The Agency for Healthcare Research and Quality (AHRQ) U.S. Department of Health and Human Services,
https://digital.ahrq.gov/sites/default/files/docs/publication/r18hs017045-lazarus-final-report-2011.pdf.

760.Official Government Reports Suggest the Fully Vaccinated Will Develop Acquired Immunodeficiency

Syndrome by Christmas, The Expose, Ocober 27, 2021, https://theexpose.uk/2021/10/27/official-government-reports-suggest-the-fully-vaccinated-will-develop-acquired-immunodeficiency-syndrome-by-christmas/.

761.Uversky VN, Redwan EM, Makis W, Rubio-Casillas A. IgG4 Antibodies Induced by Repeated Vaccination May Generate Immune Tolerance to the SARS-CoV-2 Spike Protein. Vaccines (Basel). 2023 May 17;11(5):991. doi: 10.3390/vaccines11050991. PMID: 37243095; PMCID: PMC10222767, https://www.ncbi.nlm.nih.gov/pmc/articles/PMC10222767/.

762.Uversky VN, supra.

763.Uversky VN, supra.

764.Uversky VN, supra.

765.Uversky VN, supra.

766.Tiffany Meier, More Die After Vaccination Than From COVID-19 in Taiwan, China In Focus, NTD News, October 13, 2021, https://www.ntd.com/more-die-after-vaccination-than-from-covid-19-in-taiwan_688004.html.

767.Official Government Reports Suggest the Fully Vaccinated Will Develop Acquired Immunodeficiency Syndrome by Christmas, The Expose, Ocober 27, 2021, https://theexpose.uk/2021/10/27/official-government-reports-suggest-the-fully-vaccinated-will-develop-acquired-immunodeficiency-syndrome-by-christmas/.

768.Id.

769.Id.

770.COVID-19 Vaccine Emergency Use Authorization (EUA) Fact Sheets for Recipients and Caregivers, August 6, 2021, https://www.cdc.gov/vaccines/covid-19/eua/index.html .

771.Fact Sheet for Recipients and Caregivers Emergency Use Authorization (EUA) of The Janssen COVID-19 Vaccine to Prevent Coronavirus Disease 2019 (COVID-19) in Individuals 18 Years of Age and Older, August 27, 2021, https://www.janssenlabels.com/emergency-use-authorization/Janssen+COVID-19+Vaccine-Recipient-fact-sheet.pdf.

772.Vaccines and Related Biological Products Advisory Committee - 10/22/2020, U.S. Food and Drug Administration, at 2:33:40, https://www.youtube.com/watch?v=1XTiL9rUpkg&t=9220s.

773.A Comparison of Official Government Reports Suggests the Fully Vaccinated Are Suffering Antibody Dependent Enhancement, The Expose, January 23, 2022, https://dailyexpose.uk/2022/01/23/world-government-data-shows-covid-vaccinated-suffering-ade/.

774.Antibody-Dependent Enhancement (ADE) and Vaccines, Children's Hospital of Philidelphia, https://www.chop.edu/centers-programs/vaccine-education-center/vaccine-safety/antibody-dependent-enhancement-and-vaccines (last visited on August 26, 2021).

775.New Strain? Or Antibody Dependent Enhancement?, Everly Report, December 21, 2020, https://everlyreport.com/new-strain-or-antibody-dependent-enhancement/.

776.Joseph Mercla, How COVID-19 Vaccine Can Destroy Your Immune System, Signs of the Times, 11 November 2020, https://www.sott.net/article/445095-How-COVID-19-vaccine-can-destroy-your-immune-system.

777.Nobel Prize Winner French Virologist Luc Montagnier Explains How COVID-19 Vaccines Are Creating Variants, March 21, 2021, https://greatgameindia.com/covid-19-vaccines-creating-variants/.

778.Larry Johnson, Inventor of mRNA Vaccine: Some Covid Vaccines Make the Virus More Dangerous, Gateway Pundit, July 28, 2021, https://www.thegatewaypundit.com/2021/07/inventor-mrna-vaccine-covid-vaccines-make-virus-dangerous/.

779.Yen-Der Li, et. al., Coronavirus Vaccine Development: from SARS and MERS to COVID-19, NIH, 20 December 2020, https://www.ncbi.nlm.nih.gov/pmc/articles/PMC7749790/.

780.Ken Garber, Coronavirus Vaccine Developers Wary of Errant Antibodies, 5 June 2020, https://www.nature.com/articles/d41587-020-00016-w, found at https://www.airlinepilotforums.com/covid19/130189-we-need-plan-b-no-vaccine-33.html.

781.Nobel Prize Winner French Virologist Luc Montagnier Explains How COVID-19 Vaccines Are Creating Variants, March 21, 2021, https://greatgameindia.com/covid-19-vaccines-creating-variants/.

782.Timothy Cardozo, et al., Informed Consent Disclosure to Vaccine Trial Subjects of Risk of COVID-19 Vaccines Worsening Clinical Disease, NIH, Int J Clin Pract., March 2021, vol. 75, Issue 3, https://pubmed.ncbi.nlm.nih.gov/33113270/.

783.Wen Shi Lee, et. al., Antibody-dependent Enhancement and SARS-CoV-2 Vaccines and Therapies, NIH, September 9, 2020, https://pubmed.ncbi.nlm.nih.gov/32908214/.

784.Ann M. Arvin, A Perspective on Potential Antibody-Dependent Enhancement of SARS-CoV-2, 2020 July 13, https://pubmed.ncbi.nlm.nih.gov/32659783/.

785.Beattie, Kyle. (2021). Worldwide Bayesian Causal Impact Analysis of Vaccine Administration on Deaths and Cases Associated with COVID-19: A BigData Analysis of 145 Countries. 10.13140/RG.2.2.34214.65605, https://www.researchgate.net/publication/356248984_Worldwide_Bayesian_Causal_Impact_Analysis_of_Vaccine_Administration_on_Deaths_and_Cases_Associated_with_COVID-19_A_BigData_Analysis_of_145_Countries.

786.Beattie, Kyle, supra

787.New Strain? Or Antibody Dependent Enhancement?, Everly Report, December 21, 2020, https://everlyreport.com/new-strain-or-antibody-dependent-enhancement/.

788.Id.

789.Steven Li, Hospital Fully Vaccinated, Doctor Calls Mandates 'Diabolic', Vision Times, August 8, 2021, https://www.visiontimes.com/2021/08/08/israel-hospital-vaccinated.html.

790.Vaccines and Related Biological Products Advisory Committee Meeting, December 10, 2020, FDA Briefing Document Pfizer-BioNTech COVID-19 Vaccine, at 49,
https://www.fda.gov/media/144245/download.

791.Id.

792.Larry Johnson, Inventor of mRNA Vaccine: Some Covid Vaccines Make the Virus More Dangerous, Gateway Pundit, July 28, 2021, https://www.thegatewaypundit.com/2021/07/inventor-mrna-vaccine-covid-vaccines-make-virus-dangerous/.

793.Vaccines and Related Biological Products, supra.

794.Vaccines and Related Biological Products, supra.

795.Pfizer admits in Confidential Documents that its Covid-19 Vaccine may cause Vaccine-Associated Enhanced Disease; and real-world data now proves it definitely does, The Expose, February 3, 2022, https://dailyexpose.uk/2022/02/03/pfizer-admits-covid-vaccine-causes-ade/.

796.5.3.6 CUMULATIVE ANALYSIS OF POST-AUTHORIZATION ADVERSE EVENT REPORTS OF PF-07302048 (BNT162B2)

RECEIVED THROUGH 28-FEB-2021, https://drtrozzi.org/wp-content/uploads/2022/01/Pfizer-Cumulative-Analysis-of-Post-authorization-Adverse-Event-Reports.pdf.

797.VAERS COVID Vaccine Data, August 13, 2021, https://www.openvaers.com/covid-data.

798.Lazarus, Ross, et al., Grant ID: R18 HS 017045, Final Report, Electronic Support for Public Health–Vaccine Adverse Event Reporting System (ESP:VAERS), at 6, 2/01/07 - 09/30/10, Submitted to: The Agency for Healthcare Research and Quality (AHRQ) U.S. Department of Health and Human Services, https://digital.ahrq.gov/sites/default/files/docs/publication/r18hs017045-lazarus-final-report-2011.pdf.

799.Megan Redshaw, Latest VAERS Data Show Reports of Blood Clotting Disorders After All Three Emergency Use Authorization Vaccines, The Defender, April 16, 2021, https://childrenshealthdefense.org/defender/vaers-reports-clotting-disorders-all-three-emergency-use-authorization-vaccines/?itm_term=home. See also Tyler Durden, What The CDC's VAERS Database Reveals About "Adverse" Post-Vaccine Reactions, April 18, 2021, https://www.zerohedge.com/covid-19/what-cdcs-vaers-database-reveals-about-adverse-post-vaccine-reactions.

800.Report of Toddler's Death Disappears from Vaers and CDC Has No Records as to Why!, ICAN, March 4, 2022, https://icandecide.org/press-release/report-of-toddlers-death-disappears-from-vaers-and-cdc-has-no-records-as-to-why/.

801.VAERS Detail, VEARS ID: 1887456, https://icandecide.org/wp-content/uploads/2022/02/Missing-VAERS-Report.pdf

802.Justice Department Announces Largest Health Care Fraud Settlement in Its History, Pfizer to Pay $2.3 Billion for Fraudulent Marketing, September 2, 2009, https://www.justice.gov/opa/pr/justice-department-announces-largest-health-care-fraud-settlement-its-history.

803.Id.

804.Sammy Almashat, et. al., Twenty-Seven Years of Pharmaceutical Industry Criminal and Civil Penalties: 1991 Through 2017, Public Citizen, March 14, 2018, https://www.citizen.org/wp-content/uploads/2408.pdf.

805.Sammy Almashat, March 14, 2018, supra.

806.VAERS COVID Vaccine Data, August 13, 2021, COVID Vaccine Reported Mortality Breakdowns, https://www.openvaers.com/covid-data/mortality.

807.Id.

808.Court Orders CDC to Release Data Showing 18 Million Vaccine Injuries in America, American Liberty Report, https://www.americanlibertyreportnews.com/articles/court-orders-cdc-to-release-data-showing-18-million-vaccine-injuries-in-america/ (last visited on November 11, 2022).

809.Vaccines for COVID-19, https://www.cdc.gov/coronavirus/2019-ncov/vaccines/index.html (last visited on November 11, 2022).

810.V-safe Data, Informed Consent Network, https://icandecide.org/v-safe-data/ (last visited on November 11, 2022).

811.Id.

812.Inova Health to require employees be vaccinated against COVID-19, June 25, 2022, https://www.insidenova.com/headlines/inova-health-to-require-employees-be-vaccinated-against-covid-19/article_b7b54cec-d438-11eb-a8ba-7736e356c2fd.html. See also Mandatory COVID Vaccination Information, https://www.inova.org/sites/default/files/education/gme/policies_procedures/mandatory_covid_vaccination_information_rev.pdf (last visited on November 11, 2022).

813.COVID-19 Vaccine & Booster Information from Inova, https://www.inova.org/COVID19/vaccine-scheduling#accordion-149336 (last visited on November 11, 2022).

814.V-safe Data, Informed Consent Network, https://icandecide.org/v-safe-data/ (last visited on November 11, 2022).

815.Majority of Physicians Decline COVID Shots, according to Survey, AAPS, June 16, 2021, https://aapsonline.org/majority-of-physicians-decline-covid-shots-according-to-survey/.

816.Medicare and Medicaid Programs; Omnibus COVID-19 Health Care Staff Vaccination, Federal Register, publication date November 5, 2021, https://www.federalregister.gov/documents/2021/11/05/2021-23831/medicare-and-medicaid-programs-omnibus-covid-19-health-care-staff-vaccination.

817.Biden-Harris Administration Issues Emergency Regulation Requiring COVID-19 Vaccination for Health Care Workers, CMS Newsroom Press Release, November 4, 2021.

818.Fact Sheet: Majority of Hospital Payments Dependent on Medicare or Medicaid, AHA, https://www.aha.org/fact-sheets/2022-05-25-fact-sheet-majority-hospital-payments-dependent-medicare-or-medicaid (last visited on February 21, 2023).

819.Barrows v. Becerra, 24 F.4th 116 (2d Cir. 2022).

820.Mission Hospital Agrees to Pay $89,000 To Settle EEOC Religious Discrimination Lawsuit, Asheville Hospital Fired Employees for Declining Flu Vaccination, Federal Agency Charged, January 12, 2018, https://www.eeoc.gov/newsroom/mission-hospital-agrees-pay-89000-settle-eeoc-religious-discrimination-lawsuit.

821.Letter from Jason Miyars, Attorney General of Virginia to Dr. J. Stephen Jones, CEO, Inova Health Systems, July 22, 2022.

822. Letter from Jason Miyars, Attorney General of Virginia to Dr. J. Stephen Jones, CEO, Inova Health Systems, July 22, 2022.

823.Debra Heine, Dr. McCullough: COVID Vaccines Have Already Killed Up to 50,000 Americans, According to Whistleblowers, American Greatness, June 15, 2021, https://amgreatness.com/2021/06/15/dr-mccullough-covid-vaccines-have-already-killed-up-to-50000-americans-according-to-whistleblowers/.

824.Id.

825.Edward Hendrie, The FDA and Pfizer Concealed Evidence That COVID-19 Vaccines Will Cause Myocarditis in Children, November 7, 2021, https://greatmountainpublishing.com/2021/11/07/the-fda-and-pfizer-concealed-evidence-that-covid-19-vaccines-will-cause-myocarditis-in-children/.

826.The COVID Vaccines; Are they Safe and Effective? Presented by Dr. Peter A. McCullough At the United For Healthcare Summit 2022, published July 24, 2022, https://rumble.com/v1dgd7p-dr.-peter-a.-mccullough-united-for-healthcare-summit-2022.html.

827.Covid-19 Vaccine Pharmacovigilance Report, World Council For Health, June 16, 2022, https://worldcouncilforhealth.org/resources/covid-19-vaccine-pharmacovigilance-report.

828.Dr. Katarina Lindley, Independent Pharmacovigilance Report Confirms Evidence for Recall of Covid-19 Vaccines, World Council For Health, July 11, 2022, https://worldcouncilforhealth.org/news/independent-pharmacovigilance-report-recall-of-covid-19-vaccines.

829.Dr. Katarina Lindley, July 11, 2022, supra.

830.Lazarus, Ross, et al., Grant ID: R18 HS 017045, Final Report, Electronic Support for Public Health–Vaccine Adverse Event Reporting System (ESP:VAERS), at 6, 2/01/07 - 09/30/10, Submitted to: The Agency for Healthcare Research and Quality (AHRQ) U.S. Department of Health and Human Services, https://digital.ahrq.gov/sites/default/files/docs/publication/r18hs017045-lazarus-final-report-2011.pdf.

831.Kimberly Blumenthal, Acute Allergic Reactions to mRNA COVID-19 Vaccines, Journal of the American Medical Association, March 8, 2021, https://jamanetwork.com/journals/jama/fullarticle/2777417.

832. Tom T. Shimabukuro, Reports of Anaphylaxis After Receipt of mRNA COVID-19 Vaccines in the US—December 14, 2020-January 18, 2021, Journal of the American Medical Association, https://jamanetwork.com/journals/jama/fullarticle/2776557.

833.Selected Adverse Events Reported after COVID-19 Vaccination, CDC, March 30, 2021, https://web.archive.org/web/20210405130532/https://www.cdc.gov/coronavirus/2019-ncov/vaccines/safety/adverse-events.html.

834.Kimberly Blumenthal, Acute Allergic Reactions to mRNA COVID-19 Vaccines, Journal of the American Medical Association, March 8, 2021, https://jamanetwork.com/journals/jama/fullarticle/2777417.

835.Letter from Elizabeth A. Brehm to Dr. Rochelle P. Walensky, Director, Centers for Disease Control and Prevention, March 17, 2021, https://www.icandecide.org/wp-content/uploads/2021/03/Letter-to-Dr.-Walensky-re-anaphylaxis.pdf.

836.Id.

837.Id.

838.Megan Redshaw, Latest VAERS Data Show Reports of Blood Clotting Disorders After All Three Emergency Use Authorization Vaccines, The Defender, April 16, 2021, https://childrenshealthdefense.org/defender/vaers-reports-clotting-disorders-all-three-emergency-use-authorization-vaccines/?itm_term=home. See also Tyler Durden, What The CDC's VAERS Database Reveals About "Adverse" Post-Vaccine Reactions, April 18, 2021, https://www.zerohedge.com/covid-19/what-cdcs-vaers-database-reveals-about-adverse-post-vaccine-reactions.

839.Covid-19 Vaccine Pharmacovigilance Report, World Council For Health, June 16, 2022, https://worldcouncilforhealth.org/resources/covid-19-vaccine-pharmacovigilance-report.

840.Covid-19 Vaccine Pharmacovigilance Report, World Council For Health, June 16, 2022, https://worldcouncilforhealth.org/resources/covid-19-vaccine-pharmacovigilance-report.

841.Lazarus, Ross, et al., Grant ID: R18 HS 017045, Final Report, Electronic Support for Public Health–Vaccine Adverse Event Reporting System (ESP:VAERS), at 6, 2/01/07 - 09/30/10, Submitted to: The Agency for Healthcare Research and Quality (AHRQ) U.S. Department of Health and Human Services, https://digital.ahrq.gov/sites/default/files/docs/publication/r18hs017045-lazarus-final-report-2011.pdf.

842.Scott McLachlan, et al., Analysis of COVID-19 vaccine death reports from the Vaccine Adverse Events Reporting System (VAERS) Database Interim: Results and Analysis, ResearchGate, June 2021, https://www.researchgate.net/publication/352837543_

Analysis_of_COVID-19_vaccine_death_reports_from_the_Vaccine_Adverse_Events_Reporting_System_VAERS_Database_Interim_Results_and_Analysis.

843.BREAKING – The Covid-19 Vaccines have killed at least 150,000 people in the USA including 574 children according to new Scientific Study, The Expose , September 20, 2021, https://expose-news.com/2021/09/20/covid-19-vaccines-have-killed-at-least-150000-people-in-the-usa/.

844.Ben Armstrong, CDC Data & Scientific Study suggest 1.2 million Americans may already have died due to COVID Vaccination, The Expose, October 4, 2022, https://expose-news.com/2022/10/04/cdc-12-million-americans-dead-covid-vaccination/.

845.Open VEARS, https://www.openvaers.com/ (last visited on July 28, 2022).

846.Megan Redshaw, Latest VAERS Data Show Reports of Blood Clotting Disorders After All Three Emergency Use Authorization Vaccines, The Defender, April 16, 2021, https://childrenshealthdefense.org/defender/vaers-reports-clotting-disorders-all-three-emergency-use-authorization-vaccines/?itm_term=home. See also Tyler Durden, What The CDC's VAERS Database Reveals About "Adverse" Post-Vaccine Reactions, April 18, 2021, https://www.zerohedge.com/covid-19/what-cdcs-vaers-database-reveals-about-adverse-post-vaccine-reactions.

847.Fact Sheet for Recipients and Caregivers Emergency Use Authorization (EUA) of The Janssen COVID-19 Vaccine to Prevent Coronavirus Disease 2019 (COVID-19) in Individuals 18 Years of Age and

Older, August 27, 2021, https://www.janssenlabels.com/emergency-use-authorization/Janssen+COVID-19+Vaccine-Recipient-fact-sheet.pdf.

848.See COVID-19 Vaccine Emergency Use Authorization (EUA) Fact Sheets for Recipients and Caregivers, CDC, August 6, 2021, https://www.cdc.gov/vaccines/covid-19/eua/index.html.

849.Vaccines and Related Biological Products Advisory Committee - 10/22/2020, U.S. Food and Drug Administration, at 2:33:40, https://www.youtube.com/watch?v=1XTiL9rUpkg&t=9220s.

850.Shari Roan, Swine Flu 'Debacle' of 1976 Is Recalled, Los Angeles Times, April 27, 2009, https://www.latimes.com/archives/la-xpm-2009-apr-27-sci-swine-history27-story.html#:~:text=Waiting%20in%20long%20lines%20at,receiving%20the%20vaccine%3B%2025%20died.

851.Vaccines and Related Biological Products Advisory Committee - 10/22/2020, U.S. Food and Drug Administration, at 2:33:40, https://www.youtube.com/watch?v=1XTiL9rUpkg&t=9220s.

852.Remarks by President Biden on Fighting the COVID-19 Pandemic, August 18, 2021, https://www.whitehouse.gov/briefing-room/speeches-remarks/2021/08/18/remarks-by-president-biden-on-fighting-the-covid-19-pandemic-2/.

853.Remarks by President Biden Laying Out the Next Steps in Our Effort to Get More Americans Vaccinated and Combat the Spread of the Delta Variant, July 29, 2021, 4:23 p.m. EDT, https://www.whitehouse.gov/briefing-room/speeches-remarks/2021/07/29/remarks-by-president-biden-laying-out-the-next-steps-in-our-effort-to-get-more-americans-vaccinated-and-combat-the-spread-of-the-delta-variant/. See also Executive Order 14043 of September 9, 2021, Requiring Coronavirus Disease 2019 Vaccination for Federal Employees, https://www.federalregister.gov/documents/2021/09/14/2021-19927/requiring-coronavirus-disease-2019-vaccination-for-federal-employees.

854.VAERS COVID Vaccine Data, August 13, 2021, https://www.openvaers.com/covid-data.

855.COVID Vaccine Reported Mortality Breakdowns, August 13, 2021, https://www.openvaers.com/covid-data/mortality.

856.American Frontline Doctors v. Xavier Becerra, Secretary of the U.S. Department of Health and Human Services, Petition For Temporary Restraining Order, United States District Court for The Northern District of Alabama, Case 2:21-cv-00702-CLM, May 20, 2021, at 46, https://americasfrontlinedoctors.org/files/tro/. See also CDC: as Many People Have Died from COVID-19 Vaccines as All Vaccines in Last 20 Years Combined, World News Daily, May 8, 2021, https://www.wnd.com/2021/05/cdc-many-people-died-covid-19-vaccines-vaccines-last-20-years-combined/.

857.Id. at 47.

858.Id. at 46.

859.Id.

860.Id.

861.Ethan Huff, Government Caught "Scrubbing" Covid-19 Vaccine Injuries and Deaths, Natural News, May 6, 2021, https://www.naturalnews.com/2021-05-06-government-caught-scrubbing-covid19-vaccine-injuries-deaths.html.

862.Debra Heine, Dr. McCullough: COVID Vaccines Have Already Killed Up to 50,000 Americans, According to Whistleblowers, American Greatness, June 15, 2021, https://amgreatness.com/2021/06/15/dr-mccullough-covid-vaccines-have-already-killed-up-to-50000-americans-according-to-whistleblowers/.

863.Declaration of Jane Doe, Executed on July 13, 2021, Case 2:21-cv-00702-CLM, United States District Court, Northern District of Alabama, Filed 07/19/21.

864.Id.

865.Lazarus, Ross, et al., Grant ID: R18 HS 017045, Final Report, Electronic Support for Public Health–Vaccine Adverse Event Reporting System (ESP:VAERS), at 6, 2/01/07 - 09/30/10, Submitted to: The Agency for Healthcare Research and Quality (AHRQ) U.S. Department of Health and Human Services, https://digital.ahrq.gov/sites/default/files/docs/publication/r18hs017045-lazarus-final-report-2011.pdf.

866.Open VEARS, https://www.openvaers.com/ (last visited on July 28, 2022).

867.The Expose, COVID Vaccines are at least 75x deadlier than all other Vaccines combined according to Medicine Regulators, August 19, 2022, https://expose-news.com/2022/08/19/covid-jabs-75x-deadlier-than-all-vaccines/.

868.Id.

869.AFLDS suit seeks to immediately revoke emergency COVID vaccine use based on disturbing new mortality data, AFLDS Frontline News, November 23, 2021, https://americasfrontlinenews.com/post/aflds-suit-seeks-to-immediately-revoke-emergency-covid-vaccine-use-based-on-disturbing-new-mortality-data. See also Alabama TRO/Complaint/Preliminary Injunction, SFLDS, https://americasfrontlinedoctors.org/2/legal/tro/ (last visited on July 28, 2022).

870.Robert Malone, et al., Cationic Liposome-mediated RNA Transfection, Proc. Nati. Acad. Sci. USA Vol. 86, pp. 6077-6081, August 1989, https://www.pnas.org/content/pnas/86/16/6077.full.pdf. See also Jon A. Wolfe, Robert Malone, et. al., Direct Gene Transfer into Mouse Muscle in Vivo, Science, Vol. 247, Issue 4949, pp. 1465-1468, DOI: 10.1126/science.1690918, 23 March 1990, https://science.sciencemag.org/content/247/4949/1465.abstract.

871.Spike Protein Is Very Dangerous, It's Cytotoxic (Robert Malone, Steve Kirsch, Bret Weinstein), June 13, 2021, https://www.youtube.com/watch?v=Du2wm5nhTXY.

872.Id.

873.Karen Weintraub, The first 22M Americans have been vaccinated for COVID-19, and initial safety data shows everything is going well, CDC says, USA Today, January 28, 2021, https://www.usatoday.com/story/news/health/2021/01/28/covid-19-vaccines-cdc-safety-data-pfizer-moderna-coronavirus/4281434001/.

874.Karen Weintraub, January 28, 2022, supra.

875.VAERS COVID Vaccine Adverse Event Reports, December 16, 2022, https://web.archive.org/web/20221231001252/https://openvaers.com/covid-data.

876.Karen Weintraub, January 28, 2022, supra.

877.Karen Weintraub, January 28, 2022, supra.

878.Karen Weintraub, January 28, 2022, supra.

879.Karen Weintraub, January 28, 2022, supra.

880.Denis G. Rancourt, et al., Age-stratified COVID-19 vaccine-dose fatality rate for Israel and Australia, Correlation Research in the Public Interest, 9 February 2023, https://correlation-canada.org/report-age-stratified-covid-19-vaccine-dose-fatality-rate-for-israel-and-australia/.

881.Health Alert on mRNA COVID-19 Vaccine Safety, Florida Department of Health, February 15, 2023, https://www.floridahealth.gov/newsroom/2023/02/20230215-updated-health-alert.pr.html.

882.Florida Surgeon General, Joseph Ladapo, Letter to Robert M. Calif, Commissioner, FDA and Rochelle P. Walensky, Director, (CDC), February 15, 2023, https://www.floridahealth.gov/_documents/newsroom/press-releases/2023/02/20230215-updated-health-alert-letter.pdf?utm_source=floridahealth.gov&utm_medium=referral&utm_campaign=newsroom&utm_content=article&url_trace_7f2r5y6=https%3A%2F%2Fwww.floridahealth.gov%2Fnewsroom%2F2023%2F02%2F20230215-updated-health-alert.pr.html.

883.Id.

884.Fraiman J, Erviti J, Jones M, Greenland S, Whelan P, Kaplan RM, Doshi P. Serious adverse events of special interest following mRNA COVID-19 vaccination in randomized trials in adults. Vaccine. 2022 Sep 22;40(40):5798-5805. doi: 10.1016/j.vaccine.2022.08.036. Epub 2022 Aug 31. PMID: 36055877; PMCID: PMC9428332. https://pubmed.ncbi.nlm.nih.gov/36055877/.

885.Sun CLF, Jaffe E, Levi R. Increased emergency cardiovascular events among under-40 population in Israel during vaccine rollout and third COVID-19 wave. Sci Rep. 2022 Apr 28;12(1):6978. doi: 10.1038/s41598-022-10928-z. PMID: 35484304; PMCID: PMC9048615. https://pubmed.ncbi.nlm.nih.gov/35484304/.

886.Dag Berild J, Bergstad Larsen V, Myrup Thiesson E, et al. Analysis of Thromboembolic and Thrombocytopenic Events After the AZD1222, BNT162b2, and MRNA-1273 COVID-19 Vaccines in 3 Nordic Countries. JAMA Netw Open. 2022;5(6):e2217375. doi:10.1001/jamanetworkopen.2022.17375.

https://jamanetwork.com/journals/jamanetworkopen/fullarticle/2793348?utm_source=floridahealth.gov&utm_medium=referral&utm_campaign=newsroom&utm_content=article&url_trace_7f2r5y6=https://www.floridahealth.gov/newsroom/2023/02/20230215-updated-health-alert.pr.html.

887.Cindy Krischer Goodman and Caroline Catherman, CDC Says Florida Surgeon General Draws Wrong Conclusion From COVID Data In His Vaccine Warning, South Florida SunSentinel, February 17, 2023, https://www.sun-sentinel.com/health/fl-ne-ladapo-covid-vaccine-warning-cdc-data-response-20230217-3zufwdbgrbc4fovew3yca2osji-story.html.

888.Dr. Katarina Lindley, Independent Pharmacovigilance Report Confirms Evidence for Recall of Covid-19 Vaccines, World Council For Health, July 11, 2022, https://worldcouncilforhealth.org/news/independent-pharmacovigilance-report-recall-of-covid-19-vaccines.

889.Dr. Katarina Lindley, July 11, 2022, supra.

890.Sam Ogozalek and Kirby Wilson, Florida surgeon general, again questioning COVID vaccines, sends letter to CDC, FDA, Tampa Bay Times, February 17, 2023, https://www.tampabay.com/news/health/2023/02/17/ladapo-surgeon-general-coronavirus-vaccines-mrna-vaers-safety/.

891.Sam Ogozalek and Kirby Wilson, Florida surgeon general, again questioning COVID vaccines, sends letter to CDC, FDA, Tampa Bay Times, February 17, 2023, https://www.tampabay.com/news/health/2023/02/17/ladapo-surgeon-general-coronavirus-vaccines-mrna-vaers-safety/.

892.Arek, Sarkissian, DeSantis calls for grand jury to investigate Covid-19 vaccines, Politico, December 12, 2022,
https://www.politico.com/news/2022/12/13/desantis-grand-jury-covid-19-vaccines-00073718.

893.Ron Desantis, Governor of Florida, Petition for Order to Impanel
A Statewide Grand Jury, In Re Statewide Grand Jury, Case No. SC22-_____, December 13, 2022,
https://www.flgov.com/wp-content/uploads/2022/12/Vaccine-Grand-Jury-Petition.pdf.

894.Sucharit Bhakdi MD,
https://www.chelseagreen.com/writer/sucharit-bhakdi-md/ (last visited on February 21, 2023).

895.COVID Shots to "Decimate World Population," Warns Dr. Bhakdi,
https://rumble.com/vfpgoh-dr.-bhakdi-interview.html (last visited on February 21, 2023).

896.Steve Kirsch, Survey shows over 500,000 killed by the COVID vaccines so far, May 13, 2022,
https://stevekirsch.substack.com/p/jackpot-over-500000-killed-by-the#%C2%A7the-bradford-hill-criteria.

897.MacIntyre, C.R., 2021. Using the Bradford-Hill criteria to assess causality in the association between CHADOX1 NCOV-19 vaccine and thrombotic immune thrombocytopenia. Global Biosecurity, 3(1), p.null.DOI: https://doi.org/10.31646/gbio.109.

898.Aarstad, J.; Kvitastein, O.A. Is there a Link between the 2021 COVID-19 Vaccination Uptake in Europe and 2022 Excess All-Cause Mortality?. Preprints 2023, 2023020350. https://doi.org/10.20944/preprints202302.0350.v1.

899.Aarstad, J.; Kvitastein, supra.

900.Mortality and life expectancy statistics, Eurostat, December 14, 2021, http://web.archive.org/web/20211214113409/https://ec.europa.eu/eurostat/statistics-explained/index.php?title=Mortality_and_life_expectancy_statistics#Number_of_deaths.

901.CDC coding error led to overcount of 72,000 Covid deaths, The Guardian, https://www.theguardian.com/world/2022/mar/24/cdc-coding-error-overcount-covid-deaths (last visited on March 28, 2023).

902.Deaths and Mortality, CDC, https://www.cdc.gov/nchs/fastats/deaths.htm (last visited on March 22, 2023).

903.OECD, https://stats.oecd.org/index.aspx?queryid=104676 (last visited on March 28, 2023).

904.Deaths and Mortality, CDC, https://www.cdc.gov/nchs/fastats/deaths.htm (last visited on March 22, 2023).

905.OECD, https://stats.oecd.org/index.aspx?queryid=104676 (last visited on March 28, 2023).

906.U.S. and World Population Clock, United States Census Bureau, https://www.census.gov/popclock/ (last visited on March 29, 2023).

907.OECD, https://stats.oecd.org/index.aspx?queryid=104676 (last visited on March 28, 2023).

908.U.S. and World Population Clock, United States Census Bureau, https://www.census.gov/popclock/ (last visited on March 29, 2023).

909.OECD, https://stats.oecd.org/index.aspx?queryid=104676 (last visited on March 28, 2023).

910.U.S. and World Population Clock, United States Census Bureau, https://www.census.gov/popclock/ (last visited on March 29, 2023).

911.The Expose calculated the U.S. excess death figure from the beginning of the COVID-19 vaccine rollout on 12/14/2020, until week 38 of 2022 to be 1,106,019. Secret CDC Report confirms over 1.1m Americans have 'Died Suddenly' since the COVID Vaccine Roll-Out; & further Government reports confirm the Vaccines are to blame, The Expose, April 23, 2023, https://expose-news.com/2023/04/23/over-6-million-americans-dead-covid-vaccine/?cmid=4ea57df8-d67e-458f-ad4f-8292f27ad868.

912.Government publishes shocking figures on COVID Vaccine Deaths: 1 in every 73 Vaccinated people died by June 2022 compared to just 1 in every 172 Not-Vaccinated People, The Expose, March 21, 2023, https://expose-news.com/2023/03/21/1-in-73-covid-va

ccinated-died-by-june-22/?cmid=91f62e17-7553-4a2c-95c0-f160c94a2e50.

913.The Expose, 1 in every 73, March 21, 2023, supra.

914.The Expose, 1 in every 73, March 21, 2023, supra.

915.Jawad, M., Hone, T., Vamos, E.P. et al. Estimating indirect mortality impacts of armed conflict in civilian populations: panel regression analyses of 193 countries, 1990–2017. BMC Med 18, 266 (2020). https://doi.org/10.1186/s12916-020-01708-5. Also available at https://bmcmedicine.biomedcentral.com/articles/10.1186/s12916-020-01708-5.

916.European Centre for Disease Prevention and Control, COVID-19 Vaccine Tracker, https://vaccinetracker.ecdc.europa.eu/public/extensions/COVID-19/vaccine-tracker.html#uptake-tab (last visited on March 22, 2023).

917.John Campbell, Vaccination v excess deaths, correlation study, March 21, 2023, https://www.youtube.com/watch?v=iyo2UNQcdpQ&t=3s.

918.Igor Chudov, PROVEN RELATIONSHIP: COVID Boosters and Excess Mortality in 2022, August 30, 2022, https://igorchudov.substack.com/p/proven-relationship-covid-boosters?utm_source=substack&utm_campaign=post_embed&utm_medium=email.

919.Igor Chudov, August 30, 2022, supra.

920.Excess Mortality in England, Office for Health Improvements and Disparities, https://app.powerbi.com/view?r=eyJrIjoiYmUwNmFhMjYtNGZhYS00NDk2LWFlMTAtOTg0OGNhNmFiNGM0IiwidCI6ImVlNGUxNDk5LTRhMzUtNGIyZS1hZDQ3LTVmM2NmOWRlODY2NiIsImMiOjh9 (last visited on March 30, 2023).

921.Igor Chudov, Is UK's Depopulation Caused by Covid Vaccines?, October 15, 2022, https://igorchudov.substack.com/p/is-uks-depopulation-caused-by-covid?utm_source=substack&utm_campaign=post_embed&utm_medium=web.

922.T. Coddington, UK Birth Data- the need to continue following up, October 11, 2022, https://inumero.substack.com/p/uk-birth-data-the-need-to-continue?utm_source=substack&utm_campaign=post_embed&utm_medium=web.

923.Igor Chudov, October 15, 2022, supra.

924.Secret Government Documents confirm COVID-19 Vaccine roll-out caused Excess Deaths in Australia to increase by 5,162%, The Expose, March 23, 2023, https://expose-news.com/2023/03/23/secret-government-documents-confirm-covid-19-vaccine-roll-out-caused-excess-deaths-in-australia-to-increase-by-5162/?cmid=006a759f-21c8-4d4f-837e-e76b83e849a1.

925.Secret Government Documents, The Expose, March 23, 2023, supra.

926.Denis Rancourt, There Was No Pandemic, July 2, 2023, https://denisrancourt.substack.com/p/there-was-no-pandemic.

927.Denis Rancourt, supra.

928.Denis Rancourt, supra.

929.Rancourt, D.G., Baudin, M., Hickey, J., Mercier, J. "COVID-19 vaccine-associated mortality in the Southern Hemisphere". CORRELATION Research in the Public Interest, Report, 17 September 2023. https://correlation-canada.org/covid-19-vaccine-associated-mortality-in-the-Southern-Hemisphere/.

930.Megan Redshaw, Researchers Find COVID Vaccines Causally Linked to Increased Mortality, Estimate 17 Million Deaths, Epoch Times, September 28, 2023, quoting Rancourt, D.G., supra.

931.Rancourt, supra.

932.Will Jones, Lancet Study on Covid Vaccine Autopsies Finds 74% Were Caused by Vaccine – Study is Removed Within 24 Hours, July 6, 2023, https://dailysceptic.org/2023/07/06/lancet-study-on-covid-vaccine-autopsies-finds-74-were-caused-by-vaccine-journal-removes-study-within-24-hours/.

933.Hulscher, Nicolas and Alexander, Paul E. and Amerling, Richard and Gessling, Heather and Hodkinson, Roger and Makis, William and Risch, Harvey A. and Trozzi, Mark and McCullough, Peter A., A Systematic Review of Autopsy Findings in Deaths after COVID-19 Vaccination. Available at SSRN: https://ssrn.com/abstract=4496137 or http://dx.doi.org/10.2139/ssrn.4496137.

934.Debra Heine, Dr. McCullough: COVID Vaccines Have Already Killed Up to 50,000 Americans, According to Whistleblowers, American Greatness,

June 15, 2021, https://amgreatness.com/2021/06/15/dr-mccullough-covid-vaccines-have-already-killed-up-to-50000-americans-according-to-whistleblowers/.

935.Classen JB. COVID-19 RNA Based Vaccines and the Risk of Prion Disease. Microbiol Infect Dis. 2021; 5(1): 1-3, ISSN 2639-9458, February 8, 2021, https://scivisionpub.com/pdfs/covid19-rna-based-vaccines-and-the-risk-of-prion-disease-1503.pdf.

936.Id.

937.Jean-Claude PerezEmergence of a New Creutzfeldt-Jakob Disease: 26 Cases of the Human Version of Mad-Cow Disease, Days After a COVID-19 Injection, January 2023, https://www.researchgate.net/publication/367167725_Emergence_of_a_New_Creutzfeldt-Jakob_Disease_26_Cases_of_the_Human_Version_of_Mad-Cow_Disease_Days_After_a_COVID-19_Injection.

938.Jeff Childers, Prion Shells, Coffee and COVID, DOI:10.5281/zenodo.7540331, January 31, 2023, https://www.coffeeandcovid.com/p/prion-shells-tuesday-january-31-2023?utm_source=post-email-title&publication_id=463409&post_id=100021796&isFreemail=true&utm_medium=email.

939.Classen JB. COVID-19 RNA Based Vaccines and the Risk of Prion Disease. Microbiol Infect Dis. 2021; 5(1): 1-3, ISSN 2639-9458, February 8, 2021, https://scivisionpub.com/pdfs/covid19-rna-based-vaccines-and-the-risk-of-prion-disease-1503.pdf.

940.COVID Shots Could Cause 'Crippling' Neurodegenerative Disease in Young People, MIT

Scientist Warns, The Defender, January 14, 2022, https://childrenshealthdefense.org/defender/mit-scientist-stephanie-seneff-neurodegenerative-disease-young-people-covid-shots/.

941.Id.

942.Id.

943.Id.

944.Rose & McCullough, A Report on Myocarditis Adverse Events in the U.S. Vaccine Adverse Events Reporting System (VAERS) in Association with COVID-19 Injectable Biological Products, October 1, 2021, https://www.ncbi.nlm.nih.gov/pmc/articles/PMC8483988/.

945.Lazarus, Ross, et al., Grant ID: R18 HS 017045, Final Report, Electronic Support for Public Health–Vaccine Adverse Event Reporting System (ESP:VAERS), at 6, 2/01/07 - 09/30/10, Submitted to: The Agency for Healthcare Research and Quality (AHRQ) U.S. Department of Health and Human Services, https://digital.ahrq.gov/sites/default/files/docs/publication/r18hs017045-lazarus-final-report-2011.pdf.

946.Jessica Rose and Peter A. McCullough, A Report on Myocarditis Adverse Events in the U.S. Vaccine Adverse Events Reporting System (VAERS) in Association with COVID-19 Injectable Biological Products, October 1, 2021, https://web.archive.org/web/20211002192421/https://www.ncbi.nlm.nih.gov/pmc/articles/PMC8483988/.

947.Rose & McCullough, A Report on Myocarditis Adverse Events in the U.S. Vaccine Adverse Events Reporting System (VAERS) in Association with COVID-19 Injectable Biological Products, October 1, 2021, https://www.ncbi.nlm.nih.gov/pmc/articles/PMC8483988/.

948.Stay Up to Date with COVID-19 Vaccines Including Boosters, CDC, October 4, 2022, https://www.cdc.gov/coronavirus/2019-ncov/vaccines/stay-up-to-date.html#children.

949.Oster ME, Shay DK, Su JR, et al. Myocarditis Cases Reported After mRNA-Based COVID-19 Vaccination in the US From December 2020 to August 2021. JAMA. 2022;327(4):331–340. doi:10.1001/jama.2021.24110.

950.Heart disease risk skyrockets 13,200% following covid injections, CDC admits, Natural News, June 21, 2023, https://www.naturalnews.com/2023-06-21-heart-disease-risk-13200-percent-covid-vaccination.html.

951.Joseph A. Ladapo, M.D., Ph.D., State Surgeon General, Guidance for mRNA COVID-19 Vaccines, October 7, 2022, https://floridahealthcovid19.gov/wp-content/uploads/2022/10/20221007-guidance-mrna-covid19-vaccines-doc.pdf.

952.Toby Rogers, Ten red flags in the FDA's risk-benefit analysis of Pfizer's EUA application to inject American children 5 to 11 with its mRNA product, October 25, 2021, https://tobyrogers.substack.com/p/ten-red-flags-in-the-f

das-risk-benefit.

953.Toby Rogers, October 25, 2021, supra.

954.Toby Rogers, October 25, 2021, supra.

955.Toby Rogers, October 25, 2021, supra.

956.Jessica Rose and Peter A. McCullough, A Report on Myocarditis Adverse Events in the U.S. Vaccine Adverse Events Reporting System (VAERS) in Association with COVID-19 Injectable Biological Products, October 1, 2021, https://web.archive.org/web/20211002192421/https://www.ncbi.nlm.nih.gov/pmc/articles/PMC8483988/.

957.Jessica Rose and Peter A. McCullough, supra.

958.Toby Rogers, October 25, 2021, supra.

959.Toby Rogers, October 25, 2021, supra.

960.Aaron Kheriaty, Twitter, November 15, 2021, https://twitter.com/akheriaty/status/1460135683561963520?lang=en.

961.Terrence Fraser, Myocarditis is often mild, contrary to online claims, AP, November 18, 2021, https://apnews.com/article/fact-checking-552859079506.

962.Edward Hendrie, The FDA and Pfizer Concealed Evidence That COVID-19 Vaccines Will Cause Myocarditis in Children, Great Mountain Publishing, November 7, 2021, https://greatmountainpublishing.com/2021/11/07/the-fda-and-pfizer-concealed-evidence-that-covid-19-vaccines-will-cause-myocarditis-in-children/.

963.Doctor Warns How COVID mRNA 'Vaccines' Will Cause Delayed Strokes & Heart Attacks — 'The Worst Is Yet To Come', Christians for Truth, July 14, 2021, https://christiansfortruth.com/doctor-warns-how-covid-mrna-vaccines-will-soon-cause-strokes-heart-attacks-the-worst-is-yet-to-come/.

964.FAQ on Sudden Death and Myocarditis, Myocarditis Foundation, https://www.myocarditisfoundation.org/research-and-grants/faqs/sudden-death-and-myocarditis/ (last visited on February 2, 2023).

965.Michael Kang, Viral Myocarditis, NIH, September 6, 2022, https://www.ncbi.nlm.nih.gov/books/NBK459259/.

966.Terrence Fraser, Myocarditis is often mild, contrary to online claims, AP, November 18, 2021, https://apnews.com/article/fact-checking-552859079506.

967.Terrence Fraser, November 18, 2021, supra.

968.Michael Kang, Viral Myocarditis, NIH, September 6, 2022, https://www.ncbi.nlm.nih.gov/books/NBK459259/.

969.Terrence Fraser, November 18, 2021, supra.

970.Michael Kang, September 2, 2022, supra.

971.Michael Kang, September 2, 2022, supra.

972.Covid: The Path not Taken - DarkHorse Podcast with Dr. Peter McCullough, December 6, 2021, https://www.youtube.com/watch?v=-zg1j7Zquoc&t=2

959s.

973.Tennis world shocked after scores of players drop out of Miami Open, Free West Media, April 2, 2022, https://freewestmedia.com/2022/04/02/tennis-world-shocked-after-scores-of-players-drop-out-of-miami-open/.

974.E.g., Riley Morgan, 'What's going on': Tennis world stunned after Miami Open carnage, Yahoo Sports, 30 March 2022, https://au.sports.yahoo.com/tennis-2022-viewers-shocked-bizarre-miami-open-carnage-004007552.html.

975.J.D. Ruccker, March Was Not a Good Month for "Vaccinated" Cyclists, March 31, 2022, https://endmedicaltyranny.substack.com/p/march-was-not-a-good-month-for-vaccinated.

976.J.D. Rucker, Buried Bombshell: Tennis World Rocked as FIFTEEN "Fully Vaccinated" Players Unable to Finish Miami Open, The Liberty Daily, April 2, 2022, https://thelibertydaily.com/buried-bombshell-tennis-world-rocked-as-fifteen-fully-vaccinated-players-unable-to-finish-miami-open/.

977.Jeff Childers, Prion Shells, Coffee and COVID, January 31, 2023, https://www.coffeeandcovid.com/p/prion-shells-tuesday-january-31-2023?utm_source=post-email-title&publication_id=463409&post_id=100021796&isFreemail=true&utm_medium=email.

978.Yumiko Urasaki and Yuko Nomura, 1.6m Moderna Doses Withdrawn in Japan over Contamination, Nikkei, August 26, 2021, https://asia.nikkei.com/Spotlight/Coronavirus/COVID-vaccines/1.6m-Moderna-doses-withdrawn-in-Japan-over-contamination.

979.Owen Shroyer, Yumiko Urasaki and Yuko Nomura, 1.6m Moderna Doses Withdrawn in Japan over Contamination, Nikkei, August 26, 2021, https://asia.nikkei.com/Spotlight/Coronavirus/COVID-vaccines/1.6m-Moderna-doses-withdrawn-in-Japan-over-contamination.

980.Jongdarm Yi, et. al., Graphene Oxide-Incorporated Hydrogels for Biomedical Applications, Polymer Jounal, 8 May 2020, https://www.nature.com/articles/s41428-020-0350-9.

981.Xubo Zhao, et al., Biocompatible Graphene Oxide Nanoparticle-Based Drug Delivery Platform for Tumor Microenvironment-Responsive Triggered Release of Doxorubicin, ACS Publications, August 10, 2014, https://pubs.acs.org/doi/abs/10.1021/la502952f.

982.Tyler Durden, Japan Suspects Contaminant In Moderna Vaccines Is Metallic, 'Reacts To Magnets', Zero Hedge, August 27, 2021, https://www.zerohedge.com/covid-19/japan-withdraws-16-million-moderna-doses-over-contaminant-reacts-magnets.
https://www.zerohedge.com/covid-19/japan-withdraws-16-million-moderna-doses-over-contaminant-reacts-magnets

983.Jongdarm Yi, et al., 8 May 2020, supra.

984.Stephanie Pappas, Rare Magnetism Found in the World's Strongest Material, Live Science, October 14, 2020, https://www.livescience.com/graphene-hides-rare-magnetism.html.

985.Angus Liu, An mRNA Vaccine Delivered in Hydrogel Shows Promise as a Durable Cancer Immunotherapy, Fierce Biotech, February 17, 2020, https://www.fiercebiotech.com/research/mrna-vaccine-delivered-hydrogel-shows-promise-as-a-durable-cancer-immunotherapy.

986.Yue Yin, et. al., *In Situ* Transforming RNA Nanovaccines from Polyethylenimine Functionalized Graphene Oxide Hydrogel for Durable Cancer Immunotherapy, ACS Publications, February 17, 2021, https://pubs.acs.org/doi/abs/10.1021/acs.nanolett.0c05039.

987.Angus Liu, February 17, 2021, supra.

988.Robert Young, Scanning & Transmission Electron Microscopy Reveals Graphene Oxide in CoV-19 Vaccines, August 20, 2021, https://www.drrobertyoung.com/post/transmission-electron-microscopy-reveals-graphene-oxide-in-cov-19-vaccines.

989.Edward Hendrie, Expert Reportedly Killed After He Publicly Revealed that Graphene Hydroxide is in COVID-19 Vaccines and Warned of Its Dangers, December 2, 2021, https://greatmountainpublishing.com/2021/12/02/expert-reportedly-killed-after-he-publicly-revealed-that-graphene-hydroxide-is-in-covid-19-vaccines-and-warned-of-its-dangers/.

990.Edward Hendrie, December 2, 2021, supra.

991.Doctor Warns How COVID mRNA ‘Vaccines’ Will Cause Delayed Strokes & Heart Attacks — ‘The Worst Is Yet To Come’, Christians For Truth, July 14, 2021, https://christiansfortruth.com/doctor-warns-how-covid-mrna-vaccines-will-soon-cause-strokes-heart-attacks-the-worst-is-yet-to-come/.

992.Id.

993.Id.

994.Richard Harris, Long-Term Studies Of COVID-19 Vaccines Hurt By Placebo Recipients Getting Immunized, NPR, February 19, 2021, https://www.npr.org/sections/health-shots/2021/02/19/969143015/long-term-studies-of-covid-19-vaccines-hurt-by-placebo-recipients-getting-immuni.

995.Richard Harris, February 19, 2021, supra.

996.Lance Johnson, Moderna and Pfizer Vaccine Trials RIGGED by Vaccinating the Control Group…Blatant Science FRAUD exposed, August 10, 2021, https://www.naturalnews.com/2021-08-10-moderna-and-pfizer-vaccine-trials-rigged-vaccinating-control-group.html.

997.Vaccines and Related Biological Products Advisory Committee Meeting, December 10, 2020, FDA Briefing Document Pfizer-BioNTech COVID-19 Vaccine, at 42, https://www.fda.gov/media/144245/download.

998.Vaccines and Related Biological Products Advisory Committee Meeting December 17, 2020,

FDA Briefing Document, Moderna COVID-19 Vaccine, at 10, https://www.fda.gov/media/144434/download. Vaccines and Related Biological Products Advisory Committee Meeting, December 10, 2020, FDA Briefing Document Pfizer-BioNTech COVID-19 Vaccine, at 10, https://www.fda.gov/media/144245/download.

999.The Pfizer Inoculations for COVID-19 More Harm Than Good, https://www.canadiancovidcarealliance.org/wp-content/uploads/2021/12/The-COVID-19-Inoculations-More-Harm-Than-Good-REV-Dec-16-2021.pdf (last visited on February 8, 2023).

1000.Pfizer-BioNTech COVID-19 Vaccine Frequently Asked Questions, FDA, August 23, 2021, https://web.archive.org/web/20210830124725/https://www.fda.gov/emergency-preparedness-and-response/coronavirus-disease-2019-covid-19/pfizer-biontech-covid-19-vaccine-frequently-asked-questions.

1001.Interim Public Health Recommendations for Fully Vaccinated People, CDC, March 8, 2021, https://web.archive.org/web/20210312000532/https://www.cdc.gov/coronavirus/2019-ncov/vaccines/fully-vaccinated-guidance.html.

1002.Interim Public Health Recommendations for Fully Vaccinated People, CDC, March 8, 2021, https://web.archive.org/web/20210312000532/https://www.cdc.gov/coronavirus/2019-ncov/vaccines/fully-vaccinated-guidance.html.

1003.FDA Takes Key Action in Fight Against COVID-19 By Issuing Emergency Use Authorization for First COVID-19 Vaccine, FDA, December 11, 2020, https://www.fda.gov/news-events/press-announcements/fda-takes-key-action-fight-against-covid-19-issuing-emergency-use-authorization-first-covid-19. See also Pfizer-BioNTech COVID-19 Vaccine Frequently Asked Questions, FDA, August 23, 2021, https://web.archive.org/web/20210830124725/https://www.fda.gov/emergency-preparedness-and-response/coronavirus-disease-2019-covid-19/pfizer-biontech-covid-19-vaccine-frequently-asked-questions.

1004.Edward Hendrie, CDC Says Vaccines Are Ineffective in Stopping Infection and Spread of COVID-19, March 13, 2021, https://greatmountainpublishing.com/2021/03/13/cdc-says-vaccines-are-ineffective-in-stopping-infection-and-spread-of-covid-19/.

1005.Interim Public Health Recommendations for Fully Vaccinated People, CDC, March 8, 2021, https://web.archive.org/web/20210312000532/https://www.cdc.gov/coronavirus/2019-ncov/vaccines/fully-vaccinated-guidance.html.

1006.Id.

1007.FDA Takes Key Action in Fight Against COVID-19 By Issuing Emergency Use Authorization for First COVID-19 Vaccine, FDA, December 11, 2020, https://www.fda.gov/news-events/press-announcements/fda-takes-key-action-fight-against-covid-19-issuing-emergency-use-authorization-first-covid-19. See also Pfizer-BioNTech COVID-19 Vaccine Frequently Asked Questions, FDA, August 23, 2021, https://web.archive.org/web/20210830124725/https://

www.fda.gov/emergency-preparedness-and-response/coronavirus-disease-2019-covid-19/pfizer-biontech-covid-19-vaccine-frequently-asked-questions.

1008.Interim Public Health Recommendations for Fully Vaccinated People, CDC, March 8, 2021, https://web.archive.org/web/20210312000532/https://www.cdc.gov/coronavirus/2019-ncov/vaccines/fully-vaccinated-guidance.html.

1009.Id.

1010.Id.

1011.Id.

1012.Id.

1013.Id.

1014.Statement from CDC Director Rochelle P. Walensky, MD, MPH on Today's MMWR, CDC, July 30, 2021, https://www.cdc.gov/media/releases/2021/s0730-mmwr-covid-19.html.

1015.Outbreak of SARS-CoV-2 Infections, Including COVID-19 Vaccine Breakthrough Infections, Associated with Large Public Gatherings — Barnstable County, Massachusetts, July 2021, Morbidity and Mortality Weekly Report, CDC, August 6, 2021, https://www.cdc.gov/mmwr/volumes/70/wr/mm7031e2.htm?s_cid=mm7031e2_w.

1016.Rochelle Walensky Statement, July 30, 2021, supra.

1017.Dr Birx admits they oversold vaccines- “I knew these vaccines were not going to prevent infection”, Natural News, August 1, 2022, https://www.naturalnews.com/2022-08-01-dr-birx-admits-they-oversold-vaccines.html#. See also https://100percentfedup.com/dr-birx-admits-they-oversold-vaccines-i-knew-these-vaccines-were-not-going-to-prevent-infection/, July 22, 2022.

1018.Meg Cunningham, Dr. Birx on her relationship with Trump: 'Respectful in public but very clear in private', December 16, 2020, https://abcnews.go.com/Politics/dr-birx-relationship-trump-respectful-public-clear-private/story?id=74760598.

1019.Meg Cunningham, Dr. Birx on her relationship with Trump: 'Respectful in public but very clear in private', December 16, 2020, https://abcnews.go.com/Politics/dr-birx-relationship-trump-respectful-public-clear-private/story?id=74760598.

1020.Lawrence Smith, Dr. Deborah Birx applauds Beshear's 'proactive' handling of the coronavirus, WDRB, December 15, 2020, https://www.wdrb.com/news/dr-deborah-birx-applauds-beshears-proactive-handling-of-the-coronavirus/article_72b4f436-3f18-11eb-ac9d-4be187f7f7a6.html.

1021.Immunity. (n.d.) Farlex Partner Medical Dictionary. (2012). Retrieved September 9, 2022, from https://medical-dictionary.thefreedictionary.com/immunity.

1022.Immunity, Merriam-Webster Dictionary, https://www.merriam-webster.com/dictionary/immunit

y (last visited on September 9, 2022).

1023.Immunity. (n.d.) McGraw-Hill Concise Dictionary of Modern Medicine. (2002). Retrieved September 9, 2022, from https://medical-dictionary.thefreedictionary.com/immunity.

1024.Immunity, Merriam-Webster Dictionary, https://www.merriam-webster.com/dictionary/immunity (last visited on September 9, 2022).

1025.Remarks by President Biden on the Importance of COVID-?19 Vaccine Requirements, Data Center, Clayco Construction Site Elk Grove Village, Illinois, October 7, 2021, https://www.whitehouse.gov/briefing-room/speeches-remarks/2021/10/07/remarks-by-president-biden-on-the-importance-of-covid-19-vaccine-requirements/.

1026.Special Committee on COVID-19 Pandemic, European Parliament, October 10, 2022, at 15:23:00, https://multimedia.europarl.europa.eu/en/webstreaming/special-committee-on-covid-19-pandemic_20221010-1430-COMMITTEE-COVI.

1027.Id.

1028. Joseph Choi, Fauci: Vaccinated people become ‘dead ends' for the coronavirus, The Hill, May 16, 2021, https://thehill.com/homenews/sunday-talk-shows/553773-fauci-vaccinated-people-become-dead-ends-for-the-coronavirus/.

1029.Mark Connors, Barney S. Graham, H. Clifford Lane, et al; SARS-CoV-2 Vaccines: Much

Accomplished, Much to Learn. Ann Intern Med.2021;174:687-690. [Epub 19 January 2021]. doi:10.7326. Article posted in May 2021 at: https://www.acpjournals.org/doi/full/10.7326/M21-0111.

1030.Joseph Choi, Pfizer chairman: We're not sure if someone can transmit virus after vaccination, The Hill, December 3, 2020, https://thehill.com/news-by-subject/healthcare/528619-pfizer-chairman-were-not-sure-if-someone-can-transmit-virus-after/.

1031.Pfizer Inc. Tweet, @Pfizer, January 13, 2020, https://twitter.com/pfizer/status/1349421959222853633?lang=en.

1032.Albert Bourla, @AlbertBourla, Twitter, June 8, 2021, from archive dated June 19, 2021, https://web.archive.org/web/20210619045416/https://twitter.com/AlbertBourla.

1033.Dr. John Campbell, Simple questions for Pfizer, YouTube, August 5, 2023, https://www.youtube.com/watch?v=hN4o3lJR0yM&t=125s.

1034.Sally Fallon Morell, Dr. Thomas Cowan, and Dr. Andrew
Kaufman, Statement on Virus Isolation (SOVI). "SARS-CoV-2 Has Never Been Isolated or Purified", Global Research, May 17, 2022.

1035.Peter Andrews, *Landmark Legal Ruling Finds That Covid Tests Are Not Fit for Purpose. So What Do the MSM Do? They Ignore It*, RT, 27 November 2020, https://www.rt.com/op-ed/507937-covid-pcr-test-fail/.

1036.A Comparison of Official Government Reports Suggests the Fully Vaccinated Are Suffering Antibody Dependent Enhancement, The Expose, January 23, 2022, https://dailyexpose.uk/2022/01/23/world-government-data-shows-covid-vaccinated-suffering-ade/.

1037.Edward Hendrie, The COVID-19 Gambit, Edward Hendrie's Newsletter, October 16, 2022, https://hendrie.substack.com/p/the-covid-19-gambit.

1038.Vaccines and Related Biological Products Advisory Committee - 10/22/2020, U.S. Food and Drug Administration, at 2:33:40, https://www.youtube.com/watch?v=1XTiL9rUpkg&t=9220s.

1039.Id.

1040.Denise M. Hinton, Chief Scientist, FDA, Letter to Pfizer Inc., Attention: Ms. Elisa Harkins, August 23, 2021, https://www.fda.gov/media/150386/download.

1041.FDA Approves First COVID-19 Vaccine, FDA, August 23, 2021, https://www.fda.gov/news-events/press-announcements/fda-approves-first-covid-19-vaccine.

1042.Anjalee Khemlani, Fauci: Early COVID-19 Vaccines Will Only Prevent Symptoms, Not Block the Virus, Yahoo Finance, October 20, 2020, https://www.yahoo.com/now/fauci-vaccines-will-only-prevent-symptoms-not-block-the-virus-195051568.html.

1043.Vaccines and Related Biological Products Advisory Committee - 10/22/2020, U.S. Food and

Drug Administration, at 2:33:40, https://www.youtube.com/watch?v=1XTiL9rUpkg&t=9220s.

1044.AXIOS on HBO: Moderna Chief Medical Officer Tal Zaks (Clip) | HBO, November 23, 2020, https://www.youtube.com/watch?v=po7qt9BZz0s&t=65s.

1045.Vaccines and Related Biological Products Advisory Committee Meeting December 17, 2020, FDA Briefing Document, Moderna COVID-19 Vaccine, https://www.fda.gov/media/144434/download.

1046.Fact Sheet for Healthcare Providers Administering Vaccine (Vaccination Providers) Emergency Use Authorization (Eua) of the Pfizer-biontech COVID-19 Vaccine to Prevent Coronavirus, Disease 2019 (Covid-19), 12 August 2021, https://www.fda.gov/media/144413/download.

1047.Id.

1048.Id.

1049.Frequently Asked Questions about COVID-19 Vaccination, FDA, updated November 23, 2021, archive page from December 1, 2021, https://web.archive.org/web/20211201021445/https://www.cdc.gov/coronavirus/2019-ncov/vaccines/faq.html.

1050.Id.

1051.Frequently Asked Questions about COVID-19 Vaccination, FDA, updated April 19, 2023, https://www.cdc.gov/coronavirus/2019-ncov/vaccines/f

aq.html.

1052.Benefits of Getting A COVID-19 Vaccine, CDC, Updated December 22, 2022, https://www.cdc.gov/coronavirus/2019-ncov/vaccines/vaccine-benefits.html.

1053.Andrew Court, Democrat Congressman Stephen Lynch, 65, Tests Positive to COVID-19 after Receiving Both Doses of Pfizer's Vaccine, The Daily Mail, January 30, 2021, https://www.dailymail.co.uk/news/article-9205321/Rep-Stephen-Lynch-65-tests-positive-COVID-19-receiving-doses-Pfizer-vaccine.html?ito=push-notification&ci=73039&si=23070647.

1054.Andrew Court, Democrat Congressman Stephen Lynch, 65, Tests Positive to COVID-19 after Receiving Both Doses of Pfizer's Vaccine, The Daily Mail, January 30, 2021, https://www.dailymail.co.uk/news/article-9205321/Rep-Stephen-Lynch-65-tests-positive-COVID-19-receiving-doses-Pfizer-vaccine.html?ito=push-notification&ci=73039&si=23070647.

1055.Pfizer-BioNTech COVID-19 Vaccine Frequently Asked Questions, FDA, https://www.fda.gov/emergency-preparedness-and-response/mcm-legal-regulatory-and-policy-framework/pfizer-biontech-covid-19-vaccine-frequently-asked-questions (last visited on August 20, 2021).

1056.Id.

1057.60% of People Being Admitted to UK Hospitals Are Unvaccinated - Adviser, Reuters, July 19, 2021, https://www.reuters.com/business/healthcare-pharmace

uticals/60-people-being-admitted-uk-hospitals-had-two-covid-jabs-adviser-2021-07-19/.

1058.Pfizer-BioNTech COVID-19 Vaccine Frequently Asked Questions, FDA, https://www.fda.gov/emergency-preparedness-and-response/mcm-legal-regulatory-and-policy-framework/pfizer-biontech-covid-19-vaccine-frequently-asked-questions (last visited on August 20, 2021). See also Pfizer-BioNTech COVID-19 Vaccine Frequently Asked Questions, FDA, August 23, 2021, https://web.archive.org/web/20210830124725/https://www.fda.gov/emergency-preparedness-and-response/coronavirus-disease-2019-covid-19/pfizer-biontech-covid-19-vaccine-frequently-asked-questions.

1059.Interim Public Health Recommendations for Fully Vaccinated People, CDC, August 19, 2021, https://www.cdc.gov/coronavirus/2019-ncov/vaccines/fully-vaccinated-guidance.html.

1060.Pien Huang, et al., COVID Booster Shots Are Coming. Here's What You Need To Know, NPR, August 19, 2021, https://www.npr.org/sections/health-shots/2021/08/19/1028594715/covid-booster-shots-are-coming-heres-what-you-need-to-know.

1061.Emily Kopp, CDC report shows vaccinated people can spread COVID-19, Roll Call, July 30, 2021, https://www.rollcall.com/2021/07/30/cdc-report-shows-vaccinated-people-can-spread-covid-19/.

1062.SARS-CoV-2 Variants of Concern and Variants under Investigation in England, Technical Briefing, Public Health England, 18 June 2021, 16https://assets.publishing.service.gov.uk/government/

uploads/system/uploads/attachment_data/file/1001359/Variants_of_Concern_VOC_Technical_Briefing_16.pdf.

1063.Id. at 12.

1064.Suzanne Humphries, Dissolving Illusions, at 74 (2013).

1065.Interim Clinical Considerations for Use of COVID-19 Vaccines Currently Approved or Authorized in the United States, CDC, Last Reviewed by the CDC on March 17, 2023, https://www.cdc.gov/vaccines/covid-19/clinical-considerations/interim-considerations-us.html.

1066.Helen Millar, COVID-19 vaccine: Does it stop people getting the virus?, Medical News Today, October 27, 2022, https://www.medicalnewstoday.com/articles/mucus-in-chest-that-wont-come-up-covid#is-a-productive-cough-common.

1067.Helen Millar, October 27, 2022, supra.

1068.Ensuring COVID-19 Vaccine Safety in the US, CDC, Updated Dec. 22, 2022, https://www.cdc.gov/coronavirus/2019-ncov/vaccines/safety.html#print.

1069.Dr. John Campbell, Staff increased 20 fold, March 28, 2023, https://www.youtube.com/watch?v=kELiEGA3q4I.

1070.Dr. John Campbell, March 28, 2023, supra.

1071.Dr. John Campbell, March 28, 2023, supra.

1072.Dr. John Campbell, March 28, 2023, supra.

1073.Dr. John Campbell, March 28, 2023, supra.

1074.Gabor David Kelen, M.D., Lisa Maragakis, M.D., M.P.H., COVID-19 Vaccine: What You Need to Know, Johns Hopkins, March 30, 2021, archived version of article, https://web.archive.org/web/20210330002308/https://www.hopkinsmedicine.org/health/conditions-and-diseases/coronavirus/covid-19-vaccine-what-you-need-to-know.

1075.Id.

1076.UK Government quietly confirms Triple+ Vaccinated accounted for 92% of COVID Deaths in 2022, The Expose, March 26, 2023, https://expose-news.com/2023/03/26/uk-gov-confirms-vaccinated-accounted-for-92-percent-of-covid-deaths-in-2022/.

1077.Gabor David Kelen, M.D., Lisa Maragakis, M.D., M.P.H., COVID-19 Vaccine: What You Need to Know, Johns Hopkins, Updated on November 1, 2022, https://www.hopkinsmedicine.org/health/conditions-and-diseases/coronavirus/covid-19-vaccine-what-you-need-to-know#:~:text=Yes%2C%20evidence%20continues%20to%20indicate,had%20COVID%2D19%20or%20not.

1078.E.g., Richard Gray, This is how new Covid-19 variants are changing the pandemic, BBC, 27 January 2021, https://www.bbc.com/future/article/20210127-covid-19-variants-how-mutations-are-changing-the-pandemic.

1079.E.g., CDC Admits They Have No Records of Any Person with Recovered Immunity Every Trasnmitting The COVID-19 Virus, The Last Refuge, November 11, 2021, https://theconservativetreehouse.com/blog/2021/11/11/cdc-admits-they-have-no-records-of-any-person-with-recovered-immunity-ever-transmitting-the-covid-19-virus/, quoting November 5, 2021 Letter to Elizabeth Brenm from Roger Andoh, CDC/ATSDR FOIA Officer. See also Aaron Siri, CDC Admits Crushing Rights of Naturally Immune Without Proof They Transmit the Virus, November 11, 2021, https://aaronsiri.substack.com/p/cdc-admits-crushing-rights-of-naturally.

1080.The World's Best Hospitals 2023, Newsweek, 2023, https://www.newsweek.com/rankings/worlds-best-hospitals-2023.

1081.Gabor David Kelen, M.D., Lisa Maragakis, M.D., M.P.H., COVID-19 Vaccine: What You Need to Know, Johns Hopkins, Updated on November 1, 2022, https://www.hopkinsmedicine.org/health/conditions-and-diseases/coronavirus/covid-19-vaccine-what-you-need-to-know#:~:text=Yes%2C%20evidence%20continues%20to%20indicate,had%20COVID%2D19%20or%20not.

1082.Andrew Pekosz, What You Need to Know About COVID-19 Variants, https://publichealth.jhu.edu/2021/what-you-need-to-know-about-covid-19-variants (last visited on May 5, 2023).

1083.Frequently Asked Questions about COVID-19 Vaccination, CDC, updated March 30, 2022, archived page from April 1, 2022, https://web.archive.org/web/20220401064853/https://www.cdc.gov/coronavirus/2019-ncov/vaccines/faq.html.

1084.Letter from Peter Marks, MD, PhD, Director, FDA Center for Biologics Evaluation and Research to Linda Wastila, Coalition Advocating for Adequately Labeled Medicines (CAALM), April 18, 2023, https://www.regulations.gov/document/FDA-2023-P-0360-019.

1085.Ensuring COVID-19 Vaccine Safety in the US, CDC, Updated Dec. 22, 2022, https://www.cdc.gov/coronavirus/2019-ncov/vaccines/safety.html#print.

1086. Joseph Choi, Fauci: Vaccinated people become 'dead ends' for the coronavirus, The Hill, May 16, 2021, https://thehill.com/homenews/sunday-talk-shows/553773-fauci-vaccinated-people-become-dead-ends-for-the-coronavirus/.

1087.CDC: 'Vaccinated People Do Not Carry the Virus', Totality of Evidence, https://totalityofevidence.com/timeline/cdc-vaccinated-people-do-not-carry-the-virus/ (last visited on May 5, 2023).

1088.Id.

1089.Id.

1090.Susan Wollersheim, MD and Ann Schwartz, MD, STN:125742, BLA Clinical Review Memorandum, FDA, August 23, 2021, https://www.fda.gov/media/152256/download#page=95. See also Linda Wastila, BSPharm, MSPH, PhD, Citizen Petition, Coalition Advocating for Adequately Labeled Medicines (CAALM), January 31, 2023, https://totalityofevidence.com/wp-content/uploads/2023/04/caalm-citizen-petition-to-fda.pdf.

1091.Letter from Peter Marks, MD, PhD, Director, FDA Center for Biologics Evaluation and Research to Linda Wastila, Coalition Advocating for Adequately Labeled Medicines (CAALM), April 18, 2023, https://www.regulations.gov/document/FDA-2023-P-0360-019.

1092.Vaccines and Related Biological Products Advisory Committee October 26, 2021 Meeting Document, BNT162B2 [COMIRNATY (COVID-19 Vaccine, MRNA)] Vaccines and Related Biological Products Advisory Committee Briefing Document, https://www.fda.gov/media/153409/download#page=16.

1093.Special Committee on COVID-19 Pandemic, European Parliament, October 10, 2022, at 15:23:00, https://multimedia.europarl.europa.eu/en/webstreaming/special-committee-on-covid-19-pandemic_20221010-1430-COMMITTEE-COVI.

1094.Letter from Peter Marks, April 18, 2023, supra.

1095.Your vaccination questions answered, Moderna, archived page from January 7, 2023, http://web.archive.org/web/20230107040800/https://www.makeityourvaccine.com/faqs.

1096.Denise M. Hinton, Chief Scientist, FDA, Letter to Pfizer Inc., Attention: Ms. Elisa Harkins, August 23,

2021, https://www.fda.gov/media/150386/download.

1097.Id.

1098.Id.

1099.Comirnaty and Pfizer-BioNTech COVID-19 Vaccine, August 23, 2021, https://www.fda.gov/coronavirus-disease-2019-covid-19/comirnaty-and-pfizer-biontech-covid-19-vaccine.

1100.Understanding Investigational Drugs. FDA, https://www.fda.gov/patients/learn-about-expanded-access-and-other-treatment-options/understanding-investigational-drugs#:~:text=An%20investigational%20drug%20can%20also,drug%20is%20safe%20and%20effective. (last visited on November 19, 2022).

1101.Investigational vaccine, https://www.cdc.gov/vaccines/terms/glossary.html (last visited on July 31, 2021).

1102.Investigational Product, NIH, March 14, 2013, https://www.niaid.nih.gov/research/dmid-investigational-product.

1103.FDA Approves First COVID-19 Vaccine, FDA, August 23, 2021, https://www.fda.gov/news-events/press-announcements/fda-approves-first-covid-19-vaccine.

1104.Id.

1105.COVID-19 Vaccine Explainer, 18 January 2021, https://www.who.int/publications/m/item/comirnaty-covid-19-mrna vaccine. See also Comirnaty, Summary of Product Characteristics, https://www.ema.europa.eu/en/documents/product-info

rmation/comirnaty-epar-product-information_en.pdf.

1106.Denise M. Hinton, Chief Scientist, FDA, Letter to Pfizer Inc., Attention: Ms. Elisa Harkins, August 23, 2021, https://www.fda.gov/media/150386/download.

1107.21 U.S.C. § 360bbb–3(c)(3).

1108.Pfizer-BioNTech COVID-19 Vaccine Comirnaty® Receives Full U.S. FDA Approval for Individuals 16 Years and Older, Pfizer Press Release, August 23, 2021, https://www.pfizer.com/news/press-release/press-release-detail/pfizer-biontech-covid-19-vaccine-comirnatyr-receives-full.

1109.Remarks by President Biden on Fighting the COVID-?19 Pandemic, September 9, 2021, https://www.whitehouse.gov/briefing-room/speeches-remarks/2021/09/09/remarks-by-president-biden-on-fighting-the-covid-19-pandemic-3/.

1110.Kayal Rivas, FDA Grants Pfizer-BioNTech COVID-19 Vaccine Full Approval, Fox Business, https://www.foxbusiness.com/healthcare/fda-grants-pfizer-covid-19-vaccine-full-approval

1111.Lauran Neergaard and Matthew Perrone, US Regulators Give Full Approval to Pfizer COVID-19 Vaccine, Associated Press, August 23, 2021, https://apnews.com/article/coronavirus-vaccine-pfizer-approval-1361ff61d06b815652a08a7cc0683a72.

1112.Zachary Stieber, Few, If Any, Doses of Spikevax or Comirnaty Available in United States, Despite FDA Approvals, The Epoch Times, February 2, 2022, https://archive.ph/Ry0Xh. See also SpikeVax

COVID-19 Vaccine (Moderna), Updated May 28, 2022, https://www.precisionvaccinations.com/vaccines/spikevax-covid-19-vaccine-moderna. “As of July 11, 2022, Moderna's SpikeVax was **available** in Poland, Czech Republic, Caribbean, Denmark, Romania, Hungary, Bulgaria, Slovenia, Slovakia, Croatia, Estonia, Latvia, Lithuania, Serbia, Ukraine, Moldova, Albania, Bosnia-Herzegovina, Kosovo, North Macedonia, Montenegro, Israel, France, the African Union, Australian, Spain, Switzerland, South Korea, the United Kingdom, Switzerland, and was **Approved in the U.S.**” Id.

1113.Vaccine Information Fact Sheet for Recipients and Caregivers About the Pfizer-biontech Covid-19 Vaccine to Prevent Coronavirus Disease 2019 (Covid-19) for Use in Individuals 5 Through 11 Years of Age, October 29, 2021, https://www.fda.gov/media/153717/download.

1114.Id.

1115.Spike Protein Is Very Dangerous, It's Cytotoxic (Robert Malone, Steve Kirsch, Bret Weinstein), June 13, 2021, https://www.youtube.com/watch?v=Du2wm5nhTXY.

1116.Denise M. Hinton, Chief Scientist, FDA, Letter to Pfizer Inc., Attention: Ms. Elisa Harkins, August 23, 2021, https://www.fda.gov/media/150386/download.

1117.Countermeasures Injury Compensation Program, Request for Benefits Form Instructions, OMB Control No. 0915-0334, Expiration Date: 3/31/2023, https://www.hrsa.gov/sites/default/files/hrsa/cicp/cicp-request-form-instructions.pdf.

1118.42 U.S. C. § 300aa–16.

1119.McKenzie Sigalos, You Can't Sue Pfizer or Moderna If You Have Severe Covid Vaccine Side Effects. The Government Likely Won't Compensate You for Damages Either, CNBC, December 17, 2020, https://www.cnbc.com/2020/12/16/covid-vaccine-side-effects-compensation-lawsuit.html.

1120.McKenzie Sigalos, December 17, 2020, supra.

1121.Megan Redshaw, Injured by a COVID Vaccine? Want Financial Compensation? Too Bad, Says Injury Compensation Law Firm, The Defender, July 1, 2021, https://childrenshealthdefense.org/defender/covid-vaccine-injury-no-compensation-program/.

1122.Megan Redshaw, July 1, 2021, supra.

1123.Vaccine Injury Fund: Lessons From a Vaccine Lawyer-"Covered" Vaccines in the Court (and the DtaP), Widman Law Firm, https://www.widmanlawfirm.com/vaccine-injury-fund-lessons-from-a-vaccine-lawyer-covered-vaccin.html (last visited on August 28, 2021).

1124.HRSA, Covered Vaccines, COVID-19 Claims, https://www.hrsa.gov/vaccine-compensation/covered-vaccines/index.html (last visited on August 28, 2021).

1125.VAERS COVID Vaccine Data, August 13, 2021, https://www.openvaers.com/covid-data.

1126.FDA Approves First COVID-19 Vaccine, FDA, August 23, 2021, https://www.fda.gov/news-events/press-announcements/fda-approves-first-covid-19-vaccine.

1127.COVID Vaccine Reported Mortality Breakdowns, August 13, 2021, https://www.openvaers.com/covid-data/mortality.

1128.Lazarus, Ross, et al., Grant ID: R18 HS 017045, Final Report, Electronic Support for Public Health–Vaccine Adverse Event Reporting System (ESP:VAERS), at 6, 2/01/07 - 09/30/10, Submitted to: The Agency for Healthcare Research and Quality (AHRQ) U.S. Department of Health and Human Services, https://digital.ahrq.gov/sites/default/files/docs/publication/r18hs017045-lazarus-final-report-2011.pdf.

1129.Report an Adverse Event to VAERS, HHS, https://vaers.hhs.gov/reportevent.html (last visited on September 12, 2021).

1130.Id.

1131.VACCINE INFORMATION FACT SHEET FOR RECIPIENTS AND CAREGIVERS, June 17, 2022, https://eua.modernatx.com/covid19vaccine-eua/eua-fact-sheet-recipients.pdf?tc=ps_stqbut0&cc=4003&utm_source=google&utm_medium=search&utm_campaign=unb+eua&gclsrc=aw.ds&&gclid=CjwKCAiArNOeBhAHEiwAze_nKGKcF1Z00sKmtvjxZkMQJeZpY7fVCqINBfGT6EvlchVv_0T9iVYG5BoCkTkQAvD_BwE.

1132.Overview of COVID-19 Vaccines, CDC, https://www.cdc.gov/coronavirus/2019-ncov/vaccines/different-vaccines/overview-COVID-19-vaccines.html?s_cid=11758:moderna%20shots:sem.ga:p:RG:GM:gen:PTN:FY22 (last visited on January 28, 2023).

1133.Zachary Stieber, Few, If Any, Doses of Spikevax or Comirnaty Available in United States, Despite FDA Approvals, The Epoch Times, February 2, 2022, https://archive.ph/Ry0Xh. See also SpikeVax COVID-19 Vaccine (Moderna), Updated May 28, 2022, https://www.precisionvaccinations.com/vaccines/spikevax-covid-19-vaccine-moderna. "As of July 11, 2022, Moderna's SpikeVax was **available** in Poland, Czech Republic, Caribbean, Denmark, Romania, Hungary, Bulgaria, Slovenia, Slovakia, Croatia, Estonia, Latvia, Lithuania, Serbia, Ukraine, Moldova, Albania, Bosnia-Herzegovina, Kosovo, North Macedonia, Montenegro, Israel, France, the African Union, Australian, Spain, Switzerland, South Korea, the United Kingdom, Switzerland, and was **Approved in the U.S.**" Id.

1134.COVID-19: Vaccinator Guidance for Moderna (Spikevax) Vaccine, Wisconsin Department of Health Services, https://www.dhs.wisconsin.gov/covid-19/vaccinator-moderna.htm (last visited on January 28, 2023).

1135.CDC Recommends the First Updated COVID-19 Booster, CDC, September 1, 2022, https://www.cdc.gov/media/releases/2022/s0901-covid-19-booster.html.

1136.Booster Doses of Moderna COVID-19 Vaccines in Adults, Adolescents & Children, September 1. 2022, https://www.cdc.gov/vaccines/acip/meetings/downloads/slides-2022-09-01/06-COVID-Miller-508.pdf.

1137.Kena Swanson, Pfizer/BioNTech COVID-19 Omicron-Modified Vaccine Options, Vaccines and Related Biological Products Advisory Committee, June

28, 2022,
https://www.fda.gov/media/159496/download.

1138.Kena Swanson, June 28, 2022, supra.

1139.Igor Chudov, Bivalent Booster's "8-Mice Trial" Actually FAILED, August 31, 2022, https://igorchudov.substack.com/p/ba5-boosters-8-mice-trial-actually?utm_source=substack&utm_campaign=post_embed&utm_medium=web.

1140.COVID-19 Vaccine & Booster Information from Inova, https://www.inova.org/COVID19/vaccine-scheduling#accordion-149336 (last visited on November 11, 2022).

1141.Should People Who Have Recovered from COVID Take a Vaccine?, The Vaccine Reaction, July 12, 2021, https://thevaccinereaction.org/2021/07/should-people-who-have-recovered-from-covid-take-a-vaccine/#_edn24.

1142.Nabin K. Shrestha, et al., Necessity of COVID-19 vaccination in previously infected individuals, June 5, 2020, https://www.medrxiv.org/content/10.1101/2021.06.01.21258176v2.

1143.Nabin K. Shrestha, et al., June 5, 2020, supra.

1144.Lasting immunity found after recovery from COVID-19, January 26, 2021, https://www.nih.gov/news-events/nih-research-matters/lasting-immunity-found-after-recovery-covid-19.

1145.Dr. Scot Youngblood at San Diego City Council Meeting, September 20, 2022, https://www.bitchute.com/video/H3onzCie2198/.

1146.Id.

1147.Baruch Fischoff, et al., (editors), FDA, 2011, Communicating Risks and Benefits: An Evidence-Based User's Guide, https://www.fda.gov/media/81597/download.

1148.Toby Rogers, Pfizer COVID Vaccine Fails Risk-Benefit Analysis in Children 5 to 11, The Defender, November 5, 2021, https://childrenshealthdefense.org/defender/fda-pfizer-covid-vaccine-risk-benefit-analysis-nntv-children/.

1149.Toby Rogers, November 5, 2021, supra.

1150.Toby Rogers, November 5, 2021, supra.

1151.Edward Dowd, "Cause Unknown," The Epidemic of Sudden Deaths in 2021 and 2022, at 33 (2022).

1152.Edward Dowd, "Cause Unknown," The Epidemic of Sudden Deaths in 2021 and 2022, at 33 (2022).

1153.E.g., Kevin Airs, Shattered wife relives the horrific moment her fit husband, 35, dropped dead in front of her from a condition linked to Sudden Adult Death Syndrome - and shares the ONE test that could have saved him, Daily Mail, June 18, 2022, https://www.dailymail.co.uk/news/article-10918281/SADS-Sudden-Adult-Death-Syndrome-Moment-young-mums-husband-dropped-dead-her.html.

1154.Ethan Huff, Sudden Adult Death Syndrome is the new name for vaccine deaths in the medical establishment's play-pretend reality, Natural News, June 10, 2022, https://www.naturalnews.com/2022-06-10-sads-new-name-vaccine-deaths-medical-establishment.html.

1155.Ethan Huff, June 10, 2022, supra.

1156.Ethan Huff, June 10, 2022, Supra.

1157.Vaccines and Related Biological Products Advisory Committee Meeting, FDA Briefing Document, Moderna COVID-19 Vaccine,December 17, 2020, https://www.fda.gov/media/144434/download.

1158.Id.

1159.Ronald Brown, Outcome Reporting Bias in COVID-19 mRNA Vaccine Clinical Trials, 26 February 2021, https://www.mdpi.com/1648-9144/57/3/199/htm.

1160.Dr. Ron Brown Discusses Outcome Reporting Bias in COVID-19 mRNA Clinical Trials | Interview, TrialSite News, April 10, 2021, https://www.youtube.com/watch?v=Jkwn5I8tLmE.

1161.Ronald Brown, February 2021, supra.

1162.Presenting Quantitative Efficacy and Risk Information in Direct-to-Consumer Promotional Labeling and Advertisements Guidance for Industry DRAFT GUIDANCE, FDA, Center for Biologics Evaluation and Research (CBER), October 2018, https://www.fda.gov/media/117573/download.

1163.Id..

1164.Ronald Brown, February 2021, supra.

1165.Butterfly of the Week, 22 February '21: Now You See Me, Now You Don't, David Martin World, February 23, 2021, https://www.youtube.com/watch?v=qtPy7Qrd1mg&t=1389s.

1166.Vaccines and Related Biological Products Advisory Committee Meeting December 17, 2020, FDA Briefing Document, Moderna COVID-19 Vaccine, https://www.fda.gov/media/144434/download.

1167.Id. at 13.

1168.Id. at 13.

1169.Lindsey R. Baden, et al., Efficacy and Safety of the mRNA-1273 SARS-CoV-2 Vaccine, N Engl J Med 2021; 384:403-416, DOI: 10.1056/NEJMoa2035389, February 4, 2021, https://www.nejm.org/doi/full/10.1056/NEJMoa2035389.

1170.Peter Doshi, Pfizer and Moderna's "95% Effective" Vaccines—we Need More Details and the Raw Data, BMJ, January 4, 2021, https://blogs.bmj.com/bmj/2021/01/04/peter-doshi-pfizer-and-modernas-95-effective-vaccines-we-need-more-details-and-the-raw-data/.

1171.Peter Doshi, BMJ, January 4, 2021, supra.

1172.Peter Doshi, BMJ, January 4, 2021, supra.

1173.Vaccines and Related Biological Products Advisory Committee Meeting, December 10, 2020, FDA Briefing Document Pfizer-BioNTech COVID-19 Vaccine, at 42, https://www.fda.gov/media/144245/download.

1174.Id.

1175.80% of the Nuns in this Kentucky Convent Got COVID 2 Days after Vaccine, Life Site News, February 25, 2021, https://www.lifesitenews.com/news/several-nuns-die-after-taking-first-shot-of-covid-vaccine/.

1176.The Pfizer Inoculations for COVID-19 More Harm Than Good, https://www.canadiancovidcarealliance.org/wp-content/uploads/2021/12/The-COVID-19-Inoculations-More-Harm-Than-Good-REV-Dec-16-2021.pdf (last visited on February 8, 2023).

1177.Id.

1178.Id.

1179.What Really Happened Inside the COVID-19 Vaccine Trials?, A Midwestern Doctor, March 13, 2023, https://amidwesterndoctor.substack.com/p/what-really-happened-inside-the-covid?utm_source=substack&utm_medium=email.

1180.A Midwestern Doctor, March 13, 2023, supra.

1181.A Midwestern Doctor, March 13, 2023, supra.

1182.Megan Redshaw, U.S. Sen. Johnson Holds News Conference With Families Injured by COVID Vaccines, Ignored by Medical Community, The Defender, June 29, 2021, https://childrenshealthdefense.org/defender/sen-johnson-ken-ruettgers-press-conference-families-injured-covi d-vaccines/.

1183.The Pfizer Inoculations for COVID-19 More Harm Than Good, https://www.canadiancovidcarealliance.org/wp-content/uploads/2021/12/The-COVID-19-Inoculations-More-Harm-Than-Good-REV-Dec-16-2021.pdf (last visited on February 8, 2023).

1184.Megan Redshaw, June 29, 2021, supra.

1185.Comment from de Garay, Stephanie
Posted by the Food and Drug Administration on Nov 6, 2021,
https://www.regulations.gov/comment/FDA-2021-N-1088-12 9763.

1186.The Pfizer Inoculations for COVID-19 More Harm Than Good, https://www.canadiancovidcarealliance.org/wp-content/uploads/2021/12/The-COVID-19-Inoculations-More-Harm-Than-Good-REV-Dec-16-2021.pdf (last visited on February 8, 2023).

1187.Jared Hopkins, Pfizer, BioNTech Get $1.95 Billion Covid-19 Vaccine Order From U.S. Government, The Wall Street Jounal, July 22, 2020, https://www.wsj.com/articles/pfizer-biontech-get-1-95-billion-covid-19-vaccine-order-from-u-s-government-11595418221?mod=searchresults&page=1&pos=2.

1188.Jared Hopkins, WSJ, July 22, 2020, supra.

1189.Jared Hopkins, WSJ, July 22, 2020, supra.

1190.Jared Hopkins, WSJ, July 22, 2020, supra.

1191.Jared Hopkins, WSJ, July 22, 2020, supra.

1192.Jared Hopkins, WSJ, July 22, 2020, supra.

1193.Jared Hopkins, WSJ, July 22, 2020, supra.

1194.Katie Adams, Pfizer's COVID-19 vaccine becomes highest-selling pharmaceutical in history, Becker's Hospital Review, February 9, 2022, https://www.beckershospitalreview.com/pharmacy/pfizer-s-covid-19-vaccine-becomes-highest-selling-pharmaceutical-in-history.html#:~:text=Pfizer%20on%20Feb., %2429%20billion%20in%20international%20sales.

1195.Matt Grossman, Johnson & Johnson to Begin Human Trials of Covid-19 Vaccine by September, The Wall Street Jounal, March 30, 2020, https://www.wsj.com/articles/johnson-johnson-to-begin-human-trials-on-covid-19-vaccine-by-september-11585569380.

1196.Peter Loftus and Matt Grossman, Johnson & Johnson Readies to Start Covid-19 Vaccine Studies, The Wall Street Journal, July 15, 2020, https://www.wsj.com/articles/johnson-johnson-raises-2020-earnings-guidance-11594897686?mod=searchresults&page=1&pos=7.

1197.Andrew Court, Democrat Congressman Stephen Lynch, 65, Tests Positive to COVID-19 after Receiving Both Doses of Pfizer's Vaccine, The Daily Mail, January 30, 2021, https://www.dailymail.co.uk/news/article-9205321/Rep-Stephen-Lynch-65-tests-positive-COVID-19-receiving-doses-Pfizer-vaccine.html?ito=push-notification&ci=73039&si=23070647.

1198.Carolyn Crist, Early Vaccines Will Prevent Symptoms, Not Virus, WebMD, October 28, 2020, https://www.webmd.com/vaccines/covid-19-vaccine/news/20201027/early-vaccines-wil-prevent-symptoms-not-virus.

1199.Sarah Jacoby, Early COVID-19 Vaccines May Prevent Symptoms but Not the Infection, Dr. Fauci Says, Self, October 29, 2021, https://www.self.com/story/early-covid-19-vaccines-prevent-symptoms.

1200.See, e.g., Vaccines and Related Biological Products Advisory Committee Meeting December 17, 2020, FDA Briefing Document, Moderna COVID-19 Vaccine, at 13, https://www.fda.gov/media/144434/download.

1201.HCQ for COVID-19, https://c19hcq.com (last visited on August 27, 2021).

1202.Denise M. Hinton, Chief Scientist Food and Drug Administration, Revocation of EUA for Hydroxychloroquine, June 15, 2020, https://www.fda.gov/media/138945/download.

1203.Stéphane Bancel, Chief Executive Officer, Moderna 2019 Shareholder Letter, https://web.archive.org/web/20200913054217/https:/www.modernatx.com/moderna-blog/moderna-2019-shareholder-letter (last visited on August 22, 2021).

1204.Denise M. Hinton, FDA, June 15, 2020, supra.

1205.Mandeep R Mehra, Frank Ruschitzka, Amit N Patel. Retraction—Hydroxychloroquine or chloroquine with or without a macrolide for treatment of COVID-19: a multinational registry analysis The Lancet Published: June 5, 2020 Available at:

https://www.thelancet.com/journals/lancet/article/PIIS 0140-6736(20)31324-6/fulltext

1206.Melissa Davey, et. al., The Suspicious Funding and Characters Behind That Study and How it Got Published Is an Interesting Study but Is Beyond the Scope of this Memorandum., The Guardian, June 3, 2020, https://www.theguardian.com/world/2020/jun/03/covid-19-surgisphere-who-world-health-organization-hydroxychloroquine.

1207.Catherine Offord, The Scientist, WHO Halts Hydroxychloroquine Testing Over Safety Concerns, May 27, 2020, https://www.the-scientist.com/news-opinion/who-halts-hydroxychloroquine-testing-after-safety-warning-67573.

1208.Lancet Editor Spills the Beans and Britain's PM Surrenders to the Gates Vaccine Cartel, Alliance for Human Research Protection, June 5, 2020, https://ahrp.org/lancet-editor-spills-the-beans-and-britains-pm-surrenders-to-the-gates-vaccine-cartel/.

1209.Updated: Lancet Published a Fraudulent Study: Editor Calls it "Department of Error," Alliance for Human Research Protection, June 2, 2020, https://ahrp.org/the-lancet-published-a-fraudulent-study-editor-calls-it-department-of-error/.

1210.Id.

1211.Vera, Sharav, Lancet Editor Spills the Beans, Health Impact News, June 5, 2020, https://healthimpactnews.com/2020/editors-of-the-lancet-and-the-new-england-journal-of-medicine-pharmace utical-companies-are-so-financially-powerful-they-pressure-us-to-accept-papers/.

1212.Id.

1213.Id.

1214.Denise M. Hinton, FDA, June 15, 2020, supra.

1215.Meryl Nass, MD, WHO "Solidarity" and UK "Recovery" Clinical Trials of Hydroxychloroquine using Potentially Fatal Doses, https://www.ageofautism.com/2020/06/who-solidarity-and-uk-recovery-clinical-trials-of-hydroxychloroquine-using-potentially-fatal-doses.html (last visited on August 22, 2021).

1216.Id.

1217.Denise M. Hinton, Chief Scientist, Food and Drug Administration, Letter to Pfizer Inc., Attention: Ms. Elisa Harkins, May 10, 2021, https://www.fda.gov/media/144412/download.

1218.PCR Pandemic: Interview with Virus Mania's Dr Claus Köhnlein, https://www.bitchute.com/video/t80IONwUSUXP/ (last visited on August 22, 2021).

1219.Hongchao Pan, et. al., Repurposed antiviral drugs for COVID-19–interim WHO SOLIDARITY trial results, WHO Solidarity trial, October 15, 2020 version, https://www.medrxiv.org/content/10.1101/2020.10.15.20209817v1.full.pdf.

1220.Hongchao Pan, et. al., October 15, 2020, supra.

1221.Hongchao Pan, et. al., October 15, 2020, supra.

1222.Treating Lupus with Anti-Malarial Drugs, Johns Hopkins Lupus Center, https://www.hopkinslupus.org/lupus-treatment/lupus-medications/antimalarial-drugs/ (last visited on February 7, 2023).

1223.Id. at 9.

1224.RADM Denise M. Hinton, FDA Chief Scientist, letter to Elisa Harkins, Pfizer Inc., May 10, 2021, https://www.fda.gov/media/144412/download.

1225.Gates Foundation announces new funds to develop COVID-19 vaccines and increase access to affordable vaccines in low-income countries, Bill and Melinda Gates Foundation, November 12, 2020, https://www.gatesfoundation.org/Ideas/Media-Center/Press-Releases/2020/11/Gates-Foundation-announces-new-funds-to-develop-COVID-19-vaccines.

1226.Policy Brief, COVID-19 and mandatory vaccination: Ethical considerations, WHO, 30 May 2022.

1227.Policy Brief, WHO, 30 May 2022, supra.

1228.Policy Brief, WHO, 30 May 2022, supra.

1229.Policy Brief, WHO, 30 May 2022, supra.

1230.Policy Brief, WHO, 30 May 2022, supra.

1231.Jeremy R. Hammond, Yes, Fauci and Gates Do Have Ties to COVID-19 Vaccine Maker, September 16, 2020, https://www.jeremyrhammond.com/2020/09/16/fauci-g

ates-moderna/.

1232.Foundations Advancing mRNA Science and Research, https://www.modernatx.com/ecosystem/strategic-collaborators/foundations-advancing-mrna-science-and-research (last visited on August 22, 2021).

1233.Id.

1234.Watch Bill Gates Admitting That His $10 Billion Investment in Vaccines Brought Him $200 BILLIONS (A Return of 20:1), January 4, 2021, https://humansarefree.com/2021/01/bill-gates-his-10-billion-investment-in-vaccines-brought-him-200-billions.html.

1235.The Bill & Melinda Gates Foundation, GAVI, https://www.gavi.org/investing-gavi/funding/donor-profiles/bill-melinda-gates-foundation (last visited on February 10, 2023).

1236.Shirmila Ramasamy, COVID-19 (coronavirus): Ensuring equal access to vaccines through advanced market, World Bank Blog, May 20, 2021, https://blogs.worldbank.org/health/covid-19-coronavirus-ensuring-equal-access-vaccines-through-advanced-market-commitments.

1237.Our Pledge to the Developing World, Pfizer, https://www.pfizer.com/science/focus-areas/vaccines/pledge (last visited on February 10, 2023).

1238.Jared Hopkins, WSJ, July 22, 202, supra.

1239.Edward Hendrie, Bill Gates Used a Stand-In to Pretend to be Him Getting a COVID-19 Vaccination, January 26, 2921, https://greatmountainpublishing.com/2021/01/26/bill-gates-used-a-stand-in-to-pretend-to-be-him-getting-a-covid-19-vaccination/.

1240.Bill Gates @BillGates, Twitter, https://twitter.com/BillGates/status/1352662770416664577?s=20.

1241.Gael Fashingbauer Cooper, Bill Gates shares photo of his coronavirus vaccine, says 'I feel great', CNET, January 22, 2021, https://www.cnet.com/culture/bill-gates-shares-photo-of-his-coronavirus-vaccine-says-i-feel-great/.

1242.Bill Gates, What I'm thinking about this New Year's Eve, GatesNotes, December 30, 2019, https://www.gatesnotes.com/Year-in-Review-2019.

1243.Dr. Archie Kalokerinos, Interview---- International Vaccine Newsletter June 1995, http://www.whale.to/v/kalokerinos.html.

1244.Crime: after the Don: A Donnybrook?, Time, November 1, 1976, https://content.time.com/time/subscriber/article/0,33009,914624,00.html.

1245.The Charlie Kirk Show: 9 Frontline Doctors Speak out on HCQ and Censorship, August 10, 2020, https://www.bitchute.com/video/2JPy7qZiXvNr/.

1246.The Charlie Kirk Show, August 10, 2020, supra.

1247.Jon Passantino and Oliver Darcy, Social media giants remove viral video with false coronavirus claims that Trump retweeted, CNN, July 28, 2020, https://www.cnn.com/2020/07/28/tech/facebook-youtube-coronavirus/index.html.

1248.Christopher Zara, 'America's Frontline Doctors' website goes dark as platforms scramble to scrub misinformation, Fast Company, July 28, 2020, https://www.fastcompany.com/90533570/americas-frontline-doctors-website-goes-dark-as-platforms-scramble-to-scrub-misinformation.

1249.Everett Piper, How Democrats' Trump Derangement Syndrome is literally killing people, Washington Times, August 7, 2020, https://www.washingtontimes.com/news/2020/aug/7/how-trump-derangement-syndrome-is-literally-killin/.

1250.Why You Should Not Use Ivermectin to Treat or Prevent COVID-19, https://www.fda.gov/consumers/consumer-updates/why-you-should-not-use-ivermectin-treat-or-prevent-covid-19 (last visited on September 8, 2021).

1251.Id.

1252.Ivermectin for COVID-19: Real-Time Meta Analysis of 63 Studies, September 7, 2021, https://ivmmeta.com/.

1253.Id.

1254.Why You Should Not Use Ivermectin to Treat or Prevent COVID-19, https://www.fda.gov/consumers/consumer-updates/why-you-should-not-use-ivermectin-treat-or-prevent-covid-19 (last visited on September 8, 2021).

1255.Amicus Curiae Brief of the Association of American Physicians and Surgeons, Robert L. Apter v. HHS, Case No. 3:22-cv-184 (JVB), https://aapsonline.org/judicial/aaps-amicus-apter-v-hhs

-09-29-2022.pdf.

1256.Apter v. U.S. Dep't of Health & Hum. Servs., No. 3:22-CV-184, 2022 WL 17578869 (S.D. Tex. 2022), rev'd and remanded sub nom. Apter v. Dep't of Health & Hum. Servs., No. 22-40802, 2023 WL 5664191 (5th Cir. 2023).

1257.Apter v. Dep't of Health & Hum. Servs., ___ F.4th ___, No. 22-40802, 2023 WL 5664191 (5th Cir. 2023)

1258.Andrew White, Rolling Stone Forced To Correct Story That Falsely Claimed Oklahoma Hospital Was Overrun With Ivermectin Overdoses, National File, September 5, 2021, https://nationalfile.com/rolling-stone-caught-running-sham-story-about-oklahoma-hospital-ivermectin-overdoses/.

1259.Katelyn Ogle, Patients overdosing on ivermectin backing up rural Oklahoma hospitals, ambulances, KFOR, September 1, 2021, https://kfor.com/news/local/patients-overdosing-on-ivermectin-backing-up-rural-oklahoma-hospitals-ambulances/.

1260.One Hospital Denies Oklahoma Doctor's Story of Ivermectin Overdoses Causing ER Delays for Gunshot Victims, Rolling Stone, September 5, 2021, https://www.rollingstone.com/politics/politics-news/gunshot-victims-horse-dewormer-ivermectin-oklahoma-hospitals-covid-1220608/.

1261.Andrew White, Rolling Stone Forced To Correct Story That Falsely Claimed Oklahoma Hospital Was Overrun With Ivermectin Overdoses, National File,

September 5, 2021, https://nationalfile.com/rolling-stone-caught-running-sham-story-about-oklahoma-hospital-ivermectin-overdoses/.

1262.21 U.S. Code § 360bbb–3.

1263.Why You Should Not Use Ivermectin to Treat or Prevent COVID-19, https://www.fda.gov/consumers/consumer-updates/why-you-should-not-use-ivermectin-treat-or-prevent-covid-19 (last visited on September 8, 2021).

1264.Id.

1265.Ivermectin for COVID-19: Real-Time Meta Analysis of 63 Studies, September 7, 2021, https://ivmmeta.com/.

1266.Did CIA Director William Casey Really Say 'We'll Know Our Disinformation Program Is Complete When Everything the American Public Believes Is False'?, Infinite Unknown, http://www.infiniteunknown.net (last visited on March 17, 2016).

1267.Did William Casey (CIA Director) really say, "We'll know our disinformation program is complete when everything the American public believes is false."?, https://www.quora.com/Did-William-Casey-CIA-Director-really-say-Well-know-our-disinformation-program-is-complete-when-everything-the-American-public-believes-is-false (last visited on April 28, 2016).

1268.MOCKINGBIRD: The Subversion Of The Free Press By The CIA, www.whatreallyhappened.com (last visited on April 24, 2016).

1269.Id.

1270.Michael Collins Piper, Final Judgement, 6th Edition, at 260 (2007).

1271.David Wise, The American Police State: The Government Against the People. (New York: Random House, 1976), pp. 200-201, quoted in Michael Collins Piper, Final Judgement, 6th Edition, at 260 (2007).

1272.David Wise, supra, at 200-201.

1273.Alex Constantine, The Depraved Spies and Moguls of the CIA's Operation MOCKINGBIRD, www.whatreallyhappened.com (last visited on April 24, 2016), citing Deborah Davis, Katharine The Great, New York: Sheridan Square Press, at 119-132, 1991, and Carl Bernstein, The CIA and the Media, October 20, 1977.

1274.Carl Bernstein, The CIA and the Media, October 20, 1977, http://www.carlbernstein.com/magazine_cia_and_media.php.

1275.Carl Bernstein, supra.

1276.Carl Bernstein, supra.

1277.Carl Bernstein, supra.

1278.MOCKINGBIRD: The Subversion Of The Free Press By The CIA, www.whatreallyhappened.com (last visited on April 24, 2016).

1279.Edward Bernays, Propaganda, at 37 (1928).

1280.Bernays at 38.

1281.Cong. Rec. 2947-2948 (February 9, 1917) (speech of Rep. Callaway), http://www.iahf.com/media.html (current as of October 3, 2001).

1282.Granville Williams, *Bestriding The World, Campaign for Press and Broadcasting Freedom*, New Internationalist magazine, http://www.mediachannel.org/ownership/granville.shtml (last visited on May 25, 2008). Christopher Bollyn, *Arnon Milchan & Israeli Control of the Media*, http://www.bollyn.com/index/?id=10568 (September 1, 2007).

1283.Cong. Rec. 2947-2948 (February 9, 1917) (speech of Rep. Callaway), http://www.iahf.com/media.html (current as of October 3, 2001).

1284.ERIC JON PHELPS, VATICAN ASSASSINS: "WOUNDED IN THE HOUSE OF MY FRIENDS," p. 465 (2001) (quoting A U.S. Police Action: Operation Vampire Killer, pp. 18-19 (1992)).

1285.Joseph Mercola, US Government gave $1billion of Tax Payers Money to the Mainstream Media to falsely promote Covid-19 Vaccines, The Expose, March 26, 2022, https://expose-news.com/2022/03/26/us-gov-1-billion-to-falsely-promote-covid-vaccine/.

1286.Joseph Mercola, March 26, 2020, supra.

1287.Joseph Mercola, March 26, 2020, supra.

1288.Theresa Thamkins and Dan Vergano, Do You Need A COVID Booster? The Essential Facts About Who Can Get One Right Now, BuzzFeed News, October 20, 2021, updated January 5. 2022, https://www.buzzfeednews.com/article/theresatamkins/covid-vaccine-boosters.

1289.Dr. Anthony Fauci on positive signs from coronavirus drug study on remdesivir, CBS News, April 29, 2020, https://www.youtube.com/watch?v=LWyC4Q4l49g.

1290.Newsmax Opposes Vaccine Mandate, Here's Why, NewsMax, 7 November 2021, https://www.newsmax.com/newsfront/vaccine-mandates-constitution-overreach-privacy/2021/11/07/id/1043635/.

1291.Jessica Roy, How to convince someone to get the vaccine, Los Angeles Times, May 17, 2021, https://www.latimes.com/science/story/2021-05-17/tips-how-to-convince-someone-to-get-vaccinated.

1292.Frances Stead Sellers and Bonnie Berkowitz, These are the pro-vaccine messages people want to hear, Washington Post, April 22, 2021, https://www.washingtonpost.com/health/interactive/2021/covid-vaccine-messages/.

1293.Edward Hendrie, Statistical Proof that COVID-19 Vaccines are Worse than Ineffective—They Are Causing Most of the COVID-19 Hospitalizations, November 12, 2021, https://greatmountainpublishing.com/2021/11/12/statistical-proof-that-covid-19-vaccines-are-worse-than-ineffective-they-are-causing-most-of-the-covid-19-hospitalizations/.

1294.Dr. Nass's Orwellian Nightmare: Med License Suspended for COVID "Misinformation," March 4, 2022, https://www.bitchute.com/video/t6TYVYmivlTV/.

1295.Meryl Nass, https://www.justiceclearinghouse.com/resource/meryl-nass/ (last visited on February 7, 2023).

1296.Dr. Nass's Orwellian Nightmare: Med License Suspended for COVID "Misinformation," March 4, 2022, https://www.bitchute.com/video/t6TYVYmivlTV/.

1297.Steve Kirsch, ACIP committee approves mRNA vaccines for the childhood schedule 15-0, Substack, October 20, 2022, https://stevekirsch.substack.com/p/acip-committee-approves-mrna-vaccines.

1298.Edward Hendrie, The COVID-19 Gambit, Substack, Ocober 16, 2022, https://hendrie.substack.com/p/the-covid-19-gambit.

1299.Meryl Nass, CDC's advisory committee on immunization practices will vote at 1:20 pm today to put the covid vaccines on the childhood schedule. Expect a unanimous yes vote, Substack, October 20, 2022, https://merylnass.substack.com/p/cdcs-advisory-committee-on-immunization.

1300.Steve Kirsch, ACIP committee approves mRNA vaccines for the childhood schedule 15-0, Substack, October 20, 2022, https://stevekirsch.substack.com/p/acip-committee-approves-mrna-vaccines.

1301.Steve Kirsch, October 20, 2022, supra.

1302.Steve Kirsch, October 20, 2022, supra.

1303.Coronavirus (COVID-19) Update: FDA Authorizes Moderna, Pfizer-BioNTech Bivalent COVID-19 Vaccines for Use as a Booster Dose, FDA, August 31, 2022, https://www.fda.gov/news-events/press-announcements/coronavirus-covid-19-update-fda-authorizes-moderna-pfizer-biontech-bivalent-covid-19-vaccines-use.

1304.Kena A. Swanson, Ph.D, Vice President, Viral Vaccines, Vaccine Research and Development, Pfizer Inc., Pfizer/BioNTech COVID-19 Omicron-Modified Vaccine Options, Vaccines and Related Biological Products Advisory Committee, Presentation Outline, June 28, 2022, https://www.fda.gov/media/159496/download. See also Joseph Mercola, The new COVID vaccines have only been tested on mice, Signs of the Times, 6 September 2022, https://www.sott.net/article/471833-The-new-COVID-vaccines-have-only-been-tested-on-mice.

1305.Igor Chudov, Bivalent Booster's "8-Mice Trial" Actually FAILED, Substack, August 31, 2022, https://igorchudov.substack.com/p/ba5-boosters-8-mice-trial-actually.

1306.Sara Oliver, COVID-19 vaccines in Children, ACIP Meeting, CDC, October 19, 2022, https://www.cdc.gov/vaccines/acip/meetings/downloads/slides-2022-10-19-20/05-COVID-Oliver-508.pdf.

1307.Igor Chudov, All "Bivalent Boosted" Mice Got Covid When Challenged, Substack, September 1,

2022,
https://igorchudov.substack.com/p/all-bivalent-boosted-mice-got-covid?utm_source=substack&utm_campaign=post_embed&utm_medium=web.

1308.Exclusive – 100% of COVID-19 Vaccine Deaths Were Caused by Just 5% of the Batches Produced According to Official Government Data, The Expose, October 31, 2021,
https://theexpose.uk/2021/10/31/100-percent-of-covid-19-vaccine-deaths-caused-by-just-5-percent-of-the-batches-produced/.

1309.Id.

1310.Dr Mike Yeadon – "The Findings That 100% of COVID-19 Vaccine Deaths Have Been Caused by Just 5% of the Batches Produced Are Unprecedented," The Expose, November 1, 2021,
https://theexpose.uk/2021/11/01/dr-mike-yeadon-just-when-you-though-things-couldnt-get-any-worse/.

1311.Dr Mike Yeadon, November 1, 2021, supra.

1312.Dr Mike Yeadon, November 1, 2021, supra.

1313.Dr Mike Yeadon, November 1, 2021, supra.

1314.Dr Mike Yeadon, November 1, 2021, supra.

1315.Karl Denninger, Uh, That's Not A Conspiracy Theory, The Market Ticker, November 2, 2021, https://market-ticker.org/akcs-www?post=244109.

1316.Karl Denninger, November 2, 2021, supra.

1317.Karl Denninger, November 2, 2021, supra.

1318.Blaylock RL. COVID UPDATE: What is the truth? Surg Neurol Int. 2022 Apr 22;13:167. doi: 10.25259/SNI_150_2022. PMID: 35509555; PMCID: PMC9062939, https://www.ncbi.nlm.nih.gov/pmc/articles/PMC9062939/.

1319.Schmeling M, Manniche V, Hansen PR. Batch-dependent safety of the BNT162b2 mRNA COVID- 19 vaccine. Eur J Clin Invest. 2023;00:e13998. https://doi.org/10.1111/eci.13998.

1320.Dr. John Campbell, Viral Vaccine Paper, July 5, 2023, https://www.youtube.com/watch?v=IZAso_eLJLI.

1321.Josh Guetzkow, FOIA'd Contracts Show CDC Expected up to 1,000 VAERS Reports per Day for COVID Vaccines, December 10, 2022, https://jackanapes.substack.com/p/foiad-contracts-show-cdc-expected.

1322.Josh Guetzkow, December 10, 2022, supra.

1323.Josh Guetzkow, December 10, 2022, supra.

1324.Jared Hopkins, Pfizer, BioNTech Get $1.95 Billion Covid-19 Vaccine Order From U.S. Government, The Wall Street Jounal, July 22, 2020, https://www.wsj.com/articles/pfizer-biontech-get-1-95-billion-covid-19-vaccine-order-from-u-s-government-11595418221?mod=searchresults&page=1&pos=2.

1325.Jared Hopkins, Pfizer, BioNTech Get $1.95 Billion Covid-19 Vaccine Order From U.S. Government, The Wall Street Jounal, July 22, 2020, https://www.wsj.com/articles/pfizer-biontech-get-1-95-

billion-covid-19-vaccine-order-from-u-s-government-11595418221?mod=searchresults&page=1&pos=2.

1326.Remarks by President Biden on Fighting the COVID-19 Pandemic, The White House, September 9, 2021, https://www.whitehouse.gov/briefing-room/speeches-remarks/2021/09/09/remarks-by-president-biden-on-fighting-the-covid-19-pandemic-3/.

1327.Fact Sheet: Biden Administration Announces Details of Two Major Vaccination Policies, The White House, November 4, 2021, https://www.whitehouse.gov/briefing-room/statements-releases/2021/11/04/fact-sheet-biden-administration-announces-details-of-two-major-vaccination-policies/.

1328.Remarks by President Biden on Fighting the COVID-19 Pandemic, The White House, September 9, 2021, https://www.whitehouse.gov/briefing-room/speeches-remarks/2021/09/09/remarks-by-president-biden-on-fighting-the-covid-19-pandemic-3/.

1329.Id.

1330.Id.

1331.Id.

1332.Eric Katz, Federal Court Orders Nationwide Pause on Biden's Federal Employee Vaccine Mandate, Government Executive, January 21, 2022, https://www.govexec.com/workforce/2022/01/federal-court-orders-nationwide-pause-bidens-federal-employee-vaccine-mandate/361010/.

1333.Edward Hendrie, CDC Data Reveals That the COVID-19 Vaccines are 18,000% More Deadly Than the Flu Vaccines, February 17, 2021, https://greatmountainpublishing.com/2021/02/17/cdc-data-reveals-that-the-covid-19-vaccines-are-18000-more-deadly-than-the-flu-vaccines/.

1334.Interim Infection Prevention and Control Recommendations for Healthcare Personnel During the Coronavirus Disease 2019 (COVID-19) Pandemic, CDC, September 23, 2022, https://www.cdc.gov/coronavirus/2019-ncov/hcp/infection-control-recommendations.html#.

1335.Milton J. Rosenau, M.D., Experiments to Determine Mode of Spread of Influenza, Journal of the American Medical Association, Volume 73, Number 5, August 2, 1919, https://zenodo.org/record/1505669#.X4DQ0y1q3mo.

1336.Milton J. Rosenau, supra.

1337.Eleanor McBean, The Poisoned Needle (1957).

1338.Fredericks L. Gates, M.D., A Report on Antimeningitis Vaccination and Observations on Agglutinins in the Blood of Chronic Meningococcus Carriers, July 20, 2018, https://www.ncbi.nlm.nih.gov/pmc/articles/PMC2126288/pdf/449.pdf.

1339.The 1918 "Spanish Flu": Only The Vaccinated Died, May 29, 2020, https://salmartingano.com/the-1918-spanish-flu-only-the-vaccinated-died/.

1340.Eleanor McBean, Swine Flu Exposed, 1977, http://www.whale.to/a/mcbean2.html.

1341.Eleanor McBean, Swine Flu Exposed, 1977, Chap. 2: Vaccination Condemned, https://www.mnwelldir.org/docs/vaccines/vaccinations_condemned_McBean.htm.

1342.E.g., Gabor David Kelen, M.D., Lisa Maragakis, M.D., M.P.H., COVID-19 Vaccine: What You Need to Know, Johns Hopkins, Updated on November 1, 2022, https://www.hopkinsmedicine.org/health/conditions-and-diseases/coronavirus/covid-19-vaccine-what-you-need-to-know#:~:text=Yes%2C%20evidence%20continues%20to%20indicate,had%20COVID%2D19%20or%20not.

1343.E.g., Richard Gray, This is how new Covid-19 variants are changing the pandemic, BBC, 27 January 2021, https://www.bbc.com/future/article/20210127-covid-19-variants-how-mutations-are-changing-the-pandemic.

1344.Christine Massey, CDC confesses: our DHCPP "experts" have never obtained scientific evidence of any alleged "virus"... including "hantavirus", August 26, 2024, https://christinemasseyfois.substack.com/p/cdc-confesses-our-dhcpp-experts-have.

1345.Id.

1346.Sally Fallon Morell, Dr. Thomas Cowan, and Dr. Andrew Kaufman, Statement on Virus Isolation (SOVI). “SARS-CoV-2 Has Never Been Isolated or Purified”, Global Research, May 17, 2022.

1347.Sally Fallon, May 17, 2022, supra.

1348.Affidavit of Christine Massey, November 30. 2021, https://drive.google.com/file/d/1axe-YpJIFlV0NRtm47XvYzhQAski_oac/view.

1349.Christine Massey, FOIs reveal that health/science institutions around the world (208 and counting!) have no record of SARS-COV-2 isolation/purification, anywhere, ever, https://www.fluoridefreepeel.ca/fois-reveal-that-health-science-institutions-around-the-world-have-no-record-of-sars-cov-2-isolation-purification/ (last visited on September 2, 2022).

1350.Pieter Borger, et al., Review report Corman-Drosten et al. Eurosurveillance 2020, November 27, 2020, https://cormandrostenreview.com/report/.

1351.Kary B. Mullis, The Nobel Prize, https://www.nobelprize.org/prizes/chemistry/1993/mullis/facts/ (last visited on September 27, 2022).

1352.Inventor of COVID test calls Fauci a liar, says it 'doesn't tell you that you're sick'. Narural News, March 17, 2021, https://www.naturalnews.com/2021-03-17-inventor-calls-fauci-a-liar.html#.

1353.Id.

1354.Apoorva Mandavilli, Your Coronavirus Test Is Positive. Maybe It Shouldn't Be, The New York Times, August 29, 2020, https://www.nytimes.com/2020/08/29/health/coronavir

us-testing.html.

1355.Amandha Vollmer, PCR Tests Show Positive Because They Respond to Genetic Material Present in All Humans, G. Edward Griffin's Need to Know, August 28, 2020, https://needtoknow.news/2020/08/pcr-tests-show-positive-because-they-respond-to-genetic-material-present-in-all-humans/?utm_source=rss&utm_medium=rss&utm_campaign=pcr-tests-show-positive-because-they-respond-to-genetic-material-present-in-all-humans.

1356.Protocol: Real-time RT-PCR assays for the detection of SARS-CoV-2 Institut Pasteur, Parishttps://www.who.int/docs/default-source/coronaviruse/real-time-rt-pcr-assays-for-the-detection-of-sars-cov-2-institut-pasteur-paris.pdf?sfvrsn=3662fcb6_2 (last visited on September 2, 2022).

1357.Homo sapiens chromosome 8, GRCh38.p14 Primary Assembly, https://www.ncbi.nlm.nih.gov/nucleotide/NC_000008.11?report=genbank&log%24=nuclalign&from=63648346&to=63648363 (last visited on September 2, 2022).

1358.CDC 2019-Novel Coronavirus (2019-nCoV) Real-Time RT-PCR Diagnostic Panel, Instructions for Use, at page 35, 7/21/2021, https://www.fda.gov/media/134922/download.

1359.Edward Hendrie, The PCR Test is Generating False-Positive COVID-19 Results, November 19, 2020, https://greatmountainpublishing.com/2020/11/19/the-pcr-test-is-generating-false-positive-covid-19-results/.

1360.Apoorva Mandavilli, *supra*.

1361.Apoorva Mandavilli, *supra.*

1362.Id.

1363.Peter Andrews, *Landmark Legal Ruling Finds That Covid Tests Are Not Fit for Purpose. So What Do the MSM Do? They Ignore It*, RT, 27 November 2020, https://www.rt.com/op-ed/507937-covid-pcr-test-fail/.

1364.Id.

1365.Potential for False Positive Results with Antigen Tests for Rapid Detection of SARS-CoV-2 - Letter to Clinical Laboratory Staff and Health Care Providers, https://www.fda.gov/medical-devices/letters-health-care-providers/potential-false-positive-results-antigen-tests-rapid-detection-sars-cov-2-letter-clinical-laboratory (last visited on September 2, 2022).

1366.Id.

1367.*Potential for False Positive Results with Antigen Tests for Rapid Detection of SARS-CoV-2 - Letter to Clinical Laboratory Staff and Health Care Providers*, U.S. Food and Drug Administration, November 3, 2020, https://www.fda.gov/medical-devices/letters-health-care-providers/potential-false-positive-results-antigen-tests-rapid-detection-sars-cov-2-letter-clinical-laboratory.

1368.Edward Hendrie, Authoritative Study Shows Zero Transmission of COVID-19 by Asymptomatic Carriers, December 22, 2020, https://greatmountainpublishing.com/2020/12/22/authoritative-study-shows-zero-transmission-of-covid-19-by-asymptomatic-carriers/.

1369.Edward Hendrie, Proof that COVID-19 Statistics are Being Padded With Influenza Cases, February 3, 2021, https://greatmountainpublishing.com/2021/02/03/proof-that-covid-19-statistics-are-being-padded-with-influenza-cases/.

1370.Edward Hendrie, February 3, 2021, supra.

1371.Edward Hendrie, February 3, 2021, supra.

1372.Edward Hendrie, World Council For Health Calls for Immediate Recall of All COVID-19 Vaccines, July 30, 2022, https://greatmountainpublishing.com/2022/07/30/world-council-for-health-calls-for-immediate-recall-of-all-covid-19-vaccines/.

1373.David Zweig, The Most Important Test You've Never Heard Of, Substack, May 8, 2023, https://davidzweig.substack.com/p/the-most-important-test-youve-never.

1374.Allyson M. Pollock, et al., Asymptomatic transmission of covid-19, The BMJ, 21 December 2020, https://www.bmj.com/content/371/bmj.m4851?utm_source=twitter&utm_medium=social&utm_term=hootsuite&utm_content=sme&utm_campaign=usage.

1375.Cao, S., Gan, Y., Wang, C. et al. Post-lockdown SARS-CoV-2 nucleic acid screening in nearly ten million residents of Wuhan, China. Nat Commun 11, 5917 (2020). https://doi.org/10.1038/s41467-020-19802-w.

1376.David Zweig, May 8, 2023, supra.

1377.Catherine A. Hogan, et al., Strand-Specific Reverse Transcription PCR for Detection of Replicating SARS-CoV-2, CDC, Emerging Infectious Diseases, Volume 27, Number 2, February 2021, https://wwwnc.cdc.gov/eid/article/27/2/20-4168_article .

1378.David Zweig, May 8, 2023, supra.

1379.David Zweig, May 8, 2023, supra.

1380.Chuck Callesto, CHD interview of Michael Yeadon, Twitter, May 8, 2023, https://twitter.com/ChuckCallesto/status/1655735185206329345.

1381.Leading Report, Twitter, May 11, 2023, https://twitter.com/LeadingReport/status/1656654739659018240.

1382.Thomas S. Cowan, M.D., The Contagion Myth, at 68 (2020), https://pattoverascienza.com/wp-content/uploads/2020/08/The_Contagion-MITH_W.pdf.

1383.Derek M. Yellon and Sean M. Davidson, Exosomes, Nanoparticles Involved in Cardioprotection?, AHA Journals, 17 January 2014, https://www.ahajournals.org/doi/10.1161/circresaha.113.300636#pane-pcw-references.

1384.Stefan Lanka, The Virus Misconception, WISSENSCHAFFTPLUS magazin 01/2020, https://truthseeker.se/wp-content/uploads/The-Virus-Misconception-Part-1-Measles-as-an-example-By-Dr-Stefan-Lanka.pdf.

1385.The Contagion Myth, at 69 (2020).

1386.The Contagion Myth, at 70 (2020).

1387.The Contagion Myth, at 72 (2020).

1388.Interim Operational Considerations for Implementing the Shielding Approach to Prevent COVID-19 Infections in Humanitarian Settings, CDC, https://www.cdc.gov/coronavirus/2019-ncov/global-covid-19/shielding-approach-humanitarian.html (last visited on February 14, 2023).

1389.Id.

1390.Nada Abdelmagid, et al., Guidance for the prevention of COVID-19 infections among high-risk individuals in camps and camp-like settings, London School of Hygiene & Tropical Medicine, Health in Humanitarian Crisis Centre, 30 March 2020, https://www.lshtm.ac.uk/sites/default/files/2020-04/Guidance%20for%20the%20prevention%20of%20COVID-19%20infections%20among%20high-risk%20individuals%20in%20camps%20and%20camp-like%20settings.pdf.

1391.Nada Abdelmagid, 30 March 2020, supra.

1392.Nada Abdelmagid, 30 March 2020, supra.

1393.Nada Abdelmagid, 30 March 2020, supra.

1394.Nada Abdelmagid, 30 March 2020, supra.

1395.Nada Abdelmagid, 30 March 2020, supra.

1396.Interim Operational Considerations, supra.

1397.42 C.F.R. § 70.6.

1398.42 C.F.R. § 70.6.

1399.AFLD et al., v. Xavier Becerra, et al., Complaint, United States District Court for the Northern District of Alabama, Case 2:21-cv-00702-CLM, http://www.opensourcetruth.com/wp-content/uploads/2021/06/Doc-10-Original-AFLDs-Complaint.pdf.

1400.Coronavirus Task Force Press Breifing, White House, April 7, 2020, https://www.whitehouse.gov/briefings-statements/remarks-president-trump-vice-president-pence-members-coronavirus-task-force-press-briefing-april-7-2020/.

1401.Coronavirus Task Force Press Breifing, supra.

1402.Illinois Department of Public Health Director Dr. Ngozi Ezike Explains How Covid Deaths Are Classified, Published August 14, 2021, https://www.bitchute.com/video/vsEScGB2ifHx/.

1403.Greg Piper, Lawmakers seek federal grand jury investigation for COVID-19 statistical manipulation, Just the News, October 10, 2021, https://justthenews.com/government/federal-agencies/lawmakers-seek-federal-grand-jury-investigation-covid-19-statistical.

1404.Oregon Senators Kim Thatcher and Dennis Linthicum, Formal Federal Grand Jury Petition Rights To Petition Protected By 18 USC §3332 & Case Law, August 16, 2021, https://standforhealthfreedom.com/wp-content/uploads/2021/09/0-Senate-Letterhead-Grand-Jury-Petition-AUSA.pdf.

1405.Weekly Updates by Select Demographic and Geographic Characteristics, Comorbidities and other conditions, CDC, https://www.cdc.gov/nchs/nvss/vsrr/covid_weekly/index.htm#Comorbidities.

1406.Tyler Durden, Florida Man Who Died In Motorcycle Wreck Labeled As COVID-19 Death By State, July 19, 2020, https://www.zerohedge.com/political/florida-man-20s-who-died-motorcycle-wreck-labeled-covid-19-death-state.

1407.Danielle Lama, FOX 35 INVESTIGATES: Questions raised after fatal motorcycle crash listed as COVID-19 death, July 18, 2020, https://www.fox35orlando.com/news/fox-35-investigates-questions-raised-after-fatal-motorcycle-crash-listed-as-covid-19-death.

1408.Edward Hendrie, How the Federal Government Has Turned Hospitals into Death Chambers, February 25, 2022, https://greatmountainpublishing.com/2022/02/25/how-the-federal-government-has-turned-hospitals-into-death-chambers/.

1409.Kristin Herd, *COVID-19 Stats Betray the Facts and the American People*, July 20,2020, https://krisheldmd.wordpress.com/2020/07/20/covid-19-stats-betray-the-facts-and-the-american-people/.

1410.Kristin Herd, July 20, 2020, supra.

1411.Number of new cases of coronavirus (COVID-19) in the United States from January 20, 2020 to January 13, 2021, by day*, Statista, January

14, 2021, http://web.archive.org/web/20210114220926/https://www.statista.com/statistics/1102816/coronavirus-covid19-cases-number-us-americans-by-day/.

1412.Kristin Herd, July 20, 2020, supra.

1413.*Dr Scott Jensen With Laura Ingraham | The Ridiculous CDC Guidlines*, April 9, 2020, https://www.youtube.com/watch?v=_qWmiWf81zI&feature=emb_logo.

1414.Former gubernatorial candidate Dr. Scott Jensen under investigation by Minnesota Board of Medical Practice, NBC, KTTC, January 30, 2023, https://www.kttc.com/2023/01/31/former-gubernatorial-candidate-dr-scott-jensen-under-investigation-by-minnesota-board-medical-practice/.

1415.Id.

1416.*Vital Statistics Reporting Guidance, Guidance for Certifying Deaths Due to Coronavirus Disease 2019 (COVID–19)*, U.S. Department of Health and Human Services • Centers for Disease Control and Prevention • National Center for Health Statistics • National Vital Statistics System, Report No. 3, April 2020, https://www.cdc.gov/nchs/data/nvss/vsrg/vsrg03-508.pdf.

1417.Id.

1418.Guidance for Certifying Deaths Due to Coronavirus Disease 2019 (COVID-19), Report No. 3, U.S. Department of Health and Human Services, Centers for Disease Control and Prevention, National

Center for Health Statistics, National Vital Statistics System, Released April 2020 – Expanded February 2023, https://www.cdc.gov/nchs/data/nvss/vsrg/vsrg03-508.pdf.

1419.Danielle Waugh, I-Team: Deaths incorrectly attributed to COVID-19 in Palm Beach County, CBS 12 News, July 23, 2020, https://cbs12.com/news/local/i-team-deaths-incorrectly-attributed-to-covid-19-in-palm-beach-county.

1420.*COVID-19 In Virginia*, Dashboard Updated November 5, 2020, Department of Health, https://www.vdh.virginia.gov/coronavirus/covid-19-in-virginia/.

1421.*Coronavirus Disease 2019 (COVID-19) 2020 Interim Case Definition*, Approved August 5, 2020, Centers for Disease Control, https://wwwn.cdc.gov/nndss/conditions/coronavirus-disease-2019-covid-19/case-definition/2020/08/05/.

1422.*Five Things to Remember When Interpreting Epidemiologic Data*, Virginia Department of Health, May 1, 2020, https://www.vdh.virginia.gov/coronavirus/2020/05/01/interpreting-epidemiologic-data/.

1423.Id.

1424.Id.

1425.COVID-19 cases surpass 70,000 in Virginia | Positivity rate increases to 6.6%, NBC12 Newsroom | March 30, 2020 at 9:04 AM EDT - Updated July 12 at 5:39 PM, http://web.archive.org/web/20200713000744/https://www.nbc12.com/2020/07/11/new-covid-cases-up-by-virginia-positivity-rate-increases/.

1426.Michelle Rogers, Fact Check: Hospitals Get Paid More If Patients Listed as COVID-19, on Ventilators, USA TODAY, April 24, 2020, https://www.usatoday.com/story/news/factcheck/2020/04/24/fact-check-medicare-hospitals-paid-more-covid-19-patients-coronavirus/3000638001/.

1427.Michelle Rogers, April 24, 2020, supra.

1428.Michelle Rogers, April 24, 2020, supra.

1429.Michelle Rogers, April 24, 2020, supra.

1430.Andrew Mark Miller, CDC Director Acknowledges Hospitals Have a Monetary Incentive to Overcount Coronavirus Deaths, Washington Examiner, August 1, 2020, https://www.washingtonexaminer.com/news/cdc-director-acknowledges-hospitals-have-a-monetary-incentive-to-overcount-coronavirus-deaths?fbclid=IwAR0v4RCPBA5WAPyfUoDF1ZbV_MYFStCRKYhs1TBxwAgSbbgr5foBGrrdg3U.

1431.Andrew Mark Miller, August 1, 2020 supra.

1432.Edwin Mora, CDC Chief Agrees There's 'Perverse' Economic 'Incentive' for Hospitals to Inflate Coronavirus Deaths, Breitbart, July 31, 2020, https://www.breitbart.com/politics/2020/07/31/cdc-chief-agrees-theres-perverse-economic-incentive-for-hospitals-to-inflate-coronavirus-deaths/.

1433.Alya Ellison, State-by-state Breakdown of Federal Aid per COVID-19 Case, Becker's Hospitial

CFO Report, April 14, 2020, https://www.beckershospitalreview.com/finance/state-by-state-breakdown-of-federal-aid-per-covid-19-case.html.

1434.Id.

1435.AFLD, et. al., v, Xavier Becerra, et al., Motion For Preliminary Injunction, United States District Court for the Northern District of Alabama, Civil Action No. 2:21-cv-00702-CLM, July 19, 2021.

1436.Brian Shilhavy, CENSORED: COVID19 PCR Tests are Scientifically Meaningless – Everything We've Been Told about COVID is a HOAX!, Health Impact News, June 27, 2020, https://healthimpactnews.com/2020/censored-covid19-pcr-tests-are-scientifically-meaningless-everything-weve-been-told-about-covid-is-a-hoax/.

1437.Id.

1438.Lab Alert: Changes to CDC RT-PCR for SARS-CoV-2 Testing, July 21, 2021, https://www.cdc.gov/csels/dls/locs/2021/07-21-2021-lab-alert-Changes_CDC_RT-PCR_SARS-CoV-2_Testing_1.html.

1439.*Data and Surveillance, How is VDH counting COVID-19 deaths?*, Virginia Department of Health, Page Last Updated: October 22, 2020, https://www.vdh.virginia.gov/coronavirus/data-and-surveillance/.

1440.*Weekly Updates by Select Demographic and Geographic Characteristics*, Centers for Disease Control, Page last reviewed: November 4, 2020, https://www.cdc.gov/nchs/nvss/vsrr/covid_weekly/index.htm#Comorbidities.

1441.Chris Vanderveen, Colorado coroner says death listed by state as COVID-19 related has much more to do with alcohol, NBC, 9News, May 14, 2020, https://www.9news.com/article/news/investigations/colorado-coroner-says-death-listed-by-state-as-covid-19-related-has-much-more-to-do-with-alcohol/73-eec4517a-13dd-45bc-bc59-7e50cedf2272.

1442.Chris Vanderveen, May 14, 2020, supra.

1443.Chris Vanderveen, May 14, 2020, supra.

1444.Chris Vanderveen, May 14, 2020, supra.

1445.Kyle Clark and Erin Powell, GOP rep alleges falsified COVID-19 records, calls for indictment of Colorado's top health official, NBC 9News, May 14, 2020, https://www.9news.com/article/news/local/next/gop-rep-alleges-falsified-covid-19-records-calls-for-indictment-of-colorados-top-health-official/73-bf02452f-4615-4efe-9413-a4826a8105b2.

1446.State-by-State Breakdown: Delivery of Initial $30 Billion of CARES Act Public Health and Social Services Emergency Fund, https://www.hrsa.gov/sites/default/files/hrsa/provider-relief/state-state-breakdown-delivery-initial-30-billion-cares-act.pdf (last visited on May 7, 2023).

1447.COVID-19 CARES Act Funds, Maricopa County, https://www.maricopa.gov/5744/COVID-19-Cares-Act-Funds (last visited on May 7, 2023).

1448.Noah Higgins Dunn, *Fauci Debunks Theories of Low CDC Coronavirus Death Toll: 'There Are 180,000-plus Deaths' in U.S.*, CNBC, September 1, 2020, https://www.msn.com/en-us/health/medical/fauci-debunks-theories-of-low-cdc-coronavirus-death-toll-there-are-180-000-plus-deaths-in-u-s/ar-BB18B8of?ocid=msedgntp.

1449.Id.

1450.*They Finally Admitted It!!!*, July 8, 2020, https://youtu.be/dtpYi1uC_Iw.

1451.Infra.

1452.Infra.

1453.Yanni Gu, A Closer Look at U.S. Deaths Due to COVID-19, Johns Hopkins News-Letter, November 22, 2020, https://web.archive.org/web/20201126223119/https://www.jhunewsletter.com/article/2020/11/a-closer-look-at-u-s-deaths-due-to-covid-19 (retracted).

1454.Infra.

1455.Infra.

1456.Infra.

1457.Yanni Gu, A closer look at U.S. deaths due to COVID-19, Johns Hopkins News-Letter, November 27, 2020, https://www.jhunewsletter.com/article/2020/11/a-closer-look-at-u-s-deaths-due-to-covid-19.

1458.Yoon K Loke and Carl HeneghanWhy no-one can ever recover from COVID-19 in England – a statistical anomaly, The Centre for Evidence-Based Medicine, July 16, 2020, https://www.cebm.net/covid-19/why-no-one-can-ever-recover-from-covid-19-in-england-a-statistical-anomaly/.

1459.Yoon K Loke and Carl Heneghan, supra.

1460.John Johnson, Matt Hancock orders urgent review into 'misleading' PHE coronavirus death statistics, Politics Home, July 17, 2020, https://www.politicshome.com/news/article/matt-hancock-orders-urgent-review-into-misleading-phe-coronavirus-death-statistics.

1461.John Johnson, July 17, 2020, supra.

1462.John Johnson, July 17, 2020, supra.

1463.*Tracking Dr. Anthony Fauci's Comments On Coronavirus*, CNBC, March 26, 2020, comments at 4:55 of video, https://www.youtube.com/watch?v=ShiwHR5OvtM&feature=emb_logo.

1464.*Dr. Fauci and Other CDC & NIH Officials Testify on Coronavirus – March 11*, Rev Transcripts, March 11, 2020, https://www.rev.com/blog/transcripts/dr-fauci-and-other-cdc-nih-officials-testify-on-coronavirus-march-11. *See Also, Coronavirus "10 Times More Lethal than Seasonal Flu": Fauci*, posted March 12, 2020, https://www.youtube.com/watch?v=Ono3BcbTX4Q&feature=youtu.be.

1465.Anthony S. Fauci, M.D., H. Clifford Lane, M.D., and Robert R. Redfield, M.D., *Covid-19 — Navigating the Uncharted*, New England Journal of Medicine, March 26, 2020, https://www.nejm.org/doi/full/10.1056/NEJMe2002387.

1466.Ronald Brown, Public Health Lessons Learned From Biases in Coronavirus Mortality Overestimation, Cambridge University Press, 12 August 2020, https://www.cambridge.org/core/journals/disaster-medicine-and-public-health-preparedness/article/public-health-lessons-learned-from-biases-in-coronavirus-mortality-overestimation/7ACD87D8FD2237285EB667BB28DCC6E9#.

1467.*Tracking Dr. Anthony Fauci's Comments On Coronavirus*, CNBC, March 26, 2020, comments at 4:55 of video, https://www.youtube.com/watch?v=ShiwHR5OvtM&feature=emb_logo.

1468.Anthony S. Fauci, M.D., H. Clifford Lane, M.D., and Robert R. Redfield, M.D., *Covid-19 — Navigating the Uncharted*, New England Journal of Medicine, March 26, 2020, https://www.nejm.org/doi/full/10.1056/NEJMe2002387.

1469.Caterina Andreano, Dr. Fauci: Wear Goggles or Eye Shields to Prevent Spread of Covid-19; Flu Vaccine a Must, ABC News, July 29, 2020, https://abcnews.go.com/US/dr-fauci-wear-goggles-eye-shields-prevent-spread/story?id=72059055.

1470.Id. Video of interview of Dr. Fauci by ABC News commentator Dr. Jen Ashton imbedded in

Caterina Andreano's ABC News article, supra.

1471.Lisa Krieger, *Stanford Researcher Says Coronavirus Isn't as Fatal as We Thought; Critics Say He's Missing the Point*, The Mercury News, May 20, 2020, https://www.mercurynews.com/2020/05/20/stanford-researcher-says-coronavirus-isnt-as-fatal-as-we-thought-critics-say-hes-missing-the-point/.

1472.Trump and coronavirus task force brief from White House | NBC News (Live Stream Recording), Streamed live on Mar 23, 2020, https://www.youtube.com/watch?v=Fx8oJCzRJUk.

1473.Average life expectancy in Europe for those born in 2019, by gender and region, https://www.statista.com/statistics/274514/life-expectancy-in-europe/ (last visited on June 19, 2020).

1474.Tommaso Ebhardt, Chiara Remondini, and Marco Bertacche, 99% of Those Who Died From Virus Had Other Illness, Italy Says, Bloomberg, Bloomberg, March 18, 2020, https://www.bloomberg.com/news/articles/2020-03-18/99-of-those-who-died-from-virus-had-other-illness-italy-says.

1475.See supra.

1476.U.S. Death Rate 1950-2023, Chart and table of the U.S. death rate from 1950 to 2023, https://www.macrotrends.net/countries/USA/united-states/death-rate.

1477.*Weekly Updates by Select Demographic and Geographic Characteristics*, CDC, National Center for

Health Statistics, https://www.cdc.gov/nchs/nvss/vsrr/covid_weekly/index.htm#Comorbidities (last visited on November 7, 2020).

1478.Id.

1479.Id.

1480.Patrick Howley, BUSTED: CDC Inflated COVID Numbers, Accused of Violating Federal Law, National File, March 8, 2021, https://nationalfile.com/busted-cdc-inflated-covid-numbers-accused-of-violating-federal-law/.

1481.Id.

1482.Id.

1483.2003 CDC Medical Examiner's and Coroner's Handbook on Death Registration, https://www.cdc.gov/nchs/data/misc/hb_me.pdf.

1484.Id.

1485.Steven Schaartz, Ph.D., Director - Division of Vital Statistics, National Center for Health Statistics, COVID-19 Alert No. 2, National Vital Statistics System, March 24, 2020, https://www.cdc.gov/nchs/data/nvss/coronavirus/Alert-2-New-ICD-code-introduced-for-COVID-19-deaths.pdf.

1486.Id.

1487.Henry Ealy, et al., COVID-19 Data Collection, Comorbidity & Federal Law: A Historical Retrospective, Public Health Policy Initiative, October

12, 2020,
https://jdfor2020.com/wp-content/uploads/2020/11/adf864_165a103206974fdbb14ada6bf8af1541.pdf.

1488.Henry Ealy, et al., COVID-19 Data Collection, Comorbidity & Federal Law: A Historical Retrospective, Public Health Policy Initiative, October 12, 2020,
https://jdfor2020.com/wp-content/uploads/2020/11/adf864_165a103206974fdbb14ada6bf8af1541.pdf.

1489.Henry Ealy, et al., October 12, 2020, supra.

1490.COVID-19 Alert No. 2, National Vital Statistics System, March 24, 2020,
https://www.cdc.gov/nchs/data/nvss/coronavirus/Alert-2-New-ICD-code-introduced-for-COVID-19-deaths.pdf.

1491.Guidance for Certifying COVID-19 Deaths, March 4, 2020, National Vital Statistics System,
https://www.cdc.gov/nchs/data/nvss/coronavirus/alert-1-guidance-for-certifying-covid-19-deaths.pdf.

1492.Guidance for Certifying Deaths Due to Coronavirus Disease 2019 (COVID–19), National Vital Statistics System, April 2020,
https://www.cdc.gov/nchs/data/nvss/vsrg/vsrg03-508.pdf.

1493.Guidance for Certifying COVID-19 Deaths, March 4, 2020, National Vital Statistics System,
https://www.cdc.gov/nchs/data/nvss/coronavirus/alert-1-guidance-for-certifying-covid-19-deaths.pdf.

1494.Death certificate analysis shows Washington's COVID-19 death count remains inflated, Press

Release, December 16, 2020, Freedom Foundation, https://www.freedomfoundation.com/press-release/death-certificate-analysis-shows-washingtons-covid-19-death-count-remains-inflated/.

1495.Maxford Nelson, WA reduces COVID-19 deaths by 200; investigation suggests it's still too high, Freedom Foundation, December 16, 2020, https://www.freedomfoundation.com/covid-19/wa-lowers-covid-19-deaths-by-200-investigation-suggests-its-still-too-high/.

1496.Death cert. analysis, December 16, 2020, supra.

1497.Maxford Nelsen, Washington health officials: Gunshot victims counted as COVID-19 deaths, Liberty Foundation, May 21, 2020, https://www.freedomfoundation.com/washington/washington-health-officials-gunshot-victims-counted-as-covid-19-deaths/.

1498.Maxford Nelsen, May 21, 2020, supra.

1499.Death certificate analysis shows Washington's COVID-19 death count remains inflated, Press Release, December 16, 2020, Freedom Foundation, https://www.freedomfoundation.com/press-release/death-certificate-analysis-shows-washingtons-covid-19-death-count-remains-inflated/.

1500.Maxford Nelson, December 16, 2020, supra.

1501.Death cert. analysis December 16, 2020, supra.

1502.@TheOriginalSai, Twitter, January 14, 2023, https://twitter.com/TheOriginalSai/status/1614332319111970816,

1503.IT WAS ALL A LIE: NHS Director confirms Hospitals lied about Cause of Death to create illusion of COVID Pandemic, The Expose, March 20, 2023, https://expose-news.com/2023/03/20/nhs-director-confirms-hospitals-lied-about-covid-deaths/?cmid=6a508dc3-a2e4-47a3-b166-300d2b15cb67.

1504.LIE, The Expose, March 20, 2023, supra.

1505.LIE, The Expose, March 20, 2023, supra.

1506.LIE, The Expose, March 20, 2023, supra.

1507.LIE, The Expose, March 20, 2023, supra.

1508.LIE, The Expose, March 20, 2023, supra.

1509.LIE, The Expose, March 20, 2023, supra.

1510.LIE, The Expose, March 20, 2023, supra.

1511.LIE, The Expose, March 20, 2023, supra.

1512.Nicole Chavez and Artemis Moshtaghian, 48 states have ordered or recommended that schools don't reopen this academic year, CNN, https://www.cnn.com/2020/04/18/us/schools-closed-coronavirus/index.html

1513. Donohue JM, Miller E. COVID-19 and School Closures. JAMA. 2020;324(9):845–847. doi:10.1001/jama.2020.13092, July 29, 2020, https://jamanetwork.com/journals/jama/fullarticle/2769033.

1514.David Jackson, Trump says schools should reopen because children are 'virtually immune', CNN, August 5, 2020, https://www.usatoday.com/story/news/politics/2020/08/05/coronavirus-trump-pushes-reopening-saying-children-immune/3297255001/.

1515.Video Made Private, https://www.youtube.com/watch?v=kEkLwQtZd2U.

1516.Weekly Updates by Select Demographic and Geographic Characteristics, Comorbidities and other conditions, CDC, May 7, 2020, https://www.cdc.gov/nchs/nvss/vsrr/covid_weekly/index.htm#Comorbidities.

1517.Event 201, https://www.centerforhealthsecurity.org/our-work/exercises/event201/ (last visited on February 5, 2023).

1518.The Event 201 scenario, https://www.centerforhealthsecurity.org/our-work/exercises/event201/scenario.html (last visited on February 5, 2023).

1519.CAPS: The Pathogen and Clinical Syndrome, Event 201, https://www.centerforhealthsecurity.org/our-work/exercises/event201/event201-resources/CAPS-fact-sheet-191009.pdf (last visited on February 5, 2023).

1520.CAPS: The Pathogen and Clinical Syndrome, Event 201, https://www.centerforhealthsecurity.org/our-work/exercises/event201/event201-resources/CAPS-fact-sheet-191009.pdf (last visited on February 5, 2023).

1521.The Event 201 scenario, https://www.centerforhealthsecurity.org/our-work/exercises/event201/scenario.html (last visited on February

5, 2023).

1522.The Event 201 scenario, supra.

1523.Event 201 Pandemic Exercise Segment 4 Communications, https://childrenshealthdefense.org/wp-content/uploads/Event-201-Pandemic-Exercise-Segment-4-Communications-Discussion-and-Epilogue-Video-bill-gates.pdf.

1524.Players for Event 201, a pandemic exercise, include global business leaders and prominent government and public health leaders—livestream open to all, Johns Hopkins Center for Public Health, October 15, 2019, https://centerforhealthsecurity.org/2019/players-for-event-201-a-pandemic-exercise-include-global-business-leaders-and-prominent-government-and-public-health-leaders-livestream-open-to-all-0.

1525.Michael P. Senger, The Unwitting Coup: Was the Response to COVID Effectively a Coup by the Western Intelligence Community?, August 1, 2023, https://www.michaelpsenger.com/p/the-unwitting-coup-was-the-response?utm_source=share&utm_medium=android&r=3qj6.

1526.Michael Senger, How Zeynep Tufekci and Jeremy Howard Masked America, The New Normal, March 26, 2023, https://www.michaelpsenger.com/p/how-zeynep-tufekci-and-jeremy-howard.

1527.Michael Senger, The REAL Story of the Birth of 'Social Distancing' — the Western Term for Lockdown, September 9, 2022, https://www.michaelpsenger.com/p/the-real-story-of-th

e-birth-of-social.

1528.Event 201 Pandemic Exercise Segment 4 Communications, https://childrenshealthdefense.org/wp-content/uploads/Event-201-Pandemic-Exercise-Segment-4-Communications-Discussion-and-Epilogue-Video-bill-gates.pdf.

1529.Event 201 Pandemic Exercise Segment 4, supra.

1530.Event 201 Pandemic Exercise Segment 4, supra.

1531.Event 201 Pandemic Exercise Segment 4, supra.

1532.Josephine Ma, Exclusive | Coronavirus: China's first confirmed Covid-19 case traced back to November 17, 13 March 2020, https://www.scmp.com/news/china/society/article/3074991/coronavirus-chinas-first-confirmed-covid-19-case-traced-back.

1533.CDC Museum COVID-19 Timeline, https://www.cdc.gov/museum/timeline/covid19.html (last visited on February 5, 2023).

1534.U.S. Department of Defense issued a contract for 'COVID-19 Research' in Ukraine 3 months before Covid was known to even exist, The Expose, March 27, 2023, https://expose-news.com/2023/03/27/us-dod-created-covid-evidence-suggests/?cmid=3bc72fd8-9e3d-4f6b-be59-b76a261c2d04.

1535.Josephine Ma, Exclusive | Coronavirus: China's first confirmed Covid-19 case traced back to November 17, South China Morning Post, 13 March 2020, https://www.scmp.com/news/china/society/article/3074

991/coronavirus-chinas-first-confirmed-covid-19-case-traced-back

1536.Biden administration sued for censoring speech, Washington Times, October 10, 2022, https://www.washingtontimes.com/news/2022/oct/10/lawsuit-details-sprawling-biden-administration-pro/.

1537.Louisiana, Missouri Request Depositions And Add 47 Defendants To Lawsuit Against Federal Government For Alleged Collusion With Social Media Companies, Missouri and Louisiana v, Biden, https://agjefflandry.com/Article/13077 (last visited on February 5, 2023).

1538.First Amended Complaint, Missouri and Louisiana v. Joseph Biden, Jr., United States District Court For the Western District of Louisiana, Monroe Division, Case No. 3:22-cv-01213. See also Memorandum Ruling and Order, Missouri and Louisiana v. Joseph Biden, Jr., United States District Court For the Western District of Louisiana, Monroe Division, Case No. 3:22-cv-01213, https://ago.mo.gov/docs/default-source/press-releases/08916881989.pdf. Second Amended Complaint, Missouri and Louisiana v. Joseph Biden, Jr., United States District Court For the Western District of Louisiana, Monroe Division, Case No. 3:22-cv-01213-TAD-KDM, https://agjefflandry.com/Article/13077.

1539.The Parties' Joint Statement on Discovery Disputes, Missouri and Louisiana v. Joseph Biden, Jr., United States District Court For the Western District of Louisiana, Monroe Division, Case No. 3:22-cv-01213 at 5. https://ago.mo.gov/docs/default-source/press-releases/free-speech-pitch-thread-docs/doc-71---joint-statement-on-discovery-disputes.pdf?sfvrsn=3b968800_2.

1540.Joint Statement on Discovery Disputes, supra.

1541.Joint Statement on Discovery Disputes, supra.

1542.Joint Statement on Discovery Disputes, supra.

1543.Joint Statement on Discovery Disputes, supra.

1544.Joint Statement on Discovery Disputes, supra.

1545.Joint Statement on Discovery Disputes, supra.

1546.COVID-19 medical misinformation policy, YouTube, https://support.google.com/youtube/answer/9891785?hl=en (last visited on February 5, 2023).

1547.Id.

1548.Statement about nCoV and our pandemic exercise, https://www.centerforhealthsecurity.org/news/center-news/2020/2020-01-24-Statement-of-Clarification-Event201.html (February 5, 2023).

1549.The Great Reset, World Economic Forum, https://www.weforum.org/focus/the-great-reset (last visited on February 5, 2023).

1550.Ex-minister wanted to 'frighten' Brits into Covid compliance – leaked messages, RT, March 5, 2023, https://www.rt.com/news/572494-uk-hancock-text-messages-covid/.

1551.Bombshell: Gov. Officials Texts Prove Covid Was A Scam To Control You, The New American, at

5:34 of the video, March 8, 2023, https://rumble.com/v2c2wem-bombshell-gov.-officials-texts-prove-covid-was-a-scam-to-control-you.html?mref=6zof&mc=dgip3&utm_source=newsletter&utm_medium=email&utm_campaign=The+New+American&ep=2.

1552.Olivia Jones, Matt Hancock 'joked about Bill Gates Covid vaccine conspiracy theory by telling aides the Microsoft billionaire "owes me one" considering "how many people I'm getting his chips injected into",' lockdown leaks reveal, March 5, 2023, https://www.dailymail.co.uk/news/article-11823577/Matt-Hancock-joked-Bill-Gates-Covid-vaccine-conspiracy-theory.html.

1553.Olivia Jones, supra.

1554.Edward Hendrie, Dr. Fauci Inadvertently Revealed that the COVID-19 Pandemic Was Planned, July 26, 2020, https://greatmountainpublishing.com/2020/07/26/dr-fauci-inadvertently-revealed-that-the-covid-19-pandemic-was-planned/.

1555.Keynote Address by Anthony Fauci, Pandemic Preparedness in the Next Administration, The Center for Global Health Science and Security at Georgetown University Medical Center, January 10, 2017, https://ghss.georgetown.edu/pandemicprep2017/#.

1556.The Center for Global Health Science and Security at Georgetown University Medical Center, https://ghss.georgetown.edu/# (last visited on February 8, 2023).

1557.Kat Zambon, Global Health Experts Advise Advance Planning for Inevitable Pandemic, The Center for Global Health Science and Security at Georgetown University Medical Center, https://gumc.georgetown.edu/gumc-stories/global-health-experts-advise-advance-planning-for-inevitable-pandemic/#

1558.COVID-19 medical misinformation policy, YouTube, https://support.google.com/youtube/answer/9891785?hl=en (last visited on February 5, 2023).

1559.Arthur Firstenberg, The Invisible Rainbow, A History of Electricity and Life, at 2 (2020).

1560.Verizon launches first U.S. '3G' network, CNN, January 28, 2002, https://www.cnn.com/2002/TECH/ptech/01/28/verizon.3g/.

1561.SARS Basics Fact Sheet, CDC, page last reviewed December 6, 2017, https://www.cdc.gov/sars/about/fs-sars.html.

1562.Lisa Pace, 4G: History, Origin, and More, 4G Release History, December 6, 2022, https://history-computer.com/4g-guide/#:~:text=available%20shortly%20thereafter.-,4G%20reached%20the%20United%20States%20in%202012%2C%20with%20five%20companies,began%20to%20be%20rolled%20out.

1563.2009 H1N1 Pandemic (H1N1pdm09 virus), last reviewed on June 11, 2019, CDC, https://www.cdc.gov/flu/pandemic-resources/2009-h1n1-pandemic.html.

1564.When was 5G introduced?, Verizon News Center, December 6, 2019, https://www.verizon.com/about/our-company/5g/when-was-5g-introduced.

1565.CDC Museum COVID-19 Timeline, CDC, last reviewed on August 16, 2022, https://www.cdc.gov/museum/timeline/covid19.html.

1566.S. S. SEKER, "Health Effects of 5G and Millimeter Waves," 2019 11th International Conference on Electrical and Electronics Engineering (ELECO), Bursa, Turkey, 2019, pp. I16-I16, doi: 10.23919/ELECO47770.2019.8990371. https://ieeexplore.ieee.org/abstract/document/8990371.

1567.Lennart Hardell, et al., Comments on the US National Toxicology Program technical reports on toxicology and carcinogenesis study in rats exposed to whole-body radiofrequency radiation at 900 MHz and in mice exposed to whole-body radiofrequency radiation at 1,900 MHz, International Journal of Oncology, October 24, 2018, https://www.spandidos-publications.com/ijo/54/1/111?fbclid=IwAR0NncY5stN1jpPG4w63H7IeYlHbGOy_E5U4o6CaKWfrwrQbSoA13J4Adsk.

1568.Dr. Tom Cowan: 5G Millimetre Waves are a Weapon to make People sick with COVID, https://stop5g.cz/us/dr-tom-cowan-5g-millimetre-waves-are-a-weapon-to-make-people-sick-with-covid/ (last visited on February 15, 2023).

1569.Dr. Tom Cowan, 5G Millimetre Waves, supra.

1570.Dr. Tom Cowan: 5G Millimetre Waves, supra.

1571.Laruen Smiley, 27 Days in Tokyo Bay: What Happened on the Diamond Princess, Wired, April 30, 2020, https://www.wired.com/story/diamond-princess-coronavirus-covid-19-tokyo-bay/.

1572. Princess Gets Access to SES O3b mPOWER Satellite-Based Communications System, Cruise Industry News, February 3, 2020, https://cruiseindustrynews.com/cruise-news/2020/02/princess-gets-access-to-ses-o3b-mpower-satellite-based-communications-system/.

1573.Accelerating 5G roll out via satellite, SES, 22 February 2019, https://www.ses.com/newsroom/accelerating-5g-roll-out-satellite.

1574.Magda Havas, Is there an association between covid-19 cases/deaths and 5G in the United States?, April 22, 2020 (updated May 7, 2020), https://magdahavas.com/5g-and-mm-waves/is-there-an-association-between-covid-19-cases-deaths-and-5g-in-the-united-states/.

1575.Magda Havas, 5G and COVID-19 Deaths, Supra.

1576.Study Shows Direct Correlation between 5G Networks and "Coronavirus" Outbreaks, Radiation Dangers, April 24, 2020, https://radiationdangers.com/2020/04/24/study-shows-direct-correlation-between-5g-networks-and-coronavirus-outbreaks-2/.

1577.Id.

1578.Id.

1579.5G Radiation - Potential Cause of Covid-19 Pandemic, May 6, 2020, The Legal Pens, http://alchemistcook.blogspot.com/2020/05/the-potential-dangers-of-5g-radiation.html.

1580.China rolls out 'one of the world's largest' 5G networks, BBC News, 1 November 2019, https://www.bbc.com/news/business-50258287.

1581.5G network coming to Wuhan, Hubei - China, April 16, 2018, http://en.hubei.gov.cn/news/newslist/201804/t20180416_1275769.shtml.

1582.Huawei builds 5G network at Wuhan Huoshenshan Hospital, CGTN, March 13, 2020, https://news.cgtn.com/news/2020-03-13/Huawei-builds-5G-network-at-Wuhan-Huoshenshan-Hospital-OP6qhHRc1G/index.html.

1583.The Contagion Myth and Germ Theory Hoax For Dummies, August 16, 2021, https://truthscrambler.com/2021/08/16/the-contagion-myth-and-germ-theory-hoax-for-dummies/.

1584.John E. Hoover, HEROES: Tribute to Dr Scott Jensen - Part 1, https://www.youtube.com/watch?v=sVmNFoEjv90 (last visited on February 5, 2023). John E. Hoover, HEROES: Tribute to Dr Scott Jensen w/ John Cullen - Part 2, https://www.youtube.com/watch?v=4-JpcPZRU8Y (last visited on February 5, 2023). John E. Hoover, The Final Chapter: Part 3 - HEROES: A Tribute to Dr Scott Jensen, https://www.youtube.com/watch?v=2gJP-L3z6uY&t=1361s (last visited on February 5, 2023).

1585.Edward Hendrie, Proof that COVID-19 Statistics are Being Padded With Influenza Cases, February 3, 2021, Great Mountain Publishing, https://greatmountainpublishing.com/2021/02/03/proof-that-covid-19-statistics-are-being-padded-with-influenza-cases/.

1586.Peter Andrews, Flu Away: Scientists Baffled at Disappearance of Influenza... but Is it Really Gone, or Just Masked by Covid-19?, 26 October 2020, https://www.rt.com/op-ed/504625-covid19-flu-disappeared-replaced/.

1587.Jo MacFarlane, Has Covid killed off the flu? Experts pose the intriguing question as influenza cases nosedive by 98% across the globe, Daily Mail, 24 October 2020, https://www.dailymail.co.uk/health/article-8875201/Has-Covid-killed-flu.html.

1588.Vernon Coleman, https://www.vernoncoleman.com/ (last visited on March 16, 2023).

1589.Rhoda Wilson, Was Covid made in a Lab?, The Expose, March 14, 2023, https://expose-news.com/2023/03/14/was-covid-made-in-a-lab/.

1590.What's New in the Guidelines, NIH, May 12, 2020, https://web.archive.org/web/20200602022213/https://www.covid19treatmentguidelines.nih.gov/whats-new/.

1591.Edward Hendrie, Doctor Reveals that Remdesivir Was the Real Cause For Many Alleged COVID-19 Maladies, August 7, 2021, https://greatmountainpublishing.com/2021/08/07/docto r-reveals-that-remdesivir-was-the-real-cause-for-many-alleged-covid-19-maladies/#more-3877.

1592.Potential Antiviral Drugs Under Evaluation for the Treatment of COVID-19, NIH, May 12, 2020, https://web.archive.org/web/20200601162029/https:// www.covid19treatmentguidelines.nih.gov/antiviral-the rapy/.

1593.Edward Hendrie, Doctors Poisoned Test Patients to Falsely Show that Hydroxychloroquine Is Not Safe and Effective, February 15, 2021, https://greatmountainpublishing.com/2021/02/15/docto rs-poisoned-test-patients-to-falsely-show-that-hydroxy chloroquine-is-not-safe-and-effective/.

1594.Fact Sheet for Health Care Providers Emergency Use Authorization (EUA) of Remdesivir (GS-5734™), https://web.archive.org/web/20200603145642/https:// www.fda.gov/media/137566/download (last visited on February 7, 2023).

1595.Fact Sheet EUA Remdesivir, supra.

1596.Jason Goldman, et al., Remdesivir for 5 or 10 Days in Patients with Severe Covid-19, N Engl J Med 2020; 383:1827-1837, DOI: 10.1056/NEJMoa2015301, November 5, 2020, https://www.nejm.org/doi/10.1056/NEJMoa2015301?u rl_ver=Z39.88-2003&rfr_id=ori:rid:crossref.org&rfr_d at=cr_pub%20%200pubmed.

1597.Fact Sheet for Healthcare Providers Emergency Use Authorization (EUA) of Veklury® (Remdesivir) for the Treatment of Coronavirus Disease 2019

(COVID-19) in Pediatric Patients Weighing 3.5 Kg to less than 40 Kg or Pediatric Patients less than 12 Years of Age Weighing at Least 3.5 Kg, with Positive Results of Direct SARS-Cov-2 Viral Testing Who Are: Hospitalized, or Not Hospitalized and Have Mild-to-moderate Covid-19, and Are at High Risk for Progression to Severe COVID-19, Including Hospitalization or Death, https://www.fda.gov/media/137566/download, (REVOKED without explanation) (last visited on February 23, 2023).

1598.Id.

1599.Edward Hendrie, Doctor Reveals that Remdesivir Was the Real Cause For Many Alleged COVID-19 Maladies, August 7, 2021, https://greatmountainpublishing.com/2021/08/07/doctor-reveals-that-remdesivir-was-the-real-cause-for-many-alleged-covid-19-maladies/#more-3877.

1600.Fact Sheet EUA Pediatric Remdesivir, supra.

1601.Clinical Safety Data Management: Definitions and Standards for Expedited Reporting, European Medicines Agency, June 1995, https://www.ema.europa.eu/en/documents/scientific-guideline/international-conference-harmonisation-technical-requirements-registration-pharmaceuticals-human-use_en-15.pdf.

1602.Clinical Study Protocol, Gilead, February 24, 2020, https://www.aifa.gov.it/documents/20142/1131406/GS-US-540-5773_protocollo.pdf/d5a94f66-6791-252c-c705-b534fd6817dd.

1603.Jason Goldman, et al., Remdesivir for 5 or 10 Days in Patients with Severe Covid-19, N Engl J Med 2020; 383:1827-1837, DOI: 10.1056/NEJMoa2015301, November 5, 2020, https://www.nejm.org/doi/10.1056/NEJMoa2015301?url_ver=Z39.88-2003&rfr_id=ori:rid:crossref.org&rfr_dat=cr_pub%20%200pubmed.

1604.Fact Sheet EUA Pediatric Remdesivir, supra.

1605.Sabue Mulangu, et al., A Randomized, Controlled Trial of Ebola Virus Disease Therapeutics, N Engl J Med 2019; 381:2293-2303, DOI: 10.1056/NEJMoa1910993, December 12, 2019, https://www.nejm.org/doi/10.1056/NEJMoa1910993?url_ver=Z39.88-2003&rfr_id=ori:rid:crossref.org&rfr_dat=cr_pub%20%200pubmed.

1606.Ebola virus disease, WHO, 23 February 2021, https://www.who.int/news-room/fact-sheets/detail/ebola-virus-disease.

1607.FDA Approves First Treatment for COVID-19, FDA, October 22, 2020, https://www.fda.gov/news-events/press-announcements/fda-approves-first-treatment-covid-19.

1608.FDA Approves Veklury® (Remdesivir) for the Treatment of Non-Hospitalized Patients at High Risk for COVID-19 Disease Progression, Gilead, January 21, 2022, https://www.gilead.com/news-and-press/press-room/press-releases/2022/1/fda-approves-veklury-remdesivir-for-the-treatment-of-nonhospitalized-patients-at-high-risk-for-covid19-disease-progression#:~:text=(Nasdaq%3A%20GILD)%20today%20announced,to%20severe%20COVID%2D19%2C%20including.

1609.Faye Higbe, First Degree Murder: Remdesivir is Being Used to 'Kill Us', FAIR Foundation USA, January 29, 2022, https://rairfoundation.com/first-degree-murder-remdesivir-is-being-used-to-kill-us/?unapproved=11809&moderation-hash=535614b637d276be64b2c2092c8183d7.

1610.Remdesivir, Popular Timelines, https://populartimelines.com/timeline/Remdesivir#:~:text=Remdesivir%20was%20originally%20created%20and%20developed%20by%20Gilead,for%20Ebola%20virus%20disease%20and%20Marburg%20virus%20infections (last visited on February 23, 2023).

1611.Kevin Hughes, Dr. Bryan Ardis Tells Dr. Peter Breggin: Fauci Is Using Remdesivir to Mass Murder Americans, Based, January 25, 2020, https://basedunderground.com/2022/01/25/dr-bryan-ardis-tells-dr-peter-breggin-fauci-is-using-remdesivir-to-mass-murder-americans/.

1612.26% of those prescribed Remdesivir for COVID died, according to Medicare database, LifeSite News, Sep 29, 2021, https://www.lifesitenews.com/news/26-of-those-prescribed-remdesivir-for-covid-died-according-to-medicare-database/.

1613.WHO recommends against the use of remdesivir in COVID-19 patients, WHO, 20 November 2020, https://www.who.int/news-room/feature-stories/detail/who-recommends-against-the-use-of-remdesivir-in-covid-19-patients.

1614.1/19/2022 ReFounding America: Peter Breggin MD ft. Dr. Bryan Ardis, DC, https://www.brighteon.com/c098f10a-9cca-42c4-9f54-

3cb08d8e5702.

1615.New COVID-19 Treatments Add-On Payment (NCTAP), CMS, https://www.cms.gov/medicare/covid-19/new-covid-19-treatments-add-payment-nctap (last visited on February 7, 2023).

1616.Why You Should Not Use Ivermectin to Treat or Prevent COVID-19, https://www.fda.gov/consumers/consumer-updates/why-you-should-not-use-ivermectin-treat-or-prevent-covid-19 (last visited on September 8, 2021).

1617.Ivermectin for COVID-19: Real-Time Meta Analysis of 63 Studies, September 7, 2021, https://ivmmeta.com/.

1618.Coquin de Chien, Sudden kidney failure, RemDEATHivir, and hidden signals, Substack, October 20, 2022, https://coquindechien.substack.com/p/sudden-kidney-failure-remdeathivir.

1619.Coquin de Chien, October 20, 2022, supra.

1620.Hospitals Are Paid to Kill You, $100,000 per Patient! Dr. Peterson Pierre, MD, January 12, 2022, https://www.bitchute.com/video/qzBbVu1WSw62/.

1621.Mortality rate of COVID-19 patients on ventilators, Physicians Weekly, March 30, 2020, https://www.physiciansweekly.com/mortality-rate-of-covid-19-patients-on-ventilators.

1622.Id.

1623.Safiya Richardson, et al., Presenting Characteristics, Comorbidities, and Outcomes Among 5700 Patients Hospitalized With COVID-19 in the New York City Area, JAMA, April 22, 2020, https://jamanetwork.com/journals/jama/fullarticle/2765184/.

1624.Martin Gould, EXCLUSIVE: 'It's a horror movie.' Nurse working on coronavirus frontline in New York claims the city is 'murdering' COVID-19 patients by putting them on ventilators and causing trauma to the lungs, Daily Mail, 27 April 2020, https://www.dailymail.co.uk/news/article-8262351/Nurse-New-York-claims-city-killing-COVID-19-patients-putting-ventilators.html.

1625.Michelle Rogers, Fact check: Hospitals get paid more if patients listed as COVID-19, on ventilators, USA Today, April 24, 2020, https://www.usatoday.com/story/news/factcheck/2020/04/24/fact-check-medicare-hospitals-paid-more-covid-19-patients-coronavirus/3000638001/.

1626.Michelle Rogers, April 24, 2020, supra.

1627.Michelle Rogers, April 24, 2020, supra.

1628.Covid: The Path not Taken - DarkHorse Podcast with Dr. Peter McCullough, December 6, 2021, https://www.youtube.com/watch?v=-zg1j7Zquoc&t=2959s.

1629.Id.

1630.Truth.bomb.mon, Official Report: Ventilators Killed Nearly ALL COVID Patients, May 13, 2023, https://www.instagram.com/reel/CshUi1rt3Eu/?igshid=

NTc4MTIwNjQ2YQ%3D%3D.

1631.Sean Adl-Tabatabai, Official Report: Ventilators Killed Nearly ALL COVID Patients, The People's Voice, May 13, 2023, https://thepeoplesvoice.tv/official-report-ventilators-killed-nearly-all-covid-patients/.

1632.Sean Adl-Tabatabai, The People's Voice, May 13, 2023, supra.

1633.Catherine A. Gao, et al., Machine learning links unresolving secondary pneumonia to mortality in patients with severe pneumonia, including COVID-19, Journal of Clinical Investigation, April 27, 2023, https://www.jci.org/articles/view/170682.

1634.Sean Adl-Tabatabai, The People's Voice, May 13, 2023, supra.

1635.COVID-19 rapid guideline: managing symptoms (including at the end of life) in the community, National Instituted for Health and Care Excellence, April 3, 2020, https://web.archive.org/web/20200409054527/https://www.nice.org.uk/guidance/ng163/resources/covid19-rapid-guideline-managing-symptoms-including-at-the-end-of-life-in-the-community-pdf-66141899069893.

1636.National Institute for Health and Care Excellence (NICE), https://www.ncbi.nlm.nih.gov/books/NBK310330/ (lat visited on March 6, 2023).

1637.Framework Agreement Between DHSC and NICE, 2018.

1638.Ioannidis JPA. Infection fatality rate of COVID-19 inferred from seroprevalence data. Bull World Health Organ. 2021 Jan 1;99(1):19-33F. doi: 10.2471/BLT.20.265892. Epub 2020 Oct 14. PMID: 33716331; PMCID: PMC7947934. https://pubmed.ncbi.nlm.nih.gov/33716331/.

1639.WHO Coronavirus Dashboard, June 2023, https://covid19.who.int/.

1640.COVID-19 rapid guideline: managing symptoms (including at the end of life) in the community, National Instituted for Health and Care Excellence, April 3, 2020, https://web.archive.org/web/20200409054527/https://www.nice.org.uk/guidance/ng163/resources/covid19-rapid-guideline-managing-symptoms-including-at-the-end-of-life-in-the-community-pdf-66141899069893.

1641.Midazolam Injection, Medline Plus, NIH, National Library of Science, https://medlineplus.gov/druginfo/meds/a609014.html (last visited on March 26, 2023).

1642.Dr. John Campbell, Euthanasia in the pandemic?, February 13, 2023, https://www.youtube.com/watch?v=3BqbVo2sQi0.

1643.COVID-19 rapid guideline: Managing COVID-19, NICE, 27.7 published on 04.01.2023, https://www.nice.org.uk/guidance/ng191/resources/covid19-rapid-guideline-managing-covid19-pdf-51035553326.

1644.The Expose, Kill Elderly, March 25, 2023, supra.

1645.Supplies of sedative used for COVID-19 patients diverted from France to avoid potential shortages, The Pharmaceutical Journal, https://pharmaceutical-journal.com/article/news/supplies-of-sedative-used-for-covid-19-patients-diverted-from-france-to-avoid-potential-shortages (last visited on March 26, 2023).

1646.The Expose, Kill Elderly, March 25, 2023, supra.

1647.The Expose, Kill Elderly, March 25, 2023, supra.

1648.The Expose, Kill Elderly, March 25, 2023, supra.

1649.The Expose, Kill Elderly, March 25, 2023, supra.

1650.Dan Diamond, et al., Vaccine passports' are on the way, but developing them won't be easy, Wahington Post, March 28, 2021, https://archive.is/nyxyf.

1651.Tom Pappert, THEY'RE HERE: Biden Regime Is Developing 'Vaccine Passport' Americans Must Have To Engage In Commerce, March 28, 2021, https://nationalfile.com/theyre-here-biden-regime-is-developing-vaccine-passport-americans-must-have-to-engage-in-commerce/.

1652.Sonia Hickey, World Leaders Sign Declaration to Introduce COVID Vaccine Passports, Sydney Criminal Lawyers, 19 November 2022, https://www.sydneycriminallawyers.com.au/blog/world-leaders-sign-declaration-to-introduce-covid-vaccine-passports/.

1653.Sonia Hickey, World Leaders Sign Declaration to Introduce COVID Vaccine Passports, Sydney Criminal Lawyers, 19 November 2022, https://www.sydneycriminallawyers.com.au/blog/world-leaders-sign-declaration-to-introduce-covid-vaccine-passports/.

1654.Sonia Hickey, World Leaders Sign Declaration to Introduce COVID Vaccine Passports, Sydney Criminal Lawyers, 19 November 2022, https://www.sydneycriminallawyers.com.au/blog/world-leaders-sign-declaration-to-introduce-covid-vaccine-passports/.

1655.Id.

1656.Cyber Company to Supply 50M Health “COVI-PASS(TM)”, AP. May 8, 2020, https://apnews.com/article/technology-business-lifestyle-health-travel-036d8848e9f5eee78b116d3d97e9e5b5.

1657.Id.

1658.Frequently Asked Questions, Covi-Pass, Archived page dated August 31, 2020, https://web.archive.org/web/20200831154023/https://covipass.com/faq/.

1659.Id.

1660.Raul Diego, Mass-Tracking COVI-PASS Immunity Passports Slated to Roll Out in 15 Countries, June 26, 2020, Mint Press News, https://www.mintpressnews.com/mass-tracking-covi-pass-immunity-passports-slated-roll-15-countries/269006/.

1661.Ian Murphy, Tento Health gets Google and Apple app store listing, Enterprise Times, November 9, 2020, https://www.enterprisetimes.co.uk/2020/11/09/tento-health-gets-google-and-apple-app-store-listing/.

1662.Q-servi, https://qservi.com/. (last visited on February 14, 2023).

1663.Q-servi, https://qservi.com/. (last visited on February 14, 2023).

1664.Q-Servi, Your Wallet. Your Data. Your Choice., https://qservi.com/q-wallet/ (last visited on February 14, 2023).

1665.Paul Joseph Watson, Chinese Government Combines 'Track and Trace' Corona System With Social Credit Score, Summit News, 10 September 2020, https://summit.news/2020/09/10/chinese-government-combines-track-and-trace-corona-system-with-social-credit-score/.

1666.Vaccine Requirements at Brown, Healthy Brown, https://healthy.brown.edu/vaccinations#:~:text=Starting%20in%20the%20Fall%202021,level%20of%20in%2Dperson%20instruction (last visited on February 23, 2023).

1667.Id.

1668.Id.

1669.Id.

1670.Id.

1671.Robert Malone, M.D., M.S., New diagnosis codes for COVID-19 immunization status, Substack, January 25, 2023, https://rwmalonemd.substack.com/p/new-diagnosis-codes-for-covid-19.

1672.Id.

1673.CDC updates guidelines for COVID-19 underimmunization codes, National Association of Healthcar Revenue Integrity (NAHRI), Wednesday, January 26, 2022, https://web.archive.org/web/20230125235251/https://nahri.org/articles/cdc-updates-guidelines-covid-19-underimmunization-codes.

1674.Id.

1675.Robert Malone, January 25, 2023, supra.

1676.Reporting Encounters for Immunization Safety Counseling, AAP Pediatric Coding Newsletter, Volume 16, Issue 12, September 2021, https://doi.org/10.1542/pcco_book209_document002.

1677.Robert Malone, January 25, 2023, supra.

1678.Global Digital Health Certification Network, WHO, https://www.who.int/initiatives/global-digital-health-certification-network (last visited on June 11, 2023).

1679.EU Digital COVID Certificate, European Commission, https://commission.europa.eu/strategy-and-policy/coronavirus-response/safe-covid-19-vaccines-europeans/eu-digital-covid-certificate_en (last visited on June 11, 2023).

1680.Christine Rouselle, World Health Organization grants Holy See permanent observer status, Catholic News Agency, June 1, 2021, https://www.catholicnewsagency.com/news/247851/world-health-organization-grants-holy-see-permanent-ob server-status.

1681.HH Pope Francis and WHO Director-General: Health is a right and not a privilege, WHO, 23 Ocober 2018, https://www.who.int/news/item/23-10-2018-hh-pope-francis-and-who-director-general-health-is-a-right-and-not-a-privilege.

1682.On COVID vaccinations, Pope says health care is a 'moral obligation', NPR, January 10, 2022, https://www.npr.org/2022/01/10/1071785531/on-covid-vaccinations-pope-says-health-care-is-a-moral-obligation.

1683.NPR, COVID Vaccinations, January 10, 2022 supra.

1684.VISITING THE VATICAN, U.S. Embassy to the Holy See, https://va.usembassy.gov/visiting-the-vatican/ (last visited on June 11, 2023).

1685.The Jerusalem Bible, Revelation 13:18, at footnote h, (1966), *Nihil Obstat*: Lionel Swain, S.T.L., L.S.S., *Imprimatur*: John Cardinal Heenan, Westminster, July 4, 1966.

1686.*Our Sunday Visitor,* April 18, 1915. The publication is still being published today: 200 Noll Plaza, Huntington, Indiana, 46750, (800) 348-2440.

1687.D.P. SIMPSON, CASSELL'S LATIN DICTIONARY, p. 621, 1968.

1688.COLLIER'S ENCYCLOPEDIA, volume 1, p. 592-96 (1991).

1689.TEXE MARRS, PROJECT L.U.C.I.D., Living Truth Publishers (1996) (citing Antony Sutton, "Why Clinton Wants Universal Health Care," Phoenix Letter, Vol. 13, No. 10, October 1994).

1690.*Id.* at p. 88.

1691.Thomas C Greene, Feds Approve Human RFID Implants, The Register,14 Oct 2004, http://www.theregister.co.uk/2004/10/14/human_rfid_implants/.

1692.VeriChip, Our Products, http://www.verichipcorp.com/products.html (last visited on June 11, 2023).

1693.Thomas C Greene, Feds Approve Human RFID Implants, The Register,14 Oct 2004, http://www.theregister.co.uk/2004/10/14/human_rfid_implants/.

1694.Fisher, Jill A. 2006 "Indoor Positioning and Digital Management: Emerging Surveillance Regimes in Hospitals." In T. Monahan (Ed, Surveillance and Security: Technological Politics and Power in Everyday Life (pp. 77-88). New York: Routledge. Available at: http://www.jillfisher.net/papers/rfid.pdf.

1695.Id.

1696.Fisher, Jill A., supra.

1697.Countries begin negotiations on global agreement to protect world from future pandemic emergencies, WHO, 3 March 2023, https://www.who.int/news/item/03-03-2023-countries-begin-negotiations-on-global-agreement-to-protect-world-from-future-pandemic-emergencies.

1698.Global Digital Health Certification Network, supra.

1699.Peter Andrew, Big New Changes Unveiled for Credit Cards, Fox Business, March 25, 2014, http://www.foxbusiness.com/personal-finance/2014/03/24/big-new-changes-unveiled-for-credit-cards/.

1700.Remarks by President Biden on the Importance of COVID-?19 Vaccine Requirements, Data Center, Clayco Construction Site Elk Grove Village, Illinois, October 7, 2021, https://www.whitehouse.gov/briefing-room/speeches-remarks/2021/10/07/remarks-by-president-biden-on-the-importance-of-covid-19-vaccine-requirements/. See also Executive Order 14043 of September 9, 2021, Requiring Coronavirus Disease 2019 Vaccination for Federal Employees, https://www.federalregister.gov/documents/2021/09/14/2021-19927/requiring-coronavirus-disease-2019-vaccination-for-federal-employees.

1701.Fact Sheet for Recipients and Caregivers Emergency Use Authorization (EUA) of The Moderna COVID-19 Vaccine to Prevent Coronavirus Disease 2019 (Covid-19) in Individuals 18 Years of Age and Older, https://www.fda.gov/media/144638/download.

1702.21 U.S. Code § 360bbb–3(e)(1)(A)(i) (emphasis added).

1703.Emergency Use Authorization of Medical Products and Related Authorities, FDA, January 2017, https://www.fda.gov/media/97321/download.

1704.Department of Health and Human Services Centers for Disease Control and Prevention, Advisory

Committee on Immunization Practices (ACIP), Summary Report, August 26, 2020, Atlanta, Georgia, https://www.cdc.gov/vaccines/acip/meetings/downloads/min-archive/min-2020-08-508.pdf.

1705.Food and Drug Administration (FDA), Center for Biologics Evaluation and Research (CBER) 161st Vaccines and Related Biological Products Advisory Committee (VRBPAC) Meeting, October 22, 2020, https://www.fda.gov/media/143982/download.

1706.Aaron Siri, Federal Law Prohibits Employers and Others from Requiring Vaccination with a Covid-19 Vaccine Distributed under an EUA, February 23, 2021, See also 21 U.S. Code § 360bbb–3.

1707.Emergency Use Authorization of Medical Products and Related Authorities, January 2017, https://www.fda.gov/regulatory-information/search-fda-guidance-documents/emergency-use-authorization-medical-products-and-related-authorities#footnote46.

1708.Id.

1709.Emergency Use Authorization of Medical Products and Related Authorities, January 2017,https://www.fda.gov/regulatory-information/search-fda-guidance-documents/emergency-use-authorization-medical-products-and-related-authorities#eligible.

1710.Dawn Johnsen, Acting Assistant Attorney General Office of Legal Counsel, Whether Section 564 of the Food, Drug, and Cosmetic Act Prohibits Entities from Requiring the Use of a Vaccine Subject to an Emergency Use, MEMORANDUM OPINION FOR THE
DEPUTY COUNSEL TO THE PRESIDENT, July 6,

2021, Authorizationhttps://www.justice.gov/sites/default/files/opinions/attachments/2021/07/26/2021-07-06-mand-vax.pdf

1711.H.R. Rep. No. 108-354, at 782 (2003) (Conf. Rep.) (emphasis added), https://www.congress.gov/congressional-report/108th-congress/house-report/354.

1712.DOD Instruction 6200.02, § E3.4 (Feb. 27, 2008). https://www.esd.whs.mil/Portals/54/Documents/DD/issuances/dodi/620002p.pdf.

1713.Dawn Johnsen, Acting Assistant Attorney General, Office of Legal Counsel, Whether Section 564 of the Food, Drug, and Cosmetic Act Prohibits Entities from Requiring the Use of a Vaccine Subject to an Emergency Use Authorization, Memorandum Opinion for the Deputy Counsel to the President, July 6, 2021, https://www.justice.gov/sites/default/files/opinions/attachments/2021/07/26/2021-07-06-mand-vax.pdf.

1714.Authorization of Emergency Use of Anthrax Vaccine Adsorbed for Prevention of Inhalation Anthrax by Individuals at Heightened Risk of Exposure Due to Attack With Anthrax; Availability, 70 Fed. Reg. 5452, 5455 (Feb. 2, 2005), https://www.federalregister.gov/documents/2005/02/02/05-2028/authorization-of-emergency-use-of-anthrax-vaccine-adsorbed-for-prevention-of-inhalation-anthrax-by.

1715.Authorization of Emergency Use of Anthrax Vaccine Adsorbed for Prevention of Inhalation

Anthrax by Individuals at Heightened Risk of Exposure Due to Attack With Anthrax; Extension; Availability, 70 Fed. Reg. 44,657, 44,659–60 (Aug. 3, 2005).

1716.Guidance Emergency Use Authorization of Medical Products, 2007 WL 2319112, at *15.

1717.Opportunity, American Dictionary of the English Language, https://webstersdictionary1828.com/Dictionary/opportunity

1718.Eric S. Dreiband, Assistant Attorney General, The United States' Statement of Interest in Support of Plaintiff's Motion for an Injunction Pending Appeal, Lighthouse Fellowship Church V. Ralph Northam, Case No. 2:20-cv-00204-awa-rjk, United States District Court, Eastern District of Virginia, May 30, 2020, https://www.justice.gov/opa/press-release/file/1273211/download.

1719.Aaron Siri, Attorney for the Informed Consent Action Network, Letter to Dawn Johnsen, Acting Assistant Attorney General Office of Legal Counsel, August 4, 2021, https://www.icandecide.org/wp-content/uploads/2021/08/Letter-in-Response-to-DOJ-Slip-Opinion-Released-on-July-26-2021.pdf.

1720.Id.

1721.12VAC5-20-100.

1722.367 U.S. 568 (1961).

1723.Id. at 602.

1724.Id. at 603.

1725. See United States v. Harrison, 34 F.3d 886, 891 (9th Cir. 1994).

1726.Ky. Rev. Stat. Ann. § 199.011 (West).

1727.Remarks by President Biden Laying Out the Next Steps in Our Effort to Get More Americans Vaccinated and Combat the Spread of the Delta Variant, July 29, 2021, 4:23 p.m. EDT, https://www.whitehouse.gov/briefing-room/speeches-remarks/2021/07/29/remarks-by-president-biden-laying-out-the-next-steps-in-our-effort-to-get-more-americans-vaccinated-and-combat-the-spread-of-the-delta-variant/.

1728.Nightingale, S. L., Prasher, J. M., & Simonson, S. (2007). Emergency Use Authorization (EUA) to Enable Use of Needed Products in Civilian and Military Emergencies, United States. Emerging Infectious Diseases, 13(7), 1046. https://doi.org/10.3201/eid1307.061188, https://wwwnc.cdc.gov/eid/article/13/7/06-1188_article#r1.

1729.Aaron Siri, Attorney for the Informed Consent Action Network, Letter to Dawn Johnsen, Acting Assistant Attorney General Office of Legal Counsel, August 4, 2021, https://www.icandecide.org/wp-content/uploads/2021/08/Letter-in-Response-to-DOJ-Slip-Opinion-Released-on-July-26-2021.pdf.

1730.Safer Federal Workforce, GSA, https://web.archive.org/web/20210727233714/https:/www.saferfederalworkforce.gov/faq/vaccinations/.

1731.Option, Merriam-Webster Dictionary, https://www.merriam-webster.com/dictionary/option.

1732.PL 93–348 (HR 7724), PL 93–348, JULY 12, 1974, 88 Stat 342, https://www.govinfo.gov/content/pkg/STATUTE-88/pdf/STATUTE-88-Pg342.pdf.

1733.Merlin Duval, Director, Center for Disease Control, Memorandum Terminating the Tuskegee Syphilis Study, November 14, 1972, https://catalog.archives.gov/id/650716.

1734.Id.

1735.Id.

1736.The Belmont Report, Office of the Secretary, Ethical Principles and Guidelines for the Protection of Human Subjects of Research, The National Commission for the Protection of Human Subjects of Biomedical and Behavioral Research, April 18, 1979, https://www.hhs.gov/ohrp/regulations-and-policy/belmont-report/read-the-belmont-report/index.html.

1737.Id (emphasis added).

1738.Part 3 – The Belmont Report: Basic Ethical Principles and their Application, U.S. Department of Health and Human Services, June 16, 2021, Publication Date, October 9, 2018, https://www.youtube.com/watch?v=M6AKIlhoFn4.

1739.Padma Nambisan, in An Introduction to Ethical, Safety and Intellectual Property Rights Issues in Biotechnology, 2017, https://www.sciencedirect.com/topics/medicine-and-dentistry/belmont-report (last visited on August 18,

2021).

1740. Id. (emphasis added).

1741.45 C.F.R. § 46.116, https://www.ecfr.gov/cgi-bin/text-idx?SID=89a8d8aaed03e964d4a9176d34590463&mc=true&node=se45.1.46_1116&rgn=div8 (last visited on August 18, 2021).

1742. See Abdullahi v. Pfizer, 562 F.3d 163, 174-188 (2nd Cir. 2009)..

1743.290 U.S. 398 (1934).

1744.486 F. Supp. 3d 883 (W.D. Pa. 2020), complaint and district court judgment vacated as moot, 8 F.4th 226 (3rd Cir. 2021)).

1745.*City of Butler v. Wolf*, 486 F. Supp. 3d 883 (W.D. Pa. 2020), complaint and district court judgment vacated as moot, 8 F.4th 226 (3rd Cir. 2021)).

1746.Id. at 928.

1747. 197 U.S. 11 (1905).

1748.486 F. Supp. 3d. at 897.

1749.463 F. Supp. 3d 22, (D. Me. 2020).

1750.Id.

1751. 140 S.Ct. 2603 (2020) (Alito, J., dissenting).

1752.Id. at 2604.

1753.Id. at 2605.

1754.Id. at 2608.

1755. Id.

1756. 141 S. Ct. 63, 70 (2020) (Gorsuch, J., concurring).

1757. 141 S. Ct. 63, 70 (2020) (Gorsuch, J., concurring).

1758.Id. at 71.

1759.983 F.3d 620 (2d Cir. 2020).

1760.Id. at 635, citing Jacobson v. Massachusetts, 197 U.S. 11, 25 (1905).

1761.42 USC § 2000e-2.

1762.Mission Hospital Agrees to Pay $89,000 To Settle EEOC Religious Discrimination Lawsuit, Asheville Hospital Fired Employees for Declining Flu Vaccination, Federal Agency Charged, January 12, 2018, https://www.eeoc.gov/newsroom/mission-hospital-agrees-pay-89000-settle-eeoc-religious-discrimination-lawsuit.

1763.600 U.S. ___ (2023), https://www.supremecourt.gov/opinions/22pdf/22-174_k536.pdf.

1764.Saint Vincent Health Center To Pay $300,000 To Settle EEOC Religious Accommodation Lawsuit, Hospital Refused To Grant Employees Religious Belief-Based Exemptions From Flu Vaccination Requirement and Instead Fired Them, Federal Agency Charged, December 23, 2016, https://www.eeoc.gov/newsroom/saint-vincent-health-center-pay-300000-settle-eeoc-religious-accommodation

-lawsuit.

1765.450 U.S. 707 (1981).

1766.Thomas v. Rev. Bd. of Indiana, 450 U.S. 707, 714 (1981).

1767.Id. at 716.

1768.Id. at 718.

1769.508 U.S. 520 (1993).

1770.Id. at 531-32.

1771.Id. at 546.

1772.667 F.3d 727, 740 (6th Cir. 2012).

1773.Id.

1774.Id. at 546-47.

1775.170 F.3d 359 (3d Cir. 1999).

1776.497 U.S. 261 (1990).

1777.Face Masks, Including Surgical Masks, and Respirators for COVID-19, FDA, https://www.fda.gov/medical-devices/coronavirus-covid-19-and-medical-devices/face-masks-including-surgical-masks-and-respirators-covid-19 (last visited on August 19, 2021).

1778.497 U.S. at 279.

1779.497 U.S. at 279.

1780.In Vitro Diagnostics EUAs - Antigen Diagnostic Tests for SARS-CoV-2, FDA, February 17, 2023, https://www.fda.gov/medical-devices/coronavirus-disease-2019-covid-19-emergency-use-authorizations-medical-devices/in-vitro-diagnostics-euas-antigen-diagnostic-tests-sars-cov-2.

1781.Personal Protective Equipment EUAs, FDA, February 9, 2023, https://www.fda.gov/medical-devices/coronavirus-disease-2019-covid-19-emergency-use-authorizations-medical-devices/personal-protective-equipment-euas.

1782.Personal Protective Equipment EUAs, FDA, February 9, 2023, https://www.fda.gov/medical-devices/coronavirus-disease-2019-covid-19-emergency-use-authorizations-medical-devices/personal-protective-equipment-euas.

1783.Interim Infection Prevention and Control Recommendations for Healthcare Personnel During the Coronavirus Disease 2019 (COVID-19) Pandemic, CDC, updated February 2, 2022, https://www.cdc.gov/coronavirus/2019-ncov/hcp/infection-control-recommendations.html#sourcecontrol.

1784.21 USC § 321(h)(1).

1785.Personal Protective Equipment EUAs, FDA, https://www.fda.gov/medical-devices/coronavirus-disease-2019-covid-19-emergency-use-authorizations-medical-devices/personal-protective-equipment-euas (last visited on September 17, 2022).

1786.Blanket Letter of Authorization for Surgical Masks From FDA to Manufacturers of Surgical Masks, August 15, 2022, https://www.fda.gov/media/140894/download.

1787.Blanket Letter of Authorization for Surgical Masks From FDA to Manufacturers of Surgical Masks, August 15, 2022, https://www.fda.gov/media/140894/download.

1788.Requiring Coronavirus Disease 2019 Vaccination for Federal Employees, Exec. Order No. 14043, 86 FR 50989, September 9, 2021.

1789.Feds for Med. Freedom v. Biden, 581 F. Supp. 3d 826 (S.D. Tex. 2022), vacated and remanded, 30 F.4th 503 (5th Cir. 2022), reh'g en banc granted, opinion vacated, 37 F.4th 1093 (5th Cir. 2022), on reh'g en banc, No. 22-40043, 2023 WL 2609247 (5th Cir. 2023), and aff'd, No. 22-40043, 2023 WL 2609247 (5th Cir. 2023).

1790.142 S. Ct. 661 (2022).

1791. 142 S. Ct. at 665.

1792.Feds for Med. Freedom v. Biden, — F.4th ___, No. 22-40043, 2023 WL 2609247 (5th Cir. 2023) (en banc).

1793.ICAN Attorneys Secure Religious Exemption to Vaccination in Mississippi, April 17, 2023, https://icandecide.org/press-release/ican-attorneys-secure-religious-exemption-to-vaccination-in-mississippi/.

1794.Bosarge v. Edney, Verified Complaint for Declaratory and Injunctive Relief, United States District Court Southern District of Mississippi Southern Division, Civil Action No. 1:22-cv-00233-HSO-BWR, Filed September 1, 2022, https://icandecide.org/wp-content/uploads/2023/04/001

-Complaint.pdf.

1795.Tandon v. Newsom, 141 S. Ct. 1294, 1296 (2021) (per curiam).

1796.141 S. Ct. 1294, 1297 (2021) (per curiam).

1797.141 S. Ct. 63 (2020).

1798.Remarks by President Biden Laying Out the Next Steps in Our Effort to Get More Americans Vaccinated and Combat the Spread of the Delta Variant, July 29, 2021, 4:23 p.m. EDT, https://www.whitehouse.gov/briefing-room/speeches-remarks/2021/07/29/remarks-by-president-biden-laying-out-the-next-steps-in-our-effort-to-get-more-americans-vaccinated-and-combat-the-spread-of-the-delta-variant/.

1799. See De Jonge v. Oregon, 299 U.S. 353 (1937).

1800.U.S. Const., Amend. I.

1801.DeJonge, 299 U.S. at 364.

1802.Id. at 364.

1803.U.S. Const. Amend. IX.

1804.Home Building & Loan Ass'n. v. Blaisdell, 290 U.S. 398, 425 (1934).

1805. Wisconsin Legislature v. Palm, 391 Wis. 2d 497, 531, 942 N.W.2d 900, 917 (Wis. 2020).

1806. — U.S. ——, 2020 WL 4251360 (Jul. 24, 2020) (Alito, J., dissenting).

1807.*City of Butler v. Wolf*, 486 F. Supp. 3d 883 (W.D. Pa. 2020), complaint and district court judgment vacated as moot, 8 F.4th 226 (3rd Cir. 2021)).

1808.Id.

1809.Id.

1810.Id.

1811.*See generally Nicholas S. Brod, Rethinking a Reinvigorated Right to Assemble*, 63 DUKE L.J. 155 (2013).

1812.299 U.S. 353 (1937).

1813.Id. at 364.

1814.Id.

1815. Ward v. Rock Against Racism, 491 U.S. 781, 798 (1989).

1816.Id.

1817.Cao, S., Gan, Y., Wang, C. et al. Post-lockdown SARS-CoV-2 nucleic acid screening in nearly ten million residents of Wuhan, China. Nat Commun 11, 5917 (2020). https://doi.org/10.1038/s41467-020-19802-w.

1818.Olivia McCormack, On SNL, Woody Harrelson pushes popular covid-19 conspiracy theory, Washington Post, February 26, 2023, https://www.washingtonpost.com/arts-entertainment/2023/02/26/snl-harrelson-covid-vaccine-monologue/.

1819.Marlow Stern, Woody Harrelson Spreads Anti-Vax Conspiracies During 'SNL' Monologue, Rolling Stone, February 25, 2023, https://www.rollingstone.com/tv-movies/tv-movie-recaps/woody-harrelson-snl-monologue-anti-vax-rant-conspiracy-theory-1234686880/.

1820.Milton J. Rosenau, Experiments to Determine Mode of Spread of Influenza, Journal of the American Medical Association, August 2, 1919, https://zenodo.org/record/1505669#.X6WlDqpKhPZ.

1821.Ollied Reed, Jr., *Social Distancing Born in Abq Teen's Science Project,* Albequerque Journal, May 3, 2020, https://www.abqjournal.com/1450579/social-distancing-born-in-abq-teens-science-project.html.

1822.Michael Spenger, The REAL Story of the Birth of 'Social Distancing' — the Western Term for Lockdown, September 9, 2022, https://www.michaelpsenger.com/p/the-real-story-of-the-birth-of-social.

1823.Michael P. Broderick, Christian J. Hansen, Kevin L. Russell. *Exploration of the Effectiveness of Social Distancing on Respiratory Pathogen Transmission Implicates Environmental Contributions,* The Journal of Infectious Diseases, Volume 198, Issue 10, 15 November 2008, Pages 1420–1426, https://academic.oup.com/jid/article/198/10/1420/856424.

1824.Id.

1825.Id.

1826.Id.

1827.Id. (brackets and parenthesis in original).

1828.Full Transcript: Doctor Destroys 'Utterly Unfounded Public Hysteria' over COVID-19, Life Site News, November 20, 2020, https://www.lifesitenews.com/news/full-transcript-doctor-destroys-utterly-unfounded-public-hysteria-over-covid/.

1829.Great Barrington Declaration, https://gbdeclaration.org/ (last visited on August 29, 2021).

1830.Andrew White, VIDEO: Former Senior Trump HHS COVID Advisor Says Pandemic Isn't Real, 'Task Force' Deliberately Lied To America, National File, August 29, 2021, https://nationalfile.com/video-former-senior-trump-hhs-covid-advisor-says-pandemic-isnt-real-task-force-deliberately-lied-to-america/.

1831.Michael Senger, How Zeynep Tufekci and Jeremy Howard Masked America, The New Normal, March 26, 2023, https://www.michaelpsenger.com/p/how-zeynep-tufekci-and-jeremy-howard.

1832.Mark Changizi, Robert Redfield Testimony, September 16, 2020, https://youtu.be/xzgprJ7mCCw.

1833.Xiao, J., Shiu, E., Gao, H., Wong, J. Y., Fong, M. W., Ryu, S....Cowling, B. J. (2020). Nonpharmaceutical Measures for Pandemic Influenza in Nonhealthcare Settings—Personal Protective and Environmental Measures. Emerging Infectious

Diseases, 26(5), 967-975. https://doi.org/10.3201/eid2605.190994. Also available at: https://wwwnc.cdc.gov/eid/article/26/5/19-0994_article.

1834.Xiao, J., et al., 2020, supra.

1835.American Society for Testing Materials Standard Specification For Barrier Face Coverings (ASTM F3502-23a), last Updated: Apr 20, 2023, https://www.astm.org/f3502-23a.html.

1836.Kai Kisielinski, et al., Physio-metabolic and clinical consequences of wearing face masks—Systematic review with meta-analysis and comprehensive evaluation, Front. Public Health, 05 April 2023, Sec. Environmental health and Exposome, Volume 11 - 2023, https://doi.org/10.3389/fpubh.2023.1125150.

1837.Kai Kisielinski, supra.

1838.Kai Kisielinski, supra.

1839.Kai Kisielinski, supra.

1840.Kai Kisielinski, supra.

1841.Kai Kisielinski, supra.

1842.Headway, Hypoxic and anoxic brain injury, https://www.headway.org.uk/about-brain-injury/individuals/types-of-brain-injury/hypoxic-and-anoxic-brain-injury/#:~:text=If%20the%20oxygen%20supply%20is%20interrupted%2C%20consciousness%20will%20be%20lost,about%20four%20minutes%20without%20oxygen. (last visited on May 3, 2023).

1843.Kai Kisielinski, supra.

1844.Kai Kisielinski, supra.

1845.Kai Kisielinski, supra.

1846.B. Patterson, et al., Unmasking the mask: a time-series analysis of nosocomial COVID-19 rates before and after removal, ECCMID 2023, abstract 5979, April 6, 2023, https://drive.google.com/file/d/1oZ29hRam4CXGqUFxe-Lh-_l-VCqQwXFT/view.

1847.Id.

1848.*St. Michael's Hospital v Ontario Nurses' Association*, 2018 CanLII 82519 (ON LA), <http://canlii.ca/t/htsxg>, retrieved on 2020-11-03.

1849.Michael Klompas, et al., Universal Masking in Hospitals in the Covid-19 Era, New England Journal of Medicine, https://www.nejm.org/doi/full/10.1056/NEJMp2006372.

1850.Denis G. Rancourt, Ph.D., *Masks Don't Work: a Review of Science Relevant to Covid-19 Social Policy,* April 2020, https://www.rcreader.com/sites/default/files/Denis%20G.%20Rancourt%20PhD%20April%202020%20%22Masks%20Don%27t%20Work%3A%20A%20review%20of%20science%20relevant%20to%20COVID-19%20social%20policy%22.pdf.

1851.*Community and Close Contact Exposures Associated with COVID-19 Among Symptomatic Adults =18 Years in 11 Outpatient Health Care Facilities — United States, July 2020, Centers for*

Disease Control, September 11, 2020, https://www.cdc.gov/mmwr/volumes/69/wr/mm6936a5.htm.

1852.Id.

1853.Edward Hendrie, Recent CDC Mask Study is a Scam, February 22, 2022, https://greatmountainpublishing.com/2022/02/22/recent-cdc-mask-study-is-a-scam/.

1854.Vinay Prasad, Mask studies reach a new scientific low point, February 5, 2022, https://vinayprasadmdmph.substack.com/p/mask-studies-reach-a-new-scientific.

1855.Russell Blaylock, *Face Masks Pose Serious Risks To The Healthy*, Technocracy News, May 11, 2020, https://www.technocracy.news/blaylock-face-masks-pose-serious-risks-to-the-healthy/?print=pdf.

1856.Lisa M Brosseau, Sc.D., and Margaret Sietsema, Ph.D., *Masks-for-all for COVID-19 Not Based on Sound Data*, Center for Infectious Disease and Research Policy, University of Minnesota, April 1, 2020, https://www.cidrap.umn.edu/news-perspective/2020/04/commentary-masks-all-covid-19-not-based-sound-data.

1857.Id.

1858.Id.

1859.Th. Goran Tuneval, M.D., *Postoperative Wound Infections and Surgical Face Masks: a Controlled Study*, World Journal of Surgery, May 1991, https://link.springer.com/article/10.1007/BF01658736.

1860.Marilyn M. Singleton, M.D., J.D. VIA AAPS, *Association Of American Physicians And Surgeons Sounds Off On Face Masks*, Technocracy News, July 30, 2020, https://www.technocracy.news/association-of-american-physicians-and-surgeons-sounds-off-on-face-masks/.

1861.Cao, S., Gan, Y., Wang, C. et al. Post-lockdown SARS-CoV-2 nucleic acid screening in nearly ten million residents of Wuhan, China. Nat Commun 11, 5917 (2020). https://doi.org/10.1038/s41467-020-19802-w.

1862.March 2020: Dr. Anthony Fauci talks with Dr Jon LaPook about Covid-19, 60 Minutes, CBS, March 8, 2020, https://www.youtube.com/watch?v=PRa6t_e7dgI&t=1s.

1863.Two Doctors Say Wearing a Mask Hurts Your Immune System, April 25, 2020, https://www.bitchute.com/video/GxN1vsorUhk0/.

1864.Dr. Erickson COVID-19 Briefing, April 22, 2020, https://www.bitchute.com/video/NkiM9fo1Ba0h/.

1865.Katie Mettler, STOP BUYING MASKS': Health Officials Beg Americans to Stop Panic-shopping, Washington Post, March 2, 2020, https://www.washingtonpost.com/health/2020/03/02/n95-face-mask-coronavirus/.

1866.Tyler Durden, "Not Really Effective": Fauci Panned Masks For Preventing COVID-19 Infection In Email, June 02, 2021, https://www.zerohedge.com/political/not-really-effecti

ve-fauci-panned-masks-preventing-covid-19-infection-email.

1867.Katie Mettler, STOP BUYING MASKS’: Health Officials Beg Americans to Stop Panic-shopping, Washington Post, March 2, 2020, https://www.washingtonpost.com/health/2020/03/02/n95-face-mask-coronavirus/.

1868.Katie Mettler, STOP BUYING MASKS': Health Officials Beg Americans to Stop Panic-shopping, Washington Post, March 2, 2020, https://www.washingtonpost.com/health/2020/03/02/n95-face-mask-coronavirus/.

1869.Katie Mettler, STOP BUYING MASKS': Health Officials Beg Americans to Stop Panic-shopping, Washington Post, March 2, 2020, https://www.washingtonpost.com/health/2020/03/02/n95-face-mask-coronavirus/.

1870.Katie Mettler, STOP BUYING MASKS': Health Officials Beg Americans to Stop Panic-shopping, Washington Post, March 2, 2020, https://www.washingtonpost.com/health/2020/03/02/n95-face-mask-coronavirus/.

1871.Talia Kaplan, Surgeon General: Data Doesn't Back Up Wearing Masks in Public Amid Coronavirus Pandemic, Fox News, March 31, 2020, https://www.foxnews.com/media/surgeon-general-explains-masks-public-coronavirus.

1872.President Trump Goes One-On-One with Chris Wallace | Full Interview, Fox News, July 19, 2020, https://www.youtube.com/watch?v=W6XdpDOH1JA.

1873.President Trump and Surgeon General Explain New Guidance on Wearing Face Masks, CBS News, April 2, 2020, https://www.cbsnews.com/video/coronavirus-face-masks-trump-surgeon-general-explain-new-guidance/.

1874.Cao, S., Gan, Y., Wang, C. et al. Post-lockdown SARS-CoV-2 nucleic acid screening in nearly ten million residents of Wuhan, China. Nat Commun 11, 5917 (2020). https://doi.org/10.1038/s41467-020-19802-w.

1875.Russell Blaylock, *Face Masks Pose Serious Risks To The Healthy*, Technocracy News, May 11, 2020, https://www.technocracy.news/blaylock-face-masks-pose-serious-risks-to-the-healthy/?print=pdf.

1876.Russell Blaylock, *Face Masks Pose Serious Risks To The Healthy*, Technocracy News, May 11, 2020, https://www.technocracy.news/blaylock-face-masks-pose-serious-risks-to-the-healthy/?print=pdf.

1877.Russell Blaylock, *Face Masks Pose Serious Risks To The Healthy*, Technocracy News, May 11, 2020, https://www.technocracy.news/blaylock-face-masks-pose-serious-risks-to-the-healthy/?print=pdf.

1878.Blaylock, supra.

1879.Blaylock, supra.

1880.Blaylock, supra.

1881.Blaylock, *Face Masks*. Dr. Blaylock's findings confirm the discovery made by Nobel Laureate Dr. Otto Warburg in 1931.

1882.Blaylock, *Face Masks*.

1883.*Confined or Enclosed Spaces and Other Dangerous Atmospheres » Oxygen-Deficient or Oxygen-Enriched Atmospheres*, Occupational Safety & Health Administration, United States Department of Labor, https://www.osha.gov/SLTC/etools/shipyard/shiprepair/confinedspace/oxygendeficient.html.

1884.Official Letter of Standard Interpretation from Richard E. Fairfax, Director of the Directorate of Enforcement Programs to Mr. William Costello, Vice President, FirePASS Corporation, April 2, 2007, https://www.osha.gov/laws-regs/standardinterpretations/2007-04-02-0.

1885.*Confined or Enclosed Spaces and Other Dangerous Atmospheres » Oxygen-Deficient or Oxygen-Enriched Atmospheres*, Occupational Safety & Health Administration, United States Department of Labor, https://www.osha.gov/SLTC/etools/shipyard/shiprepair/confinedspace/oxygendeficient.html.

1886.*Documentary: Everything You Need to Know about Covering Breathing Airways*, at 32:00 mark of the video, July 8, 2020, https://www.bitchute.com/video/N4wevCMjpxrY/.

1887.Christina Carrega, *Driver in Crash May Have Passed out from Wearing N95 Mask Too Long: Police*, ABC News, April 25, 2020, https://abcnews.go.com/US/driver-crash-passed-wearing-n95-mask-long-police/story?id=70346532.

1888.COVID-19 Frequently Asked Questions, https://www.osha.gov/coronavirus/faqs (last visited on September 3, 2021).

1889.Official Letter of Standard Interpretation from Richard E. Fairfax, Director of the Directorate of Enforcement Programs to Mr. William Costello, Vice President, FirePASS Corporation, April 2, 2007, https://www.osha.gov/laws-regs/standardinterpretations/2007-04-02-0.

1890.Samantha Chang, Disgusting Discovery: 2 Moms Send Kids' Masks to Lab for Analysis, Learn How Dangerous They Really Are, The Western Journal, June 8, 2021, https://www.westernjournal.com/disgusting-discovery-2-moms-send-kids-masks-lab-analysis-learn-dangerous-really/. See also Jennifer Cabrera, Dangerous pathogens found on children's face masks, Rational Ground, June 16, 2021, https://rationalground.com/dangerous-pathogens-found-on-childrens-face-masks/.

1891.Jennifer Cabrera, Dangerous pathogens found on children's face masks, Rational Ground, June 16, 2021, https://rationalground.com/dangerous-pathogens-found-on-childrens-face-masks/.

1892.Dr. Margarite Griesz-Brisson M.D., Ph.D., https://www.londonneurology.com/dr-margareta-griesz-brisson.

1893.Brain Damage From Masks CANNOT BE REVERSED, Health and Money News, October 9, 2020, https://web.archive.org/web/20201111225939/https://healthandmoneynews.wordpress.com/2020/10/09/brain-damage-from-masks-cannot-be-reversed/.

1894.Sayer Ji, ALERT: Meta-Analysis of 65 Studies Reveals Face Masks Induce Mask-Induced Exhaustion Syndrome (MIES), April 25, 2021, https://www.sgtreport.com/2021/04/alert-meta-analysis-of-65-studies-reveals-face-masks-induce-mask-induced-exhaustion-syndrome-mies/. See also https://www.greenmedinfo.com/blog/alert-meta-analysis-65-studies-reveals-face-masks-induce-mask-induced-exhaustion-.

1895.Kisielinski, Kai, Paul Giboni, Andreas Prescher, Bernd Klosterhalfen, David Graessel, Stefan Funken, Oliver Kempski, and Oliver Hirsch. 2021. "Is a Mask That Covers the Mouth and Nose Free from Undesirable Side Effects in Everyday Use and Free of Potential Hazards?" International Journal of Environmental Research and Public Health 18, no. 8: 4344. https://doi.org/10.3390/ijerph18084344.

1896.Id.

1897.Id.

1898.Id.

1899.Id.

1900.Id.

1901.Id.

1902.Id.

1903.Id.

1904.Id.

1905.Id.

1906.Zacharias Fögen, The Foegen effect: A mechanism by which facemasks contribute to the COVID-19
case fatality rate, 2022, https://jdfor2024.com/wp-content/uploads/2022/05/The_Foegen_effect__A_mechanism_by_which_facemasks.60.pdf.

1907.Id.

1908.Id.

1909.Id.

1910.Id.

1911.Amanda Brown, Study finds plastics found in masks present in patients' lungs, Western Standard, April 17, 2022, https://www.westernstandard.news/features/study-finds-plastics-found-in-masks-present-in-patients-lungs/article_056590f2-0615-5bc9-aab0-730e7704634e.html.

1912.Id.

1913.Id.

1914.Lu Li, et al., COVID-19: Performance study of microplastic inhalation risk posed by wearing masks, NIH, June 5, 2021, https://www.ncbi.nlm.nih.gov/pmc/articles/PMC7773316/.

1915.Collen Huber, Collen Huber, Q Maeeta, Masks, false safety and real dangers, Part 1: Friable mask particulate and lung vulnerability, Primary Doctor Medical Journal, July 6, 2020, https://pdmj.org/papers/masks_false_safety_and_real_

dangers_part1#10.

1916.Carla Peters, Why Mask Mandates Should be Repealed Immediately, Brownstone Institute, November 15, 2021, https://brownstone.org/articles/why-mask-mandates-should-be-immediately-banned/.

1917.Id.

1918.Eveline Verleysena, et al., Titanium dioxide particles frequently present in face masks intended for general use require regulatory control, 15 February 2022, Nature, https://www.nature.com/articles/s41598-022-06605-w.

1919.Id.

1920.Id.

1921.Carla Peters, Have the Children Been Poisoned?, Brownstone Institute, March 15, 2022, https://brownstone.org/articles/have-the-children-been-poisoned/.

1922.Id.

1923.Carla Peters, Why Mask Mandates Should be Repealed Immediately, Brownstone Institute, November 15, 2021, https://brownstone.org/articles/the-health-risks-of-graphene/.

1924.Lingling Ou, et al., Toxicity of graphene-family nanoparticles: a general review of the origins and mechanisms, Particle and Fibre Toxicology, 2016, https://www.ncbi.nlm.nih.gov/pmc/articles/PMC5088662/pdf/12989_2016_Article_168.pdf.

1925.Pedro A. Ruiz, et al., Titanium dioxide nanoparticles exacerbate DSS-induced colitis: role of the NLRP3 inflammasome, Gut Online, BMJ Publishing Group, 2015, https://gut.bmj.com/content/gutjnl/early/2016/03/16/gutjnl-2015-310297.full.pdf?with-ds=yes.

1926.Carla Peters, How Masking Contributes to Long Covid, Brownstone Institute, August 12, 2022, https://brownstone.org/articles/how-masking-contributes-to-long-covid/.

1927.Edward Hendrie, States With Mask Mandates Have Greater Number of COVID-19 Cases, December 22, 2020, https://greatmountainpublishing.com/2020/12/22/states-with-mask-mandates-have-greater-number-of-covid-19-cases/.

1928.Lim EC, Seet RC, Lee KH, Wilder-Smith EP, Chuah BY, Ong BK. Headaches and the N95 face-mask amongst healthcare providers. Acta Neurol Scand. 2006 Mar;113(3):199-202. doi: 10.1111/j.1600-0404.2005.00560.x. PMID: 16441251; PMCID: PMC7159726. https://pubmed.ncbi.nlm.nih.gov/16441251/.

1929.Michela Cimberle, PPE-associated headaches increase among health care workers amid COVID-19, April 7, 2020, https://www.healio.com/news/primary-care/20200407/ppeassociated-headaches-increase-among-health-care-workers-amid-covid19.

1930.What Are Migraine Symptoms?, Cove, https://www.withcove.com/learn/what-are-migraine-symptoms (last visited on February 21, 2023).

1931.How to Avoid Migraine Triggers While Wearing Your Mask, Cove, https://www.withcove.com/learn/migraine-triggers-mask (last visited on February 21, 2023).

1932.Russell Blaylock, Blaylock: Face Masks Pose Serious Risks To The Healthy, Technocracy News & Trends, May 11, 2020, https://www.technocracy.news/blaylock-face-masks-pose-serious-risks-to-the-healthy/.

1933.Coronavirus Disease 2019 (COVID-19) 2020 Interim Case Definition, Approved April 5, 2020, CDC, April 5, 2020, https://ndc.services.cdc.gov/case-definitions/coronavirus-disease-2019-2020/.

1934.Id.

1935.Erin Anderson, Texas' New Coronavirus Criteria Could Artificially Spike Collin County Cases, Texas Scorecard, May 26, 2020, https://texasscorecard.com/local/texas-new-coronavirus-criteria-could-artificially-spike-collin-county-cases/.

1936.Coronavirus Disease 2019, April 5, 2020, supra.

1937.Erin Anderson, Texas' New Coronavirus Criteria Could Artificially Spike Collin County Cases, Texas Scorecard, May 26, 2020, https://texasscorecard.com/local/texas-new-coronavirus-criteria-could-artificially-spike-collin-county-cases/.

1938.Id.

1939.Erin Anderson, supra.

1940.Coronavirus Disease 2019, April 5, 2020, supra.

1941.Ian Miller, @IanmSC, Twitter, March 26, 2022, https://twitter.com/ianmSC/status/1507779461097279488/photo/1.

1942.Frankie Stokes, Virginia: Child COVID Cases Have Dropped by 93% Since Youngkin Lifted School Mask Mandates, National File, March 29, 2022, https://nationalfile.com/virginia-child-covid-cases-have-dropped-by-93-since-youngkin-lifted-school-mask-mandates/.

1943.Frankie Stokes. National File, supra.

1944.Mask Guidance, CDC, March 21, 2022, https://www.cdc.gov/coronavirus/2019-ncov/easy-to-read/mask-guidance.html. Order: Wearing of face masks while on conveyances and at transportation hubs, CDC, April 18, 2022, https://www.cdc.gov/quarantine/masks/mask-travel-guidance.html.

1945.Frankie Stokes, National File, supra

1946.Nicholas Wu, Fauci Wears a Mask as a 'Symbol' of What 'You Should Be Doing' amid Coronavirus Pandemic, USA Today, May 27, 2020, https://www.usatoday.com/story/news/politics/2020/05/27/coronavirus-fauci-says-he-wears-mask-symbol-what-do/5266189002/.

1947.Nicholas Wu, USA Today, May 27, 2020, supra.

1948.Nicholas Wu, USA Today, May 27, 2020, supra.

1949.Lauren Mascarenhas, Amid Coronavirus Surge, Health Officials Urge People to Wear Masks as a Symbol of Respect, CNN, July 13, 2020, https://www.cnn.com/2020/07/13/health/masks-respect

-coronavirus-wellness/index.html?utm_source=feedburner&utm_medium=feed&utm_campaign=Feed%3A+rss%2Fcnn_health+%28RSS%3A+CNN+-+Health%29.

1950.Lauren Mascarenhas, CNN, July 13, 2020, supra.

1951.Lauren Mascarenhas, CNN, July 13, 2020, supra.

1952.Lauren Mascarenhas, CNN, July 13, 2020, supra.

1953.Michael Senger, How Zeynep Tufekci and Jeremy Howard Masked America, The New Normal, March 26, 2023, https://www.michaelpsenger.com/p/how-zeynep-tufekci-and-jeremy-howard.

1954.Id.

1955.Id.

1956.Symbol, https://www.merriam-webster.com/dictionary/symbol.

1957.Symbol, https://www.merriam-webster.com/dictionary/symbol.

1958.United States v. United Foods, Inc., 533 U.S. 405, 410 (2001).

1959.Wooley v. Maynard, 430 U.S. 705, 714 (1977).

1960.Wooley v. Maynard, 430 U.S. 705, 714 (1977).

1961.Katie Mettler, STOP BUYING MASKS': Health Officials Beg Americans to Stop Panic-shopping, Washington Post, March 2, 2020, https://www.washingtonpost.com/health/2020/03/02/n95-face-mask-coronavirus/.

1962.Symbol,
https://www.merriam-webster.com/dictionary/symbol.

1963.The Functions and Forms of Masks, The Encyclopedia Britannica, https://www.britannica.com/art/mask-face-covering/The-functions-and-forms-of-masks (last visited on September 4, 2021).

1964.Gayland Hurst and Robert Marsh, Satanic Occult Awareness, National Criminal Justice Reference Service, January 27, 1993, https://www.ojp.gov/pdffiles1/Photocopy/140554NCJRS.pdf.

1965.The Wearing of Masks, The Encyclopedia Britannica, https://www.britannica.com/art/mask-face-covering/The-wearing-of-masks (last visited on September 4, 2021).

1966.The Satanic Temple Presents Satancon, https://archive.is/zf48L#selection-1389.0-1389.195 (last visited on February 22, 2023).

1967.See generally Sch. Dist. of Abington Twp., Pa. v. Schempp, 374 U.S. 203 (1963).

1968.Lauren Mascarenhas, Amid Coronavirus Surge, Health Officials Urge People to Wear Masks as a Symbol of Respect, CNN, July 13, 2020, https://www.cnn.com/2020/07/13/health/masks-respect-coronavirus-wellness/index.html?utm_source=feedburner&utm_medium=feed&utm_campaign=Feed%3A+rss%2Fcnn_health+%28RSS%3A+CNN+-+Health%29.

1969.Philip Buckler, The Book on Masks, at 672-73 (2023).

1970.Hans J. Hillerbrand, ed., The Reformation: A Narrative History Related by Contemporary Observers and Participants. New York, 1964, pp. 41-43. Retrieved from: https://archive.org/details/reformationnarra00hill/page/42/mode/2up?view=theater, quoted in Philip Buckler, The Book on Masks, at 672-73 (2023).

1971.Buckler, at 673.

1972.Buckler, at 659.

1973.508 U.S. 520 (1993).

1974.Id. at 546-47.

1975.U.S. Const. amend. I.

1976.268 U.S. 652 (1925),

1977.Wellcome Trust Centre for Neuroimaging at UCL, Centre of Functionally Integrative Neuroscience, University of Aarhus, Aarhus, Denmark, *Role of Facial Expressions in Social Interactions*, National Institutes of Health, December 12, 2020.

1978.Id.

1979.393 U.S. 503 (1969).

1980.491 U.S. 397 (1989).

1981.Id. at 404.

1982.Id. at 416.

1983.*Ward v. Rock Against Racism*, 491 U.S. 781 (1989).

1984.Blaylock RL. COVID UPDATE: What is the truth? Surg Neurol Int. 2022 Apr 22;13:167. doi: 10.25259/SNI_150_2022. PMID: 35509555; PMCID: PMC9062939, https://www.ncbi.nlm.nih.gov/pmc/articles/PMC9062939/.

1985.Blaylock RL. COVID UPDATE: What is the truth? Surg Neurol Int. 2022 Apr 22;13:167. doi: 10.25259/SNI_150_2022. PMID: 35509555; PMCID: PMC9062939, https://www.ncbi.nlm.nih.gov/pmc/articles/PMC9062939/.

1986.Ausman JI, Blaylock RL. What is the truth? United States: James I. and Carolyn R. Ausman Education Foundation (AEF); 2021. The China Virus. Blaylock RL. Covid-19 pandemic: What is the truth? Surg Neurol Inter. 2021;12(151). Parpia R. Mayo Clinic fires 700 employees for refusing to get Covid-19 vaccinations. The Vaccine Reaction. https://thevaccinereaction.org/2022/01/mayo-clinic-fires-700-employees-for-refusing-to-get-covid-19-vaccinations [Last accessed on 2022 Feb 06].

1987.Front Line Covid Critical Care Alliance. https://covid19criticalcare.com [Last accessed on 2022 Feb 06]. Kennedy R., Jr . Skyhorse Publishing; 2021. The Real Anthony Fauci. Bill Gates, Big Pharma, and the Global War on Democracy and Public Health; p. 135.

1988.Front Line Covid Critical Care Alliance. https://covid19criticalcare.com [Last accessed on 2022

Feb 06].

1989.McCullough P, Kelly R, Ruocco G, Lerma E, Tumlin J, Wheeland KR, et al. Pathophysiological basis and rationale for early outpatient treatment of SARS-CoV-2 (COVID-19) Infection. Amer J Med. 2021;134:16–22.

1990.Albright L. Medical nonconformity and its persecution. Brownstone Institute. https://brownstone.org/articles/medical-nonconformaity-and-its-persecution [Last accessed on 2022 Feb 06].

1991.Blaylock RL. Haciendia Publishing; When rejecting orthodoxy becomes a mental illness. Aug 15, 2013 https://haciendapublishing.com/when-rejecting-orthodoxy-becomes-a-mental-illness-by-russell-l-blaylock-m-d [Last accessed on 2022 Feb 06]. Saxena V. Doctors loses medical license. Ordered to have Psych Eval for Ivermectin Scrits, Sharing Covid "misinformation" BRP News. Available from: https://bizpacreview.com/2022/01/16/doctor-loses-license-orderedto-have-psych-eval-for-prescribing-ivermectin-sharining-covid-falsehoods-1189313. [Last accessed on 2022 Feb 06].

1992.Breggin PR, Breggin GR. Breggin PR, Breggin GR. Covid-19 and the Global Predators: We are the Prey. Ithaca, NY: Lake Edge Press; 2021. Top Medical Journals Sell their Souls; pp. 285–292. Ross E. How drug companies' PR tactics skew the presentation of medical research. The Guardian. https://www.theguardian.com/science/2011/may/20/drug-companies-ghost-writing-journalism [Last accessed on 2022 Feb 06].

1993.Breggin PR, Breggin GR. Breggin PR, Breggin GR. Covid-19 and the Global Predators: We are the Prey. Ithaca, NY: Lake Edge Press; 2021. Top Medical Journals Sell their Souls; p. 133. Kennedy R., Jr . Skyhorse Publishing; 2021. The Real Anthony Fauci. Bill Gates, Big Pharma, and the Global War on Democracy and Public Health; pp. 26-30, 32.

1994.Moffatt B, Elliott C. Ghost Marketing: Pharmaceutical companies and ghostwritten journal articles. Persp Biol Med. 2007;50(1):18–31. Saul S. Ghostwriters used in Vioxx studies, article says. New York Times. April 15, 2008 https://www.fpparchive.org/media/documents/public_policy/Ghostwriters%20Used%20in%20Vioxx%20studies_Stephanie%20Saul_Apr%2015,%202008_The%20New%20Times.pdf [Last accessed on 2022 Feb 06].

1995.Breggin PR, Breggin GR. Breggin PR, Breggin GR. Covid-19 and the Global Predators: We are the Prey. Ithaca, NY: Lake Edge Press; 2021. Top Medical Journals Sell their Souls; p. 133. Ross E. How drug companies' PR tactics skew the presentation of medical research. The Guardian. https://www.theguardian.com/science/2011/may/20/drug-companies-ghost-writing-journalism [Last accessed on 2022 Feb 06].

1996.Moffatt B, Elliott C. Ghost Marketing: Pharmaceutical companies and ghostwritten journal articles. Persp Biol Med. 2007;50(1):18–31. Ross E. How drug companies' PR tactics skew the presentation of medical research. The Guardian. https://www.theguardian.com/science/2011/may/20/drug-companies-ghost-writing-journalism [Last accessed on 2022 Feb 06].

1997.Bosh X, Ross JS. Ghostwriting: Research misconduct, plagiarism, or Fool's gold. Amer J Med. 2012;125(4):324–6.

1998.Bulik BS. The top 10 ad spenders in Big Pharma for 2020. Fierce Pharma Apr 19, 2021 https://www.fiercepharma.com/special-report/top-10-ad-spenders-big-pharma-for-2020 [Last accessed on 2022 Feb 06].

1999.Bulik BS. The top 10 ad spenders in Big Pharma for 2020. Fierce Pharma Apr 19, 2021 https://www.fiercepharma.com/special-report/top-10-ad-spenders-big-pharma-for-2020 [Last accessed on 2022 Feb 06]. Breggin PR, Breggin GR. Breggin PR, Breggin GR. Covid-19 and the Global Predators: We are the Prey. Ithaca, NY: Lake Edge Press; 2021. Top Medical Journals Sell their Souls; p. 133.

2000.Bulik BS. The top 10 ad spenders in Big Pharma for 2020. Fierce Pharma Apr 19, 2021 https://www.fiercepharma.com/special-report/top-10-ad-spenders-big-pharma-for-2020 [Last accessed on 2022 Feb 06].

2001.Kennedy R., Jr . Skyhorse Publishing; 2021. The Real Anthony Fauci. Bill Gates, Big Pharma, and the Global War on Democracy and Public Health; pp. 24–25. Parpia R. Mayo Clinic fires 700 employees for refusing to get Covid-19 vaccinations. The Vaccine Reaction. https://thevaccinereaction.org/2022/01/mayo-clinic-fires-700-employees-for-refusing-to-get-covid-19-vaccinations [Last accessed on 2022 Feb 06].

2002.McCullough P. "We're in the middle of a major biological catastrophe": Covid expert Dr. Peter

McCullough. 2021. Oct 6, https://www.lifesitenews.com/news/were-in-the-middle-of-a-major-biological-catastrophe-top-covid-doc-mccullough/?_kx=9EtupqemhhFXJ1kgCo9W3xUNfwrkqB5nT7V2H15fUnA%3D.WXNMR7 [Last accessed on 2022 Feb 06].

2003.Mulvany C. Covid-19 exacerbates bankruptcy for at-risk hospitals. Health Care Financial Management Association. 2020. Nov 9.

2004.Bloche MG. Corporate takeover of Teaching Hospitals. Georgetown Univ Law Center. 1992. https://scholarship.law.georgetown.edu/cgi/viewcontent.cgi?referer=https://www.google.com/&httpsredir=1&article=1731&context=facpub [Last accessed on 2022 Feb 06].

2005.Abelson R. Buoyed by federal Covid aid, big hospital chains buy up competitors. The New York Times Mat 21, 2021 (updated Oct 22, 2022) https://www.nytimes.com/2021/05/21/health/covid-bailout-hospital-merger.html. Noether M, Mat S. Hospital merger benefits: Views from hospital leaders and econometric analysis. Amer Hospital Assoc. Charles Rivers Associates. Jan, 2017 https://www.aha.org/guidesreports/2017-01-24-hospital-merger-benefits-views-hospital-leaders-and-econometric-analysis [Last accessed on 2022 Feb 06].

2006.Muoio D. How many employees have hospitals lost to vaccine mandates? Here are the numbers so far. Fierce Healthcare. 2022. Jan 13, https://www.fiercehealthcare.com/hospitals/how-many-employees-have-hospitals-lost-to-vaccine-mandates-numbers-so-far [Last accessed on 2022 Feb 06]. Parpia R. Mayo Clinic fires 700 employees for refusing to get

Covid-19 vaccinations. The Vaccine Reaction. https://thevaccinereaction.org/2022/01/mayo-clinic-fires-700-employees-for-refusing-to-get-covid-19-vaccinations [Last accessed on 2022 Feb 06].

2007.Coleman-Lochner L. U.S. Hospitals pushed to financial ruin as nurses quit during pandemic. Bloomberg. Dec 21, 2021 https://www.bloomberg.com/news/articles/2021-12-21/u-s-hospitals-pushed-to-financial-ruin-as-nurses-quit-en-masse [Last accessed on 2022 Feb 06]. Muoio D. How many employees have hospitals lost to vaccine mandates? Here are the numbers so far. Fierce Healthcare. 2022. Jan 13, https://www.fiercehealthcare.com/hospitals/how-many-employees-have-hospitals-lost-to-vaccine-mandates-numbers-so-far [Last accessed on 2022 Feb 06].

2008.Marik PE, Kory P, Varon J, Iglesias J, Meduri GU. MATH+ protocol for the treatment oof SARS-CoV-2 infection: the scientific rationale. Exp rev Ant-infective Ther. 2020 doi: 10.1080/14787210.2020.1808462. McCullough P, Kelly R, Ruocco G, Lerma E, Tumlin J, Wheeland KR, et al. Pathophysiological basis and rationale for early outpatient treatment of SARS-CoV-2 (COVID-19) Infection. Amer J Med. 2021;134:16–22.

2009.Id.

2010.Rancourt DG. Mask don't work. A review of science relevant to the covid-19 social policy. https://archive.org/details/covid-censorship-at-research-gate-2 [Last accessed on 2022 Feb 06].

2011.Chughtai AA, Stelzer-Braid S, Rawlinson W, Pontivivi G, Wang Q, Pan Y, et al. Contamination by respiratory viruses on outer surface of medical mask used by hospital healthcare workers. BMC Infect Dis. 2019. Article number 491.

2012.Lee M. University of Florida finds dangerous pathogens on children's face mask. NTD https://www.ntd.com/university-of-florida-lab-finds-dangerous-pathogens-on-childrens-face-masks_630275.html [Last accessed on 2022 Feb 06].

2013.Beder A, Buyukkocak U, Sabuncuoglu H, Keskil ZA, Keskil S. Preliminary report on surgical mask induced deoxygenation during major surgery. Neurocirugia. 2008;19. Westendorf AM, et al. Hypoxia enhances immunosuppression by inhibiting CD4+ effector T cell function and promoting Treg activity. Cell Physiol Biochem. 2017;41:1271–84. Nalivaeva NN, Turner AJ, Zhuravin IA. Role of prenatal hypoxia in brain development, cognitive functions, and neurodegeneration. Front Neurosci. 2018 doi: 10.3389/fnins.2018.00825.

2014.D'Souza K. Pandemic effects may have lowered baby's IQs, study says EdSource. https://edsource.org/2021/pandemic-may-have-lowered-baby-iq-study-says/661285.

2015.New York Post. Post Editorial Board Facebook admits the truth: "Fact checks" are just (lefty) opinion. Dec 14,2021. https://nypost.com/2021/12/14/facebook-admits-the-truth-fact-checks-are-really-just-lefty-opinion [Last accessed on 2022 Feb 06].

2016.Ioannou P, Karakonstantis S, Astrinaki E, Saplamidou S, Vitsaxaki E, Hamilos G, et al. Transmission of SARS-C0V-2 variant B1.1.7 among vaccinated health care workers. Infect Dis. 2021:1–4. Loffredo J. Fully vaccinated are Covid 'Superspreaders' Says inventor of mRNA technology. https://childrenshealthdefernce.org/defender/justin-Williams-Robert-Malone-fully-vaccinated-covid-super-spreaders [Last accessed on 2022 Feb 06]. McCullough P. Study: Fully vaccinated healthcare workers carry 251 times viral load, pose threat to unvaccinated patients, Co-workers. The Defender 08/23/21.

2017.Katz E. Postal service seeks temporary exemption from Biden's vaccine-or-test mandate. Government Executive. 2022. Jan 22, https://www.govexec.com/workforce/2022/01/postal-service-seeks-temporary-exemption-bidens-vaccine-or-test-mandate/360376 [Last accessed on 2022 Feb 06]. Roche D. Boston Herald. 2021. Sept 14, Members of Congress and their staff are exempt from Biden's vaccine mandate, Newsweek 9/10/21 Boston Herald Editorial Staff. Editorial: Political elites exempt from vax mandates.

2018.Redshaw M. As reports of injuries after Covid vaccines near 1 million mark. CDC, FDA clear Pfizer, Moderna boosters for all adults. The Defender 11/19/21.

2019.Children's Health Defense Team Harvard experts critique cozy FDA-Pharma relationship. The Defender. Jan 28, 2020. Sen. Ron Johnson on Covid-19 vaccine injuries to test subjects. https://www.youtube.com/watch?v=6mxqC9SiRh8 [Last accessed on 2022 Feb 06].

2020.Kennedy R., Jr . Skyhorse Publishing; 2021. The Real Anthony Fauci. Bill Gates, Big Pharma, and the Global War on Democracy and Public Health; pp.

24–29. Marik PE, Kory P, Varon J, Iglesias J, Meduri GU. MATH+ protocol for the treatment oof SARS-CoV-2 infection: the scientific rationale. Exp rev Ant-infective Ther. 2020 doi: 10.1080/14787210.2020.1808462.

2021.Kennedy R., Jr . Skyhorse Publishing; 2021. The Real Anthony Fauci. Bill Gates, Big Pharma, and the Global War on Democracy and Public Health; pp. 24–25, 35-56.

2022.Kennedy R., Jr, Fauci, supra, pp. 24–25.

2023.Front Line Covid Critical Care Alliance. https://covid19criticalcare.com [Last accessed on 2022 Feb 06].

2024.Mercola J. Bill Gates and Anthony Fauci: a 'formidable, nefarious' partnership. Mercola.com. https://childrenshealthdefense.org/defender/rfk-jr-the-real-anthony-fauci-bill-gates [Last accessed on 2022 Feb 06]. Children's Health Defense Team Harvard experts critique cozy FDA-Pharma relationship. The Defender. Jan 28, 2020.

2025.Kennedy R., Jr., Fauci, supra, pp. 26–30.

2026.Front Line Covid Critical Care Alliance. https://covid19criticalcare.com [Last accessed on 2022 Feb 06].

2027.Kennedy R., Jr . Skyhorse Publishing; 2021. The Real Anthony Fauci. Bill Gates, Big Pharma, and the Global War on Democracy and Public Health; pp. 47-56. Marik PE, Kory P, Varon J, Iglesias J, Meduri GU. MATH+ protocol for the treatment oof SARS-CoV-2 infection: the scientific rationale. Exp rev Ant-infective

Ther. 2020 doi: 10.1080/14787210.2020.1808462.

2028.Kennedy R., Jr. Fauci, supra, pp. 24–29.

2029.Coleman-Lochner L. U.S. Hospitals pushed to financial ruin as nurses quit during pandemic. Bloomberg. Dec 21, 2021 https://www.bloomberg.com/news/articles/2021-12-21/u-s-hospitals-pushed-to-financial-ruin-as-nurses-quit-en-masse [Last accessed on 2022 Feb 06]. Jimenez J, Vigdor N. Covid-19 news: Over 150 Texas hospital workers are fired or resign over vaccine mandates. The New York Times. 2021 Jun 22, https://www.nytimes.com/live/2021/06/22/world/covid-vaccine-coronavirus-mask [Last accessed on 2022 Feb 06]. Muoio D. How many employees have hospitals lost to vaccine mandates? Here are the numbers so far. Fierce Healthcare. 2022 Jan 13, https://www.fiercehealthcare.com/hospitals/how-many-employees-have-hospitals-lost-to-vaccine-mandates-numbers-so-far [Last accessed on 2022 Feb 06].

2030.Sen. Ron Johnson on Covid-19 vaccine injuries to test subjects. https://www.youtube.com/watch?v=6mxqC9SiRh8 [Last accessed on 2022 Feb 06].

2031.Schwab K, Malleret T. Cologny/Geneva: The Covid-19 Pandemic and the Great Reset. Forum Publishing 2020 World Economic Forum.

2032.Huff E. Idaho doctor reports “20 times increase” in cancer among those “vaccinated” for covid. Natural News. 2021 Sept 14, https://www.naturalnews.com/2021-09-14-idaho-doctor-20times-increase-cancer-vaccinated-covid.html [Last accessed on 2022 Feb 06].

2033.McGovern C. Thousands report developing abnormal tumors following Covid shots. LifeSite News. Nov 1, 2021 https://www.lifesitenews.com/news/thousands-report-developing-abnormal-tumors-following-covid-shots [Last accessed on 2022 Feb 06].

2034.Jiang H, Mei Y-F. SARS-CoV-2 spike protein impairs DNA damage repair and inhibits V(D)J recombination in vitro. Viruses. 2021;13:2056. doi: 10.3390/10.3390/v13102056.

2035.Kennedy R., Jr., Fauci, supra, pp. 24–29, 47-56.

2036.Marik PE, Kory P, Varon J, Iglesias J, Meduri GU. MATH+ protocol for the treatment oof SARS-CoV-2 infection: the scientific rationale. Exp rev Ant-infective Ther. 2020 doi: 10.1080/14787210.2020.1808462. [CrossRef] [Google Scholar]. McCullough P, Kelly R, Ruocco G, Lerma E, Tumlin J, Wheeland KR, et al. Pathophysiological basis and rationale for early outpatient treatment of SARS-CoV-2 (COVID-19) Infection. Amer J Med. 2021;134:16–22.

2037. James Thorpe interview by Dr. Steve Kirsch. Rumble https://rumble.com/vru732-dr.-james-thorp-on-medical-censorship.html [Last accessed on 2022 Feb 06]. McCullough P. "We're in the middle of a major biological catastrophe": Covid expert Dr. Peter McCullough. 2021. Oct 6, https://www.lifesitenews.com/news/were-in-the-middle-of-a-major-biological-catastrophe-top-covid-doc-mccullough/?_kx=9EtupqemhhFXJ1kgCo9W3xUNfwrkqB5nT7V2H15fUnA%3D.WXNMR7 [Last accessed on 2022 Feb 06].

2038.Bulik BS. The top 10 ad spenders in Big Pharma for 2020. Fierce Pharma Apr 19, 2021 https://www.fiercepharma.com/special-report/top-10-ad-spenders-big-pharma-for-2020 [Last accessed on 2022 Feb 06]. Kennedy R., Jr . Skyhorse Publishing; 2021. The Real Anthony Fauci. Bill Gates, Big Pharma, and the Global War on Democracy and Public Health; pp. 24–29.

2039.James Thorpe interview by Dr. Steve Kirsch. Rumble https://rumble.com/vru732-dr.-james-thorp-on-medical-censorship.html [Last accessed on 2022 Feb 06].

2040.US Medical, Scientific, Patient and Civic Organization Funding Report: Pfizer: Fourth Quarter 2010. https://cdn.pfizer.com/pfizercom/responsibility/grants_contributions/pfizer_us_grants_cc_q4_2010.pdf [Last accessed on 2022 Feb 06].

2041.Department of Health and Human Services: Part 1. Overview Information. https://grants.nih.gov/grants/guide/rfa-files/RFA-HD-20-013.html [Last accessed on 2022 Feb 06].

2042.Kennedy R., Jr., Fauci, supra, pp. 217.

2043.Hope JR. Sudden death by "hot lot"—Dr. Michael Yeadon sounds the alarm. The Desert review. 2022 Jan 24.

2044.Gueriero M. Restriction of autopsies during the Covid-19 epidemic in Italy. Prudence or fear? Pathologica. 2020;112:172–3.

2045.Elder C, Schroder AS, Aepfelbacher M, Fitzek A, Heinemann A, Heinrich F, et al. Dying with SARS-CoV-2 infection an autopsy study of the first consecutive 80 cases in Hamberg, Germany. Inter J Legal Med. 2020;134:1275–84.

2046.Liu Q, Wang RS, Qu GQ, Wang YY, Liu P, Zhu YZ, et al. Gross examination report of a Covid-19 death autopsy. Fa Yi Xue Za Zhi. 2020;36:21–23. Sperhake J-P. Autopsies of Covid-19 deceased? Absolutely! Legal Med. 2020 doi: 10.1016/j.legalmed.2020.101769.

2047.New York Post. Post Editorial Board Facebook admits the truth: "Fact checks" are just (lefty) opinion. Dec 14,2021. https://nypost.com/2021/12/14/facebook-admits-the-truth-fact-checks-are-really-just-lefty-opinion [Last accessed on 2022 Feb 06].

2048.Davis GG, Williamson AK. Risk of covid-19 transmission during autopsy. Arch Path Lab Med. 2020;144(12):1445a–1445.

2049.Gueriero M. Restriction of autopsies during the Covid-19 epidemic in Italy. Prudence or fear? Pathologica. 2020;112:172–3.

2050.Elder C, Schroder AS, Aepfelbacher M, Fitzek A, Heinemann A, Heinrich F, et al. Dying with SARS-CoV-2 infection an autopsy study of the first consecutive 80 cases in Hamberg, Germany. Inter J Legal Med. 2020;134:1275–84.

2051.Nicole Sirotek shares what she saw on the front lines in NYC. # Murder. https://rumble.com/vt7tnf-registered-nurse-nicole-sirot

ek-shares-what-she-saw-on-the-front-lines-in-n.html [Last accessed on 2022 Feb 06]. Nurse Colette Martin testimony to Louisiana House of Representatives. https://www.youtube.com/watch?v=cBwnIRUav5I [Last accessed on 2022 Feb 06].

2052.Bhakdi S. Presentation of autopsy findings. https://www.brighteon.com/4b6cc929-f559-4577-b4f8-3b40f0cd2f77 Pathology presentation on findings https://pathologie-konferenz.de/en [Last accessed on 2022 Feb 06].

2053.Schwab K, Malleret T. Cologny/Geneva: The Covid-19 Pandemic and the Great Reset. Forum Publishing 2020 World Economic Forum.

2054.Wood PM. Coherent Publishing; 2018. Technocracy: The Hard Road to World Order. Wood PM. Coherent Publishing; 2015. Technocracy Rising: The Trojan Horse of Global Transformation.

2055.Blaylock RL. National Health Insurance (Part 1): the socialist nightmare. Aug 19, 2009 https://haciendapublishing.com/national-health-insurance-part-i-the-socialist-nightmare-by-russell-l-blaylock-md [Last accessed on 2022 Feb 06]. Blaylock RL. Regimentation in medicine and its human price (part 1 & 2) Hacienda publishing. March 20, 2015 https://haciendapublishing.com/regimentation-in-medicine-and-its-human-price-part-2-by-russell-l-blaylock-md [Last accessed on 2022 Feb 06].

2056.Marik PE, Kory P, Varon J, Iglesias J, Meduri GU. MATH+ protocol for the treatment oof SARS-CoV-2 infection: the scientific rationale. Exp rev Ant-infective Ther. 2020 doi: 10.1080/14787210.2020.1808462. McCullough P,

Kelly R, Ruocco G, Lerma E, Tumlin J, Wheeland KR, et al. Pathophysiological basis and rationale for early outpatient treatment of SARS-CoV-2 (COVID-19) Infection. Amer J Med. 2021;134:16–22.

2057.Albright L. Medical nonconformity and its persecution. Brownstone Institute. https://brownstone.org/articles/medical-nonconformaity-and-its-persecution [Last accessed on 2022 Feb 06]. Saxena V. Doctors loses medical license. Ordered to have Psych Eval for Ivermectin Scrits, Sharing Covid "misinformation" BRP News. Available from: https://bizpacreview.com/2022/01/16/doctor-loses-license-orderedto-have-psych-eval-for-prescribing-ivermectin-sharining-covid-falsehoods-1189313. [Last accessed on 2022 Feb 06]. Vivek Saxena. Doctors loses license, ordered to have psych eval for Ivermectin scrits, sharing Covid 'misinformation' BPR News. https://www.bizpacreview.com/2022/01/16/doctor-loses-license-ordered-to-have-psych-eval-for-prescribing-ivermectin-sharing-covid-falsehoods-1189313.

2058.Durden T. Life Insurance CEO says deaths up 40% among those aged 18 to 64. Tyler Durden Report. 2022 Jan 3.

2059.McCullough P. "We're in the middle of a major biological catastrophe": Covid expert Dr. Peter McCullough. 2021. Oct 6, https://www.lifesitenews.com/news/were-in-the-middle-of-a-major-biological-catastrophe-top-covid-doc-mccullough/?_kx=9EtupqemhhFXJ1kgCo9W3xUNfwrkqB5nT7V2H15fUnA%3D.WXNMR7 [Last accessed on 2022 Feb 06]. Nurse Dani: It's the Covid-19 hospital protocols are killing pcoplc. https://rumble.com/vqs1v6-nurse-dani-its-the-covid-19-hospital-protocols-are-killing-people.html [Last accessed on 2022 Feb 06].

2060.Sen. Ron Johnson on Covid-19 vaccine injuries to test subjects.
https://www.youtube.com/watch?v=6mxqC9SiRh8
[Last accessed on 2022 Feb 06].

Other books available from Great Mountain Publishing®

The Sphere of Influence: The Heliocentric Perversion of the Gospel
Edward Hendrie
ISBN: 978-1-943056-06-4

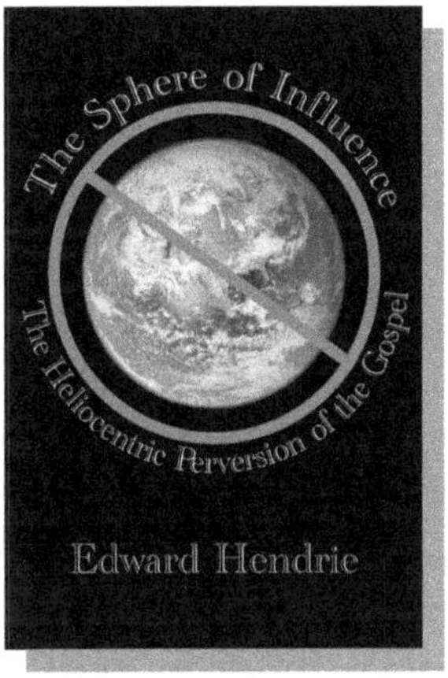

This book is a sequel to *The Greatest Lie on Earth (Expanded Edition): Proof That Our World Is Not a Moving Globe.* It will primarily focus on the infiltration into the church of the superstitious myth of heliocentrism and how that infiltration has served to undermine the gospel. The gospel is the entire Holy Bible, not just some of it. Matthew 4:4. Christian belief is an all or nothing proposition. "All scripture is given by inspiration of God, and is profitable for doctrine, for reproof, for correction, for instruction in righteousness." 2 Timothy 3:16. God's account of his creation is part and parcel of the gospel. A person with genuine faith believes what Jesus said about both heavenly and earthly things. "If I have told you earthly things, and ye believe not, how shall ye believe, if I tell you of heavenly things?" John 3:12. Jesus is God. Jesus created all things in heaven and on earth. See Colossians 1:16-18. God has revealed himself through his creation. "[T]hat which may be known of God is manifest in them; for God hath shewed it unto them. For the invisible things of him from the creation of the world are clearly seen, being understood by the things that are made, even his eternal power and Godhead; so that they are without excuse." Romans 1:19-20. If men have a misunderstanding of God's creation, they will also have a misunderstanding of who God is. If people believe in a creation that does not exist, they consequently also believe in a creator that does not exist. It is essential, therefore, to have an accurate understanding of God's creation. God did not make a movable, spherical earth. If men believe in a heliocentric creation, they will necessarily believe in a heliocentric creator. A heliocentric creation does not exist. So also, a heliocentric creator does not exist. A heliocentric creator is a false god. We have been warned to avoid the preaching of a false gospel, which presents a false Jesus. "For if he that cometh preacheth another Jesus, whom we have not preached, or if ye receive another spirit, which ye have not received, or another gospel, which ye have not accepted, ye might well bear with him." 2 Corinthians 11:4.

The Greatest Lie on Earth
Proof That Our World Is Not a Moving Globe
Edward Hendrie
ISBN-13: 978-1-943056-01-9

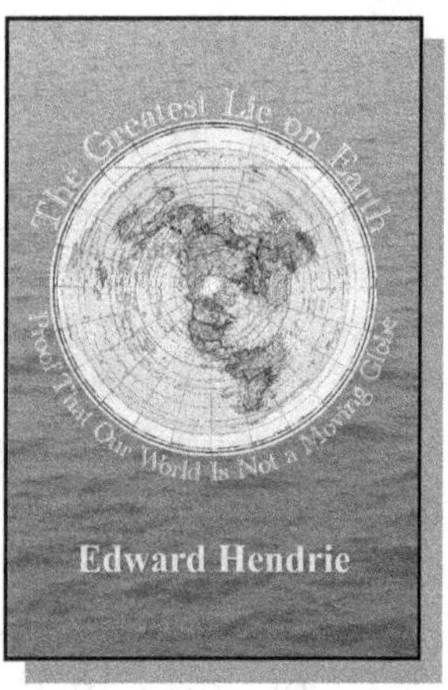

This book reveals the mother of all conspiracies. It sets forth biblical proof and irrefutable evidence that will cause the scales to fall from your eyes and reveal that the world you thought existed is a myth. The most universally accepted scientific belief today is that the earth is a globe, spinning on its axis at a speed of approximately 1,000 miles per hour at the equator, while at the same time it is orbiting the sun at approximately 66,600 miles per hour. All of this is happening as the sun, in turn, is supposed to be hurtling through the Milky Way galaxy at approximately 500,000 miles per hour. The Milky Way galaxy, itself, is alleged to be racing through space at a speed ranging from 300,000 to 1,340,000 miles per hour. What most people are not told is that the purported spinning, orbiting, and speeding through space has never been proven. In fact, every scientific experiment that has ever been performed to determine the motion of the earth has proven that the earth is stationary. Yet, textbooks ignore the scientific proof that contradicts the myth of a spinning and orbiting globe. Christian schools have been hoodwinked into teaching heliocentrism, despite the clear teaching in the Bible that the earth is not a sphere and does not move. This book reveals the evil forces behind the heliocentric deception, and why scientists and the Christian churches have gone along with it.

The Greatest Lie on Earth (Expanded Edition)
Proof That Our World Is Not a Moving Globe
Edward Hendrie
ISBN-13: 978-1943056-03-3

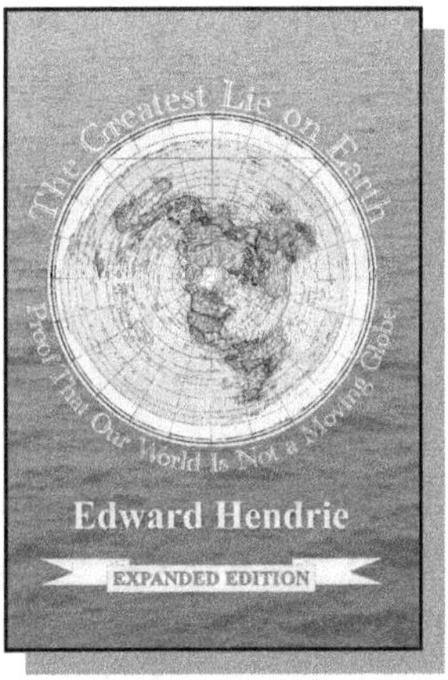

This book is an expanded edition of *The Greatest Lie on Earth*. It contains more than 1,000 pages of authoritative evidence with more than 1,300 endnotes that document proof beyond any doubt that the earth is flat and stationary. The book reveals the mother of all conspiracies. It sets forth biblical proof and irrefutable evidence that will cause the scales to fall from your eyes and reveal that the world you thought existed is a myth. The most universally accepted scientific belief today is that the earth is a globe, spinning on its axis at a speed of approximately 1,000 miles per hour at the equator, while at the same time it is orbiting the sun at approximately 66,600 miles per hour. All of this is happening as the sun, in turn, is supposed to be hurtling through the Milky Way galaxy at approximately 500,000 miles per hour. The Milky Way galaxy, itself, is alleged to be racing through space at a speed ranging from 300,000 to 1,340,000 miles per hour. What most people are not told is that the purported spinning, orbiting, and speeding through space has never been proven. In fact, every scientific experiment that has ever been performed to determine the motion of the earth has proven that the earth is stationary. Yet, textbooks ignore the scientific proof that contradicts the myth of a spinning and orbiting globe. Christian schools have been hoodwinked into teaching heliocentrism, despite the clear teaching in the Bible that the earth is not a sphere and does not move. This book reveals the evil forces behind the heliocentric deception, and why scientists and the Christian churches have gone along with it.

Antichrist: The Beast Revealed
Edward Hendrie
ISBN-13: 978-0-9832627-8-7

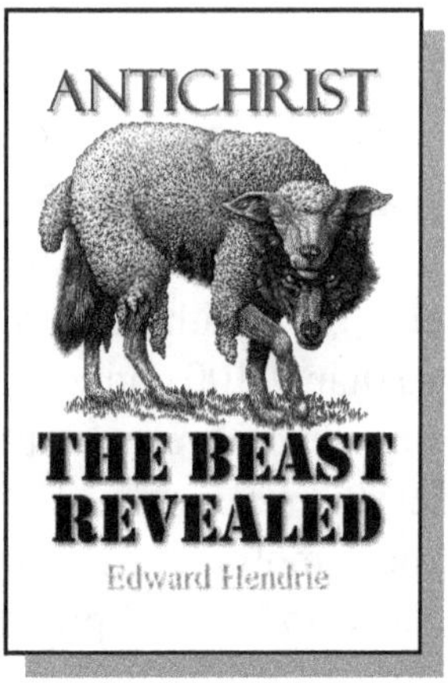

The antichrist is among us, here and now. This book proves it by comparing the biblical prophecies about the antichrist with the evidence that those prophecies have been fulfilled. This book documents the man of sin's esoteric confession that he is the antichrist. You will learn how the antichrist has changed times and laws as prophesied by Daniel, and how he is today sitting in the temple of God, "shewing himself that he is God," in fulfillment of Paul's prophecy in 2 Thessalonians 2:4. The beast of Revelation has come into the world, "after the working of Satan with all power and signs and lying wonders, and with all deceivableness of unrighteousness," as prophesied in 2 Thessalonians 2:10. The antichrist's adeptness as a hypocrite is the reason for his evil success. Indeed, to be the antichrist, his evil character must be concealed beneath a facade of piety. "And no marvel; for Satan himself is transformed into an angel of light. Therefore it is no great thing if his ministers also be transformed as the ministers of righteousness; whose end shall be according to their works." 2 Corinthians 11:14-15. The key to revealing the identity of the antichrist is to uncover his hypocrisy. Because the hypocrisy of the antichrist is so extreme, those who have been hoodwinked by his religious doctrines will be shocked to learn of it. This book exposes the concealed iniquity of the antichrist and juxtaposes it against his publicly proclaimed false persona of righteousness, thus bringing into clear relief that man of sin, the son of perdition, who is truly a ravening wolf in sheep's clothing, speaking lies in hypocrisy. See Matthew 7:15 and 1 Timothy 4:1-3.

9/11-Enemies Foreign and Domestic
Edward Hendrie
ISBN-13: 978-0983262732

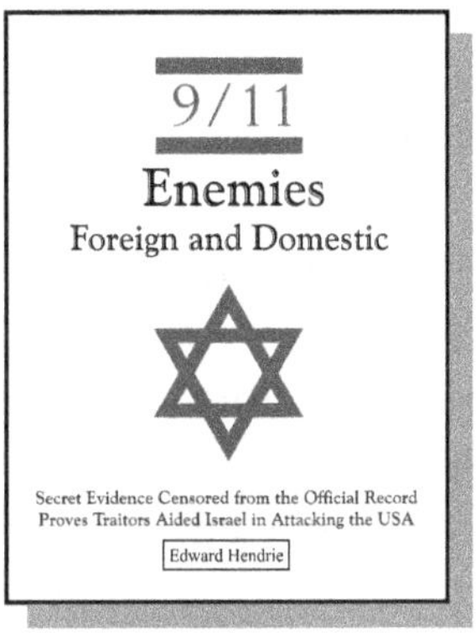

9/11-Enemies Foreign and Domestic proves beyond a reasonable doubt that the U.S. Government's conspiracy theory of the attacks on September 11, 2001, is a preposterous cover story. The evidence in 9/11-Enemies Foreign and Domestic has been suppressed from the official government reports and censored from the mass media. The evidence proves that powerful Zionists ordered the 9/11 attacks, which were perpetrated by Israel's Mossad, aided and abetted by treacherous high officials in the U.S. Government. 9/11-Enemies Foreign and Domestic identifies the traitors by name and details their subversive crimes. There is sufficient evidence in 9/11-Enemies Foreign and Domestic to indict important officials of the U.S. Government for high treason. The reader will understand how the U.S. Government really works and what Sir John Harrington (1561-1612) meant when he said: "Treason doth never prosper: what's the reason? Why if it prosper, none dare call it treason." There are millions of Americans who have taken an oath to defend the U.S. Constitution against all enemies foreign and domestic. The mass media, which is under the control of a disloyal cabal, keeps those patriotic Americans ignorant of the traitors among them. J. Edgar Hoover, former Director of the FBI, explained: "The individual is handicapped by coming face-to-face with a conspiracy so monstrous-he simply cannot believe it exists." 9/11-Enemies Foreign and Domestic erases any doubt about the existence of the monstrous conspiracy described by Hoover and arms the reader with the knowledge required to save our great nation. "My people are destroyed for lack of knowledge." Hosea 4:6.

Solving the Mystery of BABYLON THE GREAT
Edward Hendrie
ISBN-13: 978-0983262701

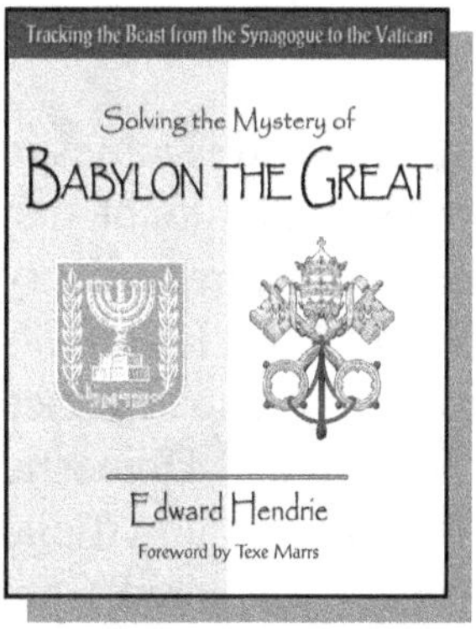

"Attorney and Christian researcher Edward Hendrie investigates and reveals one of the greatest exposés of all time. . . . a book you don't want to miss. Solving the Mystery of Babylon the Great is packed with documentation. Never before have the crypto-Jews who seized the reins of power in Rome been put under such intense scrutiny." Texe Marrs, Power of Prophecy. The evidence presented in this book leads to the ineluctable conclusion that the Roman Catholic Church was established by crypto-Jews as a false "Christian" front for a Judaic/Babylonian religion. That religion is the core of a world conspiracy against man and God. That is not a conspiracy theory based upon speculation, but rather the hard truth based upon authoritative evidence, which is documented in this book. Texe Marrs explains in his foreword to the book: "Who is Mystery Babylon? What is the meaning of the sinister symbols found in these passages? Which city is being described as the 'great city' so full of sin and decadence, and who are its citizens? Why do the woman and beast of Revelation seek the destruction of the holy people, the saints and martyrs of Jesus? What does it all mean for you and me today? Solving the Mystery of Babylon the Great answers these questions and more. Edward Hendrie's discoveries are not based on prejudice but on solid evidence aligned forthrightly with the 'whole counsel of God.' He does not condone nor will he be a part of any project in which Bible verses are taken out of context, or in which scriptures are twisted to mean what they do not say. Again and again you will find that Mr. Hendrie documents his assertions, backing up what he says with historical facts and proofs. Most important is that he buttresses his findings with scriptural understanding. The foundation for his research is sturdy because it is based on the bedrock of God's unshakeable Word."

The Anti-Gospel
Edward Hendrie
ISBN-13: 978-0983262749

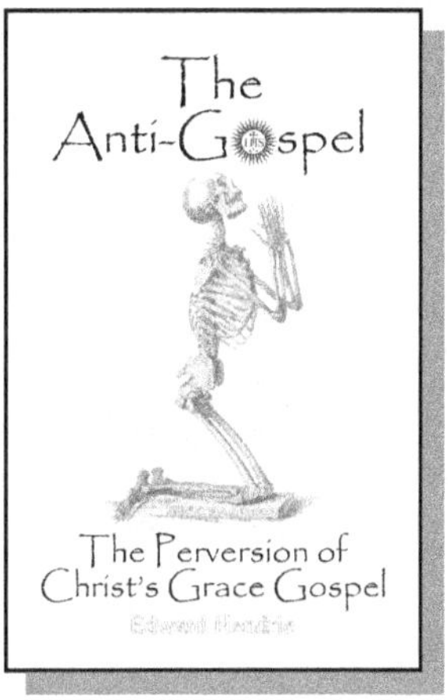

Edward Hendrie uses God's word to strip the sheep's clothing from false Christian ministers and expose them as ravening wolves preaching an anti-gospel. The anti-gospel is based on a myth that all men have a will that is free from the bondage of sin to choose whether to believe in Jesus. The Holy Bible, however, states that all men are spiritually dead and cannot believe in Jesus unless they are born again of the Holy Spirit. Ephesians 2:1-7; John 3:3-8. God has chosen his elect to be saved by his grace through faith in Jesus Christ. Ephesians 1:3-9; 2:8-10. God imbues his elect with the faith needed to believe in Jesus. Hebrews 12:2; John 1:12-13. The devil's false gospel contradicts the word of God and reverses the order of things. Under the anti-gospel, instead of a sovereign God choosing his elect, sovereign man decides whether to choose God. The calling of the Lord Jesus Christ is effectual; all who are chosen for salvation will believe in Jesus. John 6:37-44. The anti-gospel has a false Jesus, who only offers the possibility of salvation, with no assurance. The anti-gospel blasphemously makes God out to be a liar by denying the total depravity of man and the sovereign election of God. All who preach that false gospel are under a curse from God. Galatians 1:6-9.

Bloody Zion
Edward Hendrie
ISBN-13: 978-0983262763

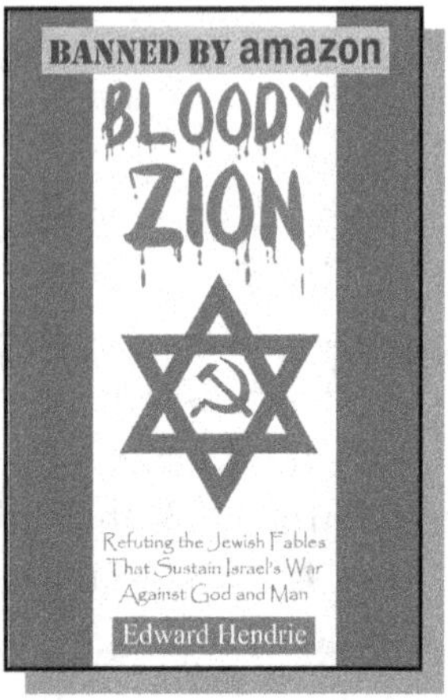

Jesus told Pontius Pilate: "My kingdom is not of this world." John 18:36. God has a spiritual Zion that is in a heavenly Jerusalem. Hebrews 12:22; Revelation 21:10. Jesus Christ is the chief corner stone laid by God in Zion. 1 Peter 2:6. Those who believe in Jesus Christ are living stones in the spiritual house of God. 1 Peter 2:5; Ephesians 2:20-22. Believers are in Jesus and Jesus is in believers. John 14:20; 17:20-23. All who are elected by God to believe in Jesus Christ are part of the heavenly Zion, without regard to whether they are Jews or Gentiles. Romans 10:12. Satan is a great adversary of God, who has created his own mystery religions. During the Babylonian captivity (2 Chronicles 36:20), an occult society of Jews replaced God's commands with Satan's Babylonian dogma. Their new religion became Judaism. Jesus explained the corruption of the Judaic religion: "Howbeit in vain do they worship me, teaching for doctrines the commandments of men." Mark 7:7. Jesus revealed the Satanic origin of Judaism when he stated: "Ye are of your father the devil, and the lusts of your father ye will do." John 8:44. Babylonian Judaism remains the religion of the Jews today. Satan has infected many nominal "Christian" denominations with his Babylonian occultism, which has given rise to "Christian" Zionism. "Christian" Zionism advocates a counterfeit, earthly Zion, within which fleshly Jews take primacy over the spiritual church of Jesus Christ. This book exposes "Christian" Zionism as a false gospel and subversive political movement that sustains Israel's war against God and man.

Murder, Rape, and Torture in a Catholic Nunnery
Edward Hendrie
ISBN-13: 978-1-943056-00-2

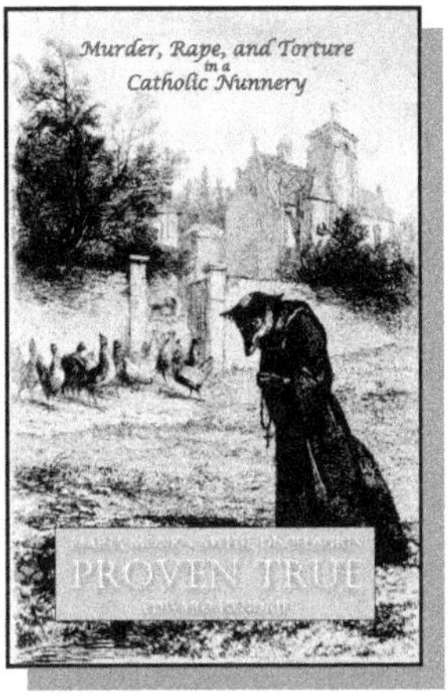

There has probably not been a person more maligned by the powerful forces of the Roman Catholic Church than Maria Monk. In 1836 she published the famous book, *Awful Disclosures of the Hotel Dieu Nunnery of Montreal*. In that book, she told of murder, rape, and torture behind the walls of the cloistered nunnery. Because the evidence was verifiably true, the Catholic hierarchy found it necessary to fabricate evidence and suborn perjury in an attempt to destroy the credibility of Maria Monk. The Catholic Church has kept up the character assassination of Maria Monk now for over 175 years. Even today, there can be found on the internet websites devoted to libeling Maria Monk. Edward Hendrie has examined the evidence and set it forth for the readers to decide for themselves whether Maria Monk was an impostor, as claimed by the Roman Catholic Church, or whether she was a brave victim. An objective view of the evidence leads to the ineluctable conclusion that Maria Monk told the truth about what happened behind the walls of the Hotel Dieu Nunnery of Montreal. The Roman Catholic Church, which is the most powerful religious and political organization in the world, has engaged in an unceasing campaign of vilification against Maria Monk. Their crusade against Maria Monk, however, can only affect the opinion of the uninformed. It cannot change the evidence. The evidence speaks clearly to those who will look at the case objectively. The evidence reveals that the much maligned Maria Monk was a reliable witness who made awful but accurate disclosures about life in a cloistered nunnery.

What Shall I Do to Inherit Eternal Life?
Edward Hendrie
ISBN-13: 978-0983262770

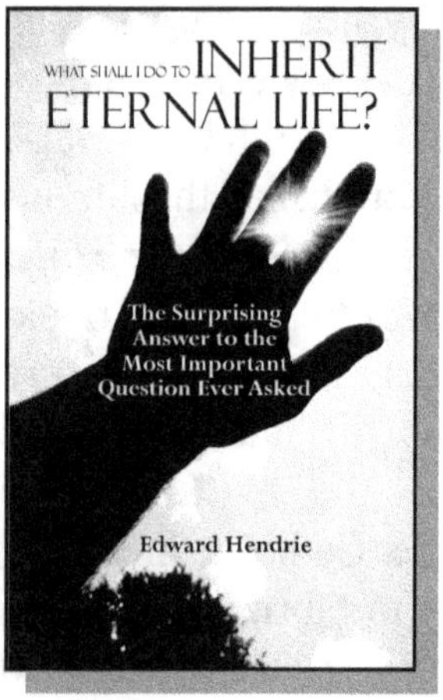

A certain ruler posed to Jesus the most important question ever asked: "Good Master, what shall I do to inherit eternal life?" (Luke 18:18) The man came to the right person. Jesus is God, and therefore his answer to that question is authoritative. This book examines Jesus' surprising answer and definitively explains how one inherits eternal life. This is a book about God's revelation to man. Except for the Holy Bible, this is the most important book you will ever read.

The Damnable Heresy Of Salvation by Dead Faith (Expanded Edition)
Edward Hendrie
ISBN 13: 978-1943056118

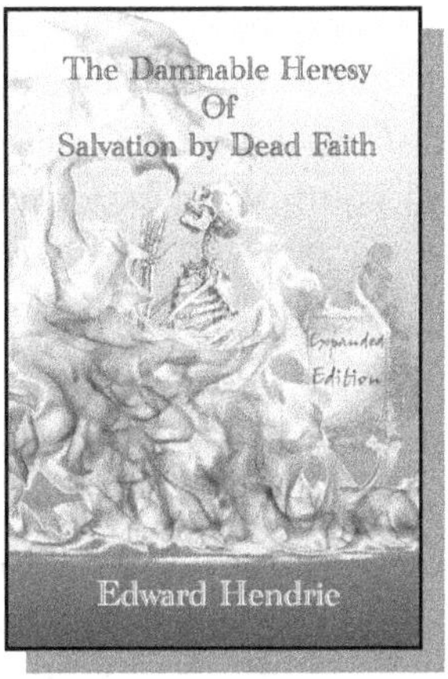

Good works follow salvation; they do not earn salvation. Good works do not save us. The works of faith are those works ordained and performed by God through the believer. They are the result of faith. It is that perfect faith that justifies the believer. "For by grace are ye saved through faith; and that not of yourselves: it is the gift of God: Not of works, lest any man should boast. For we are his workmanship, created in Christ Jesus unto good works, which God hath before ordained that we should walk in them. For we are his workmanship, created in Christ Jesus unto good works, which God hath before ordained that we should walk in them." Ephesians 2:8-10. In Romans, chapters 6 and 8, Paul explains faith without good works cannot save. Paul says that God's elect "walk not after the flesh, but after the Spirit." Romans 8:1. He states that those who do not walk in the Spirit but instead walk in the flesh "shall not inherit the kingdom of God." Galatians 5:15-25. John explains: "If we say that we have fellowship with him, and walk in darkness, we lie, and do not the truth: But if we walk in the light, as he is in the light, we have fellowship one with another, and the blood of Jesus Christ his Son cleanseth us from all sin." 1 John 1:6-7. James asks a rhetorical question: "What doth it profit, my brethren, though a man say he hath faith, and have not works? can faith save him?" James 2:14. James succinctly explains that "faith without works is dead." James 2:20. The pronouncement in James that true faith bears the fruit of good works is a theme found in the gospel. But some perniciously preach that God saves a person by faith that has no good works. That is one of the "damnable heresies" about which Peter warned. See 2 Peter 2:1-22.

Rome's Responsibility for the Assassination of Abraham

Lincoln, With an Appendix Containing Conversations Between Abraham Lincoln and Charles Chiniquy
Thomas M. Harris
ISBN-13: 978-0983262794

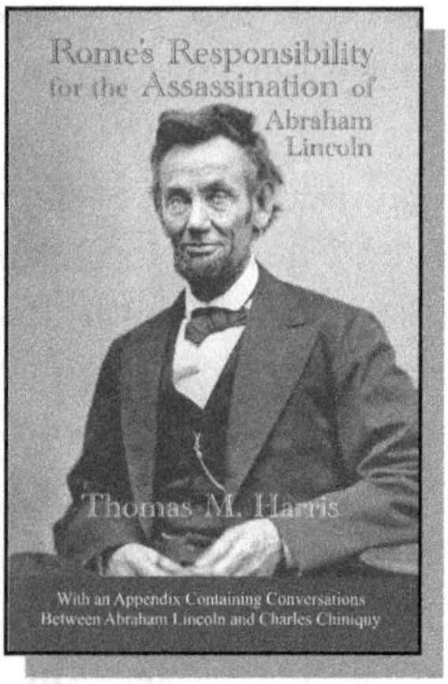

The author of this book, General Thomas Maley Harris, was a medical doctor, who recruited and served as commander of the Tenth West Virginia Volunteers during the Civil War. He rose in rank through meritorious service to become a brigadier general in the Union Army. General Harris established a reputation for faithfulness, industriousness, intelligence, and efficiency. He was noted for his leadership in preparing his troops and leading them in battle. He was brevetted a major general for "gallant conduct in the assault on Petersburg." After the Civil War, General Harris served one term as a representative in the West Virginia legislature, and was West Virginia's Adjutant General from 1869 to 1870. General Harris was a member of the Military Commission that tried and convicted the conspirators who assassinated President Abraham Lincoln. He had first hand knowledge of the sworn testimony of the witnesses in that trial. This book summarizes the salient evidence brought out during the military trial and adds information from other sources to present before the public the ineluctable conclusion that the assassination of Abraham Lincoln was the work of the Roman Catholic Church. The Roman Catholic Church has been largely successful in suppressing the circulation of this book. This book has never been given a place on bookstore shelves, as it exposed too much for the Roman Catholic hierarchy to tolerate. Any display of this book would bring an instant boycott of the bookstore. It is only now, in the age of the internet, where the marketplace of ideas has been opened wide, that this book can be found by those searching for the truth of who was behind the assassination of Abraham Lincoln.

The above books can be ordered from bookstores and from internet sites, including, but not limited to:

https://greatmountainpublishing.com
www.antichristconspiracy.com
www.911enemies.com
www.mysterybabylonthegreat.net
www.antigospel.com
https://play.google.com
www.barnesandnoble.com
www.amazon.com

Edward Hendrie
edwardhendrie@gmail.com

www.ingramcontent.com/pod-product-compliance
Lightning Source LLC
LaVergne TN
LVHW080529210926
848481LV00020B/1456
9781943056170